Acute Leukemia

Acute Leukemia

An Illustrated Guide to Diagnosis and Treatment

Editors

Ashkan Emadi, MD, PhD
Associate Professor of Medicine, Pharmacology and Experimental Therapeutics
Director, Hematology & Medical Oncology Fellowship
University of Maryland School of Medicine
Marlene and Stewart Greenebaum Comprehensive Cancer Center
Baltimore, Maryland

Judith E. Karp, MD
Professor Emerita, Oncology and Medicine
The Johns Hopkins Sidney Kimmel Comprehensive Cancer Center
Baltimore, Maryland

demosMEDICAL
An Imprint of Springer Publishing
NEW YORK

Visit our website at www.demosmedical.com

ISBN: 9781620701003
ebook ISBN: 9781617052774
Image Bank ISBN: 9780826172686

Acquisitions Editor: David D'Addona
Compositor: Exeter Premedia Services Private Ltd.

Medicine is an ever-changing science. Research and clinical experience are continually expanding our knowledge, in particular our understanding of proper treatment and drug therapy. The authors, editors, and publisher have made every effort to ensure that all information in this book is in accordance with the state of knowledge at the time of production of the book. Nevertheless, the authors, editors, and publisher are not responsible for errors or omissions or for any consequences from application of the information in this book and make no warranty, expressed or implied, with respect to the contents of the publication. Every reader should examine carefully the package inserts accompanying each drug and should carefully check whether the dosage schedules mentioned therein or the contraindications stated by the manufacturer differ from the statements made in this book. Such examination is particularly important with drugs that are either rarely used or have been newly released on the market.

Library of Congress Cataloging-in-Publication Data

Names: Emadi, Ashkan, editor. | Karp, Judith E., editor.
Title: Acute leukemia: an illustrated guide to diagnosis and treatment/
[edited by] Ashkan Emadi, Judith E. Karp.
Other titles: Acute leukemia (Emadi)
Description: New York: Demos, [2017] | Includes bibliographical references and index.
Identifiers: LCCN 2016055279 | ISBN 9781620701003 | ISBN 9781617052774 (e-book)
Subjects: | MESH: Leukemia—diagnosis | Leukemia—therapy | Acute Disease
Classification: LCC RC643 | NLM WH 250 | DDC 616.99/419—dc23
LC record available at https://lccn.loc.gov/2016055279

Printed in the United States of America by Strategic Content Imaging.
17 18 19 20 21 / 5 4 3 2 1

This book would not have happened were it not for the people who have given us knowledge, inspiration, and unwavering support in both our professional and personal lives. Ashkan thanks his PhD mentor Dr. Kenneth W. Stagliano, his wife Dr. Leili Parsa, and his son Ryan Emadi. He would like to thank Judy for her unconditional and continuous support and mentorship. Judy thanks her leukemia mentor Dr. Philip J. Burke, her husband Stanley Freedman, and Ashkan for endless inspiration and energy. We also want to "give a nod" to Catherine Lai, MD for her tremendous efforts and insights that led to a unique and comprehensive depiction of the molecular mutations that are critical to AML leukemogenesis, pathophysiology, and drug responsiveness. Finally, both of us are totally indebted to our patients and their families, and to the young caregivers who helped us to care for them. All of them have taught us how to approach challenging issues, how to realize (and attempt to deal with) what we don't know, and how to persist in the face of adversity. All of them have made us better physicians and better people than we would have been without their powerful influence.

Contents

Contributors

Anjali Advani, MD, Director, Inpatient Leukemia Unit, Staff, Department of Hematology/Oncology; Associate Professor, Cleveland Clinic Lerner College of Medicine, The Cleveland Clinic, Cleveland, Ohio

Peter D. Aplan, MD, Senior Investigator and Head, Leukemia Biology Section, Genetics Branch, National Cancer Institute, National Institutes of Health, Bethesda, Maryland

Lizamarie Bachier-Rodriguez, MD, Hematology and Oncology Fellow, Department of Medicine, Division of Hematology-Oncology, Weill Cornell Medicine, New York, New York

Maria R. Baer, MD, Professor of Medicine, University of Maryland School of Medicine; Director, Hematologic Malignancies, University of Maryland, Marlene and Stewart Greenebaum Comprehensive Cancer Center, Baltimore, Maryland

John Barrett, MD, Senior Investigator, Stem Cell Allogenic Transplantation Section, Department of Hematology Branch, National Heart, Lung, and Blood Institute, National Institutes of Health, Bethesda, Maryland

Pamela S. Becker, MD, PhD, Professor of Medicine, Division of Hematology, University of Washington; Associate Member, Clinical Research Division, Fred Hutchinson Cancer Research Center, Institute for Stem Cell and Regenerative Medicine, Seattle, Washington

Archie Bleyer, MD, Clinical Research Professor, Department of Radiation Medicine, Oregon Health and Science University, Portland, Oregon

Firas El Chaer, MD, Clinical Fellow, Hematology and Medical Oncology, Marlene and Stewart Greenebaum Comprehensive Cancer Center, University of Maryland School of Medicine, Baltimore, Maryland

Allen R. Chen, MD, PhD, MHS, Associate Professor, Oncology and Pediatrics; Vice Chair for Quality, Safety and Service, Sidney Kimmel Comprehensive Cancer Center, Johns Hopkins University School of Medicine, Baltimore, Maryland

Qing C. Chen, MD, PhD, Department of Pathology, Northwestern University Fienberg School of Medicine, Chicago, Illinois

Gordon Cohen, MD, Clinical Fellow, Pediatric Hematology/Oncology, Johns Hopkins Hospital and National Cancer Institute, Johns Hopkins Hospital, Baltimore, Maryland

Nancy Corbitt, BSN, RN, OCN, CRNI, Senior Clinical Nurse II, Department of Inpatient Nursing, University of Maryland Medical Center, Marlene and Stewart Greenebaum Comprehensive Cancer Center, Baltimore, Maryland

Lea C. Cunningham, MD, Assistant Member, Department of Bone Marrow Transplant and Cellular Therapy, St. Jude Children's Research Hospital; Faculty Advisor, St. Jude Immune Monitoring Core, St. Jude Children's Research Hospital, Memphis, Tennessee

Daniel L. Duncan, MD, Fellow, Hematopathology, Department of Pathology and Laboratory Medicine, University of North Carolina, Chapel Hill, North Carolina

Vu H. Duong, MD, MS, Assistant Professor of Medicine, University of Maryland School of Medicine, Marlene and Stewart Greenebaum Comprehensive Cancer Center, Baltimore, Maryland

Ashkan Emadi, MD, PhD, Associate Professor of Medicine, Pharmacology and Experimental Therapeutics; Director, Hematology & Medical Oncology Fellowship; University of Maryland School of Medicine; Marlene and Stewart Greenebaum Comprehensive Cancer Center, Baltimore, Maryland

Raúl Montiel Esparza, MD, Postdoctoral Fellow, Oncology, Division of Hematologic Malignancies, The Johns Hopkins Sidney Kimmel Comprehensive Cancer Center, Baltimore, Maryland

Ann T. Farrell, MD, Director, Division of Hematology Products, Office of Hematology and Oncology Products, Center for Drug Evaluation and Research, U.S. Food and Drug Administration, Silver Spring, Maryland

Amir T. Fathi, MD, Assistant Professor of Medicine, Harvard Medical School, Massachusetts General Hospital, Leukemia Program, Boston, Massachusetts

Matthew C. Foster, MD, Assistant Professor of Medicine, Division of Hematology/Oncology, Department of Medicine, Lineberger Comprehensive Cancer Center, University of North Carolina, Chapel Hill, North Carolina

Alan D. Friedman, MD, Professor, Johns Hopkins University School of Medicine, Baltimore, Maryland

Gabriel Ghiaur, MD, PhD, Assistant Professor of Oncology and Medicine, Johns Hopkins University, Sidney Kimmel Comprehensive Cancer Center, Division of Hematological Malignancies, Adult Leukemia Program, Baltimore, Maryland

Christopher D. Gocke, MD, Associate Professor of Pathology and Oncology; Director, Division of Molecular Pathology, Deputy Director for Personalized Medicine, Department of Pathology, Johns Hopkins School of Medicine, Baltimore, Maryland

Ivana Gojo, MD, Associate Professor, Oncology and Medicine, The Johns Hopkins Sidney Kimmel Comprehensive Cancer Center, Division of Hematologic Malignancies, Adult Leukemia Program, Baltimore, Maryland

Lukasz P. Gondek, MD, PhD, Assistant Professor of Oncology and Medicine, Johns Hopkins University, Sidney Kimmel Comprehensive Cancer Center, Division of Hematological Malignancies, Adult Leukemia Program, Baltimore, Maryland

Lia Gore, MD, Chief, Pediatric Hematology/Oncology/Bone Marrow Transplant, Department of Pediatrics, University of Colorado School of Medicine, Children's Hospital Colorado Center for Cancer and Blood Disorders, Aurora, Colorado

Steven D. Gore, MD, Professor of Medicine, Director of Hematologic Malignancies, Section of Hematology, Department of Internal Medicine, Yale University, New Haven, Connecticut

Steven Grant, MD, Professor of Medicine, Biochemistry, and Human and Molecular Genetics, Massey Cancer Center, Virginia Commonwealth University, Richmond, Virginia

Elizabeth A. Griffiths, MD, Associate Professor, Department of Medicine, Roswell Park Cancer Institute, Buffalo, New York

Nancy M. Hardy, MD, Associate Professor of Medicine, Medical Director, Cellular Therapeutics Laboratories; Director, Allogeneic Stem Cell Transplantation, Blood & Marrow Transplantation, Marlene and Stewart Greenebaum Cancer Center, University of Maryland, Baltimore, Maryland

Dennis D. Hickstein, MD, Senior Investigator, Experimental Transplantation and Immunology, National Cancer Institute, National Institutes of Health, Bethesda, Maryland

Noa G. Holtzman, MD, Clinical Fellow, Hematology and Medical Oncology, Marlene and Stewart Greenebaum Comprehensive Cancer Center, University of Maryland School of Medicine, Baltimore, Maryland

Christopher S. Hourigan, BM, BCh, DPhil, FACP, Tenure Track Clinical Investigator and Chief, Myeloid Malignancies Section, Hematology Branch, National Heart, Lung, and Blood Institute, National Institutes of Health, Bethesda, Maryland

Stephen P. Hunger, MD, Professor of Pediatrics, Perelman School of Medicine at the University of Pennsylvania; Chief, Division of Pediatric Oncology; Director, Center for Childhood Cancer Research, Children's Hospital of Philadelphia, Philadelphia, Pennsylvania

Sawa Ito, MD, Staff Clinician, Hematology Branch, National Heart, Lung, and Blood Institute, National Institutes of Health, Bethesda, Maryland

Craig T. Jordan, PhD, Division Chief, Division of Hematology, Nancy Carroll Allen Professor of Hematology; Professor of Medicine, University of Colorado School of Medicine, Anschutz Medical Campus, Aurora, Colorado

Farin Kamangar, MD, PhD, MPH, MHS, Professor and Chairman, Department of Public Health Analysis; Director, ASCEND Center for Biomedical Research, Morgan State University, Baltimore, Maryland

Judith E. Karp, MD, Professor Emerita, Oncology and Medicine, The Johns Hopkins Sidney Kimmel Comprehensive Cancer Center, Baltimore, Maryland

Adam R. Karpf, PhD, Associate Professor, Eppley Institute for Cancer Research, Fred and Pamela Buffett Cancer Center, University of Nebraska Medical Center, Omaha, Nebraska

Trisha Kendall, MS, RN, OCN, Clinical Nurse Specialist, Gilchrist, Hunt Valley, Maryland

Hanna A. Knaus, MD, Postdoctoral Fellow, Oncology, Division of Hematologic Malignancies, The Johns Hopkins Sidney Kimmel Comprehensive Cancer Center, Baltimore, Maryland; Hematology, Medical University of Vienna, Vienna, Austria

Jessica Knight-Perry, MD, Clinical Fellow, Pediatric Hematology/Oncology/Bone Marrow Transplant, Department of Pediatrics, University of Colorado School of Medicine, Children's Hospital Colorado Center for Cancer and Blood Disorders, Aurora, Colorado

Catherine Lai, MD, MPH, Staff Clinician and Director of Clinical Operations, Myeloid Malignancies Section, Hematology Branch, National Heart, Lung, and Blood Institute, National Institutes of Health, Bethesda, Maryland

Mark J. Levis, MD, PhD, Professor of Oncology, Medicine, and Pharmacology, Sidney Kimmel Comprehensive Cancer Center, Johns Hopkins University, Baltimore, Maryland

Timothy J. Ley, MD, Professor of Internal Medicine and Genetics, Division of Oncology, Washington University Medical School, St. Louis, Missouri

Ling Li, PhD, Assistant Professor, Division of Hematopoietic Stem Cell & Leukemia Research, Gehr Family Center for Leukemia Research, Beckman Research Institute of City of Hope, Duarte, California

Tara Lin, MD, Associate Professor, Division of Hematologic Malignancies and Cellular Therapeutics, University of Kansas Cancer Center, Westwood, Kansas

R. Coleman Lindsley, MD, PhD, Assistant Professor of Medicine, Department of Medical Oncology, Dana-Farber Cancer Institute, Boston, Massachusetts

Mark R. Litzow, MD, Professor of Medicine, Division of Hematology, Mayo Clinic; Chair, Eastern Cooperative Oncology Group-American College of Radiology Imaging Network Leukemia Committee, Rochester, Minnesota

Paul P. Liu, MD, PhD, Senior Investigator and Deputy Scientific Director, Division of Intramural Research, National Human Genome Research Institute, National Institutes of Health, Bethesda, Maryland

Aaron C. Logan, MD, PhD, Assistant Professor of Medicine, University of California San Francisco School of Medicine, San Francisco, California

Michael R. Loken, PhD, President, Hematologics, Inc., Seattle, Washington

Parvez M. Lokhandwala, MD, PhD, Fellow, Molecular Genetic Pathology, Johns Hopkins University School of Medicine, Baltimore, Maryland

Selina M. Luger, MD, Professor of Medicine, Abramson Cancer Center, University of Pennsylvania, Philadelphia, Pennsylvania

Heather J. Male, MD, Assistant Professor, Division of Hematologic Malignancies and Cellular Therapeutics, University of Kansas Cancer Center, Westwood, Kansas

Sami N. Malek, MD, Associate Professor of Medicine, University of Michigan School of Medicine, Ann Arbor, Michigan

Guido Marcucci, MD, Director and Professor, Division of Hematopoietic Stem Cell & Leukemia Research, Gehr Family Center for Leukemia Research, Beckman Research Institute of City of Hope, Duarte, California

Frank McCormick, PhD, FRS, Professor, University of California, San Francisco, UCSF Helen Diller Family Comprehensive Cancer Center, San Francisco, California

Nathan D. Montgomery, MD, PhD, Fellow, Hematopathology, Department of Pathology and Laboratory Medicine, University of North Carolina, Chapel Hill, North Carolina

Monica Reddy Muppidi, MD, Hematology Oncology Fellow, Department of Medicine, Roswell Park Cancer Institute, Buffalo, New York

Aziz Nazha, MD, Leukemia Program, Department of Hematology and Oncology, Taussig Cancer Institute, The Cleveland Clinic, Cleveland, Ohio

Yi Ning, MD, PhD, Associate Professor of Pathology; Director, Cytogenetics Laboratory, Department of Pathology, School of Medicine, Johns Hopkins University, Baltimore, Maryland

Houman Nourkeyhani, MD, Hematology and Oncology Fellow, Department of Medicine, Roswell Park Cancer Institute, Buffalo, New York

Kristen O'Dwyer, MD, Assistant Professor of Medicine and Oncology, Clinical Directory, Leukemia Program, Wilmot Cancer Institute, University of Rochester Medical Center, Rochester, New York

Priyank P. Patel, MD, Hematology Oncology Fellow, Department of Medicine, Roswell Park Cancer Institute, Buffalo, New York

Alexander E. Perl, MD, MS, Assistant Professor of Medicine at the Hospital of the University of Pennsylvania, Fellow, Institute for Translational Medicine and Therapeutics, University of Pennsylvania, Philadelphia, Pennsylvania

Daniel A. Pollyea, MD, MS, Associate Professor, Clinical Director of Leukemia Services, Assistant Professor of Medicine, University of Colorado School of Medicine, Anschutz Medical Campus, Aurora, Colorado

Keith W. Pratz, MD, Assistant Professor, Oncology and Medicine, The Johns Hopkins Sidney Kimmel Comprehensive Cancer Center, Division of Hematologic Malignancies, Adult Leukemia Program, Baltimore, Maryland

Donna Przepiorka, MD, PhD, Medical Officer, Division of Hematology Products, Office of Hematology and Oncology Products, Center for Drug Evaluation and Research, U.S. Food and Drug Administration, Silver Spring, Maryland

Mohamed Rahmani, PhD, MS, Associate Professor of Medicine, Virginia Commonwealth University, Massey Cancer Center, Richmond, Virginia

Gregory H. Reaman, MD, Associate Director for Oncology Sciences, Office of Hematology and Oncology Products, Center for Drug Evaluation and Research, U.S. Food and Drug Administration, Silver Spring, Maryland

Susan R. Rheingold, MD, Associate Professor of Clinical Pediatrics, Perelman School of Medicine at the University of Pennsylvania, Children's Hospital of Philadelphia, Philadelphia, Pennsylvania

Joseph M. Scandura, MD, PhD, Associate Professor of Medicine, Divisions of Hematology and Oncology and Regenerative Medicine, Weill Cornell Medicine, New York, New York

Sheenu Sheela, MD, Postdoctoral Research Fellow, Myeloid Malignancies Section, Hematology Branch, National Heart, Lung, and Blood Institute, National Institutes of Health, Bethesda, Maryland

Zeba N. Singh, MD, Department of Pathology, University of Maryland School of Medicine, University of Maryland Medical Center, Baltimore, Maryland

Chandrima Sinha, PhD, Postdoctoral Fellow, Department of Bone Marrow Transplant and Cellular Therapy, St. Jude Children's Research Hospital; Senior Scientist I, Department of Therapeutics Production & Quality, St. Jude Children's Research Hospital, Memphis, Tennessee

Franklin O. Smith III, MD, Adjunct Professor of Medicine and Pediatrics, University of Cincinnati College of Medicine, Cincinnati, Ohio

David H. Spencer, MD, PhD, Assistant Professor of Medicine, Section of Stem Cell Biology, Division of Oncology, Washington University Medical School, St. Louis, Missouri

Heather Symons, MD, Assistant Professor, Oncology and Pediatrics, Clinical Director, Pediatric Blood and Marrow Transplantation, Johns Hopkins Hospital, Baltimore, Maryland

Eunice S. Wang, MD, Professor of Oncology, Chief of Leukemia Service, Department of Medicine, Roswell Park Cancer Institute; Associate Professor, Department of Medicine, Jacobs School of Medicine and Biomedical Sciences, State University of New York, Buffalo, New York

Matthew J. Wieduwilt, MD, PhD, Assistant Clinical Professor, Blood and Marrow Transplantation Program, University of California, San Diego Moores Cancer Center, La Jolla, California

Amer Methqal Zeidan, MBBS, MHS, Assistant Professor of Medicine, Section of Hematology, Department of Internal Medicine, Yale University, New Haven, Connecticut

Joshua F. Zeidner, MD, Assistant Professor of Medicine, Division of Hematology/Oncology, Department of Medicine, Lineberger Comprehensive Cancer Center, University of North Carolina, Chapel Hill, North Carolina

Ying Zou, MD, PhD, Associate Professor of Pathology; Director, Clinical Cytogenetics Laboratory, School of Medicine, University of Maryland, Baltimore, Maryland

Abbreviations

6-MP	6-mercaptopurine
6-TG	thioguanine
7+3	Induction therapy regimen for acute myeloid leukemia consisting of 7 days of cytarabine and 3 days of daunorubicin
A	asparaginase
AA	amino acid
ACE	angiotensin-converting enzyme
ACR	aclarubicin
AD	automodification domain
ADE	ara-C(cytarabine), daunorubicin, etoposide
ADP	adenosine diphosphate
AEL	acute erythroid leukemia
AIEOP	Associazione Italiana Ematologia Oncologia Pediatric Group
AKT	protein kinase B
ALL	acute lymphoblastic leukemia
allo	allogeneic
allo-HSCT	allogeneic hematopoietic stem cell transplant
AML	acute myeloid leukemia
ANC	absolute neutrophil count
APC	allophycocyanin; antigen-presenting cell
APC-A	allophycocyanin-A
APL	acute promyelocytic leukemia
AraC	cytosine arabinoside or cytarabine
ara-CDP	ara-cytidine-5′-diphosphate
ara-CMP	ara-cytidine-5′-monophosphate
ara-CTP	ara-cytidine-5′-triphosphate
ara-U	uracil arabinoside
ara-UMP	ara-uridine-5′-monophosphate
ARB	angiotensin II receptor blockers
ARDS	acute respiratory distress syndrome
ASO	Allele-specific oligonucleotide

As_2O_3	arsenic trioxide
AS_4S_4	tetra-arsenic tetra-sulfide
ASCT	autologous stem cell transplantation
ASM	aggressive systemic mastocytosis
ASNS	asparagine synthetase
ASP	l-asparginase
ATO	arsenic trioxide
ATP	adenosine triphosphate
ATRA	all-trans retinoic acid
AYA	adolescent and young adult
Aza	azacitidine
BAF	B-allele frequency
BAM	binary alignment map
B-ALL	B acute lymphoblastic leukemia
BCP	B-cell precursor
bcr	breakpoint cluster region
BFM	Berlin-Frankfurt-Munster Group
BITE	bifunctional T-cell engaging
BLA	Biologics License Application
BLP	B-lymphoid progenitor
BM	bone marrow
BMT	bone marrow transplantation
bp	base-pair
BP	bisphosphate
BPDN	blastic plasmacytoid dendritic cell neoplasm
BRCT	*BRCA1* C-terminal domain
BUN/Cr	blood urea nitrogen/creatinine
C	cyclophosphamide
CAE	naphthol AS-D chloroacetate esterase
CALGB	Cancer and Leukemia Group B
CAR19	chimeric antigen receptor targeting CD19
CAR cell	CXCL12 abundant reticular cell
CARs	chimeric receptor antigens
CBC	complete blood count
CBF	core binding factor
CBF AML	core binding factor acute myeloid leukemia.

CCL3	chemokine (C-C motif) ligand 3
CCR	conventional care regimen
CD	cluster differentiation
CD44	cluster of differentiation 44
CD47	cluster of differentiation 47 ("don't eat me" signal)
CDA	cytidine deaminase
CDK	cyclin-dependent kinase
CDS	coding sequence change
CDP	cytidine diphosphate
CE	capillary electrophoresis
CFR	Code of Federal Regulations
CH_2FH_4	methylene etrahydrofolate
CHIP	clonal hematopoiesis of indeterminate potential
CHK	Checkpoint kinases
Chr	chromosome
CI	continuous infusion
CIBMTR	Center for International Blood and Marrow Transplant Research
c-KIT	c-kit receptor tyrosine kinase
CLAG-M	cladribine, ara-C, G-CSF, mitoxantrone
CLG	Children's Leukemia Group
CLL	chronic lymphocytic leukemia
CLP	common lymphoid progenitor
CML	chronic myeloid leukemia
CMML	chronic myelomonocytic leukemia
CMP	common myeloid progenitor
cMpl	cellular myeloproliferative leukemia protein (TPO-receptor)
CMV	cytomegalovirus
CN-LOH	copy neutral loss of heterozygosity
CNS	central nervous system
CNV	copy number variant
COA	coactivator complex
CoA	coenzyme A
COG	Children's Oncology Group
COSMIC	Catalogue of Somatic Mutations in Cancer
CpG	cytosine-phosphate-guanine
CPM	cyclophosphamide

CR	complete remission
CRc	Cytogenetic CR
CRi	complete remission with incomplete count recovery
CRp	complete remission with incomplete platelet recovery
CRS	cytokine release syndrome
CSF	cerebral spinal fluid
Cx43	connexin 43
CXCL12	Chemokine (C-X-C motif) ligand 12 (SDF1α – stromal derived factor 1α)
CXCL8	Chemokine (C-X-C motif) ligand 8
CXCR1	Chemokine (C-X-C motif) receptor 1 (receptor for CXCL8)
CXCR2	Chemokine (C-X-C motif) receptor 2 (receptor for CXCL8)
CXCR4	Chemokine (C-X-C motif) receptor 4 (receptor for CXCL12)
CYP	cytochrome P450
CVA	cerebrovascular accident
D	daunorubicin
DA	daunorubicin + cytarabine
DBD	DNA binding domain
dbSNP	single nucleotide polymorphism database
DCK	deoxycytidine kinase
DCOG	Dutch Childhood Oncology Group
DCTD	deoxycytidylate deaminase
dCTP	deoxycytidine triphosphate
DD	droplet digital
Dec	decitabine
Dex	dexamethasone
DEXA	bone density scanning with dual-energy x-ray absorptiometry
DexOMP	dexamethasone, vincristine, methotrexate, 6-mercaptopurine
DFCI	Dana-Farber Cancer Institute Consortium
DFS	disease-free survival
DHFR	dihydrofolate reductase
DIC	disseminated intravascular coagulation
DLI	donor lymphocyte infusion
DNMT	DNA methyltransferase
DNMT3A	DNA methyltransferase 3A
dNTP	deoxynucleotide triphosphate
DOX	doxorubicin

DRI	disease risk index
DS	Down Syndrome
DSB	double-strand break
E	etoposide
EBV	Epstein-Barr virus
ECG	electrocardiogram
ECOG	Eastern Cooperative Oncology Group
EDTA	ethylenediaminetetraacetic acid
EEG	Electroencephalogram
EFS	event-free survival
ELN	European LeukemiaNet
EOC	end of consolidation
EOI	end of induction
EORTC	European Organisation for Research and Treatment of Cancer
EPT-ALL	early precursor T-cell acute lymphoblastic leukemia
ETOP	etoposide
ETP	early T-cell precursor
FA	Fanconi anemia
FAB	French American British
FAM	6-carboxy fluorescein, the most commonly used reporter dye at the 5′ end of a TaqMan probe
FCM	flow cytometry
FCR	fludarabine, cyclophosphamide, rituximab
FDA	Food and Drug Administration
FH_2	dihydrofolate
FH_4	tetrahydrofolate
FISH	fluorescence in situ hybridization
FITC	fluorescein
FITC-A	fluorescein isothiocyanate-A
FL	FLT3 ligand
FLAG	mitoxantrone, fludarabine, cytarabine, G-CSF
FLAG-GO	gemtuzumab ozogamicin, fludarabine, cytarabine, G-CSF
FLAG-Ida	fludarabine, ara-C, G-CSF, idarubicine
FLAM	fludarabine, cytarabine, mitoxantrone
FLT3	FMS-like tyrosine kinase 3
FLT3-ITD	FMS-like tyrosine kinase 3 internal tandem duplication

FND-R	fludarabine, mitoxantrone, dexamethasone, rituximab
FSH	follicle-stimulating hormone
FWD Scatter	forward light scatter
G-CSF	granulocyte colony stimulating factor
GAS6	growth arrest specific 6
GC	guanine-cytosine
GCLAC	clofarabine, cytarabine, G-CSF
GCSF	granulocyte colony-stimulating factor
GDF15	growth differentiation factor 15
$(Glu)_n$	poly-glutamate
GLUT1/GLUT4	glucose transporter 1/4
GMALL	German Multicenter acute lymphoblastic leukemia
GM-CSF	granulocyte macrophage colony stimulating factor
GMP	granulocyte/macrophage progenitor
GO	gemtuzumab ozogamicin
GTP	guanosine triphosphate
GVHD	graft-versus-host disease
GVL	graft-versus-leukemia
HA	homoharringtonine + cytarabine
HAT	histone acetyltransferases
HCT	hematopoietic cell transplantation
HDAC	histone deacetylase
HD-AraC	high-dose cytarabine
HD-Ida	high-dose idarubicin
HD-MTX	high-dose methotrexate
HiDAC	high-dose arabinoside cytarabine
HIF-1α	hypoxia-inducible factor 1α
HLA	human leukocyte antigen
HLA-DR	human leukocyte antigen-D related
HMA	hypomethylating agent
HPC	hematopoietic progenitor cell
HR	hazard ratio; high risk
HRQoL	health-related quality of life
HSC	hematopoietic stem cell
HSCT	hematopoietic stem cell transplant
HSP90	heat shock protein 90

HSPC	hematopoietic stem/progenitor cell
HSV	herpes simplex virus
HUGO	Human Genome Organization
HVEM	herpes virus entry mediator
Hyper-CVAD	hyperfractionated cyclophosphamide, vincristine, doxorubicin, dexamethasone
IC	invasive candidiasis
ICU	intensive care unit
Ida	idarubicin
ID-AraC	intermediate-dose cytarabine
IDH	isocitrate dehydrogenase
IDO	indoleamine 2,3 dioxygenase
IFI	invasive fungal infection
IFNα	interferon alpha
IFNγ	interferon gamma
IGH	immunoglobulin heavy chain
IG/TR	immunoglobulin/T-receptor
IL	interleukin
IL-2	interleukin 2
IL1RAP	IL1 receptor accessory protein
IMI	invasive mold infection
IMIDs	immunomodulatory drugs
IND	Investigational New Drug
indel	insersion-deletion
IT	intrathecal
ITD	internal tandem duplication
IV	intravenous
JMML	juvenile myelomonocytic leukemia
JNK/AP1	c Jun N terminal kinases/activator protein 1
KIR	killer immunoglobulin-like receptor
KMT2A	lysine methyltransferase 2A
LAIP	leukemia-associated immunophenotype
LBL	lymphoblastic lymphoma
LDAC	low-dose cytosine arabinoside
LDH	lactate dehydrogenase
LFS	leukemia-free survival
LH	luteinizing hormone

LIC	leukemia-initiating cells
LOH	loss of heterozygosity
LP	lumbar puncture
LRR	log R ratio
LSC	leukemia stem cell
LT-HSC	long-term hematopoietic stem cell
M	methotrexate
MA	mitoxantrone + cytarabine
MAPK	mitogen-activated protein kinase
MCT1	monocarboxylate transporter 1
MCT4	monocarboxylate transporter 4
MDS	myelodysplastic syndrome
MDSC	myeloid-derived suppressor cell
MEC	mitomycin, etoposide, cytarabine
MEP	megakaryocytic/erythroid progenitor
MFD	matched, familial donor
MHC	major histocompatibility complex
Mit	mitoxantrone
Mito-FLAG	mitoxantrone, fludarabine, cytarabine, granulocyte colony stimulating factor
MLL	mixed lineage leukemia
MMP	matrix metalloproteinase
MOpAD	methotrexate, vincristine, pegylated asparaginase, dexamethasone
MPN	myeloproliferative neoplasm
MPO	myeloperoxidase
MPP	multipotent progenitor
MRC	Medical Research Council
MRD	minimal (or measurable) residual disease
MS	myeloid sarcoma
MSC	mesenchymal stromal cell
Mtc	mitochondria
MTD	maximal tolerated dose
mTOR	mechanistic target of rapamycin
MTX	methotrexate
MTZ	mitoxantrone
MUD	matched unrelated donor
N	asparagine

NADH	nicotinamide adenine dinucleotide (reduced)
NADPH	nicotinamide adenine dinucleotide phosphate (reduced)
N/A	not available
NCI	National Cancer Institute
NCRI	National Cancer Research Institute
NDA	new drug application
NDP	nucleoside-diphosphate
NES	nuclear export signal
NFκB	nuclear factor κB
NGS	next generation sequencing
NHL	non-Hodgkin lymphoma
NILG	Northern Italy Leukaemia Group
NK	natural killer
NLS	nuclear localization signal
NMA	nonmyeloablative
NMDP	National Marrow Donor Program
NOPHO	Nordic Society of Pediatric Hematology and Oncology
NOS	not otherwise specified
NPM	nucleophosmine
NPM1	nucleophosmine 1
NRM	nonrelapse mortality
NSAIDs	nonsteroidal antiinflammatory drugs
NSE	nonspecific esterase
OPN	osteopontin
ORR	overall response rate
OS	overall survival
P	prednisone; phosphate (or phospho)
pA	pegylated asparaginase
PAS	periodic acid-Schiff
PB	peripheral blood
PCP	pneumocystis pneumonia
PCR	pentostatin, cyclophosphamide, rituximab
PD1	programmed cell death
PDGF	platelet-derived growth factor
PDGFR	platelet-derived growth factor receptor
PE	phycoerythrin

PE-A	phycoerythrin-A
PEG	PEG-asparaginase
PerCP	peridinin chlorophyll protein
PerCP-A	peridinin-chlorophyll protein-A
Ph	Philadelphia chromosome
PK	protein kinase
PKB	Protein kinase B
PLK	Polo-like kinase
Plt	platelet
PML	promyelocytic leukemia
POMP	prednisone, vincristine, methotrexate, 6-mercaptopurine
Pos	position
PR	Partial Remission
PRD	primary refractory disease
Psl	prednisolone
PTPC	permeability transition pore complex
PT/PTT	prothrombin time/partial thromboplastin time
QA	quality assurance
R	rituximab
R/R	relapsed/refractory
RARα	retinoic acid receptor alpha
RAEB/AML	refractory anemia with excess myeloblasts/acute myeloid leukemia
ras	rat sarcoma
RBC	red blood cell
RD	Resistant Disease
RFLP	restriction fragment length polymorphism
RELP/AS-PCR	restriction fragment length polymorphism/allele-specific polymerase chain reaction
RFS	relapse-free survival
RI	reduced-intensity
RIC	reduced-intensity conditioning
RIF	realgar-indigo naturalis (an AS_4S_4-containing formulation)
RISC	RNA-induced silencing complex
RNR	ribonucleotide reductase
ROS	reactive oxygen species
RQ-PCR	real-time quantitative polymerase chain reaction
RTK	receptor tyrosine kinase

SAM	sequence alignment map
s-AML	secondary acute myeloid leukemia
SBT	sequence-based typing
SCF	stem cell factor
SCT	stem cell transplantation
SD	standard deviation
SEER	surveillance, epidemiology, and end results
SJCRH	St. Jude Children's Research Hospital
SLC1A5	solute carrier family 1 member 5
SM	solu-medrol
SNV	single nucleotide variant
SNP	single nucleotide polymorphism
SPDs	sum of the perpendicular diameters
SR	standard risk
SSC	side scatter
SSC-A	side scatter-A
SSO	sequence-specific oligonucleotide
SSP	sequence-specific priming
STRs	short tandem repeats
T	teniposide
T-ALL	T acute lymphoblastic leukemia
TAM	transient abnormal myeloid proliferations
t-AML	therapy-related acute myeloid leukemia
t-AML/t-MDS	therapy-related acute myeloid leukemia/myelodysplastic syndrome
TBI	total body irradiation
TCR	T-cell receptor
TCRB	T-cell receptors beta
TCRD	T-cell receptors delta
TCRG	T-cell receptors gamma
TdT	terminal deoxynucleotidyl transferase
TET2	ten-eleven translocation 2
TG	thioguanine
TGFβ	transforming growth factor beta
TIA	transient ischemic attack
Tie2	tunica interna endothelial cell kinase (receptor for angiopoietins)
TKI	tyrosine kinase inhibitor

TLP	T-lymphoid progenitor
TLS	tumor lysis syndrome
TMA	thrombotic microangiopathy
TMP-SMX	trimethoprim-sulfamethoxazole
TNT	tunneling nanotubules
TPO	thrombopoietin
Treg	regulatory T cell
TRM	treatment-related mortality
TSH	thyroid-stimulating hormone
UCB	unrelated cord blood
UPD	uniparental disomy
URD	unrelated donor
US	ultrasound
UTMDACC	University of Texas MD Anderson Cancer Center
V	vincristine
VCAM	vascular cell adhesion molecule
VCR	vincristine
VDJ	variable, diversity, and joining
VEGF	vascular endothelial growth factor
VEGFR	vascular endothelial growth factor receptor
VIC	variant allele-specific probe
Vind	vindesine
VOD/SOS	veno-occlusive disease and sinusoidal obstruction syndrome
VP	etoposide
VRE	vancomycin-resistant enterococci
VUS	variant of uncertain significance
WBC	white blood cell
WHO	World Health Organization
Wnt	wingless-type MMTV (mouse mammary tumor virus) integration site
WGR	tryptophan-glycine-arginine-rich domain
WT	wild-type
WT1	Wilms' tumor
Zn	zinc finger

Preface

Welcome to *Acute Leukemia: An Illustrated Guide to Diagnosis and Treatment*! When we started this project, we asked ourselves, "Who needs another textbook, especially one on acute leukemias?" After a bit of groaning and nihilism, we realized that our understanding of acute leukemias is a dynamic process, evolving in concert with our burgeoning ability to unravel the process of leukemogenesis at its most intimate molecular and cellular levels. This evolution has been taking place over at least six decades and has accelerated dramatically in the past 10 to 15 years of sophisticated genomic and other molecular technologies. With these technologies have come some powerful insights into how better to target and eradicate these devastating malignancies. So, in the end, we decided that the time might be right to create another textbook on the subject of acute leukemias, so long as we could develop something that embodied a novel approach to these very fascinating and challenging diseases.

However, traditional textbooks tend to be pretty dry—actually, very dry. Acute leukemias are anything but dry (no puns intended)! Fortunately, they lend themselves to a graphic approach, from their variegated histopathology to the depiction of new diagnostic technologies. Being able to visualize multiple intersecting molecular pathways, cellular cross-talk, and how the individual components interact provides much better understanding than a complicated text. It is so true that a picture is worth a thousand words! We certainly hope that this novel pictorial approach will afford the next generation of physicians a springboard to exert meaningful improvements for patients by exploiting cooperative cytotoxic, biologic, and immunologic treatment strategies.

While the interactive molecular and cellular components are fascinating and elegant, there is more to understanding the full impact of acute leukemias and their therapies on the host. So, in addition to the customary discussions of diagnosis, treatment, and clinical outcomes, we have included chapters on issues surrounding the epidemiology, diagnosis, treatment, and overall management in both pediatric and elderly patients; psychosexual issues that arise as a consequence of both the disease and treatment; and the complex field involving the development, approval, and regulatory aspects of new treatment strategies.

Through our pictorial approach to the broad spectrum of issues surrounding the acute leukemias and their management for patients of all ages, we have tried to blend art and science to make this resource more enjoyable and memorable than the "usual and customary" textbook. Fortunately, we were able to assemble an amazing group of clinical and basic biomedical scientists with unique, long-standing expertise in each of the subjects included in this book. We have been blessed with an amazing medical illustrator, John Ott, who has turned genes and pathways into works of art. Each contributor has given us so much more than we asked for and, as a result, we have had the joy of learning a tremendous amount while putting the book together.

And so we invite you to enjoy and learn, as we did. Our hope is that this book will stimulate you to develop new and refreshing concepts that, in turn, could lead to cures and enhanced quality of life for children and adults suffering from acute leukemias.

As simply put by Frank Gehry, "Let the experience begin!"

With our gratitude and excitement,
Ashkan Emadi, MD, PhD and Judith E. Karp, MD

1

Epidemiology

Ashkan Emadi, Farin Kamangar, and Judith E. Karp

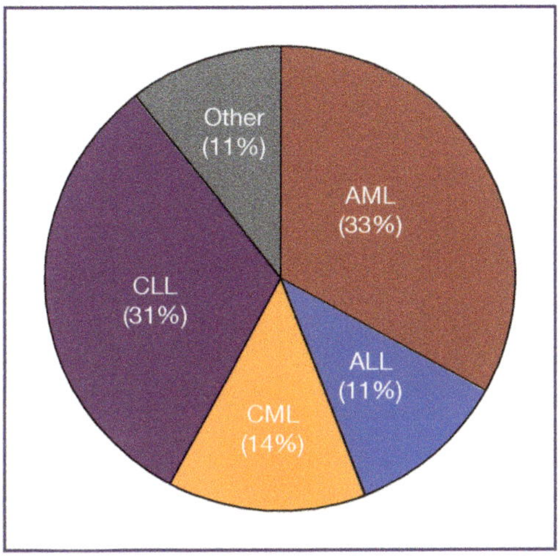

FIGURE 1-1: Estimated proportion of new cases with leukemia in 2016 in the United States by leukemia type. A total of 60,140 adults and children were diagnosed with leukemia in 2016.

ALL, acute lymphoblastic leukemia; AML, acute myeloid leukemia; CLL, chronic lymphocytic leukemia; CML, chronic myeloid leukemia.

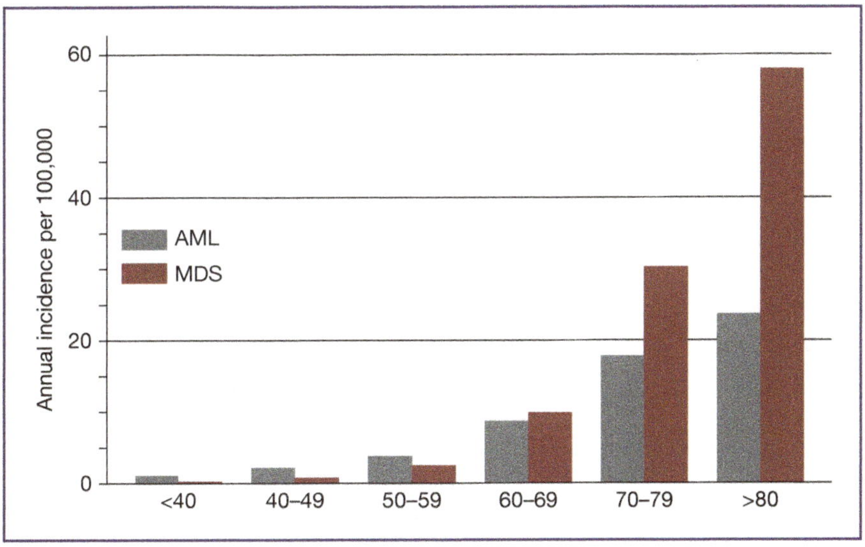

FIGURE 1-2: Incidence rates of AML and MDS by age group.

AML, acute myeloid leukemia; MDS, myelodysplastic syndrome.

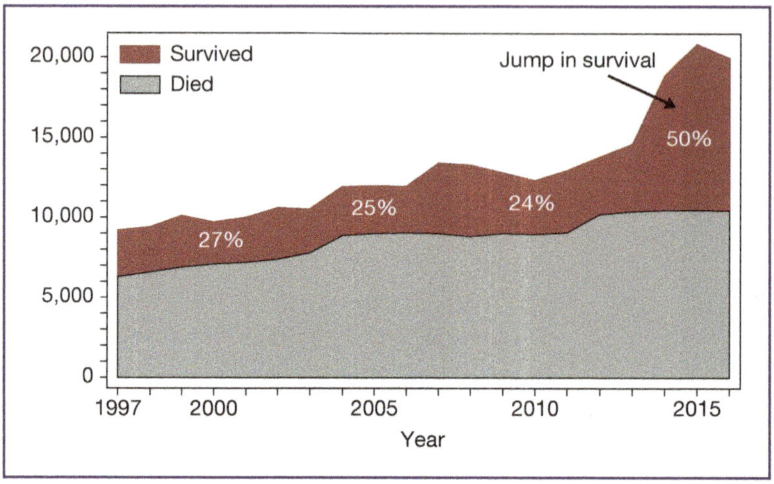

FIGURE 1-3: AML new cases and deaths by year.

AML, acute myeloid leukemia.

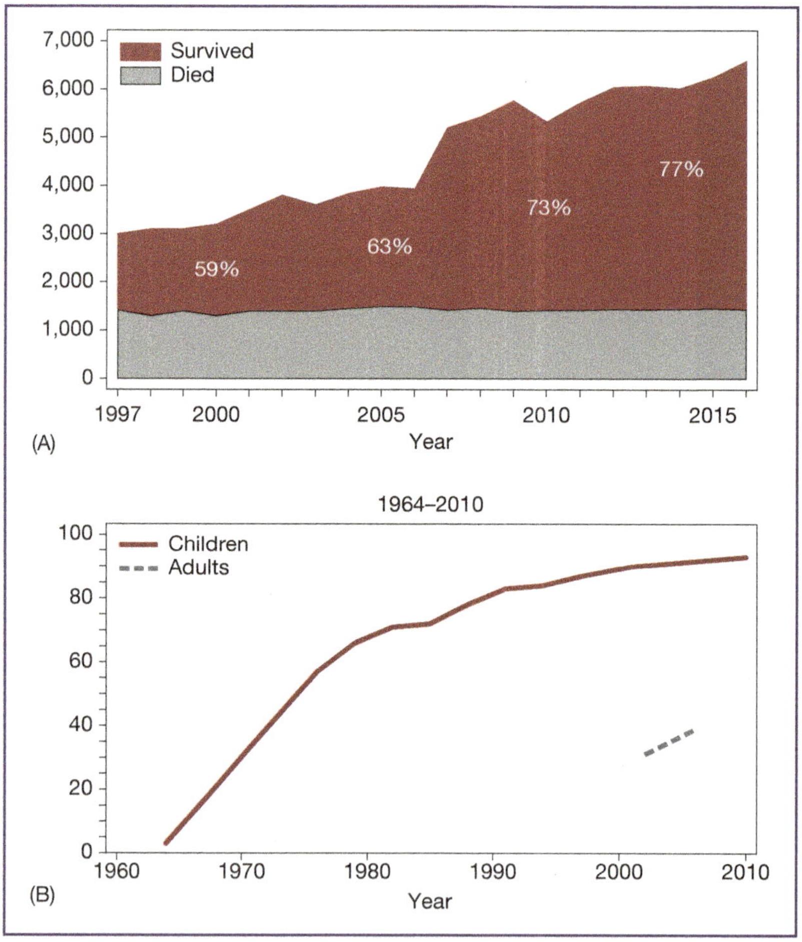

FIGURE 1-4: (A) ALL new cases (more common in children) and deaths (more common in adults) by year. (B) Five-year survival rate for ALL in children and adults (limited data available).

ALL, acute lymphoblastic leukemia.

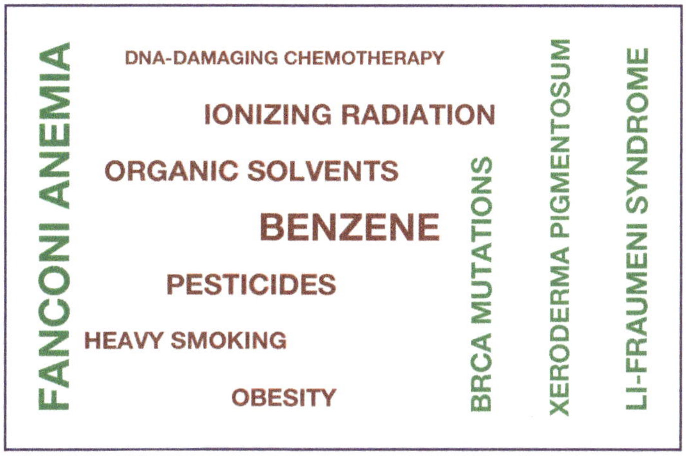

FIGURE 1-5: Environmental and genetic risk factors for acute leukemia.

Selected References

Churpek JE, Marquez R, Neistadt B, et al. Inherited mutations in cancer susceptibility genes are common among survivors of breast cancer who develop therapy-related leukemia. *Cancer*. 2016;122(2):304–311.

D'Andrea AD. Susceptibility pathways in Fanconi's anemia and breast cancer. *N Engl J Med*. 2010;362(20):1909–1919.

Emadi A, Karp JE. The state of the union on treatment of acute myeloid leukemia. *Leuk Lymphoma*. 2014;55(11):2423–2425.

Friedenson B. The BRCA1/2 pathway prevents hematologic cancers in addition to breast and ovarian cancers. *BMC Cancer*. 2007;7:152.

Golomb HM, Alimena G, Rowley JD, et al. Correlation of occupation and karyotype in adults with acute nonlymphocytic leukemia. *Blood*. 1982;60(2):404–411.

Le Beau MM, Albain KS, Larson RA, et al. Clinical and cytogenetic correlations in 63 patients with therapy-related myelodysplastic syndromes and acute nonlymphocytic leukemia: further evidence for characteristic abnormalities of chromosomes no. 5 and 7. *J Clin Oncol*. 1986;4(3):325–345.

Lindsley RC, Mar BG, Mazzola E, et al. Acute myeloid leukemia ontogeny is defined by distinct somatic mutations. *Blood*. 2015;125(9):1367–1376.

Pedersen-Bjergaard J, Rowley JD. The balanced and the unbalanced chromosome aberrations of acute myeloid leukemia may develop in different ways and may contribute differently to malignant transformation. *Blood*. 1994;83(10):2780–2786.

Siegel RL, Miller KD, Jemal A. Cancer statistics, 2016. *CA Cancer J Clin*. 2016;66(1):7–30.

Smith MT, Zhang L, Jeng M, et al. Hydroquinone, a benzene metabolite, increases the level of aneusomy of chromosomes 7 and 8 in human CD34-positive blood progenitor cells. *Carcinogenesis*. 2000;21(8):1485–1490.

Stillman WS, Varella-Garcia M, Irons RD. The benzene metabolite, hydroquinone, selectively induces 5q31- and -7 in human CD34+CD19- bone marrow cells. *Exp Hematol*. 2000;28(2):169–176.

Wolff AC, Blackford AL, Visvanathan K, et al. Risk of marrow neoplasms after adjuvant breast cancer therapy: the national comprehensive cancer network experience. *J Clin Oncol*. 2015;33(4):340–348.

Zhang L, Yang W, Hubbard AE, Smith MT. Nonrandom aneuploidy of chromosomes 1, 5, 6, 7, 8, 9, 11, 12, and 21 induced by the benzene metabolites hydroquinone and benzenetriol. *Environ Mol Mutagen*. 2005;45(4):388–396.

2

Diagnosis

Clinical Manifestations of Acute Leukemia

Daniel L. Duncan, Nathan D. Montgomery, Matthew C. Foster, and Joshua F. Zeidner

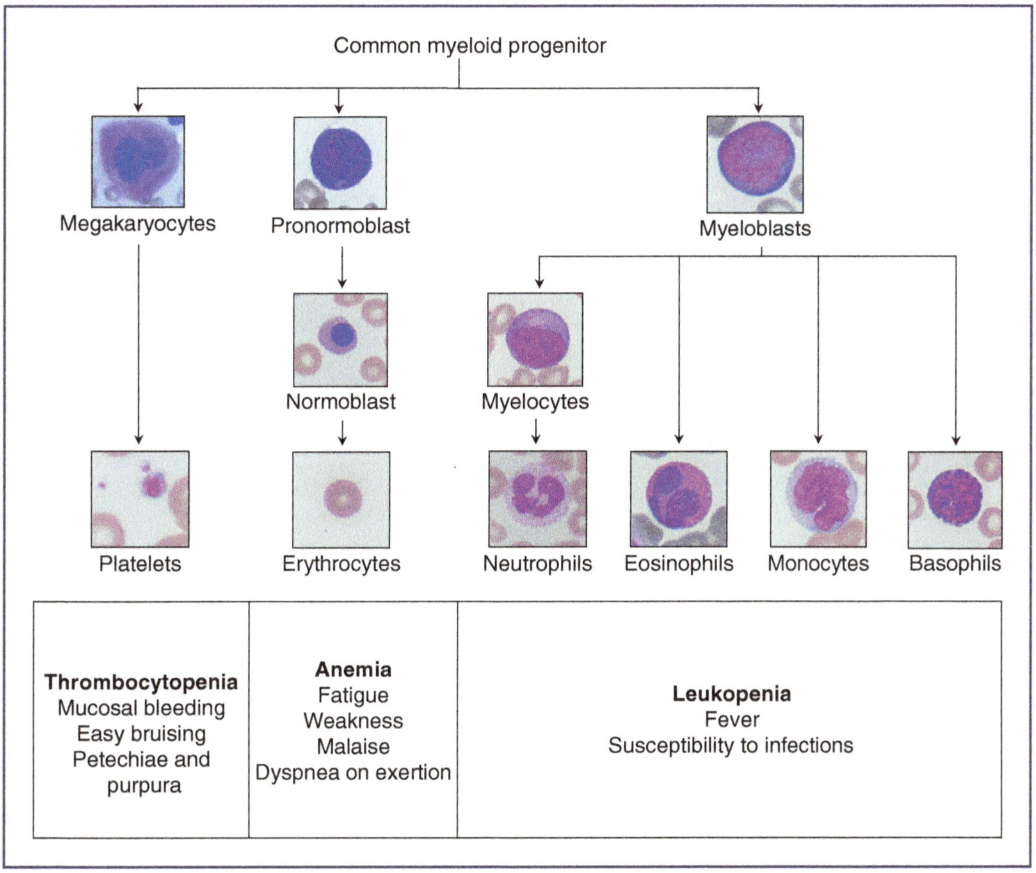

FIGURE 2-1: Lineage-specific clinical manifestations of acute leukemia. Intermediate steps in the differentiation from a primitive progenitor cell (ie, common myeloid progenitor) to mature myeloid cells. Common clinical manifestations of acute leukemia result from clonal proliferation of myeloblasts (ie, AML) or lymphoblasts (ie, ALL), which replace normal bone marrow cells, leading to the inadequate production of platelets (ie, thrombocytopenia), erythrocytes (ie, anemia), and functionally normal white blood cells (WBC) (ie, neutrophils and lymphocytes). Symptoms of thrombocytopenia include mucosal bleeding, easy bruising, and petechiae/purpura. Patients can present with spontaneous hemorrhage including intracranial, subdural, or intraabdominal hematomas. Symptoms of anemia include fatigue, weakness, pallor, malaise, and dyspnea on exertion, typically prompting patients to seek medical care. Neutropenia/lymphopenia can lead to a high risk of infections with viral, bacterial, or fungal etiologies. The earliest lymphoid cells also originate in the bone marrow but because most lymphoid maturation occurs outside of the marrow, these steps are not emphasized in Figure 2-1.

ALL, acute lymphoblastic leukemia; AML, acute myeloid leukemia.

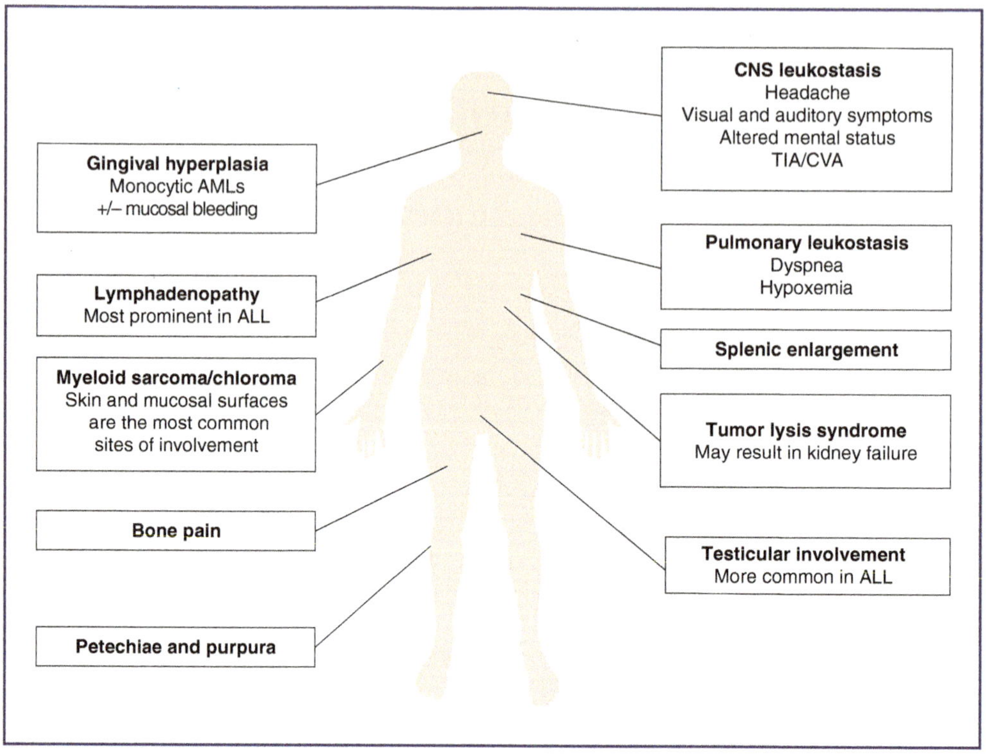

FIGURE 2-2: Anatomic sites of potential leukemic involvement. Acute leukemia can manifest in a variety of anatomic locations, as shown in Figure 2-2. The clinical presentation and site of leukemic involvement is often predicated on the nature of the leukemic blasts. For instance, lymphadenopathy can be commonly seen with ALL, whereas leukostasis is more common in AML (see Figure 2-4). It is important for the clinician to be aware of these sites during the diagnosis and management of acute leukemia.

ALL, acute lymphoblastic leukemia; AML, acute myeloid leukemia; CNS, central nervous system; TIA/CVA, transient ischemic attack/cerebrovascular accident.

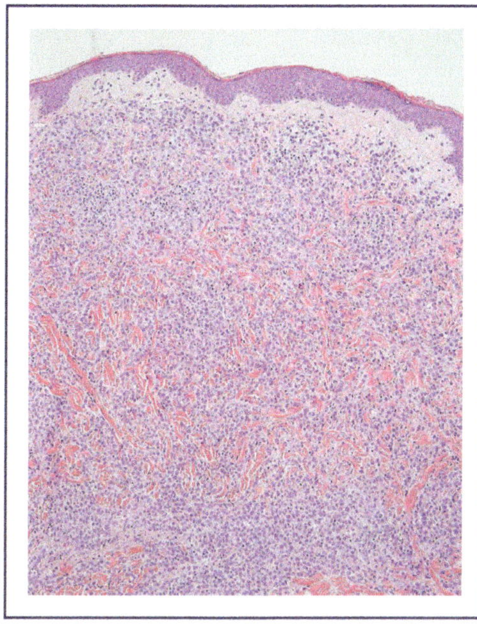

FIGURE 2-3: Myeloid sarcoma. Myeloid sarcoma (historically termed "chloroma" or "granulocytic sarcoma") refers to extramedullary accumulation of myeloblasts in AML. Rarely, these lesions may present as an isolated lesion without an antecedent diagnosis of AML. Myeloid sarcoma can involve any anatomic site, but most commonly occurs in skin (known as leukemia cutis) and mucosal surfaces. As a mass-forming hematologic lesion, myeloid sarcoma must be differentiated from lymphoma. Histologic diagnosis can be confirmed by cytochemical and immunophenotypic characterization. Commonly expressed antigens seen in cases of myeloid sarcoma include CD68 (>95%), myeloperoxidase (84%), CD117 (80%), and CD34 (<50%). Myeloid sarcomas are generally thought to confer a poor prognosis.

AML, acute myeloid leukemia.

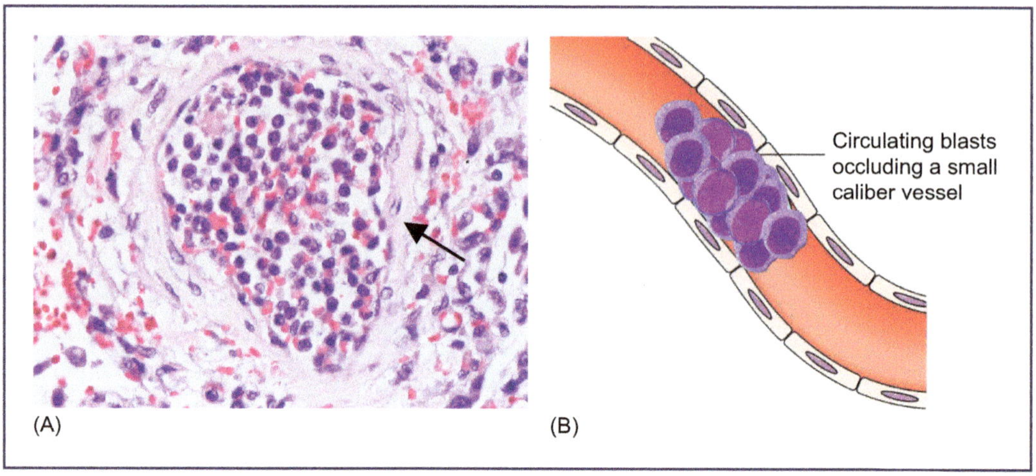

FIGURE 2-4: Leukostasis in acute leukemia. Leukostasis is the symptomatic presentation of hyperleukocytosis with the accumulation of blasts (typically myeloblasts) in blood vessels, leading to occlusion and resultant hypoxemia (Figures 2-4A and 2-4B). Although leukostasis can occur with any abnormal elevation in absolute blast count, it is more commonly seen in patients presenting with WBC counts >100,000/mcL. Leukostasis is more commonly seen in AML (5%–20%) due to the large size of myeloblasts and specific interactions with cell surface antigens such as selectins and cell adhesion molecules. Moreover, monocytic subtypes of AML (ie, FAB classification M4 and M5) present the highest risk of leukostasis compared to other AML subtypes. (A) Histologic image from the autopsy of a lung of a patient who died from leukostasis; the arrow denotes the wall of a blood vessel. The lumen of this blood vessel is filled with myeloblasts. The same concept is demonstrated schematically in (B). The resultant hypoxemia from leukostasis can manifest in a variety of ways depending on the affected tissue. The most common sites of involvement are the CNS (manifesting as mental status changes, confusion, headaches, blurred vision, cranial neuropathies) and lungs (manifesting as dyspnea and hypoxia), although renal, cardiac, and generalized vascular symptoms can occur as well. Leukostasis represents an oncologic emergency and rapid reduction in WBC count is necessary. Management options for leukostasis are discussed in Chapter 3 (Hyperleukocytosis).

AML, acute myeloid leukemia; CNS, central nervous system; FAB, French American British; WBC, white blood cell.

Selected Reference

Pileri SA, Ascani S, Cox MC, et al. Myeloid sarcoma: clinico-pathologic, phenotypic and cytogenetic analysis of 92 adult patients. *Leukemia*. 2007;21(2):340–350.

Pathology, Classification, and Methodologies

HISTOPATHOLOGY

Zeba N. Singh and Qing C. Chen

Acute leukemia is a heterogeneous group of hematopoietic neoplasms resulting from clonal proliferation of immature precursor cells (blasts). The genetic aberrations resulting in the blockage of differentiation and uncontrolled proliferation of the blasts may occur at different developmental stages, including the pluripotential stem cells, and the progenitors committed to the lymphoid or myeloid lineages.

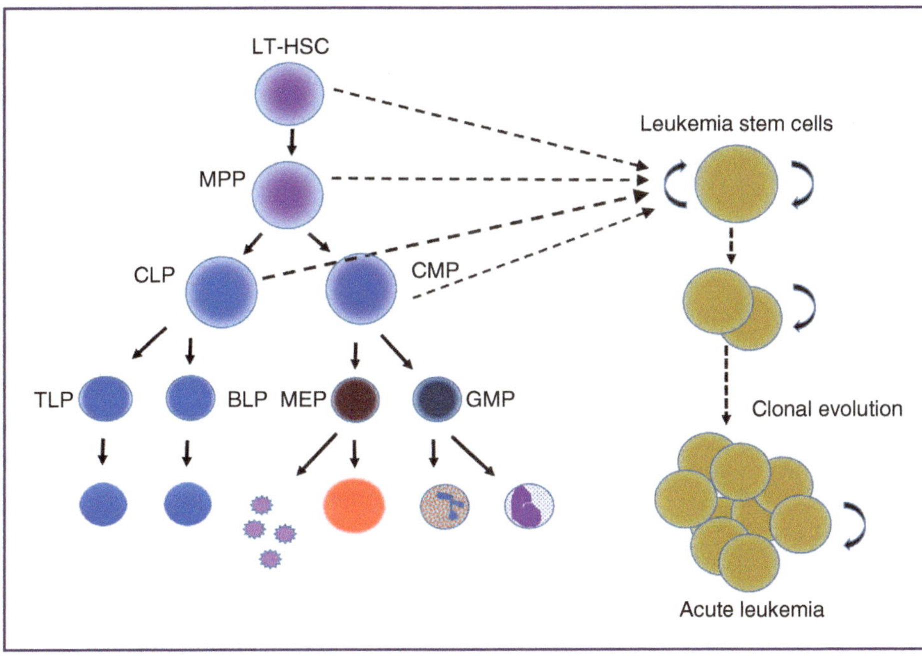

FIGURE 2-5: Pathogenesis of acute leukemia. The differentiation and phenotype of the acute leukemia varies based on the progenitors in the hematopoietic hierarchy.

BLP, B-lymphoid progenitor; CLP, common lymphoid progenitor; CMP, common myeloid progenitor; GMP, granulocyte/macrophage progenitor; LT-HSC, long-term hematopoietic stem cell; MEP, megakaryocytic/erythroid progenitor; MPP, multipotent progenitor; TLP, T-lymphoid progenitor.

The pathogenesis of acute leukemia is a cooperative effect of several genetic events—the initial event conferring self-renewal, coupled with additional mutations contributing to developmental arrest, changes in cell-cycle regulation, tumor suppression, and chromatin modification, ultimately results in the establishment of the neoplastic clone. In this chapter, we discuss the diagnostic aspects of acute leukemia. The diagnosis of acute leukemia requires the following:

1. Morphological assessment
2. Determination of cytochemical and immunophenotypic features
3. Evaluation of genetic abnormalities

Morphology

Morphology is evaluated in the peripheral blood (PB), bone marrow (BM), and less frequently in solid tissues. Different specimen types are required for a comprehensive evaluation; therefore, planning prior to the diagnostic procedure is important.

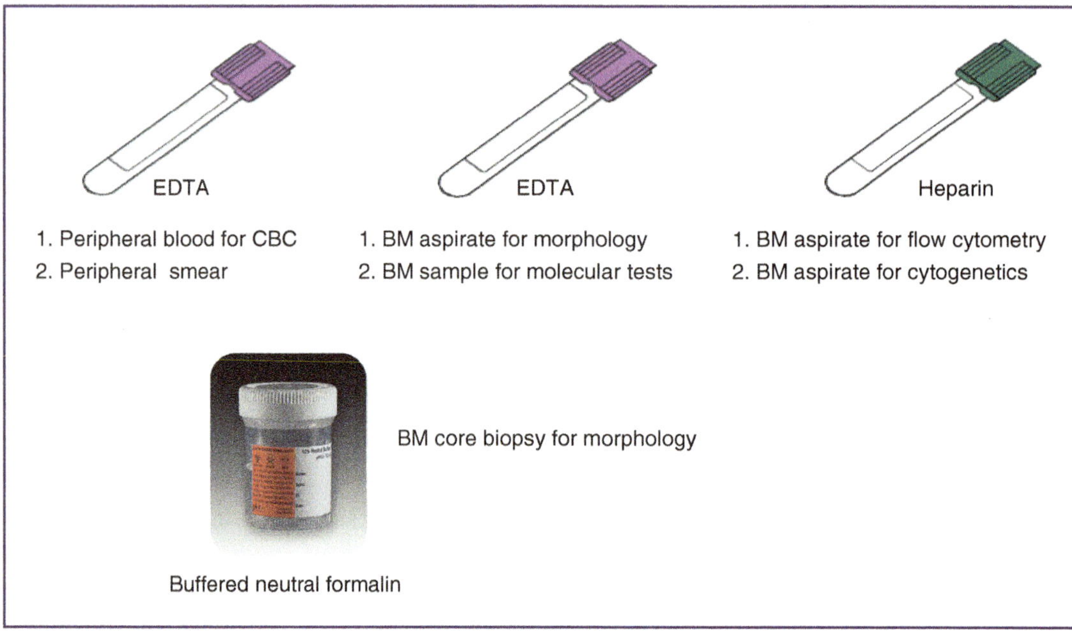

FIGURE 2-6: Sample requirement for diagnostic work-up of acute leukemia.
BM, bone marrow; CBC, complete blood count; EDTA, ethylenediaminetetraacetic acid.

PB examination should be correlated with the results of complete blood count (CBC). PB of acute leukemia patients almost always shows features of bone marrow failure, including anemia, thrombocytopenia, and neutropenia. Blasts are usually present, but the number varies widely. A manual 200-leukocyte differential is recommended unless the total count is too low to permit this. Enumeration of PB blasts, their morphology, presence of lineage-defining morphological features such as Auer rods, specific morphological features of promyelocytes, monoblasts, blasts with "Burkitt-like morphology," and dyspoietic features are important diagnostic clues that should be documented. Presence of schistocytes alerts to the possibility of associated disseminated intravascular coagulation. A preserved platelet count with giant platelets may suggest megakaryoblastic leukemia, or leukemia evolved from a prior myeloproliferative neoplasm (MPN).

BM examination: A BM differential count is performed on a Wright–Giemsa stained aspirate smear by counting 500 nucleated cells. Enumeration of the blasts is essential for diagnosis. *A diagnosis of acute leukemia requires 20% blasts in the PB or BM. The exceptions are acute myeloid leukemia with recurrent genetic abnormalities where the presence of the genetic abnormality defines acute leukemia.* For the purpose of enumeration, promonocytes are considered as "blast equivalents" in all AML, whereas promyelocytes are considered "blast equivalent" only in cases of acute promyelocytic leukemia. While flow cytometry is widely used for identification and characterization of blasts, blast percentages should be derived by morphological evaluation of the BM aspirate smears. Trephine biopsy is valuable for assessment of marrow cellularity, megakaryocyte distribution and morphology, presence of fibrosis, and other abnormal cells. In the event of a dry tap due to a packed marrow or associated marrow fibrosis, the biopsy is crucial for diagnosis of acute leukemia.

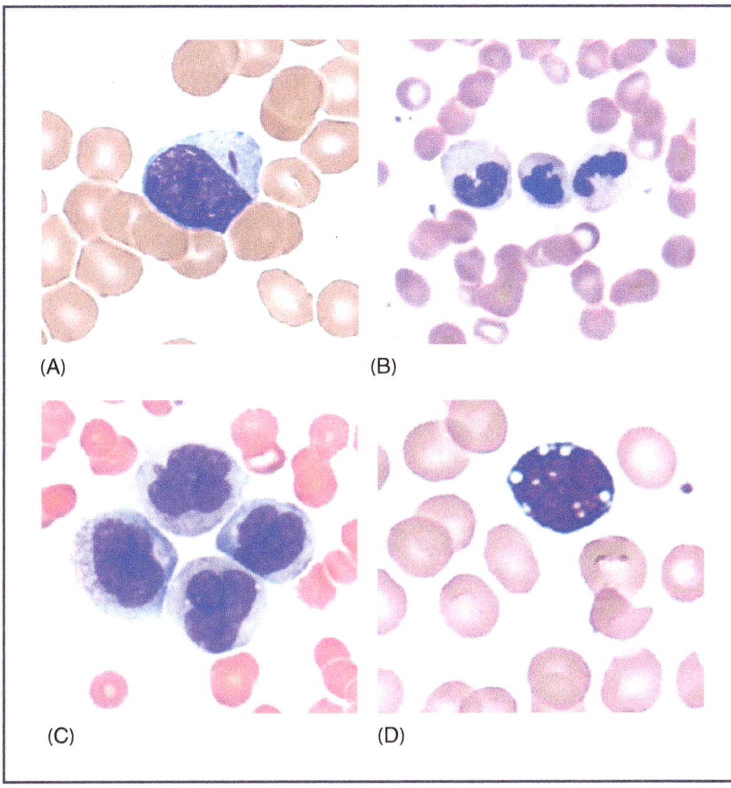

FIGURE 2-7: Peripheral blood smears (Wright stain) showing (A) Blast with Auer rod (×40), (B) Dysplastic neutrophils in AML with myelodysplasia-related changes (×20), (C) Promonocytes in acute monocytic leukemia (×40), (D) Blasts with cytoplasmic vacuoles in acute lymphoblastic leukemia with t(8;14)*MYC-IgH* (×40).

AML, acute myeloid leukemia.

Cytochemical stains are a useful adjunct to identify blast lineages. Myeloperoxidase (MPO) is specific for myeloblasts; it is usually negative or weakly positive in monoblasts and promonocytes. Lymphoid blasts, erythroid blasts, and megakaryoblasts are MPO negative. Nonspecific esterases (NSE) show diffuse reactivity in monoblasts and monocytes. Naphthol AS-D chloroacetate esterase (CAE) is a reliable specific esterase for the granulocytic lineage from the promyelocyte stage onward. A combined esterase reaction can help in identification of granulocytic (CAE positive) and monocytic (NSE positive) lineages. A positive cytochemical stain is helpful, but a negative reaction does not exclude a myeloid lineage.

Immunophenotyping is an integral part of work-up for acute leukemia. It not only defines the lineage of the leukemia cells but also identifies unusual phenotypic features that provide clues for specific types of acute leukemia. For example, expression of CD19 on myeloid blasts is often associated with AML with t(8;21), while lack of CD10 expression on B lymphoblasts is highly suggestive of B lymphoblastic leukemia with t(4;11). In suspected acute promyelocytic leukemia, the combination of lack of CD34 and HLA-DR expression plus high side scatter and bright CD33 expression is supportive of the diagnosis. Identification of the aberrant immunophenotypic characteristics of the leukemia cells is crucial for minimal residual disease evaluation. Furthermore, some of the immunophenotypic profiles may have prognostic value.

For leukemia analysis, a gating strategy based on CD45 expression and side scatter properties is routinely used. On the CD45 versus side scatter dot plot, the cells can be divided or gated into four major populations: blasts, lymphocytes, granulocytes, and monocytes. Subsequent analysis of antigen expression allows immunophenotypic characterization of the blasts and other cell populations.

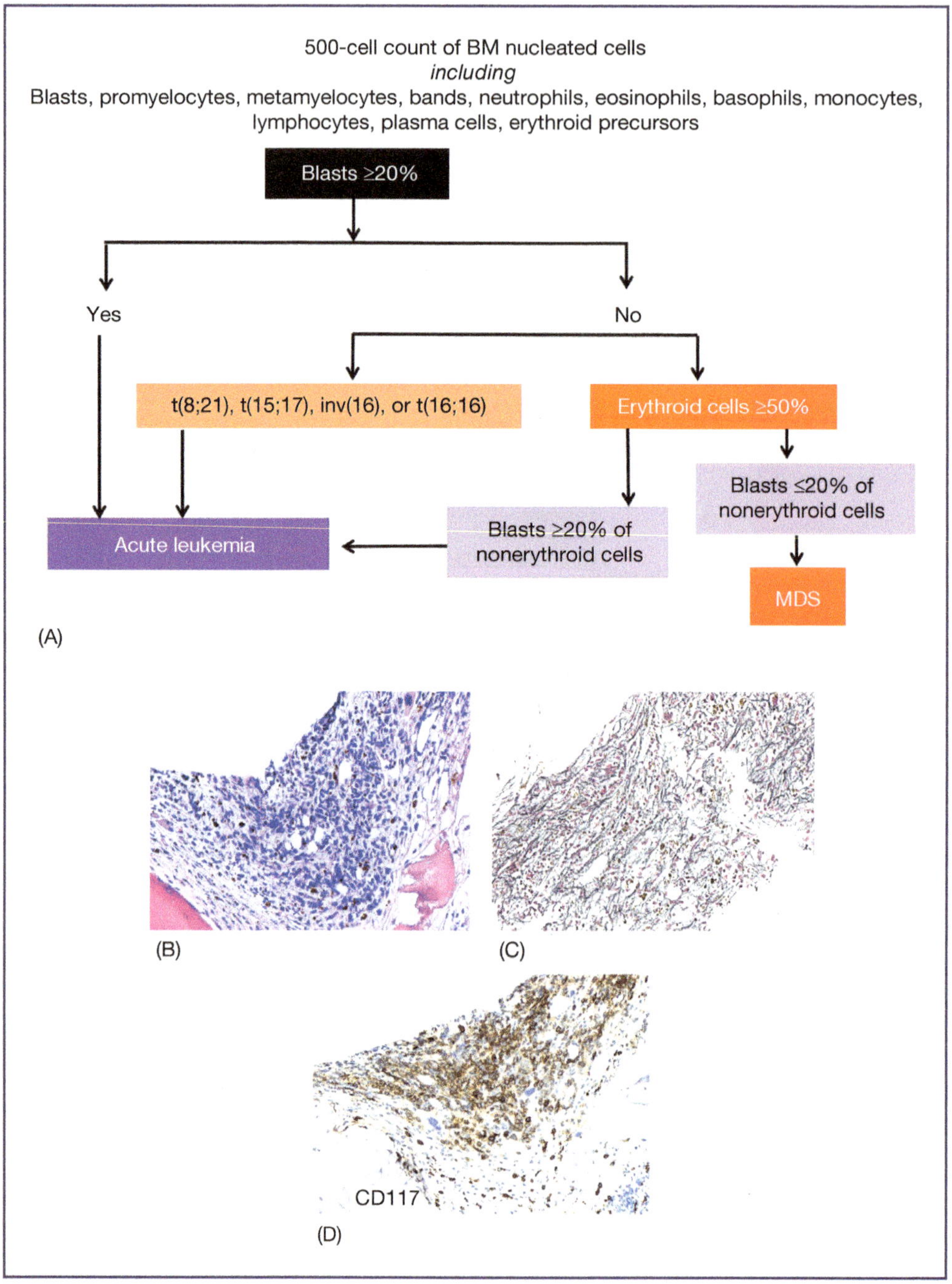

FIGURE 2-8: **(A) Algorithm for performing bone marrow differential count. A diagnosis of acute leukemia is made when blasts are ≥20% of marrow nucleated cells, or ≥20% of nonerythroid cells when the erythroid component is >50%, or at any blast percentage in the presence of recurrent cytogenetic abnormalities [t(8;21), t(15;17), or inv(16)]. The last two mentioned are applicable to AML. (B) AML with fibrosis that resulted in a dry tap. Bone marrow biopsy showing increased immature cells in a fibrotic background (Hematoxylin and Eosin ×20), (C) Reticulin stain (×20) in the same case showing Grade 2 fibrosis, (D) Immunoperoxidase stain (×20) with antibody to CD117 showing more than 20% blasts in the bone marrow.**

AML, acute myeloid leukemia; BM, bone marrow; MDS, myelodysplastic syndrome.

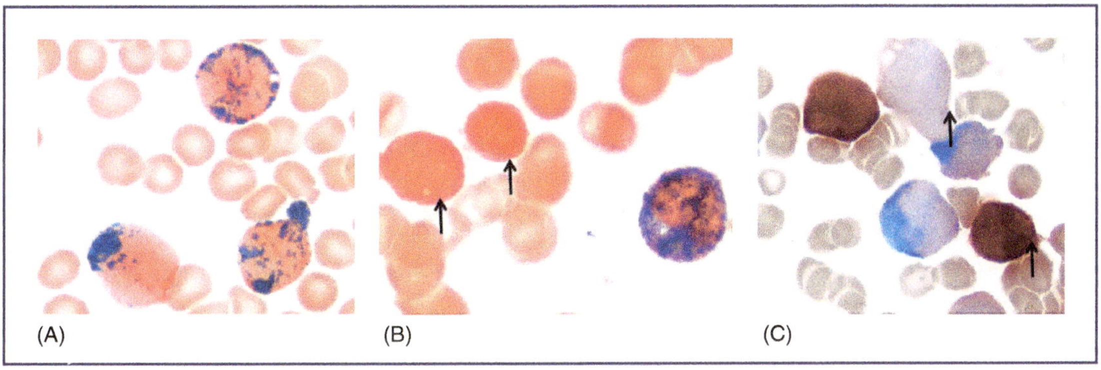

FIGURE 2-9: Cytochemical stains. (A) Myeloperoxidase (MPO). The positive reaction is seen as blue granules in the cytoplasm of the myeloid blasts. (B) Lymphoid blasts (arrow) are MPO negative. A positive neutrophil is seen in the field for comparison. (C) Double esterase stain. The monocytic lineage has a positive reaction for nonspecific esterase (red-brown) and the granulocytic lineage reacts with chloracetate esterase (blue).

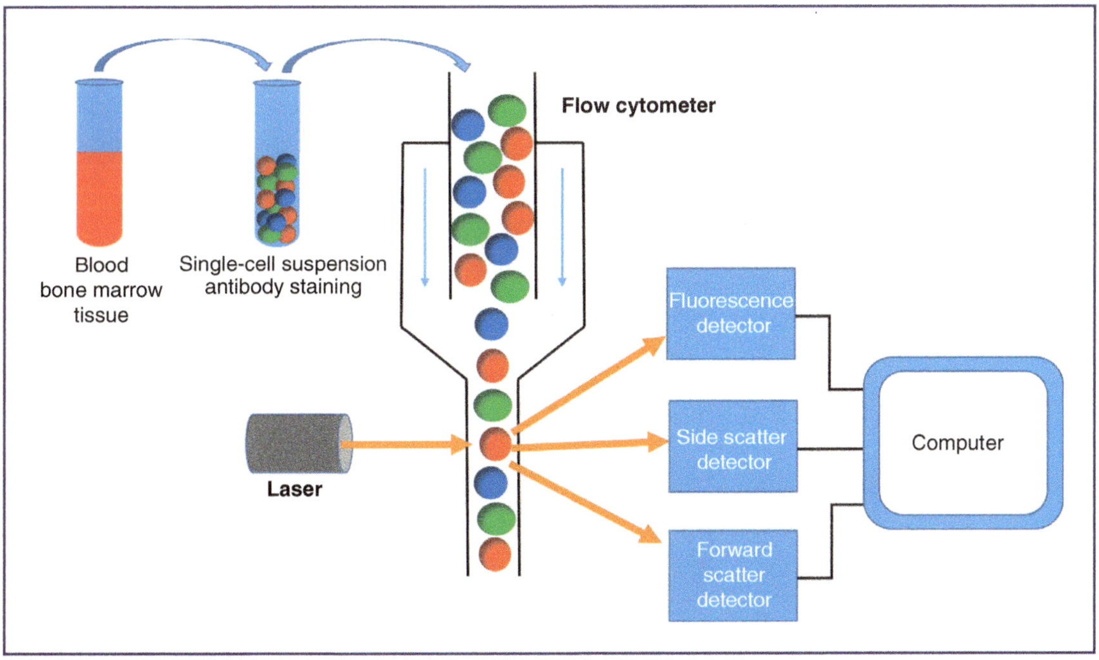

FIGURE 2-10: A schematic illustration of flow cytometry immunophenotyping. A single-cell suspension is prepared from blood, bone marrow aspirate, or solid tissue, and stained with fluorochrome-conjugated antibodies. The cells are then loaded on to the flow cytometer and run through a very narrow nozzle that allows the cells to go past the laser light one cell at a time. The light scattered by the cells and the fluorescent signal emitted by the attached antibodies are detected by a number of detectors. The data are stored and analyzed by a computer.

Immunohistochemistry can aid in the diagnosis of acute leukemia, in particular when bone marrow aspirate is inadequate due to various reasons such as marrow fibrosis (Figure 2-8), hypocellularity (Figure 2-12), or packed marrow. In cases of myeloid sarcoma or lymphoblastic lymphoma, immunohistochemical staining of tissue sections can be crucial in making the correct diagnosis.

Table 2-1 Major antigens expressed by hematopoietic cells

COMMON LEUKOCYTE	MYELOID CELL	T/NK CELL	B CELL
CD45	CD13	CD1	CD10
CD43	CD33	CD2	CD19
	CD15	CD3	CD20
PROGENITOR	***Granulocyte***	CD5	CD22
CD34	MPO	CD7	CD79a
CD117 (myeloid)	***Monocyte***	CD4	PAX-5
TdT (lymphoid)	CD14	CD8	
	CD64	CD56 (NK)	
OTHERS	***Erythrocyte***		
HLA-DR (blast, B cell, monocyte; Not promyelocyte, Not T cell)	CD235a		
	Megakaryocyte		
	CD41		
	CD61		

HLA-DR, human leukocyte antigen-D related; MPO, myeloperoxidase; NK, natural killer; TdT, terminal deoxynucleotidyl transferase.

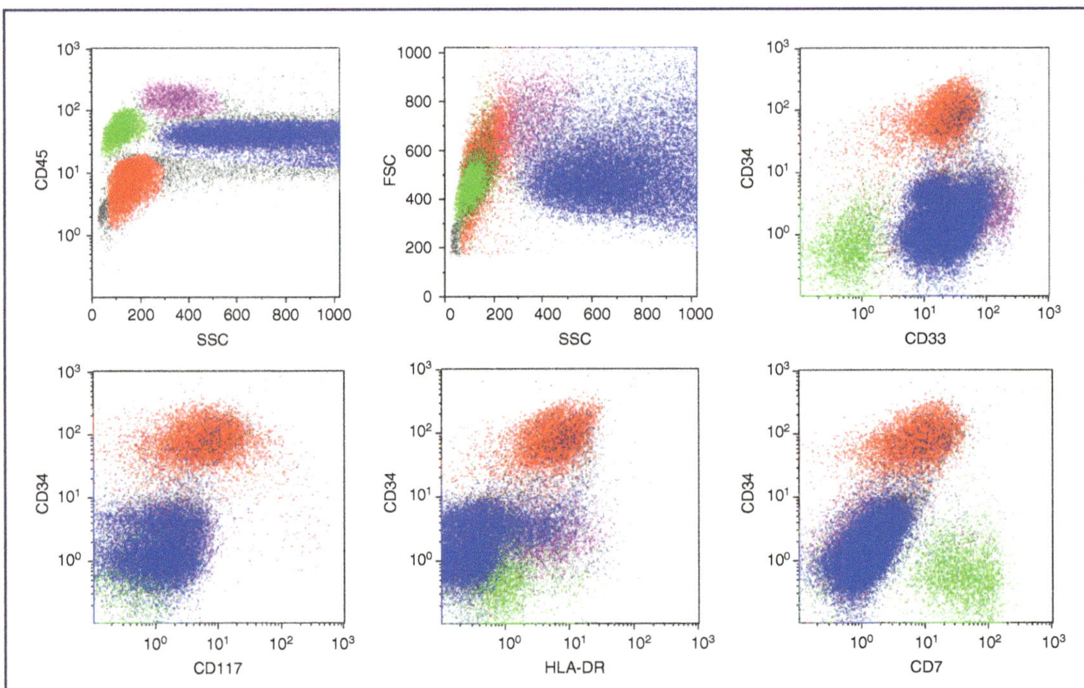

FIGURE 2-11: Flow cytometric analysis of bone marrow sample from a case of AML. The CD45 versus side scatter (SSC) plot identifies four populations of cells: blasts (red), granulocytes (blue), monocytes (magenta), and lymphocytes (green). The forward scatter (FSC) vs. SSC plot shows the sizes of the cells but does not separate blasts from lymphocytes (the blasts range from small to medium/large in size and overlap with lymphocytes). Analysis of various antigens demonstrates that the blasts express precursor markers CD34 and CD117, myeloid markers CD33 and CD117, and HLA-DR positive, and show aberrant dim expression of CD7. Also note that the majority of the lymphocytes are CD7 positive (likely T cells); the granulocytes express CD33 but not CD34, CD117, or HLA-DR; and the monocytes express bright CD33 and HLA-DR.

AML, acute myeloid leukemia; HLA-DR, human leukocyte antigen-D related.

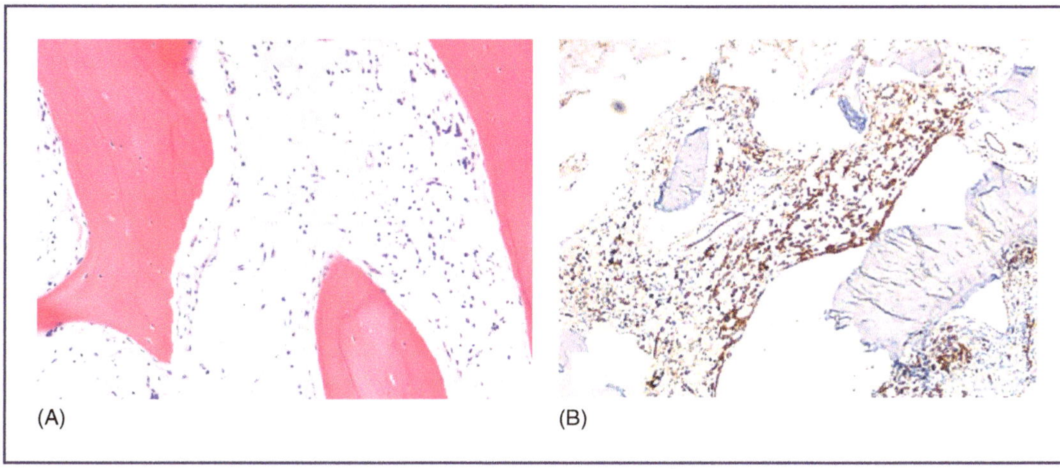

FIGURE 2-12: **A markedly hypocellular bone marrow from a 35-year-old male with pancytopenia. (A) Hematoxylin and eosin (×10), (B) Immunoperoxidase stain for CD34 (×10) shows that the majority of cells are CD34-positive blasts.**

CLASSIFICATION OF AML

The current diagnostic approach to acute leukemia is tailored around the World Health Organization (WHO) classification for hematopoietic neoplasms. The WHO classification system is based on the premise that clinically meaningful classification requires a combination of clinical, morphological, immunophenotypic, and genetic features. AML can be divided into three major groups: a genetically defined group, a biologically defined group, and a group based on cell morphology and lineage origin (Figure 2-13). Three unusual types of myeloid precursor diseases are also included under the umbrella of AML.

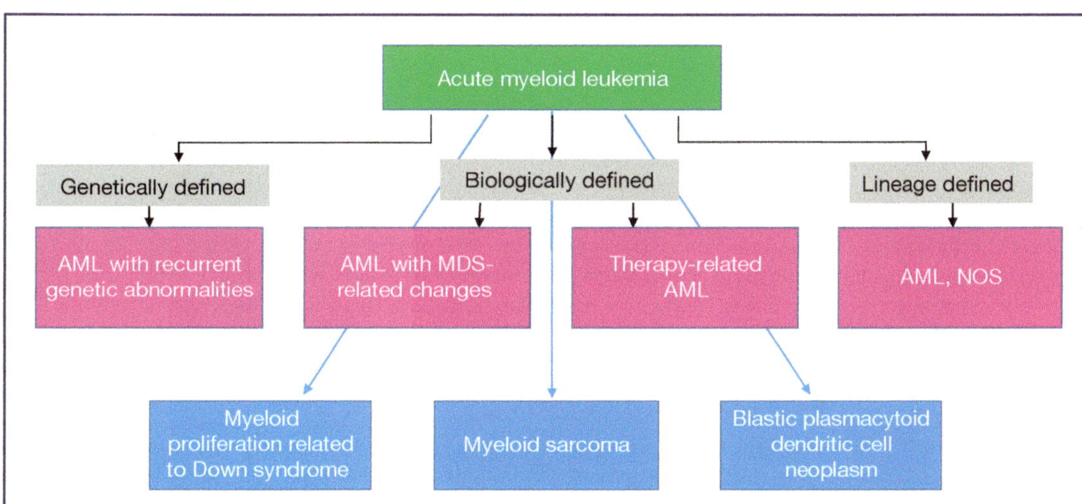

FIGURE 2-13: **Major categories of AML based on the current WHO classification (2008).**
AML, acute myeloid leukemia; MDS, myelodysplastic syndrome, NOS, not otherwise specified; WHO, World Health Organization.

AML With Recurrent Genetic Abnormalities (See Also Section Molecular Mutations in AML, page 57)

The current WHO classification identifies seven subtypes of AML with recurrent cytogenetic abnormalities (Table 2-2).

Table 2-2 AML with recurrent genetic abnormalities

SUBTYPES	INCIDENCE	PROGNOSIS	MORPHOLOGY
AML with t(8;21)*	7% adult, 15% children	Good	Large blasts
AML with inv(16)/t(16;16)*	5% adult, 5%–12% children	Good	Atypic eosinophils
APL with t(15;17)*	5%–12% adult, 8%–15% children	Good	Promyelocytes
AML with t(9;11)	1% adult, 12% children	Intermediate	Monoblasts
AML with t(6;9)	1% adult, 10% children	Poor	Basophilia, dysplasia
AML with inv(3)/t(3;3)	1%–2% adult	Poor	Atypic megakaryocytes, thrombocytosis
AML with t(1;22)	<0.5%, in infants	Poor	Megakaryoblastic

*AML with t(8;21), inv(16)/t(16;16), and t(15;17) do not require 20% blasts for diagnosis of AML.
AML, acute myeloid leukemia; APL, acute promyelocytic leukemia.

The salient features of AML with recurrent genetic abnormalities are as follows:

1. The genetic abnormalities confer a statistically significant prognosis to AML in this group. AML with t(8;21)(q22;q22), t(16;16)(p13.1;q22), or inv(16)(p13.1;q22) have a good response to chemotherapy. AML with t(15;17) is unique in its excellent response to all trans-retinoic acid (ATRA). AML with t(9;11)(p22;q23) has an intermediate prognosis.
2. *They are classified as AML regardless of the blast count.* AML with t(8;21); t(16;16) or inv(16); and t(15;17) are considered AML even if the blast count is less than 20% as the chromosomal translocations define AML in these leukemias.
3. Many of these leukemias have distinct morphological and immunophenotypic features.

*AML With t(8;21)(q22;q22)/*RUNX1-RUNX1T1

AML with t(8;21) commonly have large blasts with fine azurophil granules and long thin Auer rods (Figure 2-14A). Variable numbers of promyelocytes, myelocytes, and metamyelocytes are present. The appearance is akin to "AML with maturation." Dysgranulopoiesis is often present with abnormalities of nuclear lobation, pseudo-Pelger-Huet nuclei, and abnormal granulation, sometimes as large globular, pseudo Chediak-Higashi granules, or a homogeneous salmon pink cytoplasm of the neutrophils (Figure 2-14A). Immunophenotypically, the blasts have strong expression of CD34, HLA-DR, and CD13, and weak expression of CD33. They frequently have aberrant expression of B-lymphoid antigens CD19 (Figure 2-14B). Nearly 70% of AML with t(8;21) show additional chromosomal abnormalities such as loss of sex chromosome or del(9q); 30% of pediatric patients may have cooperating *NRAS* or *KRAS* mutations; *KIT* mutations may occur in 25% of the patients. Patients with *KIT* mutations have a high white cell count at presentation, higher incidence of extramedullary disease during the course of the disease, and a significantly higher incidence of relapse and lower overall survival at 24 months compared with those who did not have *KIT* mutations. It is therefore prudent to test for *KIT* mutations in patients who have a high white cell count at presentation or persistent disease at the end of induction chemotherapy.

*AML With inv(16)(p13.1;q22)/*CBFB-MYH11 *or t(16;16)(p13.1;q22)/*CBFB-MYH11

AML with inv(16)(p13.1;q22) or t(16;16)(p13.1;q22) involving the *CBFB* and *MYH11* genes is morphologically characterized by myelomonocytic differentiation and presence of a variable number

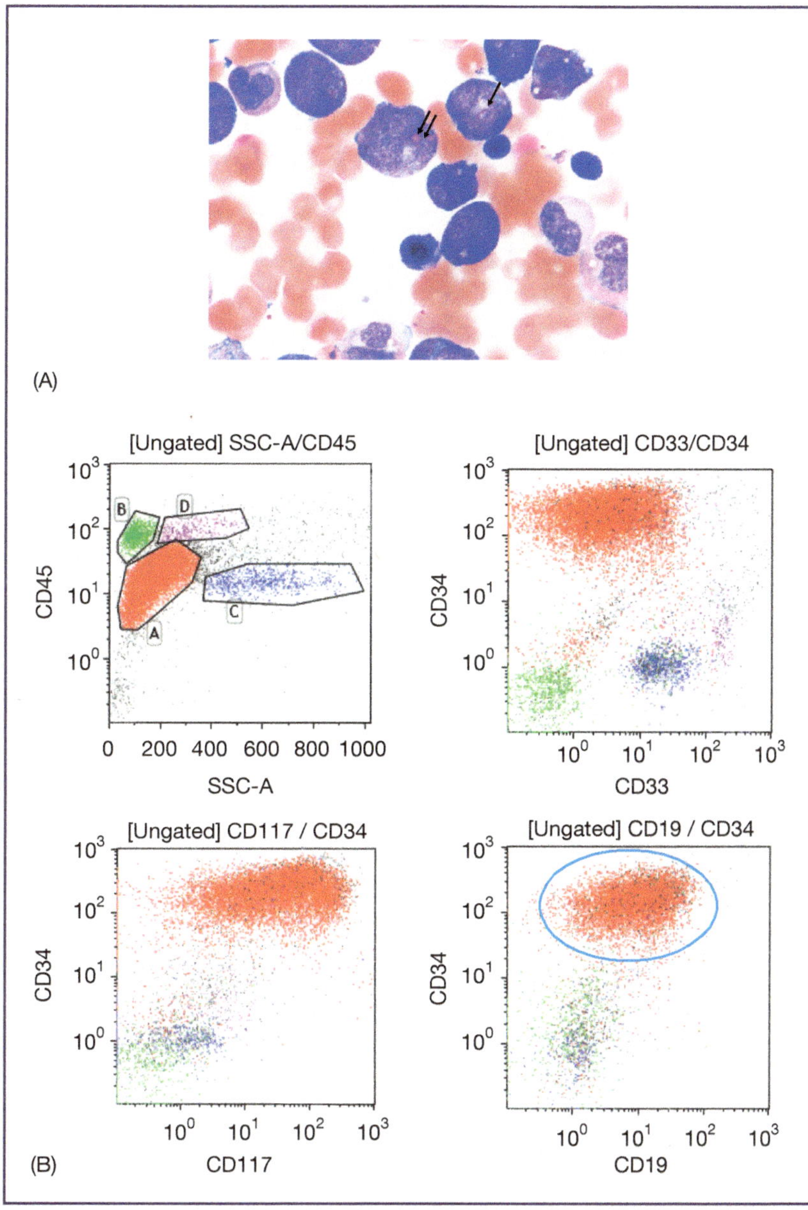

FIGURE 2-14: (A) AML with t(8;21). Note blasts with azurophil granules, thin rod-like Auer rod (single arrow), and Chediak-Higaski-like granules (double arrow). Wright stain X50, (B) Flow cytometric analysis of AML with t(8;21). The blasts (red) are positive for CD34, CD117, CD33, CD13 (not shown), MPO (not shown), HLA-DR (not shown), and have aberrant expression of B-cell marker CD19 (within blue circle).

AML, acute myeloid leukemia; HLA-DR, human leukocyte antigen-D related; MPO, myeloperoxidase; SSC-A, side scatter-A.

of abnormal eosinophils that have abnormal basophilic granules (Figure 2-15A). These abnormal granules are more frequent in the eosinophil precursors. Flow cytometric analysis typically identifies a population of myeloblasts and a population of monocytes (Figure 2-15B). The inv(16) abnormality is subtle and may be missed in metaphase preparations. Interphase FISH studies should be requested if the morphological features raise this as a possibility. Secondary cytogenetic abnormalities are present in 40% of patients, the most frequent being +22 and +8. Mutations of *KIT* occur in about 30% of the cases and can note an adverse outcome for this leukemia with an otherwise favorable outcome.

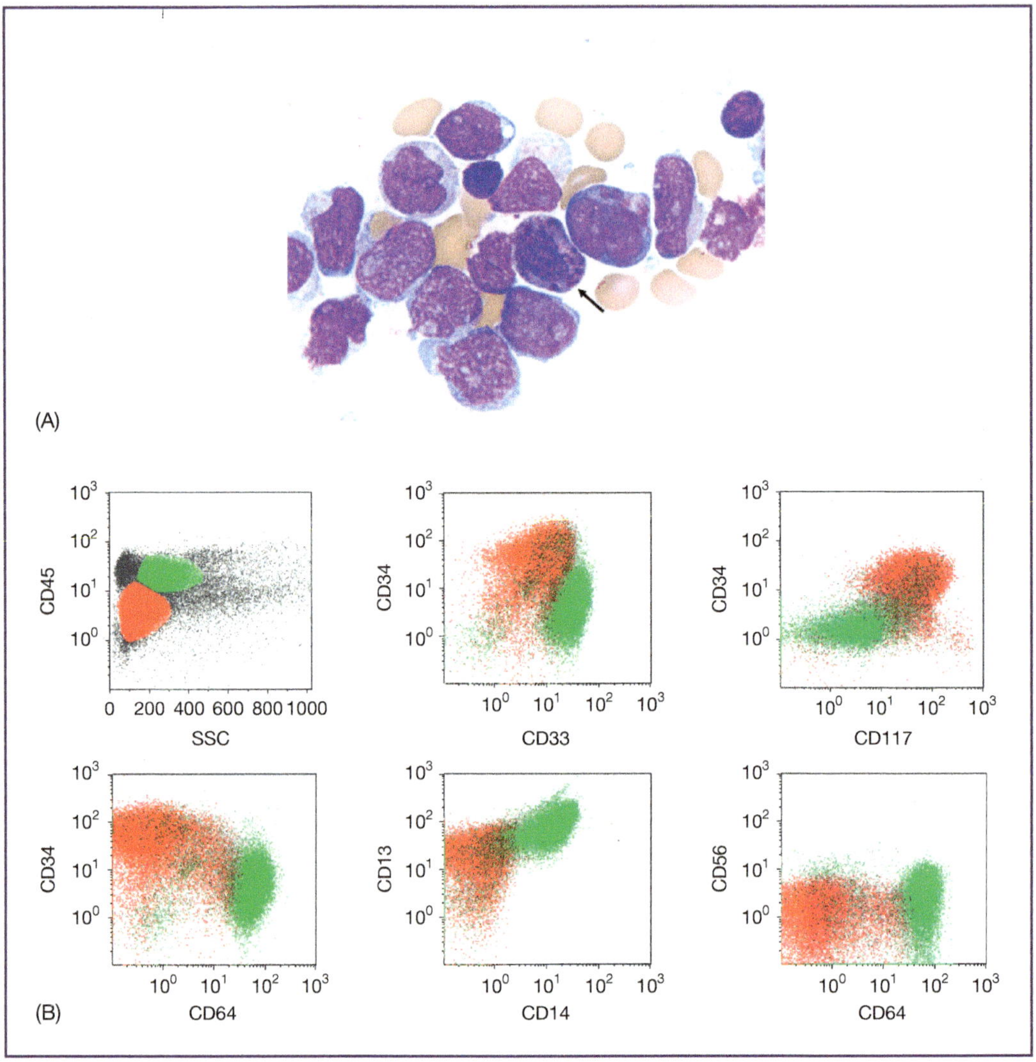

FIGURE 2-15: (A) Bone marrow aspirate from a case of AML with inv(16). Note the folded, monocytic appearance of the blasts and presence of abnormal basophilic granules in an eosinophil precursor (arrow). Wright stain X50. (B) Flow cytometric analysis of a case of AML with inv(16). There are two populations of abnormal cells, a myeloblastic population (red) and a monocytic population (green). The blasts are positive for CD13, CD33, CD34, CD117, and HLA-DR, whereas the monocytic population shows bright expression of CD13 and CD33, and is positive for CD14, CD64, and HLA-DR.
AML, acute myeloid leukemia; HLA-DR, human leukocyte antigen-D related; SSC, side scatter.

*AML With t(15;17)(q22;q22)/*PML-RARA

See Acute Promyelocytic Leukemia (APL) in Chapter 3.

*AML With t(9;11)(p22;q23)/*KMT2A-MLLT3

KMT2A, lysine methyltransferase 2A, is the current Human Genome Organization (HUGO) nomenclature for the previously known *MLL*, mixed lineage leukemia, gene at 11q23. AML cells with this genetic aberration usually have monocytic morphology as well as phenotypic markers of monocytic differentiation (Figure 2-16). Prognosis is intermediate between the previously mentioned AML with recurrent cytogenetic abnormalities and from AML that have *MLL* translocations other than t(9;11).

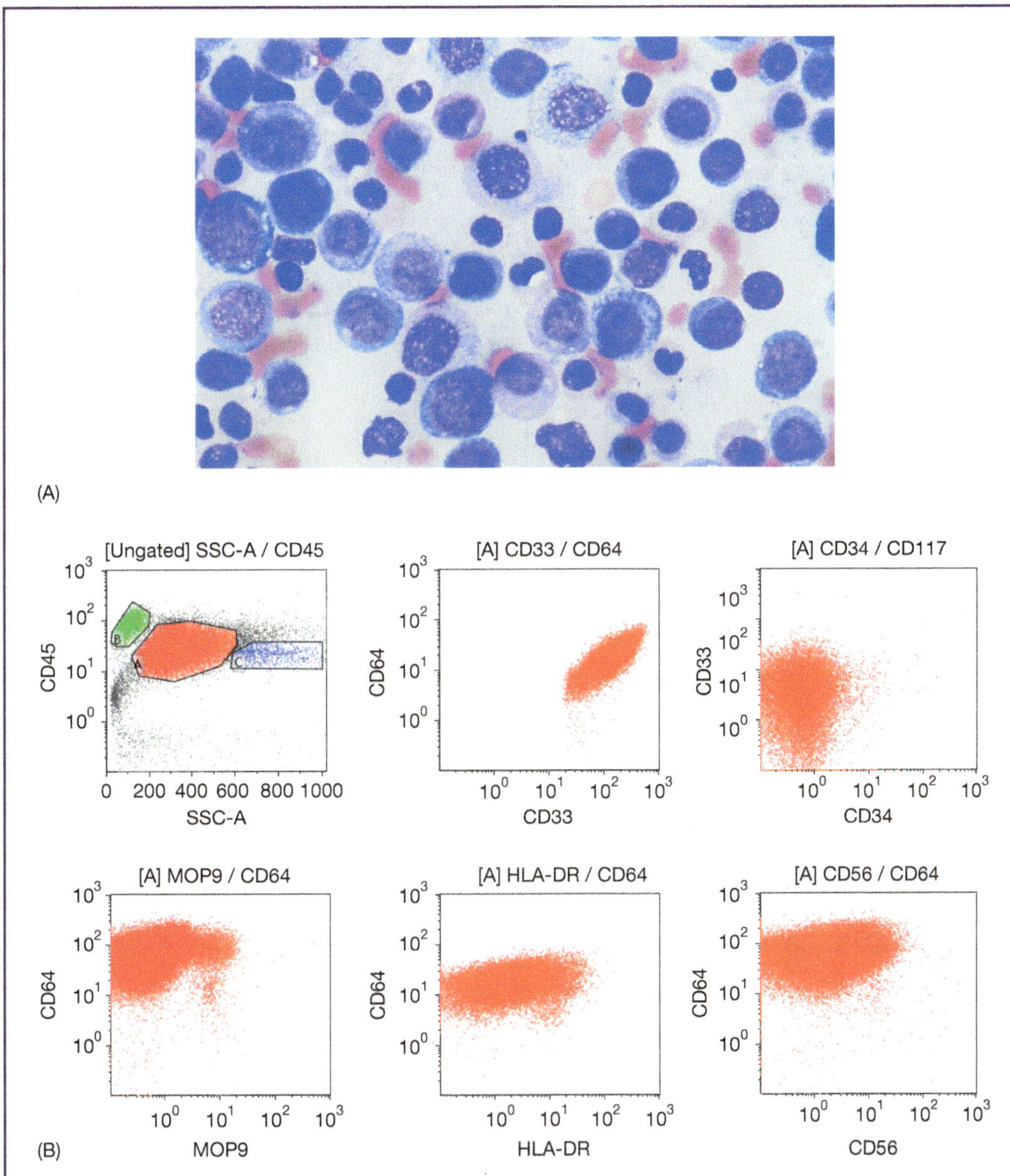

FIGURE 2-16: (A) AML with t(9;11). Bone marrow smear showing blasts with monocytic differentiation having delicately folded nuclei. Wright stain X40. (B) Flow cytometric analysis showing monoblasts (red) with a moderately bright CD45 expression, bright CD33, and CD64 expression. In contrast to mature monocytes, monoblasts do not express CD14 and have a dim expression of CD117. The blasts show aberrant CD56 expression and decreased HLA-DR expression.
AML, acute myeloid leukemia; HLA-DR, human leukocyte antigen-D related; SSC-A, side scatter-A.

*AML With inv(3)(q21q26.2) or t(3;3)(q21;q26.2)/*RPN1-EVI1

This leukemia may occur as de novo AML or arise from prior MDS, and is often associated with normal or even increased platelet count, megakaryocytic proliferation, dysmegakaryopoiesis, and often dysgranulopoiesis and dyserythropoiesis, and variable marrow fibrosis. AML with t(3;3) or inv(3) has an aggressive clinical course and a short survival.

*AML With t(1;22)(p13;q13)/*RBM15-MKL1

This type of AML shows megakaryoblastic differentiation morphologically and immunophenotypically. The megakaryoblasts are intermediate- to large-sized cells with basophilic cytoplasm that may have blebs. Immunophenotypically, the megakaryoblasts are negative for CD45, CD34, HLA-DR, and MPO, and express platelet glycoproteins CD41 and CD61.

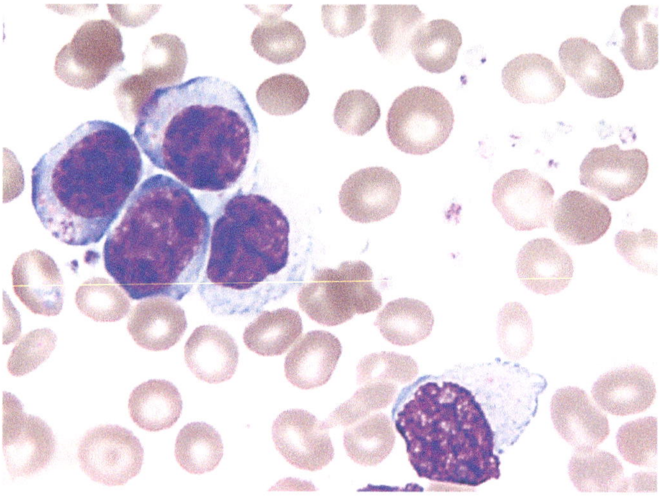

FIGURE 2-17: Acute megakaryoblastic leukemia. The megakaryoblasts have variable size and often cytoplasmic projections. The platelet count may be normal or even increased with giant thrombocytes.

AML With Myelodysplasia (MDS)-Related Changes (See Also MDS/AML in Chapter 3)

In the absence of recurrent cytogenetic abnormalities and presence of the requisite 20% blasts, after exclusion of prior cytotoxic therapy, a diagnosis of AML with MDS-related changes is made if at least one of the following three is present:

1. Multilineage dysplasia, defined as dysplasia in 50% or more cells of at least two of the hematopoietic lineages (Figure 2-18). The 50% cut-off is different from the cut-off of myelodysplastic syndrome, which requires 10% or more cells in the affected lineage to be dysplastic.
2. Prior history of MDS or MDS/MPN overlaps syndrome.
3. MDS-associated cytogenetic abnormalities. Presence of some of the cytogenetic abnormalities associated with MDS such as inv(3q) and t(6;9) is considered AML with recurrent cytogenetic abnormalities by the WHO if blast count is 20% or more.

AML with MDS-related changes is associated with a poor outcome. Data from several studies have shown that the poor prognosis is related to the common association of high-risk cytogenetics with MDS rather than the morphological features of MDS.

Therapy-Related Myeloid Neoplasms

Therapy-related myeloid neoplasms (t-MNs) encompass therapy-related MDS, therapy-related AML, and therapy-related MDS/MPN. t-MNs are late complications of cytotoxic chemotherapy or radiation therapy. Dysplasia may be observed in one or more hematopoietic lineages, often with increased blasts.

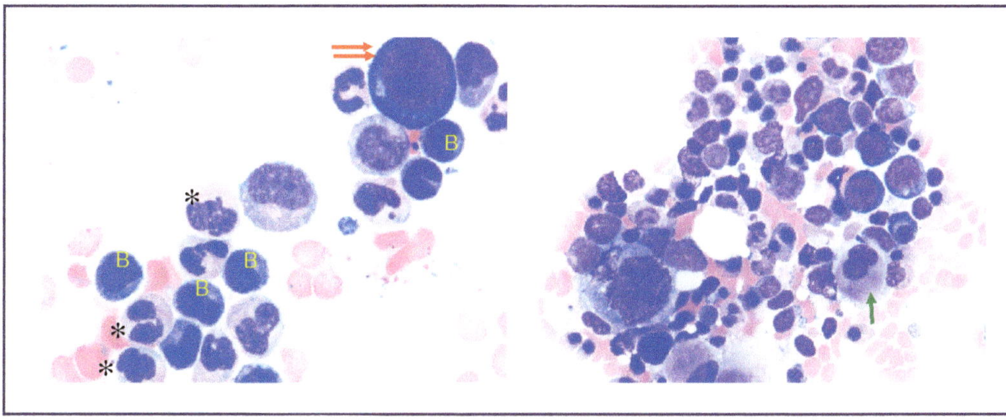

FIGURE 2-18: AML with myelodysplasia-related changes showing trilineage dysplasia: dysgranulopoiesis (asterisk), dyserythropoiesis (double red arrow), dysmegakaryopoiesis (green arrow), and increased blasts (yellow B). Wright stain ×20.

AML, acute myeloid leukemia.

Two forms of t-MN are recognized:

1. Those following therapy with alkylating agents or radiation have a latent period of 5 to 7 years and there is usually a period of bone marrow failure characterized by dysplasia and cytopenia before transforming into acute leukemia. Cytogenetic abnormalities commonly include unbalanced abnormalities of chromosomes 5 and 7 including -5/del(5q) or -7/del(7q), often as part of complex abnormalities.
2. Those that follow topoisomerase-II inhibitors have a short latency period and present as acute leukemia without a preceding myelodysplastic phase. Cytogenetic abnormalities commonly include balanced translocations or recurrent cytogenetic abnormalities similar to those occurring in de novo AML particularly involvement of chromosome 11q23.

AML, Not Otherwise Specified

AML that does not fulfill the criteria of the earlier described groups is then called AML, not otherwise specified (NOS). This group is further subclassified based on the differentiation, maturation, and lineage origin of the blasts, similar to the French American British (FAB) classification. The different subgroups and their criteria are shown in Table 2-3.

Myeloid Sarcoma

Myeloid sarcoma (MS) is an extramedullary tumor mass consisting of myeloid precursors with or without maturation, effacing the local architecture. They may occur as de novo tumors, and may precede or follow development of MDS, MDS/MPN, or MPN. Development of MS is consistent with transformation to acute leukemia. Relapse of AML may manifest itself as MS. In many cases, fresh tissue for flow cytometry may not be available. Cytochemical stains (MPO, naphthol AS-D chloroacetate esterase (CAE), and NSE) and immunohistochemical stains (CD34, CD117, CD33, lysozyme, CD68, CD163, CD123, CD99, TdT, and CD56) are valuable in identification of myeloid blasts and help to distinguish MS from lymphoblastic lymphoma, poorly differentiated carcinoma, and small round cell tumors (in children).

Myeloid Proliferations Related to Down Syndrome (DS)

Individuals with DS have an increased propensity to develop myeloid proliferations. These may be transient abnormal myeloid proliferations (TAMs) characterized by leukocytosis with circulating blasts

Table 2-3 AML, not otherwise specified

SUBGROUP	MORPHOLOGY AND DIAGNOSTIC CRITERIA	IMMUNOPHENOTYPE AND RELEVANT CYTOCHEMISTRY
AML with minimal myeloid differentiation	Blasts are agranular and have a primitive appearance.	Blasts express early markers including CD34, HLA-DR, CD38, CD13, and CD117. CD33 is found in a subset of cases; myeloid and monocytic maturation-associated antigens are absent. MPO is negative by cytochemistry, but may be expressed in a subset of blasts by flow cytometry. Aberrant T- or B-lymphoid antigens are not expressed.
AML without maturation	Blasts are ≥90% of the nonerythroid cells.	Blasts have a myeloid phenotype, with 3% or more blasts expressing MPO by cytochemistry; a population of blasts usually expresses MPO by flow cytometry.
AML with maturation	Blasts are ≥20% in PB or BM with ≥10% maturing cells of neutrophil lineage and ≤20% cells of monocytic lineage.	Myeloid phenotype.
Acute myelomonocytic leukemia	Blasts (and promonocytes) are ≥20% in PB or BM with at least 20% maturing cells each of the neutrophil and monocyte lineage.	The neutrophilic and monocytic differentiation may be present either morphologically, by cytochemistry (20% cells reactive with NSE and MPO, or dual positive cells for NSE and chloracetate (specific) esterase), or immunophenotypically with expression of monocytic antigens (CD11b, CD11c, CD14, CD15, CD36, CD64, CD68, CD163, or lysozyme) in addition to myeloid antigens.
Acute monocytic and monoblastic leukemia	>80% of leukemic cells are of the monocytic lineage, including monoblasts, promonocytes, and monocytes (see figure for morphology). In monoblastic leukemia, ≥80% of monocytic cells are monoblasts, where in acute monocytic leukemia the majority are promonocytes. Neutrophil precursors are <10%.	Blasts may be CD34 negative, but are HLA-DR positive and usually express at least two of the monocytic markers mentioned previously. MPO may be negative by flow cytometry and cytochemistry; NSE is positive.
Acute erythroid leukemia (AEL)	Two forms are identified. 1. Pure erythroleukemia is very rare. Virtually all the blasts are of erythroid lineage, with primitive appearance, deep blue cytoplasm, and cytoplasmic vacuoles. Marked erythroid proliferation and dyserythropoiesis is present. 2. In AEL, erythroid/myeloid, the erythroid component is more than 50% of marrow nucleated cells and myeloid blasts comprise ≥20% of the *non*-erythroid cells.	Blasts of pure erythroid leukemia lack MPO and other myeloid markers and express hemoglobin A, glycophorin A, and a variable amount of CD71. PAS stain shows block-like positivity in the erythroid blasts. The myeloid blasts in AEL erythroid/myeloid have a typical myeloid phenotype.
Acute panmyelosis	Marrow aspiration is often a dry tap. Biopsy shows proliferation of all the three cell lineages with left shift and collections of blasts along with markedly dysplastic small megakaryocytes. The blasts are highlighted by immunostains and are usually in the range of 20%–25%. There is significant marrow fibrosis.	Flow cytometry may not be possible due to lack of an aspirate specimen. The blasts are CD34 positive and express early myeloid antigens, but may be MPO negative.

AML, acute myeloid leukemia; BM, bone marrow; HLA-DR, human leukocyte antigen-D related; MPO, myeloperoxidase; NSE, nonspecific esterase; PAS, periodic acid-schiff; PB, peripheral blood.

and other granulocytic and erythroid precursors. TAM occurs in 10% of individuals with DS and has a high rate of spontaneous remission; in 30%, it may progress to AML. Individuals with DS have a 50- to 100-fold increased risk of acute leukemia compared with non-DS individuals. The blasts may resemble megakaryoblasts and have a distinct immunophenotype with expression of CD34, CD117, CD13, CD33, CD7, CD56, and megakaryocytic markers CD41 and CD61. They are usually negative for MPO. In addition to trisomy 21, mutations in the *GATA1* gene are present, which are pathognomonic of DS-related myeloid proliferations.

Blastic Plasmacytoid Dendritic Cell Neoplasm (BPDN)

BPDN is a rare neoplasm arising from precursors of plasmacytoid dendritic cells. The disease has a predilection for skin with BM involvement in 60% to 90%. The blasts have a primitive appearance. Immunophenotypically, they express CD43, CD4, CD56, and plasmacytoid dendritic antigens CD123, CD303, and TCL-1. They may express CD7, CD33, and TdT, but are negative for other myeloid and lymphoid antigens. They do not have rearranged T-cell receptor genes, and molecular studies may be employed to distinguish them from T-cell neoplasms if necessary.

CLASSIFICATION OF ALL

In ALL, the precursor lymphoid neoplasms are broadly categorized based on their lineage into B-lymphoblastic leukemia/lymphoma (B-ALL/LBL) and T-lymphoblastic leukemia/lymphoma (T-ALL/LBL). The disease can present as leukemia when neoplastic cells (lymphoblasts) involve blood and bone marrow (defined as >25% bone marrow blasts), or as lymphoma when blasts mainly infiltrate extramedullary tissue. ALL is the most common leukemia in children (representing 76% of leukemias among children <15 years of age), and accounts for nearly 20% of adult acute leukemia. Similar to AML, ALL is caused by a series of acquired genetic aberrations. Some of the most common genetic abnormalities in B-lymphoblastic leukemia (B-ALL) are incorporated into the current WHO classification scheme as they have important implications in disease prognosis and management (Figure 2-19).

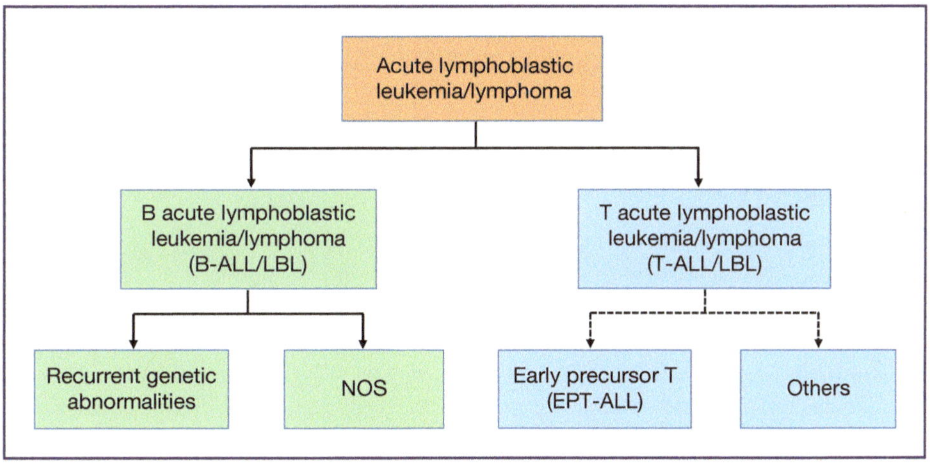

FIGURE 2-19: Overview of classification of acute lymphoblastic leukemia.
EPT-ALL, early precursor T-cell acute lymphoblastic leukemia; LBL, lymphoblastic lymphoma; NOS, not otherwise specified.

Diagnosis of Acute Lymphoblastic Leukemia

Diagnosis of ALL requires integration of information from clinical presentation; morphological examination of the peripheral blood, BM, or involved tissue; immunophenotyping by flow cytometry or immunohistochemistry; and cytogenetic and molecular testing.

Morphology: On peripheral blood and bone marrow smears, lymphoblasts vary from small cells with scant cytoplasm, condensed nuclear chromatin, and indistinct nucleoli (Figure 2-20A) to intermediate-sized cells with a moderate amount of cytoplasm, dispersed chromatin, and visible nucleoli (Figure 2-20B). Some lymphoblasts may have cytoplasmic vacuoles (Figure 2-20C). Granules are rare in ALL, and if present, they are coarse granules.

Unlike AML, Auer rods are never present. The bone marrow biopsy and tissue sections have a monotonous infiltrate of small to intermediate-sized blasts (Figure 2-20D). The blasts have finely dispersed chromatin and scant cytoplasm. Brisk mitosis and frequent apoptosis are present. Numerous tingible body macrophages may be present, giving a "starry-sky" appearance. Tumor necrosis may be seen (Figure 2-20E).

B- and T-lymphoblasts have nearly identical morphology. Therefore, it is not possible to differentiate B- from T-lymphoblasts, and sometimes myeloid from lymphoid blasts based on morphology alone. In children, in particular, the differential diagnosis also includes Ewing's sarcoma, rhabdomyosarcoma, neuroblastoma, and other small round cell tumors. The distinction can be easily made by flow cytometry or appropriate immunohistochemical stains.

Immunophenotyping by flow cytometry is the cornerstone of evaluating B- and T-ALL/LBL. In the absence of specimen availability for flow cytometry, immunophenotyping can be performed by immunohistochemistry using a panel of antibodies. The major markers expressed by B- and T-lymphoblasts are listed in Table 2-1. Although B- and T-lymphoblasts are morphologically identical, they have distinct immunophenotypes. B-ALL typically expresses B-cell-associated markers CD19, CD10, CD20, CD22, CD79a in addition to markers of stem cell or precursor cells, including CD34 and TdT (Figure 2-20F). T-ALL is usually positive for T-cell antigens CD1a, CD2, cytoplasmic CD3, CD4, CD5, CD7, CD8, and TdT (Figure 2-20G).

ALL can express myeloid-associated antigens such as CD13, CD15, or CD33. Conversely, AML may express lymphoid-associated antigens such as CD7, CD2, and CD19. In recognition of such aberrant antigen expression by leukemic cells, the current WHO classification proposes the following criteria for lineage assignment.

- To assign a blast to the B-cell lineage, expression of at least two B-cell-associated markers is required: either a strong CD19 expression with strong expression of one of the other B-cell markers (CD79a, cytoplasmic CD22, or CD10) or a weak CD19 with strong expression of two of the other B-cell markers.
- T-cell lineage assignment requires expression of cytoplasmic or surface CD3.
- To assign a blast to the myeloid lineage, expression of myeloperoxidase (MPO) or monocytic markers such as CD11c, CD14, CD64, and lysozyme is required.
- Very rarely, an acute leukemia may meet the criteria of ALL but with unequivocal expression of MPO. In this case, a diagnosis of mixed phenotype acute leukemia should be rendered.

In the case of B-ALL, distinction must be made from normal B-cell precursors or hematogones in the bone marrow. Hematogones may be especially increased in children and in individuals with iron deficiency anemia, immune thrombocytopenic purpura, regenerating bone marrow, and other etiologies. Hematogones express similar antigens as the B-ALL and can be mistaken for neoplastic blasts. This is especially so in the posttransplant BM or marrow regeneration following chemotherapy in B-ALL patients.

Leukemic blasts are distinguished from hematogones by variation in antigen expression of the leukemia population from the normal maturation sequence. The hematogones typically show a spectrum expression of CD34, TdT, CD10, CD19, and CD20 (Figure 2-21). CD34 is expressed on the earliest hematogones. With maturation, there is a drop in expression of CD34 and a gain in CD10. With further maturation, CD10 diminishes as the cells gain CD20 expression. In variance from this sequence, leukemic blasts may show under- or overexpression of antigens; asynchronous antigen expression, for example, coexpression of CD34 and CD20; or aberrant expression of antigens of a different lineage such as expression of myeloid-associated antigens CD13, CD33, CD15, and CD11b, and less commonly of T-cell-associated antigens.

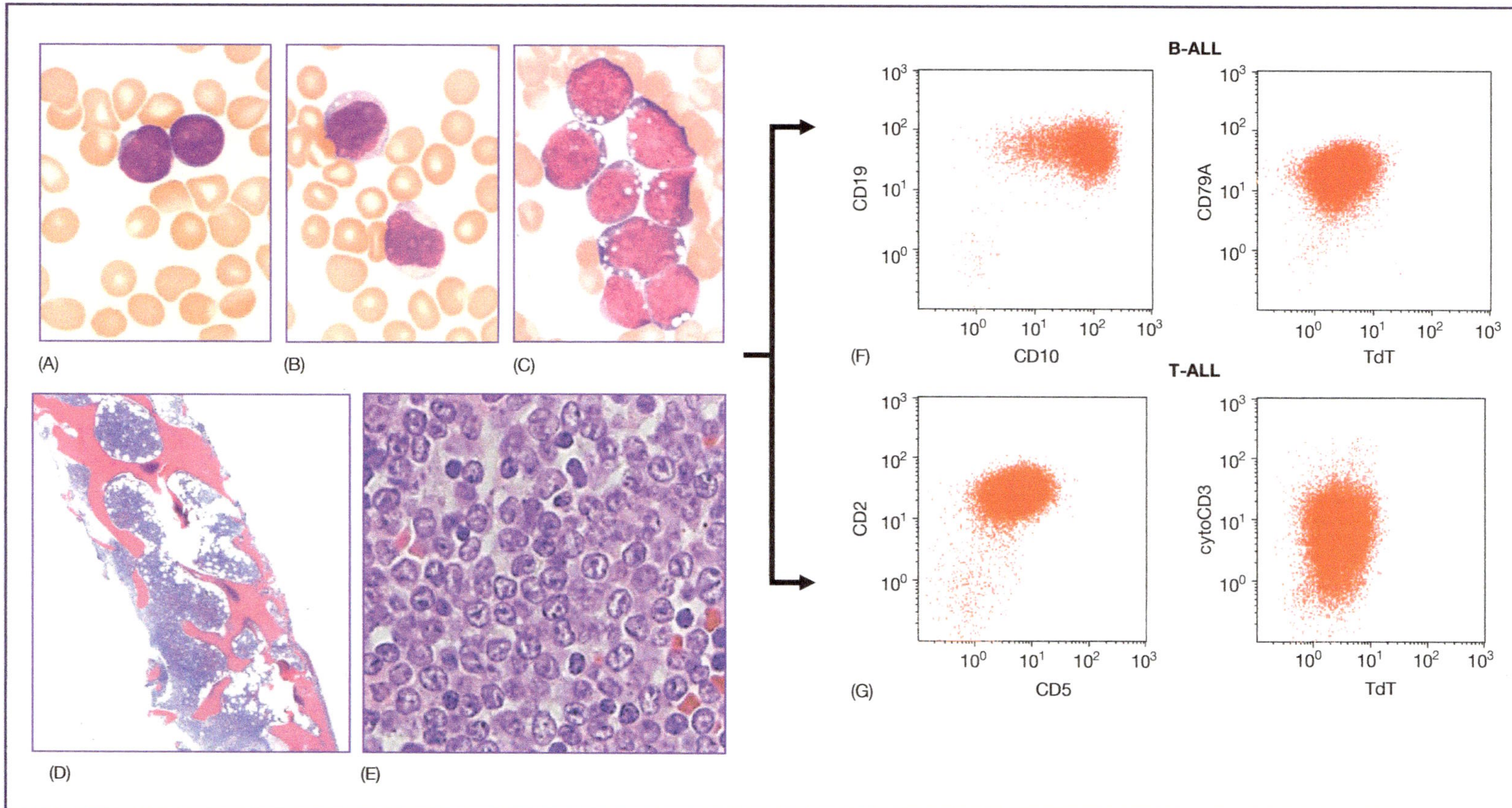

FIGURE 2-20: Precursor B- and T-lymphoblastic leukemia have similar morphology. The blasts may vary morphologically from small and homogeneous (A) to variably sized heterogeneous (B), or intermediate to large with cytoplasmic vacuoles akin to Burkitt lymphoma (C). Wright stain ×50. (D) Markedly hypercellular bone marrow in pre-B ALL (hematoxylin and eosin ×10). (E) High power of bone marrow biopsy showing monotonous infiltrate of blasts with frequent mitosis (hematoxylin and eosin ×20). (F) Typical immunophenotype of B-ALL (CD19+ CD79a+ CD10+ TdT+). (G) Typical immunophenotype of T-ALL (cytoplasmic CD3+ CD2+ CD5+ TdT+).

B-ALL, B acute lymphoblastic leukemia; T-ALL, T acute lymphoblastic leukemia; TdT, terminal deoxynucleotidyl transferase.

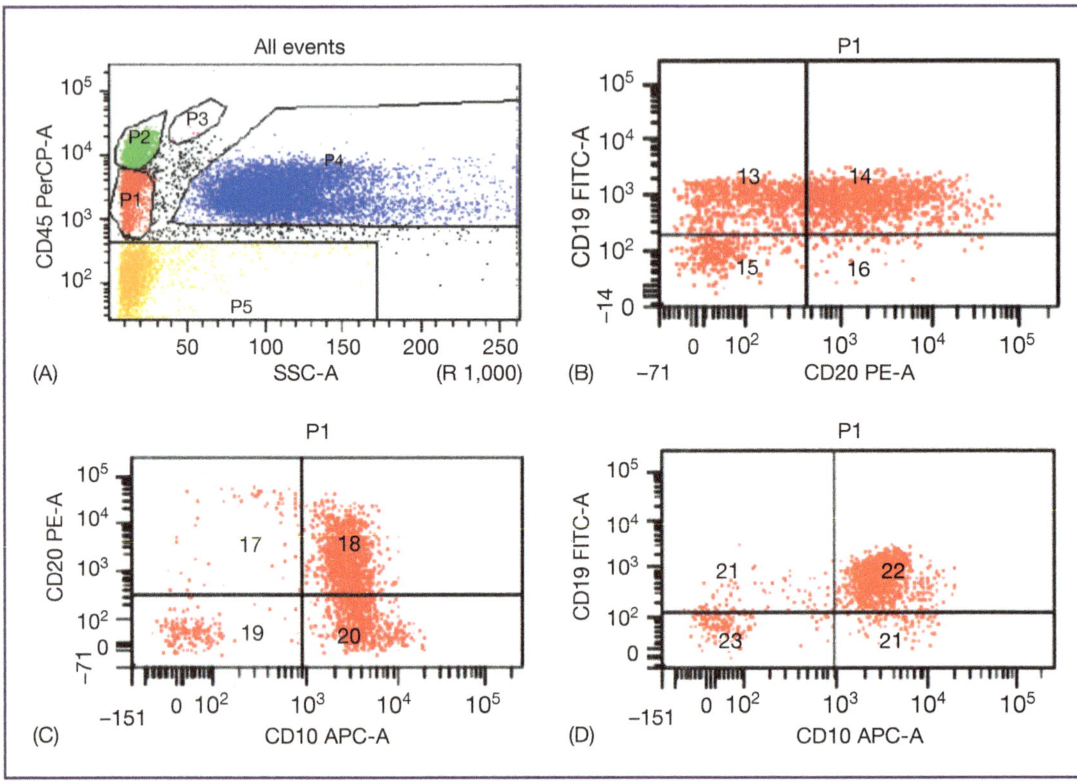

FIGURE 2-21: **Flow cytometry dot plots showing maturation pattern of hematogones. (A) The hematogones have low side scatter and dim expression of CD45 (red). (B, C, D) Analysis of this population shows variable expressions of CD10, CD19, and CD20 consistent with progressive maturation of hematogones (B-cell precursors).**

APC-A, allophycocyanin-A; FITC-A, fluorescein isothiocyanate-A; PE-A, phycoerythrin-A; PerCP-A, peridinin-chlorophyll protein-A; SSC-A, side scatter-A.

This variance from the normal phenotype is called leukemia-associated immunophenotype (LAIP). LAIP is of immense value in the follow-up of BM samples for minimal residual disease detection. Aberrant expression of myeloid antigens is an LAIP, but does not influence outcome.

Acute B-Lymphoblastic Leukemia/Lymphoma (See Also Section Molecular Mutations in ALL, page 103)

Pre-B-ALL/LBL manifests more commonly in a leukemic form. Extramedullary disease or LBL occurs most frequently in the skin (Figure 2-22), bone, lymph nodes, soft tissue, breast, and gonads. Involvement of the central nervous system is common in both ALL and LBL.

As shown in Figure 2-19, Pre-B-ALL can be classified into two major categories: B-ALL with recurrent genetic abnormalities and B-ALL, NOS. The current WHO classification lists nine groups of Pre-B-ALL with recurrent genetic abnormalities (Table 2-4). With the advent of new molecular technologies, numerous new genetic aberrations have been identified in B-ALL cases in recent years. Several such changes occur frequently and have important prognostic and therapeutic implications and warrant consideration as separate new entities.

Acute B-Lymphoblastic Leukemia/Lymphoma With t(9;22)(q34;q11.2); BCR-ABL1

Pre-B-ALL with t(9;22), *BCR-ABL1*, or Philadelphia (Ph) chromosome represents 30% of adult and 2% to 5% of pediatric B-ALL cases. While there are no unique morphologic features, the blasts of Ph+ B-ALL

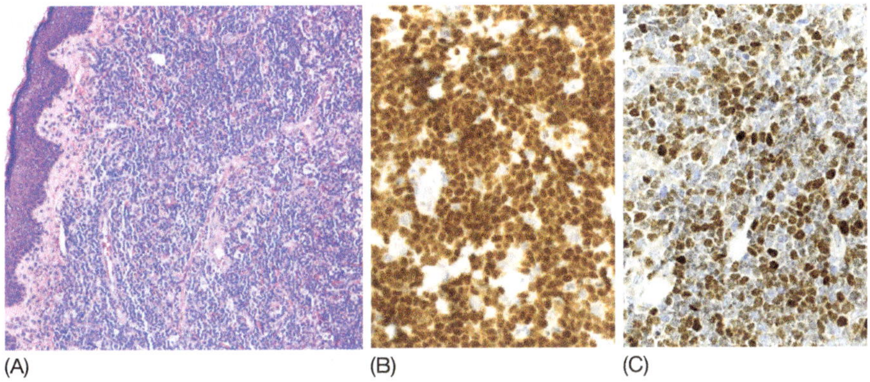

FIGURE 2-22: **Precusor B-lymphoblastic lymphoma in the skin. (A) The dermis shows sheets of blasts (hematoxylin and eosin ×20). (B) The blasts are positive for PAX-5 and (C) TdT (immunoperoxidase ×40).**
TdT, terminal deoxynucleotidyl transferase.

Table 2-4 Characteristics of B-lymphoblastic leukemia with recurrent genetic abnormalities

WHO 2008 GROUPS	INCIDENCE	PREDOMINANT IMMUNOPHENOTYPE
B-ALL with t(9;22)(q34;q11.2); *BCR-ABLI*	2%–5% children, 30% adult	CD19+ CD10+ CD34+ CD13+ CD38–/+
B-ALL with t(v;11q23); *MLL* rearrangement	60% infant, rare adult	CD19+ CD10– CD15+ C034+/–
B-ALL with t(12;21)(p13;q22); *ETV6-RUNX1*	25% children, 3% adult	CD19+ CD10+ CD34+ CD13+/–
B-ALL with t(1;19)(q23;p13.3);*E2A-PBX1*	6% children, 2% in adult	CD19+ CD10+ CD34– CD20+/–
B-ALL with t(5;14)(q31;q32); *IL3-IGH*	<1%	CD19+ CD10+; eosinophilia
B-ALL with hyperdiploidy	20%–30% children, 5% adult	CD19+ CD10+ CD34+ CD45–
B-ALL with hypodiploidy	5% all age	CD19+ CD10+
B-ALL, BCR-ABL1-like	10% children, 25% adult	CD19+ CD10+ CD34+
B-ALL with iAMP21	3%–5% older children	CD19+ CD10+

B-ALL, B acute lymphoblastic leukemia; MLL, mixed lineage leukemia.

exhibit a relatively distinct immunophenotype. They express high levels of CD19, CD10, and CD34; low level of CD38; and frequent expression of myeloid markers such as CD13 (Figure 2-23B). Additionally, expression of CD66c is reported to have a strong correlation with presence of *BCR-ABL1* translocation. Pre-B-ALL with t(9;22) is historically associated with poor prognosis, but incorporation of tyrosine kinase inhibitors into the chemotherapy regimen has greatly improved the outcome.

B-Lymphoblastic Leukemia/Lymphoma With t(v;11q23); MLL Rearrangement

Translocations involving 11q23 are most common in infants less than 1 year old, and are associated with very poor prognosis, especially in those with t(4;11)(q21;q23)/KMT2A-AFF1. B-ALL with t(4;11) is rare in older children, but up to 10% of newly diagnosed adult B-ALL patients carry this translocation, especially in those with prior cytotoxic therapy. These patients usually present with high white cell count (Figure 2-23A), frequent CNS involvement, and presence of DIC. Pre-B-ALL with t(4;11) exhibits common lymphoblastic morphology, but characteristically lacks CD10 expression (Figure 2-23C), suggesting that the blasts may be derived from B-cell precursors at a very early developmental stage (pro-B). In addition, B-ALL with t(4;11) frequently expresses myeloid-associated antigens, in particular, CD15 and CD65.

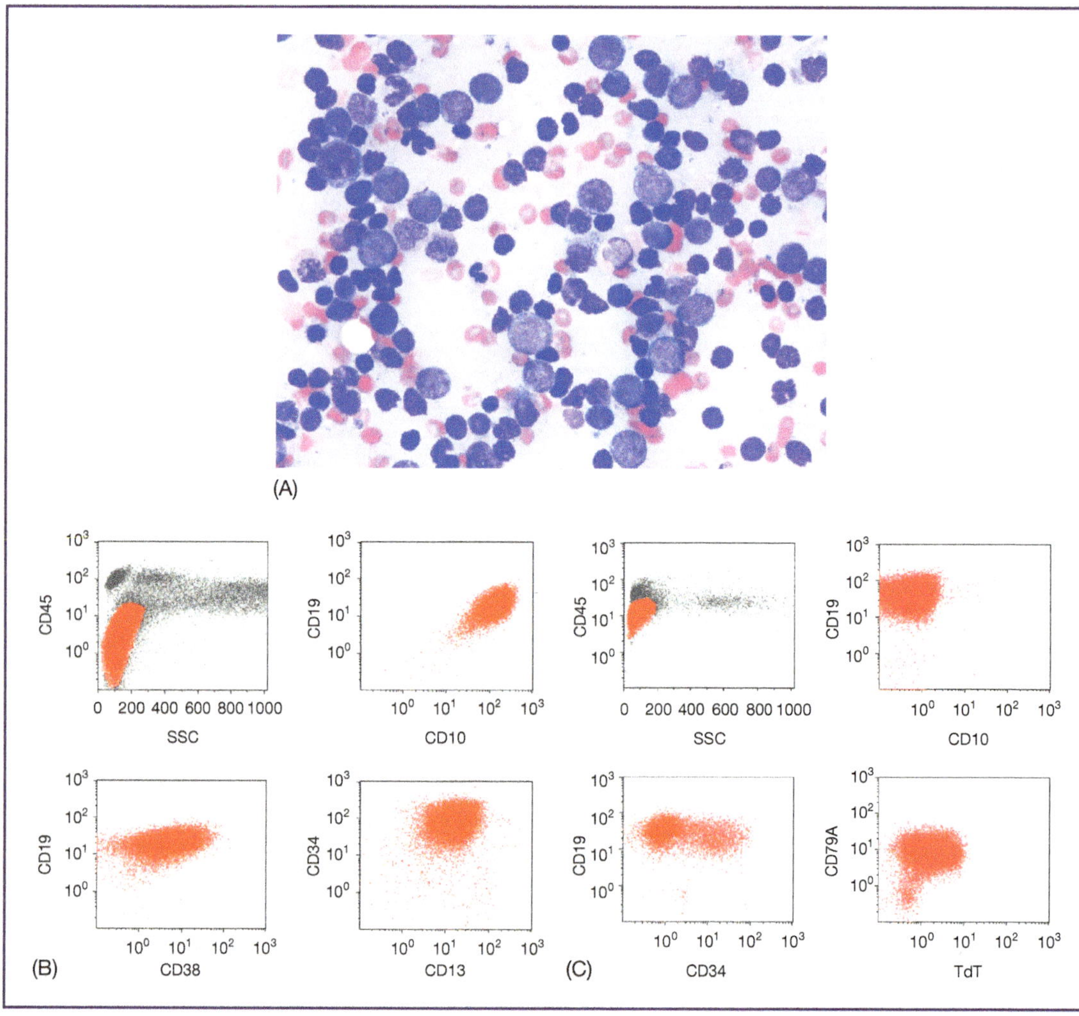

FIGURE 2-23: (A) Acute lymphoblastic leukemia with t(9;22) and t(4;11) usually has a high WBC count at presentation. Shown here is a peripheral smear from precursor B-ALL with t(4;11)(q21;q23)*KMT2A/AFF4*, Wright stain ×50. (B) Flow cytometric analysis of a case of B-ALL with t(9;22). The blasts (red) exhibit dim/negative CD45 expression and are positive for CD10, CD19, CD34, and TdT. They show aberrant dim expression of CD33 but are negative for other myeloid markers including MPO (data not shown). (C) Flow cytometric analysis of a case of B-ALL with t(4;11). The blasts (red) are positive for CD19 and CD79a, but lack expression of CD10. CD34 is expressed as a small subset of the blasts, and TdT is dim.

B-ALL, B acute lymphoblastic leukemia; MPO, myeloperoxidase; SSC, side scatter; TdT, terminal deoxynucleotidyl transferase; WBC, white blood cell.

B-Lymphoblastic Leukemia/Lymphoma With t(12;21)(p13;q22); ETV6-RUNX1

B-ALL with t(12;21), *ETV6-RUNX1* is observed in nearly 25% of children with B-ALL, but is rare in adults. This B-ALL is associated with favorable prognosis. There are no unique morphologic or immunophenotypic features associated with B-ALL with t(12;21).

B Lymphoblastic Leukemia/Lymphoma With t(1;19)(q23;p13.3); TCF3-PBX1

B-ALL with t(1;19), *TCF3-PBX1* is relatively common in children, accounting for 6% of children with B-ALL. This leukemia typically expresses cytoplasmic immunoglobulin μ heavy chain and lacks CD34 expression, indicating that the blasts are derived from a B-cell precursor at the late developmental stage (pre-B). There are no distinct morphologic features. In the past, B-ALL with t(1;19)/*TCF3-PBX1* was associated with a poor outcome, but modern intensive therapy has led to improved survival.

B-Lymphoblastic Leukemia/Lymphoma With t(5;14)(q31;q32); IL3-IGH

B-ALL with t(5;14)(q31;q32); *IL3-IGH* is a rare disease, comprising <1% of ALL cases. It is associated with eosinophilia due to the overexpression of the *IL3* gene. The blasts show typical lymphoblastic morphology and a common CD19+ CD10+ phenotype.

B-Lymphoblastic Leukemia/Lymphoma With Hyperdiploidy

Hyperdiploidy is observed in 30% to 40% of the children with B-ALL and is associated with a favorable outcome, especially in those patients with a high number of chromosomes. There is some disagreement in the prognostic role of triple trisomies of chromosomes 4, 10, and 17, considered favorable by the Pediatric Oncology Group and Children's Oncology Group, but not by the Medical Research Council of the United Kingdom (U.K.). B-ALL cases with hyperdiploidy have no specific morphologic features but typically show very low level or absence of CD45 expression.

B-Lymphoblastic Leukemia/Lymphoma With Hypodiploidy

Hypodiploidy is observed in nearly 5% of the ALL patients, in both children and adults. It can be further categorized into three subgroups:

Near-haploidy (23 to 29 chromosomes)

Low hypodiploidy (33 to 39 chromosomes)

High hypodiploidy (42 to 45 chromosomes)

All patients with hypodiploid B-ALL have poor outcome; the outcome in the near-haploid and low-hypodiploid B-ALL cases is worse than in those with high hypodiploidy. Near-diploidy is exclusively observed in children and is often associated with genetic aberrations affecting the RAS pathway and tyrosine kinase signaling. Low hypodiploidy is observed in older children and adults, and is associated with TP53 mutations. Pre-B-ALL with hypodiploidy has a typical lymphoblastic morphology and a common CD19+ CD10+ B-ALL phenotype.

BCR-ABL1*-Like B Lymphoblastic Leukemia*

BCR-ABL1-like B lymphoblastic leukemia lacks t(9;22) or *BCR-ABL1* fusion, but shares a similar gene expression profile with B-ALL with t(9;22), *BCR-ABL1*. Although the full spectrum of genetic aberrations is not completely understood, approximately 40% of the *BCR-ABL1*-like B-ALLs have a translocation involving the *CRLF2* gene. *BCR-ABL1*-like B-ALL is observed in approximately 10% of children and 25% of adults with B-ALL, and is associated with a poor prognosis. These pre-B-ALL often have a high leukocyte count and show variable lymphoblastic morphology. The blasts have a typical CD19+ CD10+ phenotype and may have expression of myeloid-associated antigens.

B-Lymphoblastic Leukemia/Lymphoma With iAMP21

Intrachromosomal amplification of chromosome 21 (iAMP21) is observed in approximately 2% of children with B-ALL. This abnormality is detected by FISH analysis using the *RUNX1* gene probe, which shows five or more *RUNX1* signals per cell. B-ALL patients with iAMP21 are usually older children and present with a low leukocyte count. This leukemia has a very poor prognosis when treated with standard risk regimens. Improved outcome can be achieved when treated as high-risk ALL. No unique morphologic or immunophenotypic features have been reported.

Acute T-Lymphoblastic Leukemia/Lymphoma

T-ALL/LBL is more common in older children and adolescents. Unlike B-ALL/LBL, which manifests more commonly in a leukemic form, T-ALL/LBL frequently presents as an anterior mediastinal or thymic mass with variable involvement of the PB and BM. In adults, the disease may present as a mediastinal mass or a lymph node-based lesion. Involvement of the central nervous system at presentation is more common in T-ALL/LBL than in B-ALL.

Flow cytometry is commonly used in the evaluation of T-ALL/LBL. In cases of tissue biopsy, immunohistochemistry is also used for the diagnosis.

The antigens expressed by T-lymphoblasts are listed in Table 2-1, including TdT, CD1a, CD2, cytoplasmic CD3, CD5, and CD7. Of these, *only cytoplasmic CD3 is T-lineage specific*. Many T-ALL cases coexpress CD4 and CD8, while others lack both. T-ALL blasts typically lack expression of surface CD3, TCR αβ, and TCR γδ. Unlike B-ALL, T-ALL is usually negative for HLA-DR. About 10% of T-ALL cases express CD10 and cytoplasmic CD79a. T-ALL/LBL may express myeloid antigens, commonly CD13 and CD33. CD117 expression, especially with the presence of other myeloid antigens, is a sensitive predictor of *FLT3* mutation, and is associated with a poor response to therapy.

While T-ALL/LBL is not further classified, several maturation stages are recognized. During normal maturation, the precursor T-cells have a sequential expression of different antigens that can be used to identify their developmental stages. Figure 2-24 shows the expression of different antigens during T-cell maturation. The WHO classification recognizes four stages of T-cell intrathymic maturation: Pro-T, Pre-T, cortical-T, and medullary-T. A T-ALL/LBL can arise from any of these stages. The pre-T and pro-T stages express cytoplasmic CD3, CD7, and TdT and may express CD34, but are double negative for CD4 and CD8 (Figure 2-24). The cortical-T stage expresses cytoplasmic CD3, CD7, CD2, CD5, TdT, and CD1a, but lacks CD34, and is double positive for CD4 and CD8. The medullary-T stage expresses surface CD3, CD7, CD2, CD5, and TdT, but is positive for either CD4 or CD8 (single positive). Expression of CD34, TdT, or CD1a distinguishes a precursor T-neoplasm from a mature T-cell neoplasm.

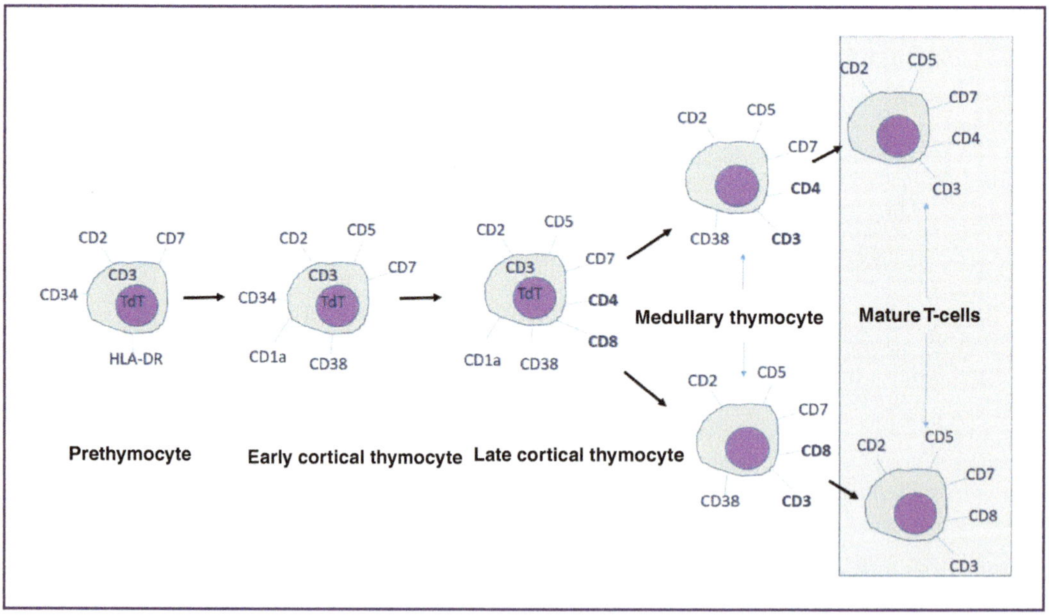

FIGURE 2-24: **Maturation stages of T-lymphoblasts. The prethymocyte and early cortical thymocytes are double negative (CD4– CD8–), the late cortical thymocytes are double positive (CD4+ CD8+), and the medullary thymocytes are positive for either CD4 or CD8. The early stages lack surface CD3. Mature T-cells express surface CD3, and either CD4 or CD8; they are negative for CD34, TdT, and CD1a.**

HLA-DR, human leukocyte antigen-D related; TdT, terminal deoxynucleotidyl transferase.

In recent years, a distinct subtype of T-ALL, the early T-cell precursor ALL (ETP-ALL), has been recognized based on the unique immunophenotype and poor prognosis. ETP-ALL is characterized by lack of CD1a and CD8 expression, weak CD5 expression (<75% of the blasts), and expression of one or more of the following myeloid and stem cell markers on at least 25% of lymphoblasts, including CD117, CD34, HLA-DR, CD13, CD33, CD11b, and/or CD65. It is thought that ETP-ALL originates from a very T cell progenitor with lineage plasticity. Indeed, ETP-ALL has a gene signature overlapping T-ALL and AML. ETP-ALL comprises about 15% of T-ALL in children, and is more common in adults. It is associated with very poor response to therapy. However, a recent UK study failed to show significant difference in 5-year event-free survival and overall survival between the ETP and non-ETP groups.

The genetics of pre T-ALL/LBL are discussed elsewhere. Briefly, the majority of pre-T-ALL/LBL show an aberrant karyotype. The most common karyotypic abnormalities involve the TCR α and TCR δ genes at 14q11. More than 50% have mutations affecting the *NOTCH1* gene. Gene expression studies have shown a correlation between expression signatures of differentiation arrest genes and those activating oncological pathways. LYL1+pre-T ALL/LBL cases are characterized by expression of early thymocyte genes, which correspond to the early-arrest double-negative stage of T-cell development. In contrast, HOX11+ and TAL1+ cases are associated with the expression of more mature thymocyte markers. Genome-wide profiling studies, including microarray analysis and genome sequencing, have revolutionized the field of diagnosis and management of ALL.

Selected References

GENERAL

Bain B, Clark DM, Lampert IA, Wilkins BS. *Bone Marrow Pathology*. 3rd ed. Oxford, UK: Blackwell Science; 2001.

Borowitz MJ, Guenther KL, Shults KE, Stelzer GT. Immunophenotyping of acute leukemia by flow cytometric analysis. Use of CD45 and right-angle light scatter to gate on leukemic blasts in three-color analysis. *Am J Clin Pathol*. 1993;100:534–540.

Greaves M, Maley CC. Clonal evolution in cancer. *Nature*. 2012;481:306–313.

Hayhoe FGJ, Quaglino D. *Haematological Cytochemistry*. 2nd ed. Edinburgh, Scotland: Churchill Livingstone; 1988.

Shlush LI, Zandi S, Mitchell A, et al. Identification of pre-leukaemic haematopoietic stem cells in acute leukaemia. *Nature*. 2014;506(7488):328–333.

Stelzer GT, Shults KE, Loken MR. CD45 gating for routine flow cytometric analysis of human bone marrow specimens. *Ann NY Acad Sci*. 1993;677:265–280.

Swerdlow SH, Campo E, Harris NL, et al. eds. *WHO Classification of Tumours of Haematopoietic and Lymphoid Tissues*. Lyon, France: IARC Press; 2008.

AML

Bueso-Ramos CE, Kanagal-Shamanna R, Routbort MJ, Hanson CA. Therapy-related myeloid neoplasms. *Am J Clin Pathol*. 2015;144:207–218.

Foucar K, Anastasi J. Acute myeloid leukemia with recurrent cytogenetic abnormalities. *Am J Clin Pathol*. 2015;144(1):6–18.

Gorczyca W, Sun ZY, Cronin W, et al. Immunophenotypic pattern of myeloid populations by flow cytometry analysis. *Methods Cell Biol*. 2011;103:221–266.

Pileri SA, Ascani S, Cox MC, et al. Myeloid sarcoma: clinico-pathologic, phenotypic and cytogenetic analysis of 92 adult patients. *Leukemia*. 2007;21(2):340–350.

Shi Y, Wang E. Blastic plasmacytoid dendritic cell neoplasm: a clinicopathologic review. *Arch Pathol Lab Med*. 2014;138(4):564–569.

Smith SM, Le Beau MM, Huo D, et al. Clinical-cytogenetic associations in 306 patients with therapy-related myelodysplasia and myeloid leukemia: the University of Chicago series. *Blood*. 2003;102:43–52.

Vardiman J, Reichard K. Acute myeloid leukemia with myelodysplasia-related changes. *Am J Clin Pathol*. 2015;144:29–43.

Wang L, Peters JM, Fuda F, et al. Acute megakaryoblastic leukemia associated with trisomy 21 demonstrates a distinct immunophenotype. *Cytometry B Clin Cytom*. 2015;88(4):244–252.

B-ALL

Dastugue N, Suciu S, Plat G, et al. Hyperdiploidy with 58-66 chromosomes in childhood B-acute lymphoblastic leukemia is highly curable: 58951 CLG-EORTC results. *Blood*. 2013;121:2415–2423.

Holmfeldt L, Wei L, Diaz-Flores E, et al. The genomic landscape of hypodiploid acute lymphoblastic leukemia. *Nat Genet*. 2013;45:242–252.

Ribeiro RC, Abromowitch M, Raimondi SC, et al. Clinical and biologic hallmarks of the Philadelphia chromosome in childhood acute lymphoblastic leukemia. *Blood*. 1987;70:948–953.

Roberts KG, Li Y, Payne-Turner D, et al. Targetable kinase-activating lesions in Ph-like acute lymphoblastic leukemia. *N Engl J Med*. 2014;371:1005–1015.

Roberts KG, Mullighan CG. Genomics in acute lymphoblastic leukaemia: insights and treatment implications. *Nat Rev Clin Oncol*. 2015;12:344–357.

Roberts KG, Pei D, Campana D, et al. Outcomes of children with *BCR-ABL1*–like acute lymphoblastic leukemia treated with risk-directed therapy based on the levels of minimal residual disease. *J Clin Oncol*. 2014;32:3012–3020.

T-ALL

Coustan-Smith E, Mullighan CG, Onciu M, et al. Early T-cell precursor leukaemia: a subtype of very high-risk acute lymphoblastic leukaemia. *Lancet Oncol*. 2009;10(2):147–156.

Han X, Bueso-Ramos CE. Precursor T-cell acute lymphoblastic leukemia/lymphoblastic lymphoma and acute biphenotypic leukemias. *Am J Clin Pathol*. 2007;127:528–544.

Haydu JE, Ferrando AA. Early T-cell precursor acute lymphoblastic leukaemia. *Curr Opin Hematol*. 2013;20(4):369–373.

Weng AP, Ferrando AA, Lee W, et al. Activating mutations of NOTCH1 in human T cell acute lymphoblastic leukemia. *Science*. 2004;306:269–271.

CLASSICAL GENETICS

Ying Zou and Yi Ning

Standard Chromosome Analyses–Karyotyping

Banding-based karyotyping is the standard method for chromosome analysis to detect chromosome abnormalities associated with malignancies. It is performed on dividing metaphase cells usually from bone marrow or peripheral blood specimens. The procedure requires the presence of spontaneously dividing cells in the specimens without mitogen stimulation.

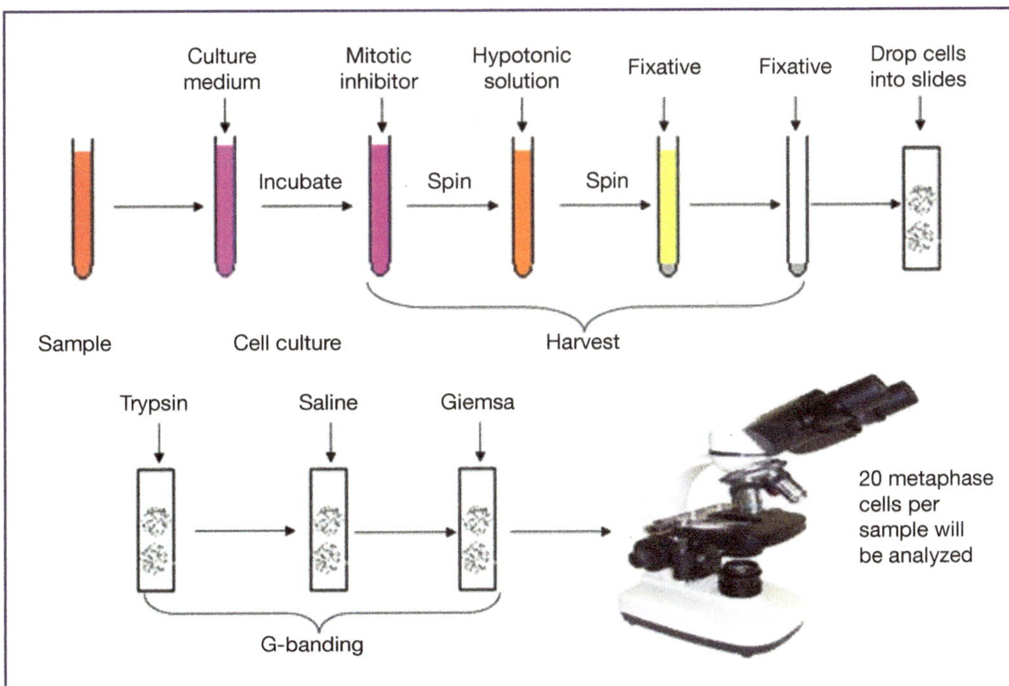

FIGURE 2-25: **The preparation for banding-based chromosome analysis. The cells are cultured for 24 hours and 48 hours without stimulation. G-banding (Giemsa staining after trypsin treatment) is the most commonly used method.**

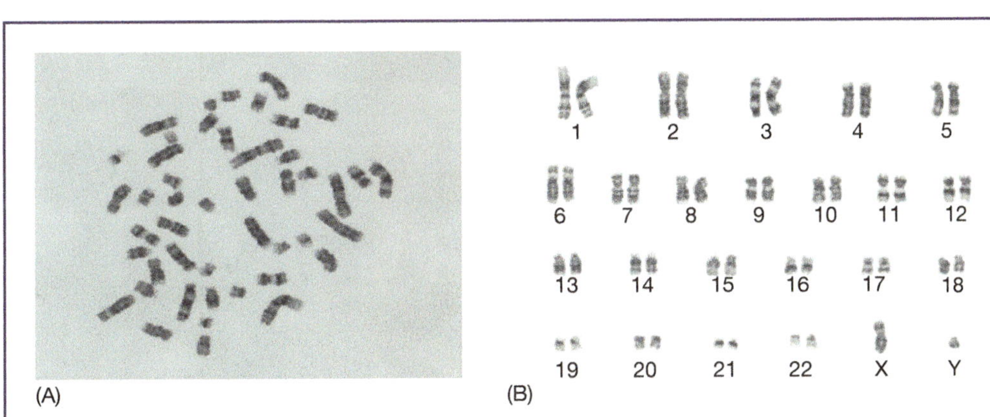

FIGURE 2-26: **(A) Metaphase spread of chromosomes that are seen under a microscope. (B) Normal male karyogram of the cell shown on the left.**

Fluorescence In Situ Hybridization (FISH)

FISH identifies a specific region of DNA with specific nucleic acid sequence in the context of the whole genome. FISH can be performed on interphase or metaphase cells from fresh or paraffin-embedded samples.

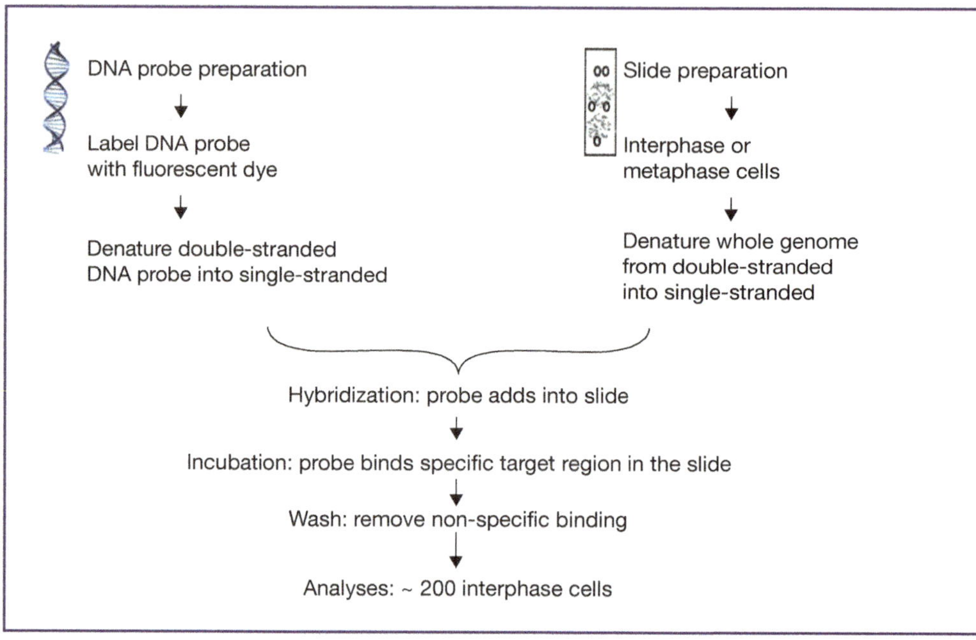

FIGURE 2-27: **FISH procedure. Different types of FISH probes include centromere probes for the detection of a specific chromosome copy number, and locus-specific probes for the detection of copy number and rearrangement of targeted oncogenes, tumor suppressor genes, or other genes of interest.**

FISH, fluorescence in situ hybridization.

Types of FISH probes:

- Whole chromosome painting probes
- Centromere probes
- Subtelomere probes
- Locus-specific probes

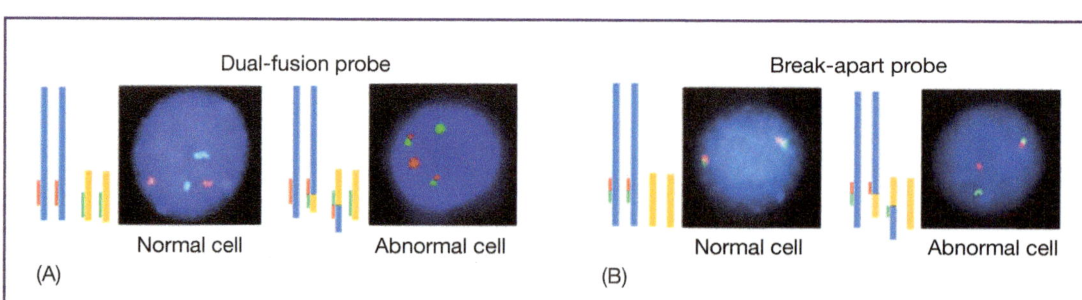

FIGURE 2-28: **FISH probes. Strategies to detect gene rearrangements with FISH include (A) dual-color dual-fusion probe set for detecting a specific reciprocal translocation or inversion, and (B) dual-color break-apart probe set for detecting a specific gene rearrangement.**

FISH, fluorescence in situ hybridization.

Table 2-5 Recurrent cytogenetic abnormalities in AML

PROGNOSIS	CYTOGENETICS	GENES INVOLVED
Better	t(8;21)	*RUNX1/RUNX1T1*
	inv(16)/t(16;16)	*CBFB*
	t(15;17)/variants	*PML/RARA, RARA*
Intermediate	Normal karyotype	
	+8	
	t(9;11)	*MLLT3/MLL*
Poor	−5/5q−; −7/7q−;	
	inv(3)/t(3;3)	*RPN1/MECOM*
	−17/17p−	*P53*
	t(6;9)	*DEK/NUP214*
	t(v;11) with MLL	*MLL*
	Complex ≥4 abnormalities	

AML, acute myeloid leukemia; MLL, mixed lineage leukemia.

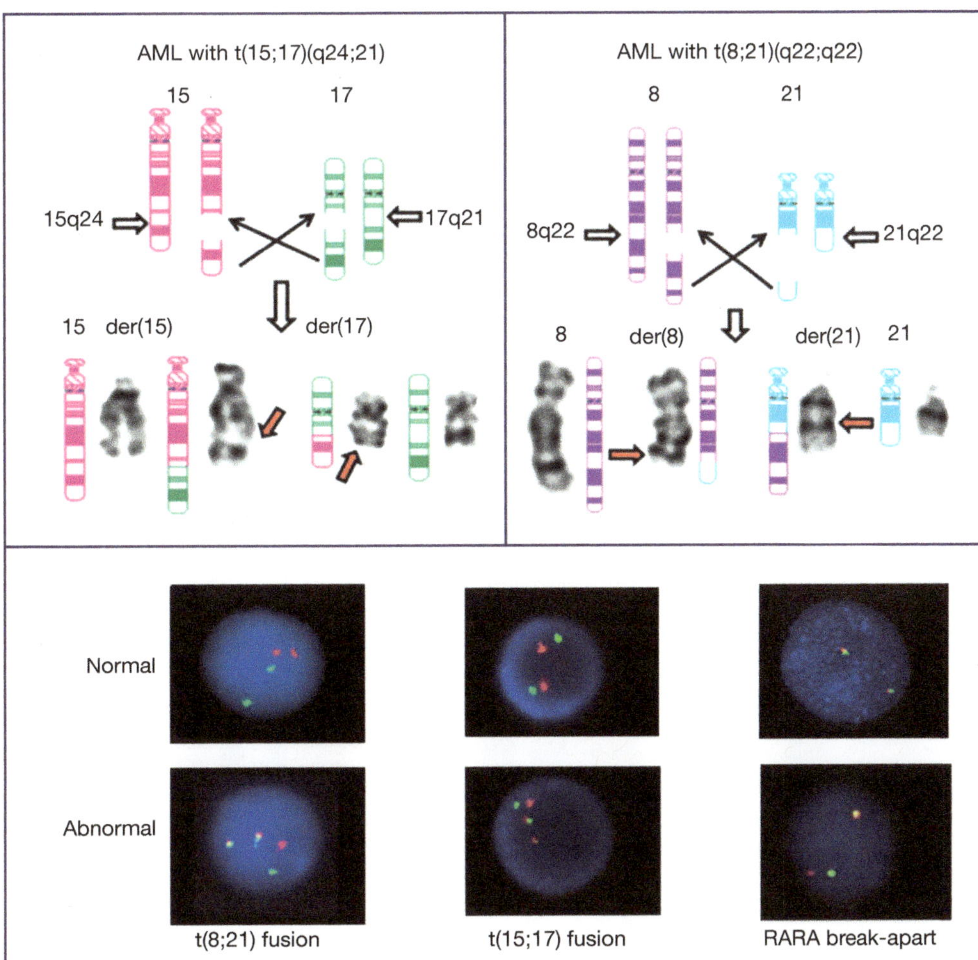

FIGURE 2-29: G-banding karyotyping (top) and FISH (bottom) showing t(15;17) and t(8;21).
AML, acute myeloid leukemia; FISH, fluorescence in situ hybridization; RARA, retinoic acid receptor alpha.

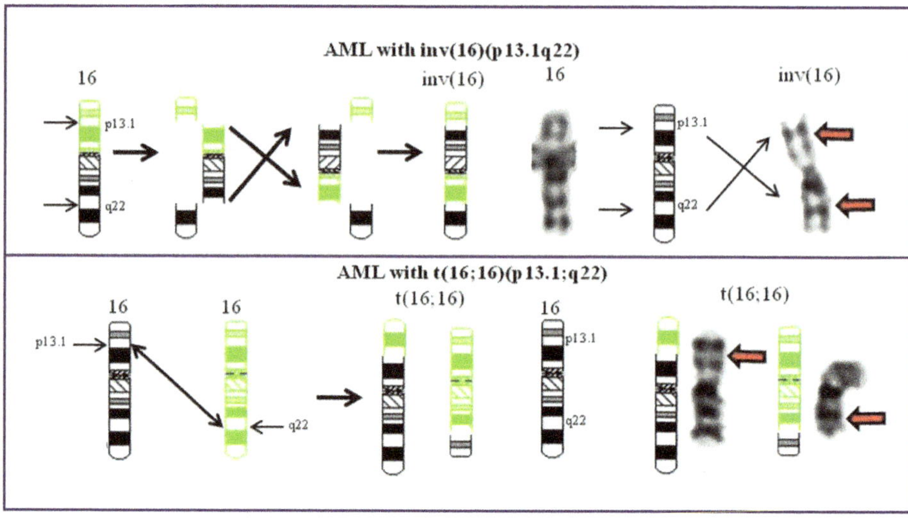

FIGURE 2-30: G-banding karyotyping showing inv(16) and t(16;16). AML, acute myeloid leukemia.

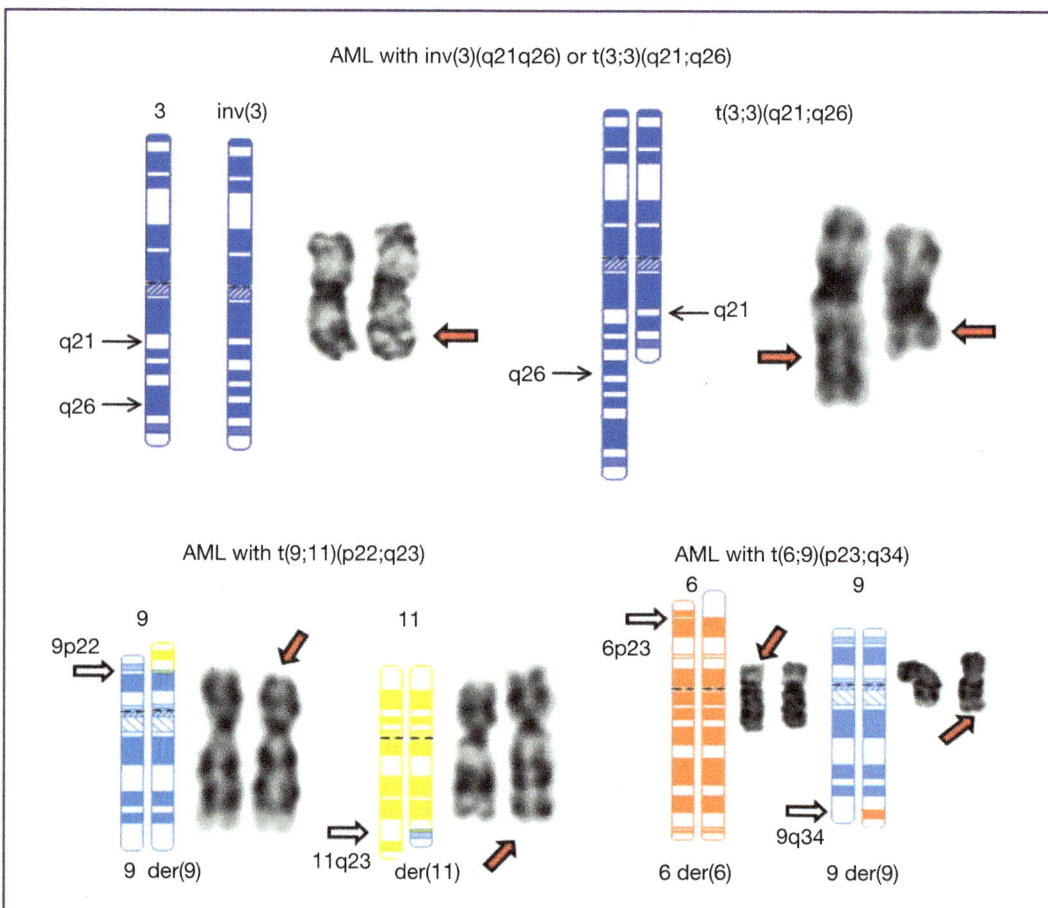

FIGURE 2-31: G-banding karyotyping showing inv(3) & t(3;3) (top), t(9;11) and t(6;9) (bottom). AML, acute myeloid leukemia.

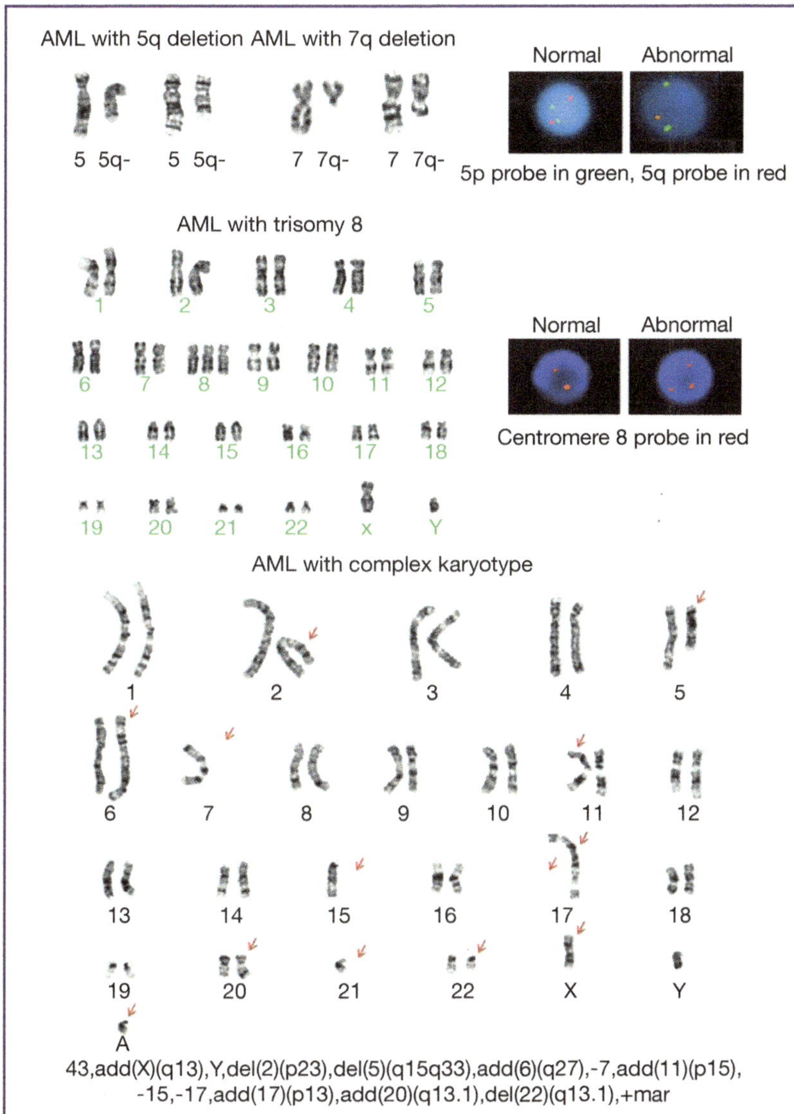

FIGURE 2-32: AML with del(5q), del(7q), +8, and complex karyotype.
AML, acute myeloid leukemia.

Table 2-6 Recurrent cytogenetic abnormalities in B-ALL

PROGNOSIS	CYTOGENETICS	GENES INVOLVED
Better	t(12;21)	*ETV6/RUNX1*
	Hyperdiploidy (≥50 chromosomes)	
Poor	Hypodiploidy (≤45 chromosomes)	
	t(9;22)	*BCR/ABL1*
	t(1;19)	*PBX1/TCF3*
	t(v;11)/del11q23/dup11q23	*MLL*
	RUNX1 amplification	*RUNX1*
	BCR-ABL1 like	Fusions involving *ABL1, ABL2, PDGFRB, JAK2, etc.*

B-ALL, B acute lymphoblastic leukemia.

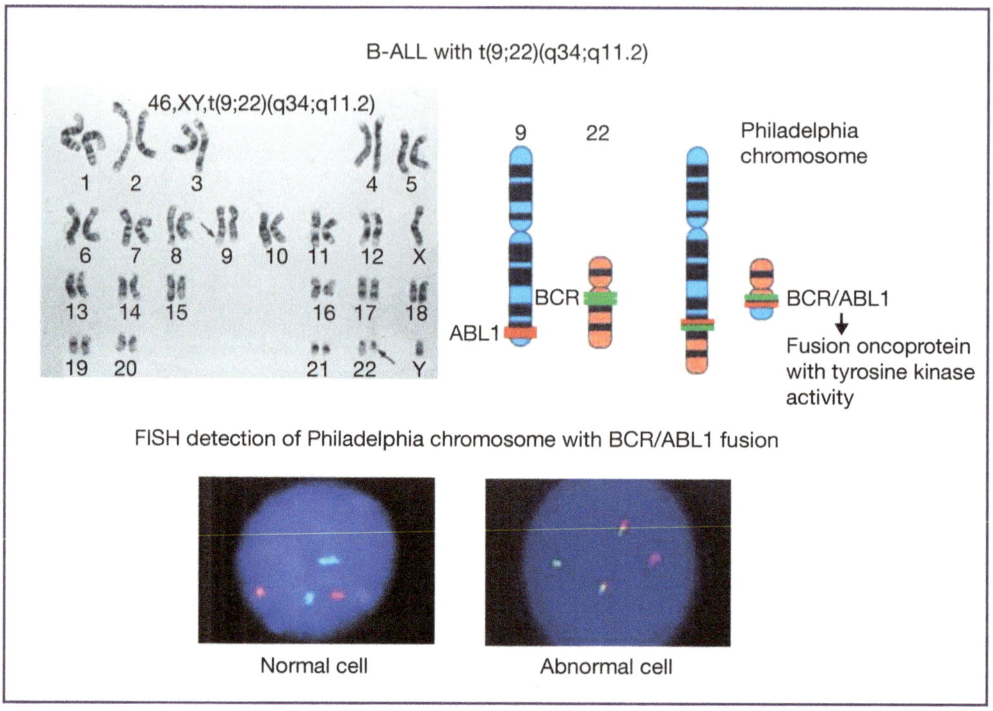

FIGURE 2-33: **Detection of Philadelphia chromosome resulting from t(9;22).**

B-ALL, B acute lymphoblastic leukemia; FISH, fluorescence in situ hybridization.

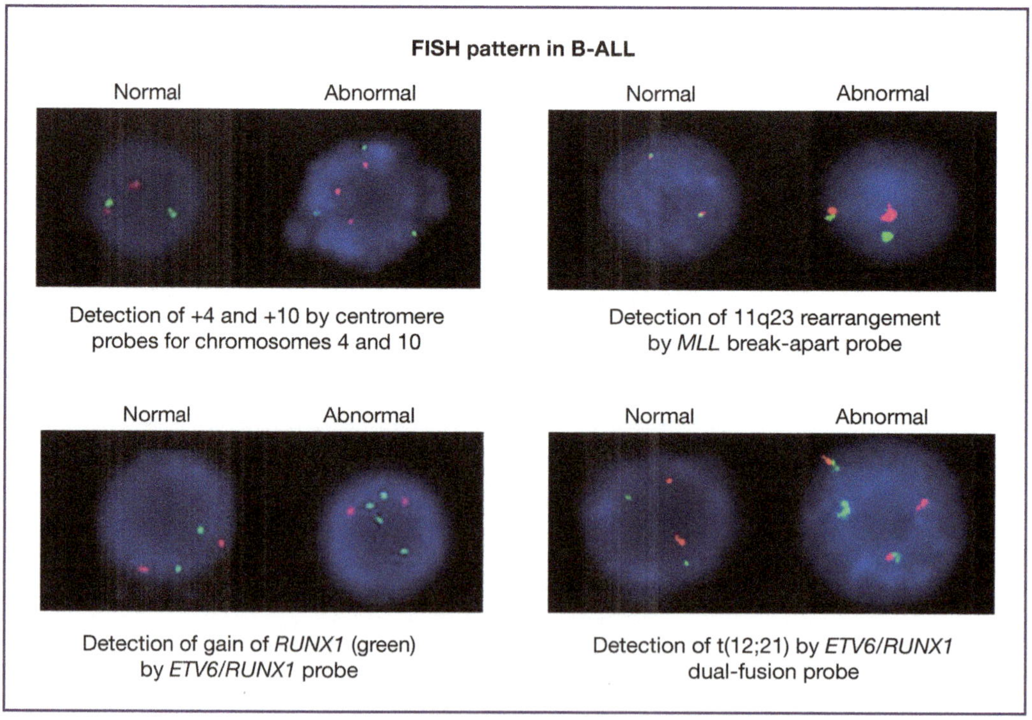

FIGURE 2-34: **FISH pattern in B-ALL.**

B-ALL, B acute lymphoblastic leukemia; FISH, fluorescence in situ hybridization; MLL, mixed lineage leukemia.

Table 2-7 Recurrent cytogenetic abnormalities in T-ALL

CYTOGENETICS	GENES INVOLVED
1p32 rearrangements, t(1;v)	*TAL1*
t(5;14)	*TLX3-BCL11B*
6q deletion	
7q34 rearrangements, t(v;7)	*TRB*
9p deletion	*CDK2NA*
12p rearrangements, t(12;v)	*ETV6*
14q11.2 rearrangements, t(v;14)	*TRA/D*
14q32 rearrangements, t(v;14)	*TCL1A*

T-ALL, T acute lymphoblastic leukemia.

Selected References

Graux C, Cools J, Michaux L, et al. Cytogenetics and molecular genetics of T-cell acute lymphoblastic leukemia: from thymocyte to lymphoblast. *Leukemia.* 2006;20:1496–1510.

Harrison CJ, Haas O, Harbott J, et al. Detection of prognostically relevant genetic abnormalities in childhood B-cell precursor acute lymphoblastic leukaemia: recommendations from the Biology and Diagnosis Committee of the International Berlin-Frankfürt-Münster study group. *Br J Haematol.* 2010;151(2):132–142.

Meijerink JP, den Boer ML, Pieters R. New genetic abnormalities and treatment response in acute lymphoblastic leukemia. *Semin Hematol.* 2009;46(1):16–23.

Mrózek K, Marcucci G, Nicolet D, et al. Prognostic significance of the European LeukemiaNet standardized system for reporting cytogenetic and molecular alterations in adults with acute myeloid leukemia. *J Clin Oncol.* 2012;30(36):4515–4523.

Mullighan CG. Molecular genetics of B-precursor acute lymphoblastic leukemia. *J Clin Invest.* 2012;122:3407–3415.

Szczepaõski T, Harrison CJ, van Dongen JJ. Review. Genetic aberrations in paediatric acute leukaemias and implications for management of patients. *Lancet Oncol.* 2010;11:880–889.

Vardiman JW, Thiele J, Arber DA, et al. The 2008 revision of the World Health Organization (WHO) classification of myeloid neoplasms and acute leukemia: rationale and important changes. *Blood.* 2009;114(5):937–951.

You MJ, Medeiros LJ, Hsi ED. T-lymphoblastic leukemia/lymphoma. *Am J Clin Pathol.* 2015;144(3): 411–422.

MODERN MOLECULAR GENETICS (SEE ALSO SECTIONS: MOLECULAR MUTATIONS IN AML AND MOLECULAR MUTATIONS IN ALL)

Parvez M. Lokhandwala and Christopher D. Gocke

Introduction

Molecular genetic testing plays an integral part in the management of patients with leukemia. The role of molecular genetic pathology in leukemia is underscored by the 2008 WHO classification, wherein molecular genetic defects form the basis of leukemia classification. Results of the molecular tests are utilized for disease diagnosis, prognosis, and targeted therapy, as well as in the follow-up of patients. Conventionally, cytogenetics, polymerase chain reaction (PCR), and FISH (Fluorescence In Situ Hybridization) have been used to gather this genetic information. However, newer methods such as next-generation sequencing (NGS) are now routinely used in conjunction with the conventional tests. The objective of this section is to give an overview of the principles, the scope, and the limitations behind the common molecular methods used in a modern laboratory.

PCR Amplification and Capillary Electrophoresis

Principle: Mutations that alter the *size* of a genetic target region can be investigated using this assay. PCR primers—one or both fluorescently labelled–are designed to amplify across the target region and the amplified products are subjected to capillary electrophoresis (CE). CE can resolve DNA molecules with as little as 1 base-pair (bp) difference. Insertion mutations yield larger PCR products, whereas deletions result in smaller PCR products when compared to the germline or wild-type (WT) DNA.

Advantages: Quick and inexpensive; high analytic limit of detection (as low as 1% mutant DNA); can be used to follow patients with detectable mutations after treatment.

Application: Ideally suited for detection of small indel (insertion-deletion) mutations; eg, *FLT3* internal tandem duplication (ITD) detection (Figure 2-35).

Limitations: Does not give the sequence of the mutant DNA; does not detect single nucleotide variants (SNVs), copy number variants (CNVs), or large indels; requires knowledge of the mutation site for flanking with PCR primers.

Modification: Restriction Fragment Length Polymorphism (RFLP) assay: If a point mutation results in gain or loss of a restriction enzyme site, then the amplified PCR product can be subjected to restriction digestion before resolving on CE. Several other modifications of the simple PCR method exist (eg, allele-specific PCR and translocation detection).

Short-Tandem Repeat Analysis/Chimerism Study

Principle: Short Tandem Repeats (STRs), or microsatellites, are DNA sequences of 1–5 bp subunits that are repeated in tandem from 5 to 50 times (eg, GCAGCAGCAGCA . . .). They are generally noncoding and are present in thousands of places in the human genome. Following Mendelian genetics, each person inherits a set of microsatellites from each parent. The number of repeats for any microsatellite can vary between individuals such that a profile of multiple microsatellites can be used to uniquely identify any individual, since only identical twins carry the same profile. In hematopoietic stem cell transplantation, it can be used to investigate engraftment of donor cells, rejection of the graft, and potentially disease relapse (Figure 2-36).

Advantages: This study is PCR-based, technically simple, inexpensive, and fast.

Application: This finds application in monitoring hematopoietic stem cell transplant engraftment.

Limitations: It requires informative loci, ie, STRs that differentiate between individuals who are often closely related; semiquantitative; the limit of detection of the minor genetic component is approximately

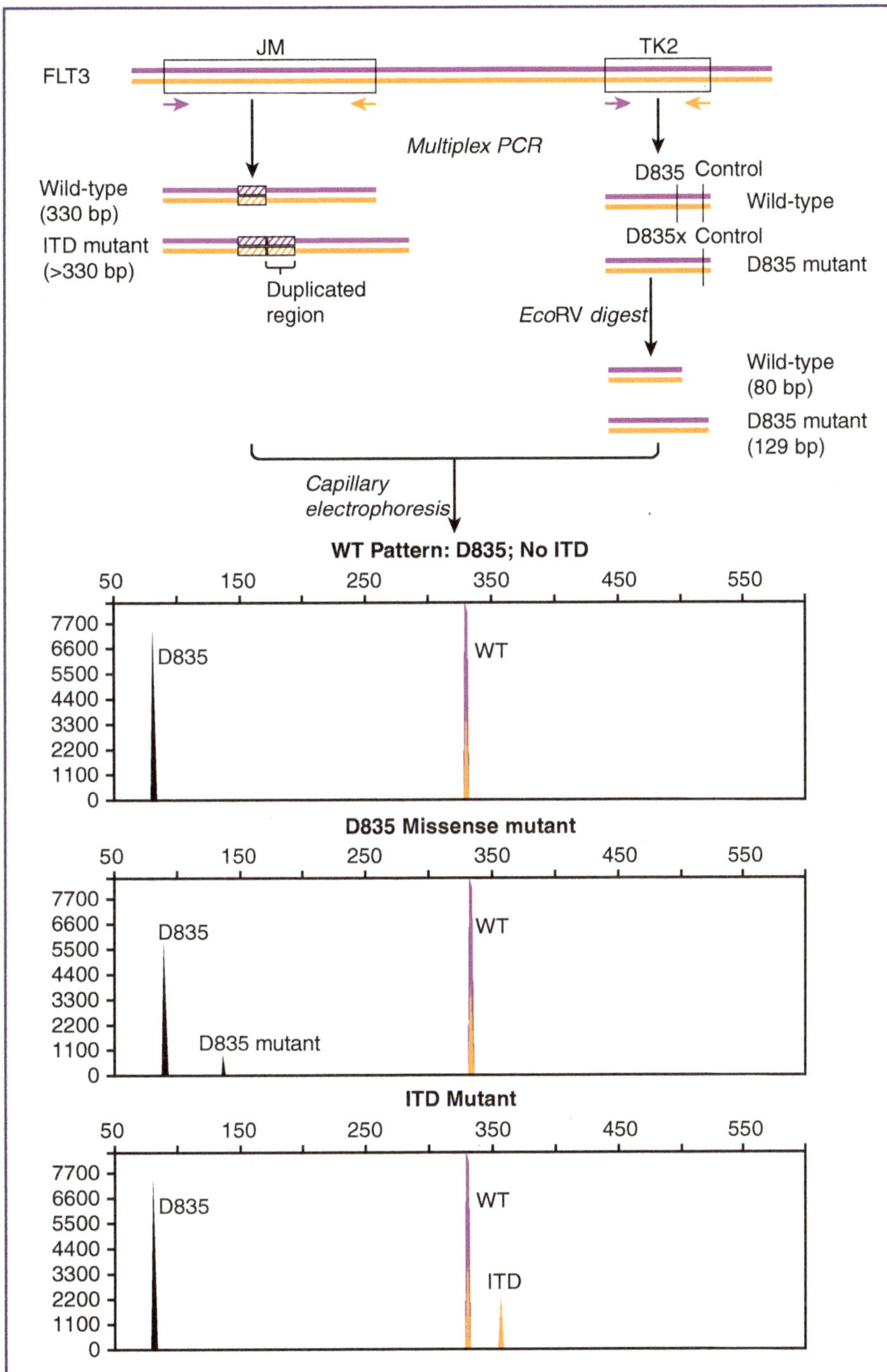

FIGURE 2-35: Two hotspot mutations are frequently tested in the *FLT3* gene: *FLT3* internal tandem duplication (ITD) mutation in the juxtamembrane (JM) domain and a D835 missense mutation in the tyrosine kinase (TK2) domain. The ITD mutation causes an increase in the size of the PCR product, while the D835 missense mutation results in a loss of the EcoRV restriction site. Fluorescently labeled PCR primers are used to amplify across the two *FLT3* regions: blue- and green-labeled primers for ITD detection and black-labeled primer for D835. The amplified PCR products are then subjected to EcoRV digestion and separated on CE. The ITD mutant results in a PCR product that is larger than the WT PCR product (330 bp). The size of the ITD product can vary depending on the mutation. The WT D835 PCR product results in a restriction fragment that is 80 bp. In contrast, the D835 missense mutant results in loss of the restriction site and yields a 129 bp product. A second artificial restriction site is engineered in the reverse primer as an internal control to ensure activity of the restriction enzyme in the reaction.

CE, capillary electrophoresis; FLT3, FMS-like tyrosine kinase 3; PCR, polymerase chain reaction; WT, wild-type.

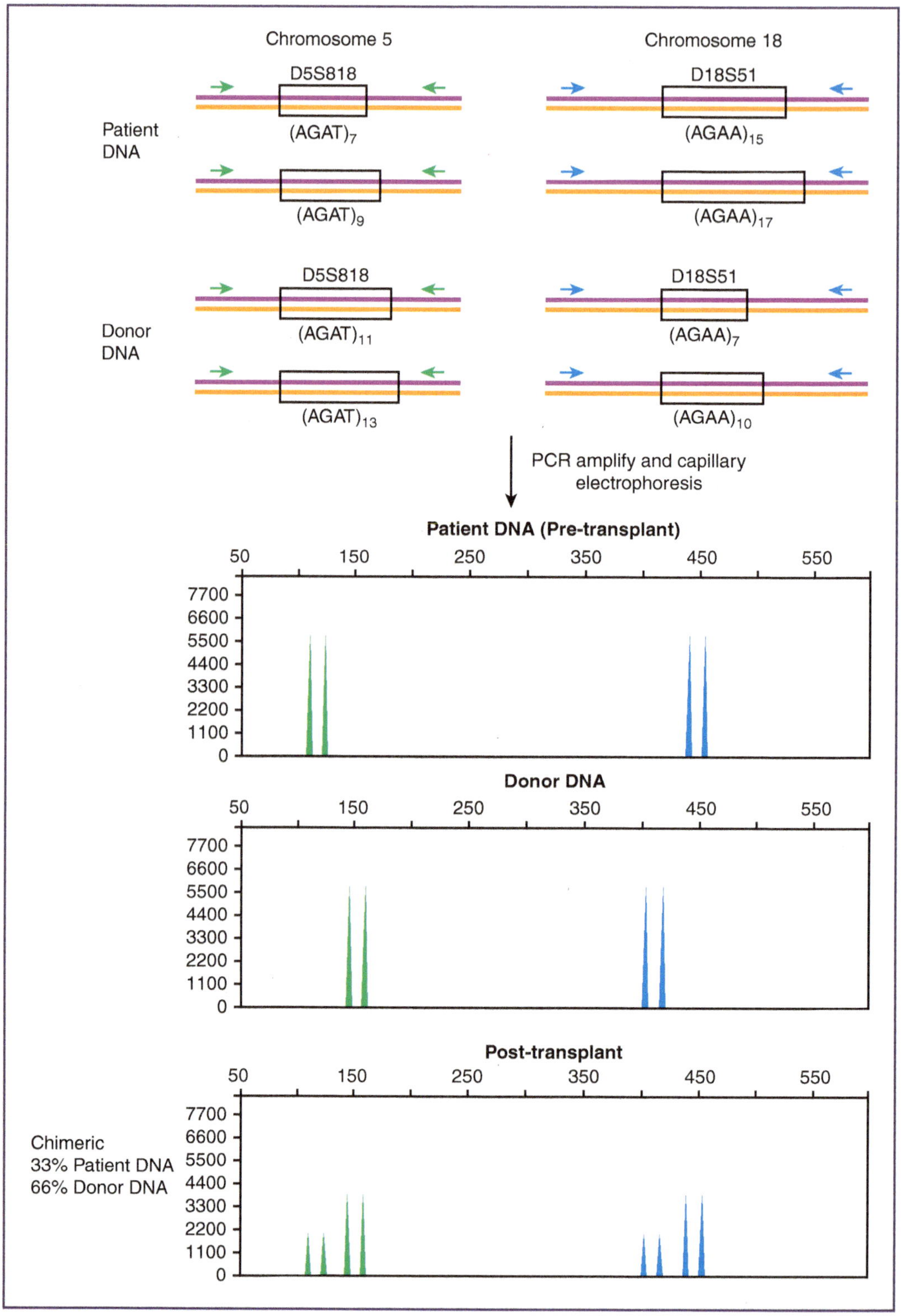

FIGURE 2-36: Genomic DNA (generally bone marrow specimen) from transplanted patient is harvested and approximately 15 different microsatellite loci are PCR amplified in a multiplex reaction using fluorescently labeled primers. Two amplified loci are seen: D5S818 labeled with orange fluorophore and D18S51 labeled with blue fluorophore. The amplified products are separated on CE and the microsatellite profile is compared to that of the donor and the patient DNA profiles prior to transplant. The bone marrow transplant status of the patient is chimeric with 33% patient DNA and 66% donor DNA.

CE, capillary electrophoresis; PCR, polymerase chain reaction.

3% to 5%, hence, this assay is not good for minimal residual disease (MRD) evaluation; genetic deletion of a region will remove any informative STR markers on it.

Modification: The chimerism analysis can be performed on bone marrow or peripheral blood specimens. A filtering or antibody-mediated selection step for T-cells or stem cells can be performed prior to STR analysis to evaluate chimerism of individual cellular fractions.

Quantitative (Real-Time) Reverse-Transcription PCR (qRT-PCR)

Principle: Reverse-transcription (RT)-PCR uses a viral reverse transcriptase enzyme to convert RNA to complementary DNA (cDNA), which is then used as a template for conventional PCR. The reverse transcription step uses an oligonucleotide primer that either is generic to convert all of the cellular RNA to cDNA, or is target specific.

Real-time PCR, also known as quantitative PCR (qPCR), is a way to detect the amount of PCR products during their synthesis (in "real-time"). One version uses dyes that nonspecifically bind to any double-stranded DNA molecules (eg, intercalating molecules like ethidium bromide or minor-groove binding

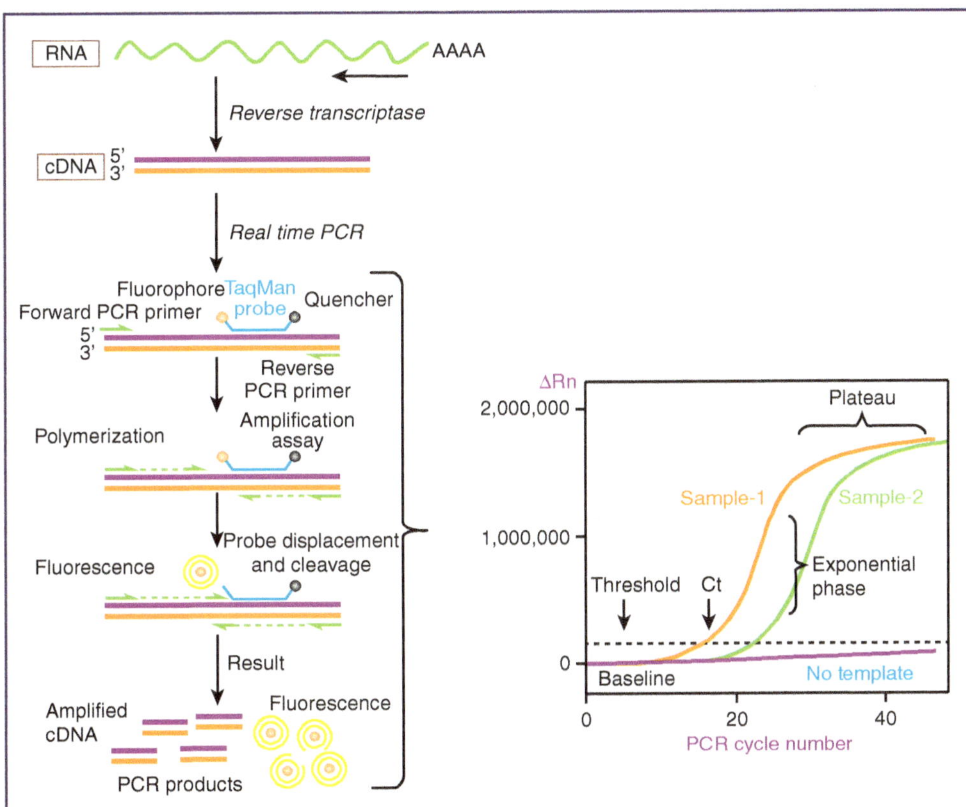

FIGURE 2-37: The target RNA molecule is converted to cDNA, which is then subjected to real-time PCR. The TaqMan version of detection is shown. The probe contains a fluorophore and a quencher. The fluorophore only emits a signal once it is separated from quencher, which occurs when the probe is cleaved by the 5′–3′ nuclease activity of the DNA polymerase during DNA synthesis. The real-time fluorescent monitoring results in a sigmoid curve, which includes base line, exponential phase, and plateau phase. The dotted line is the manually set threshold, a consistent reference point for all samples. The number of cycles it takes for a sample to cross the threshold is referred to as the threshold cycle (Ct). Sample 1 (red line) has a Ct that is three cycles lower than Sample 2 (green line). Therefore, Sample 1 has approximately 8 (2^3) times more starting target molecules compared to Sample 2. The negative control (blue line) does not cross the threshold.

PCR, polymerase chain reaction.

molecules like SYBR-green). Another approach uses a pair of fluorescently labeled sequence-specific probes, or oligonucleotides, which are designed such that they only fluoresce in the presence of complementary DNA. The amount of fluorescence in the reaction is directly proportional to the amount of target DNA amplified, allowing real-time monitoring. This method reduces nonspecific signal from primer-dimers and misprimed amplification products. A third version (TaqMan) employs a sequence-specific probe that is cleaved by the polymerase performing the PCR reaction; this probe only fluoresces after it is cleaved. The amount of starting DNA is inversely related to the number of PCR cycles required for the fluorescent signal to cross an arbitrarily set threshold, referred to as the threshold cycle (Ct). Comparing the Ct value of the target DNA to that of a prequantified standard DNA allows absolute quantification of the amount of starting target DNA (Figure 2-37).

qRT-PCR combines both the RT step and the real-time measurement.

Advantages: It is extremely sensitive and specific; quantitative with widest analytical measurement range (quantitative up to 5 logs). Real-time PCR products are detected during synthesis, thus eliminating the need to open the tube after amplification, which significantly reduces the risk of contaminating the laboratory area with amplified DNA.

Applications: It quantifies any specific RNA or DNA target; eg, *BCR-ABL1* translocation detection; it can be used for MRD measurement.

Limitations: It does not give the sequence of the mutation or the exact break-point of translocation present.

Single Nucleotide Polymorphism (SNP) Array

Principle: A healthy individual has millions of SNPs distributed throughout the genome, most of them inherited from parents. Because a somatic cell is diploid, at any given SNP locus a person may either be homozygous or heterozygous for that SNP. An SNP array probes many hundreds of thousands of SNP loci simultaneously. Genomic alterations (deletions, duplications, or uniparental disomy (UPD)) result in the loss of heterozygosity (LOH) at stretches of contiguous SNP loci, forming the basis of this assay.

Advantages: SNP array is currently the only method that can detect UPD, also known as copy-neutral LOH (CN-LOH).

Application: It detects large mutations: deletions (~>1 Mb), duplications (~>2 Mb), and CN-LOH (~>10 Mb).

Limitations: It cannot detect balanced genomic alterations, eg, reciprocal translocations or inversions; cannot detect most single-nucleotide mutations or other small mutations; does not give the precise boundaries of the mutation; relatively low limit of detection (minimum 20%–30% cells with a mutation).

Process: Genomic DNA from the tumor specimen is extracted and isothermally amplified several fold (not shown). The DNA is fragmented and hybridized to bead-bound oligonucleotide probes that are complementary to the sequence flanking the SNP loci. A synthesis step results in the production of the SNP base (either the arbitrarily named A allele, B allele, or both) depending on the individual's genotype. The synthesized SNP bases are differentially labeled with a fluorophore. The chip is scanned and the relative fluorescence intensity of A and B at each locus is measured and graphically plotted as the B-allele frequency (BAF) (blue dots). Also, the total fluorescence signal (A+B) for an SNP locus is compared to all other SNP loci through a formula resulting in the log R ratio (LRR) (red line). For a given SNP locus, a healthy individual will have three tracks for BAF approximating 0% (A/A), 50% (A/B), and 100% (B/B), and a LRR of 0. The loci that are homozygous (either A/A or B/B) are not informative with regard to chromosomal alterations (Figure 2-38).

If one of the informative alleles is deleted, the BAF for that locus will become either 0% (A/-) or 100% (B/-), but not 50%. However, because a leukemia specimen is generally a mix of tumor and normal DNA, the BAF of such a heterogeneous sample results in four tracks for all SNPs in the deleted region. Recall that the B allele fraction is the proportion of B alleles in the total pool of DNA: if there are

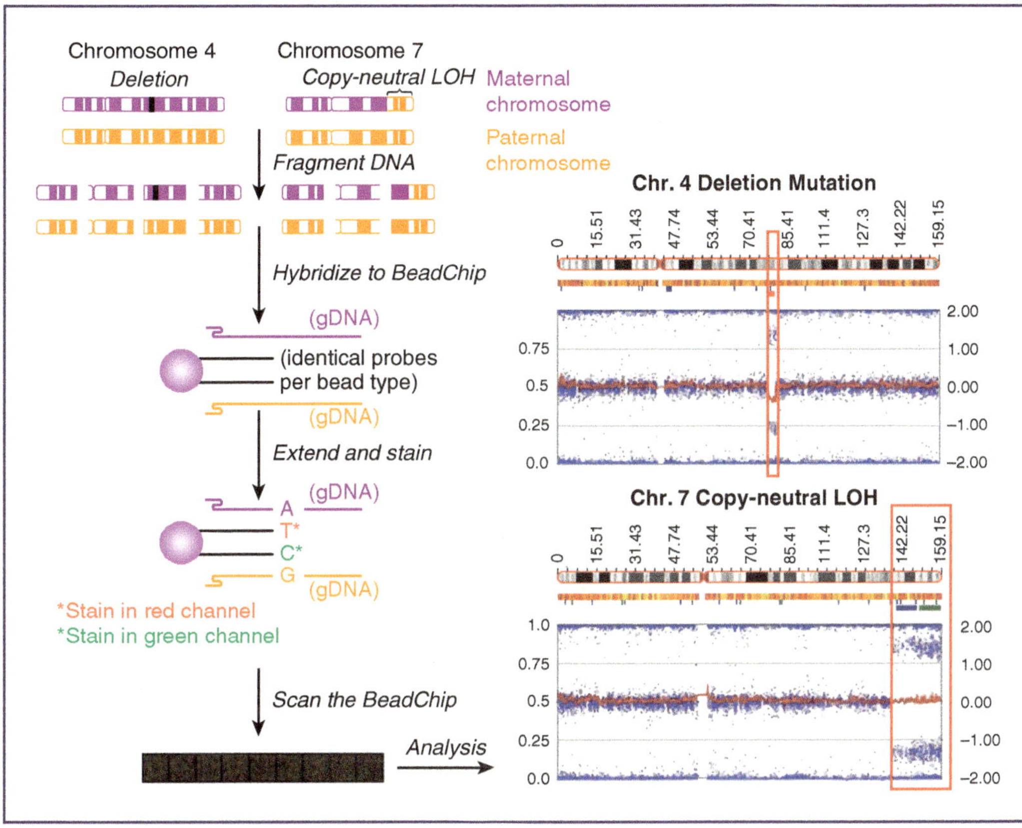

FIGURE 2-38: Demonstration of two different examples of mutations. The orange and purple chromosomes represent the maternal and paternal chromosomes. On the left is an example of a 3.5 Mb interstitial deletion in chromosome 4q (including the *TET2* gene) in approximately 60% of cells. Note the absence of the 50% BAF blue track, the presence of two additional BAF tracks, and the decreased red LRR <0. The second example on the right has an approximately 20 Mb CN-LOH in chromosome 7q in approximately 70% of cells. Note the absence of the 50% BAF track, the presence of two additional BAF tracks, and an LRR of 0. Also notice that the two blue middle tracks are slightly more separated than in Case 1.

BAF, B-allele frequency; LOH, loss of heterozygosity; LRR, log R ratio.

half-tumor cells (A/-) and half-normal cells (A/B) at a given locus, then the proportion of B in the total is one-third (A/-/A/B). The higher the tumor cell percentage in a sample, the further away the two middle genotype (A/A/B and A/B/B) tracks will be from 50%. The four tracks in this scenario will be 0% (A/A/A), between 0% and 50% (A/A/B), between 50% and 100% (A/B/B), and 100% (B/B/B), but importantly missing the mid-line 50% track. The LRR of the deleted region will be lower than 0 (A+B fluorescence for the region lower than the genomic average). Similarly, for CN-LOH and genetic amplification mutations, the 50% BAF track is lost. However, the LRR remains equal to 0 in CN-LOH, and is greater than 0 in genetic gains.

Next-Generation Sequencing (NGS)

Principle: NGS is a method to sequence several million individual DNA molecules simultaneously, each sequence in theory representing the contribution of a single cell. NGS is also referred to as massively parallel sequencing. The individual sequencing reads (from tens to a hundred bases in length) are then computationally aligned to the reference human genome to generate a consensus sequence for all of the targeted regions; the variations may represent mutations.

Because each patient DNA is labeled with a uniquely identifiable barcode, multiple patient samples can be pooled together prior to sequencing using either sequencing platform. This allows multiple patient samples to be sequenced simultaneously and the sequencing reads to be computationally decoded after the fact to determine which patient they belong to. Doing so increases the throughput of the method and reduces cost.

A typical NGS workflow can be divided into three parts: (A) library preparation (a few hours to a few days) (Figure 2-39), (B) amplification and sequencing of DNA (4–26 hours) (Figure 2-40), and (C) bioinformatics or data analysis (several hours) (Figure 2-41).

Advantages: It allows detection of SNVs, CNVs, translocations, and small indels.

Application: Sequencing entire single gene, sequencing several hot-spot mutation regions, sequencing several exons, whole exome sequencing, and whole genome sequencing.

Limitations: Large indels may be missed by current bioinformatics pipelines. The analytic sensitivity of mutation detection depends on the depth of coverage. The significance of most true (nonartifactual) variants is currently unknown.

Modifications: RNASeq is parallel sequencing of many RNA molecules; MethSeq allows investigation of the genomic methylation profile.

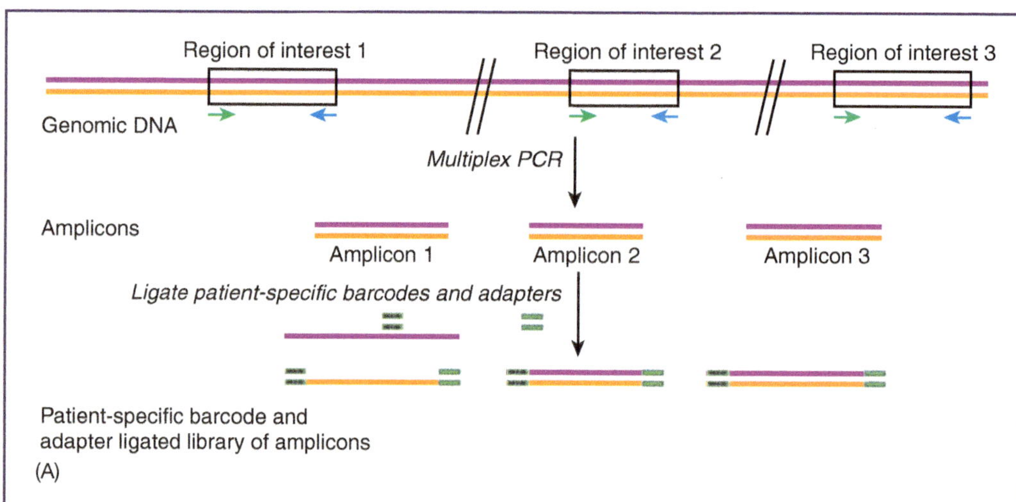

FIGURE 2-39: The two most commonly employed methods of library preparation are illustrated in this figure: (A) *Amplicon-based method:* This method is used to investigate hot-spot regions for mutations. A multiplex PCR with a couple of hundred primer-sets is used to amplify across multiple genomic targets simultaneously. In the figure, only three amplicons are shown for simplification. A small generic adapter DNA sequence and a patient-specific barcode adapter are ligated at the ends of each amplicon, creating a library of amplicons. This method is simpler than the capture method and is inexpensive, but is limited in the number of target regions that can be amplified simultaneously. Also, this method can be used to amplify very low amounts of input DNA. (*continued*)

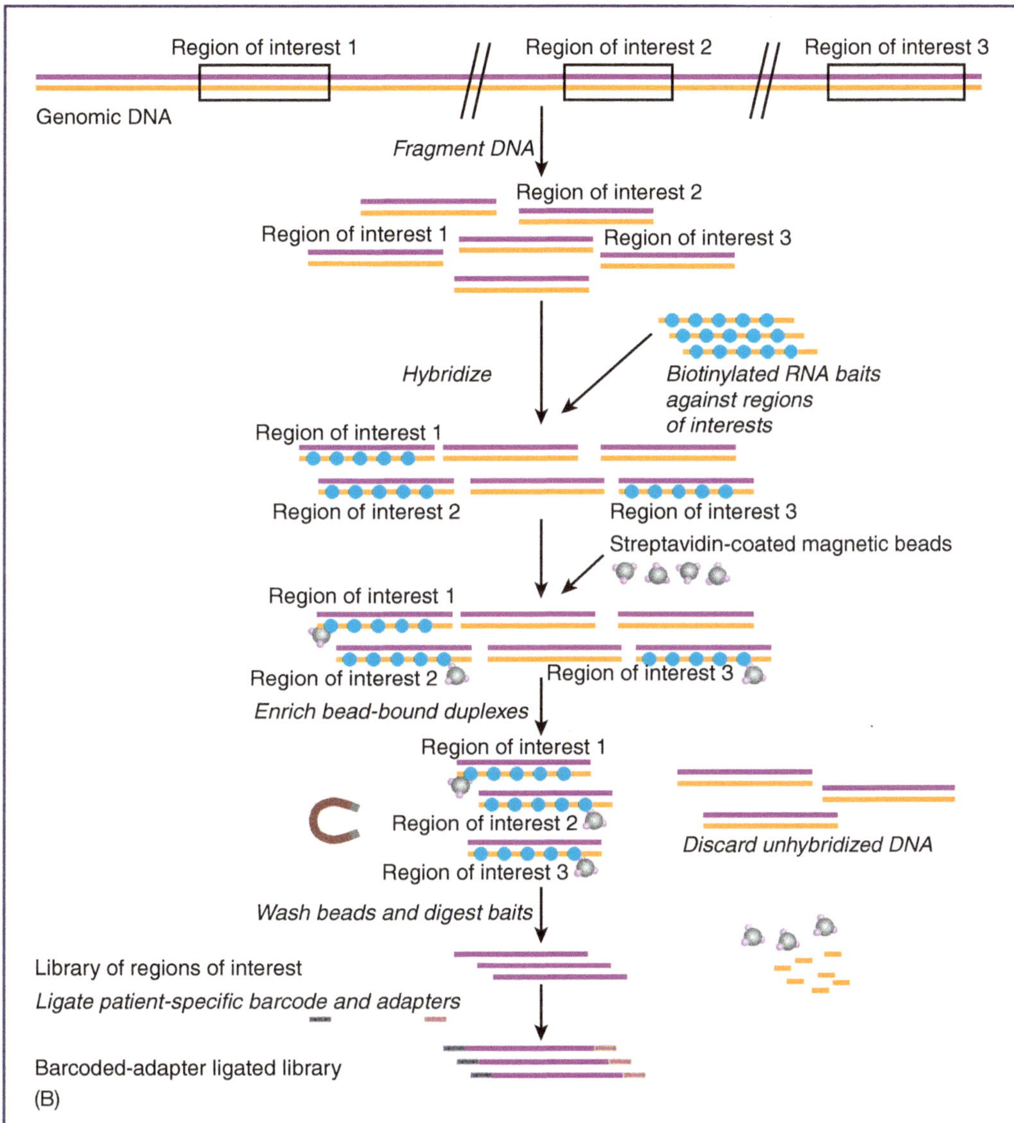

FIGURE 2-39: (*continued*) (B) ***Hybrid-capture method:*** **The genomic DNA is fragmented using sonication or enzymatic digestion. The target regions are hybridized to a pool of biotinylated complementary RNA probes that are used as baits. Streptavidin-coated magnetic beads bind to the biotin in the probe-target, forming RNA–DNA heteroduplexes (the "hybrids"). The targets are captured using a magnet and the RNA baits are subsequently digested. A generic and a patient-specific adapter are ligated onto the ends of the single-stranded DNA molecules to create a library of targets. This method allows capture of any number of target regions and is therefore the method of choice for whole exome sequencing. Some highly GC-rich regions are difficult to capture because the bait probes can bind nonspecifically to other GC-rich genomic regions.**

GC, guanine-cytosine; PCR, polymerase chain reaction.

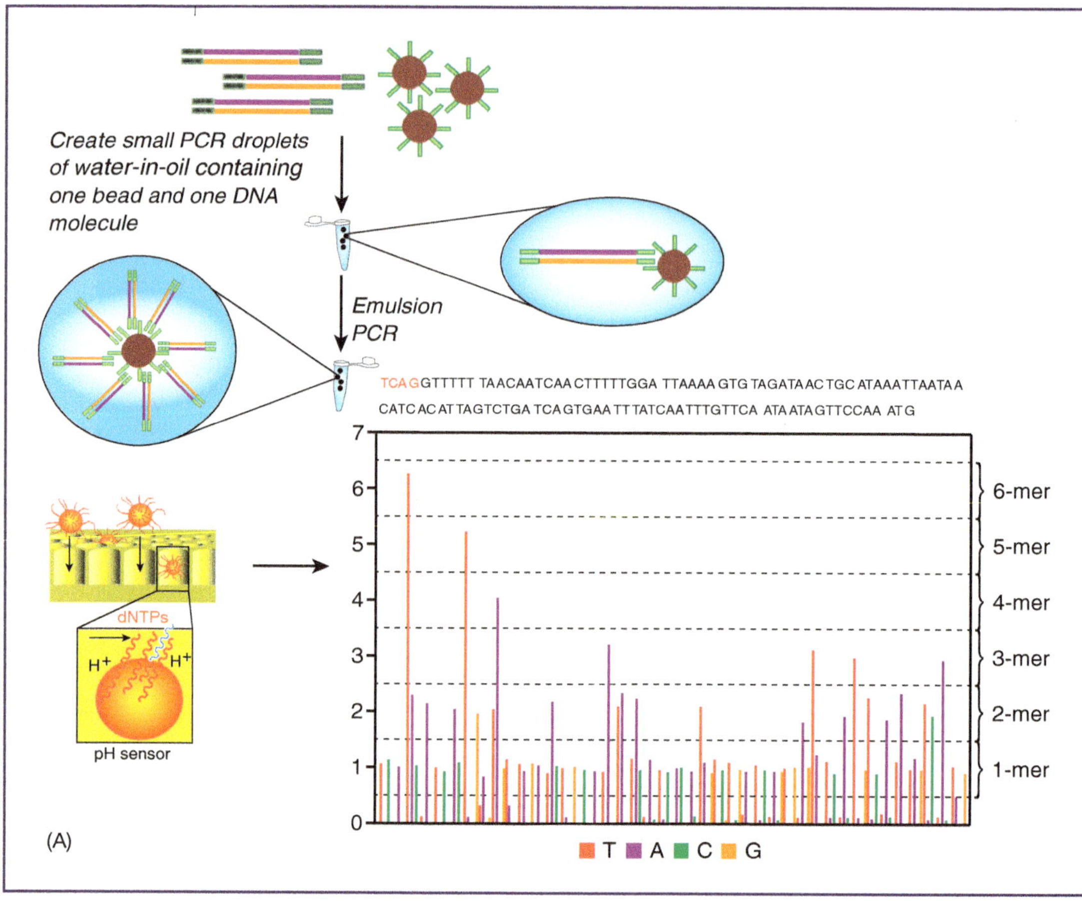

FIGURE 2-40: There are multiple sequencing platforms available currently. The two most popular methods used clinically are illustrated in this figure: (A) ***Emulsion PCR and semiconductor sequencing:*** This method uses the amplicon-based adapter-ligated library from the previous step and creates several million individual picoliter PCR reactions. Each PCR reaction is a water-in-oil droplet consisting of a single DNA molecule, one oligonucleotide-bound bead (with the oligonucleotide complementary to the generic adapter from Figure 2-39. (A), and necessary PCR reagents (dNTPs, polymerase, etc.). Emulsion PCR results in clonal amplification of each DNA molecule attached to the surface of the beads, resulting in the formation of "hairy beads." The emulsion is broken and the "hairy beads" are loaded onto a sequencing chip. The sequencing chip contains several million small wells that can accommodate one bead each. A generic sequencing primer is hybridized to the molecules on the bead. Each of four dNTPs is cyclically added to the chip in a sequential order, followed by a wash step. If a complementary dNTP is added to the growing DNA chain, an H^+ ion is released during the condensation reaction. This released H^+ ion in a given well results in a change in the pH of that well, which is measured by a pH sensor. The simultaneous measurement of voltage changes across many millions of wells uses semiconductor technology. The change in pH is converted to a graphical representation known as an ionogram, which gives the raw sequence data for that particular well (or DNA clone). (*continued*)

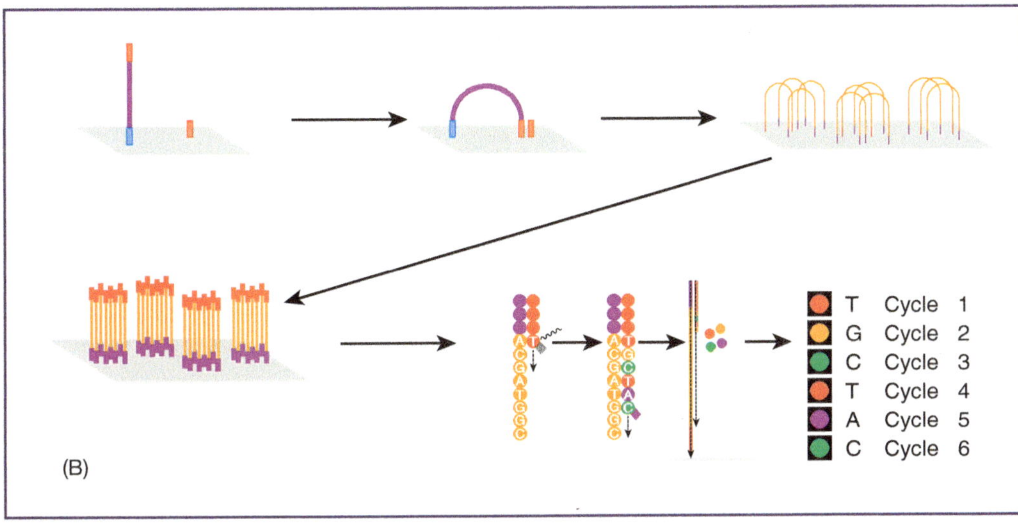

FIGURE 2-40: (*continued*) (B) ***Bridge-amplification and sequencing by synthesis:*** **This method can use either of the two libraries from Figure 2-39. The library is hybridized to oligonucleotides on a flow cell that are complementary to the adapters. The adapter-probe binding at both ends results in formation of a molecular "bridge." Bridge-PCR creates localized clonal populations of each DNA molecule, referred to as a cluster. Sequencing primers are added and fluorescently labeled reversible chain-terminator dNTPs are flowed across the cell sequentially. If a complementary dNTP is added, a fluorescent signal will be emitted, which is captured by real-time imaging of the flow cell. The chain-terminator is removed, the next nucleotide is added, and the flow cell is scanned again. The end result is a series of images of the flow cell, with each image representing a snapshot of the sequence of all the clusters on the flow cell. Following the fluorescent signal of each cluster from the beginning to the end of the sequencing process gives the raw read for that DNA clone.**

dNTP, deoxynucleotide triphosphate; PCR, polymerase chain reaction.

Droplet Digital PCR (DD-PCR)

Principle: Droplet digital PCR is useful to detect extremely low levels of mutant DNA in a background of wild-type DNA (WT-DNA). DD-PCR works by creating millions of small water-in-oil emulsions with each droplet preferably consisting of one DNA molecule. Differentially labeled sets of PCR primers are used to amplify targeted regions to discover a mutation. After PCR amplification, each droplet is evaluated for the level and the type of fluorescence to determine the number of droplets with mutant DNA versus WT-DNA molecules. This affords an absolute quantitation of the number of mutant DNA molecules in the sample (Figure 2-42).

Advantages: It is extremely sensitive (can detect very low levels of mutant DNA, as low as 1:1,000,000), relatively easy from a technical standpoint, and easy to interpret.

Application: It has application in minimal disease and molecular relapse testing.

Limitations: Mutation testing must be targeted (eg, *BRAF* V600E mutant); limited ability to multiplex.

Modification: DD-PCR can be used to create amplicon-based libraries for sequencing-by-synthesis platforms. This modification expands the role of DD-PCR from targeted mutation testing to genomic sequencing.

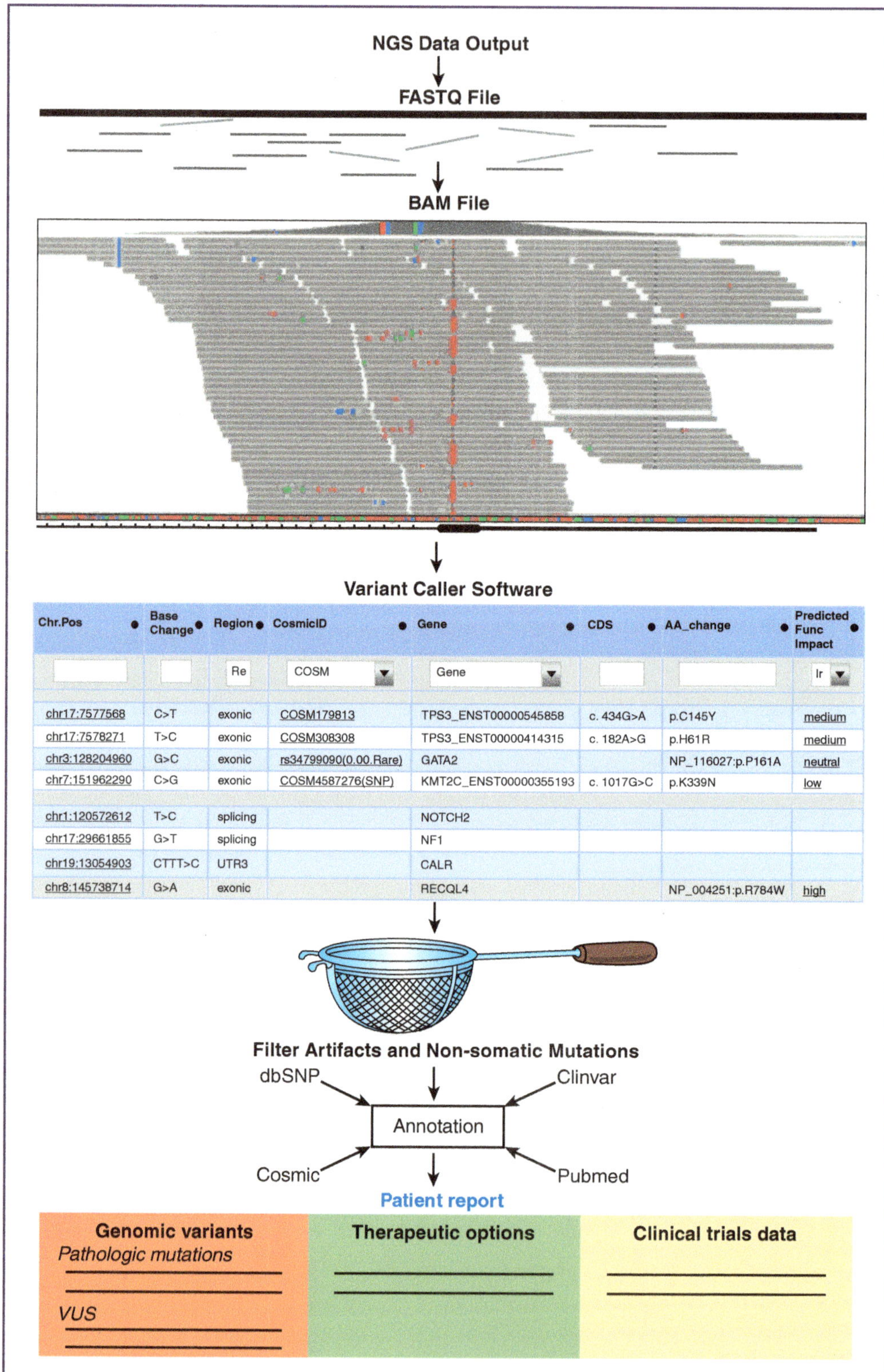

Chr.Pos	Base Change	Region	CosmicID	Gene	CDS	AA_change	Predicted Func Impact
		Re	COSM	Gene			lr
chr17:7577568	C>T	exonic	COSM179813	TPS3_ENST00000545858	c. 434G>A	p.C145Y	medium
chr17:7578271	T>C	exonic	COSM308308	TPS3_ENST00000414315	c. 182A>G	p.H61R	medium
chr3:128204960	G>C	exonic	rs34799090(0.00.Rare)	GATA2		NP_116027:p.P161A	neutral
chr7:151962290	C>G	exonic	COSM4587276(SNP)	KMT2C_ENST00000355193	c. 1017G>C	p.K339N	low
chr1:120572612	T>C	splicing		NOTCH2			
chr17:29661855	G>T	splicing		NF1			
chr19:13054903	CTTT>C	UTR3		CALR			
chr8:145738714	G>A	exonic		RECQL4		NP_004251:p.R784W	high

FIGURE 2-41: Bioinformatics. The sequencing methods have evolved so rapidly that currently the bioinformatics portion is more challenging than the wet-lab portion of NGS. The process of taking the sequence from raw data files to the detection of variants (mutations) is referred to as a bioinformatics pipeline. (*continued*)

FIGURE 2-41: (*continued*) The bioinformatics process can be arbitrarily thought of as primary, secondary, and tertiary analyses. The primary analysis takes the raw sequence data (ionographs or images) and converts each read to a sequence representation (eg, ATGCTAAGGT) with an associated quality score for each base, collectively referred to as a FASTQ file. The primary analysis generally occurs on the sequencing platform. Next, the secondary analysis alignment software aligns individual reads to a reference genome, resulting in a SAM file (or BAM file, the binary equivalent). In tertiary analysis, variant caller software compares the aligned sequences to the reference genome to identify genetic variants. The pipeline uses several filters to exclude artifacts (eg, variants that are present preferentially on either plus-strand or minus-strand, variants in genomic areas with low sequence coverage, variants in areas with poor sequence quality data, or variants that have been curated as artifacts during validation). Some laboratories use a matching normal specimen from the patient to remove germline variants. Other labs rely on the mutant allele frequency (approx. 50% or 100%) and a database of benign SNPs (eg, dbSNP) to exclude known germline variants. Once mutations/variants are identified, the final step is evaluating their clinical significance. Certain databases (eg, COSMIC, Clinvar, and dbSNP) along with published peer-reviewed articles and prediction software (to predict the effect of mutations on proteins) are all used in conjunction with medical information to determine the clinical significance of each variant. The variants are then classified into those that are pathologic versus those that have unknown clinical significance, often in a tiered fashion to indicate levels of uncertainty. Ideally, the report also includes data regarding targeted therapeutic options and potential clinical trials available to the patient.

AA, amino acid; BAM, binary alignment map; CDS, coding sequence change; Chr, chromosome; COSMIC, Catalogue of Somatic Mutations in Cancer; dbSNP, single nucleotide polymorphism database; NGS, next generation sequencing; Pos, position; SAM, sequence alignment map; VUS, variant of uncertain significance.

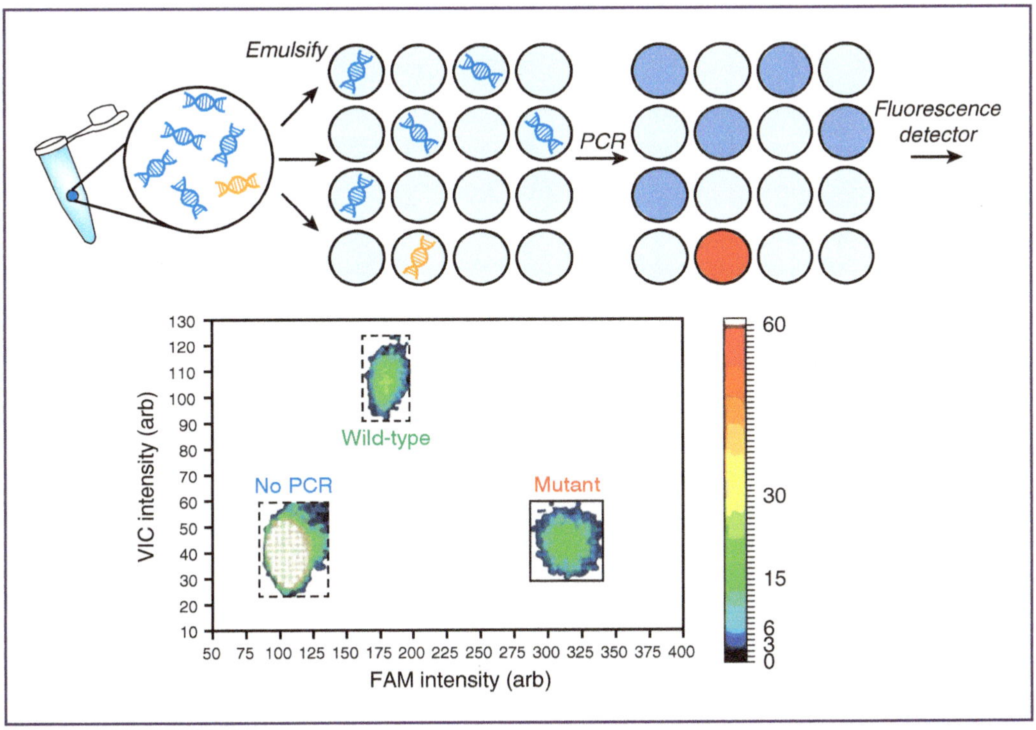

FIGURE 2-42: Droplet digital PCR. Extracted or circulating (ie, cell-free) genomic DNA from a patient sample is emulsified into small, uniformly sized pico-droplets, represented as circles. The droplets contain, on average, one or fewer target DNA molecules. The red DNA molecule represents a mutant, whereas blue represents WT-DNA and clear have no DNA. Post-PCR amplification, the droplets with mutant sequence yield a different fluorescent signal (red fluorescence) compared to droplets with WT-DNA (blue fluorescence). Droplets are evaluated one at a time in a flow cytometer for the intensity and type of fluorescence. Software graphically separates the populations based on their fluorescence intensity and gives the absolute number of mutant and WT-DNA molecules in the sample.

FAM, 6-carboxy fluorescein, the most commonly used reporter dye at the 5′ end of a TaqMan probe; PCR, polymerase chain reaction; VIC, variant allele-specific probe; WT, wild-type.

Gene Expression Array

Principle: In tumor cells, some genes are over- or underexpressed relative to normal cells. For example, pro-growth genes may be up-regulated, while checkpoint and apoptotic genes may be down-regulated. Additionally, depending on the cell of origin of the tumor, tissue-specific genes may be differentially expressed. The overall expression of the tumor is compared to normal cells to create a gene expression profile of the tumor. This information may be used for accurate diagnosis, appropriate classification, and potentially to make therapeutic decisions (Figure 2-43).

Advantages: Several genes are regulated by epigenetic mechanisms (eg, methylation and acetylation), which are not detected by conventional DNA sequencing methods. Gene expression arrays evaluate RNA profiles and therefore incorporate the epigenetic influences.

Application: It provides a gene expression profile of the tumor.

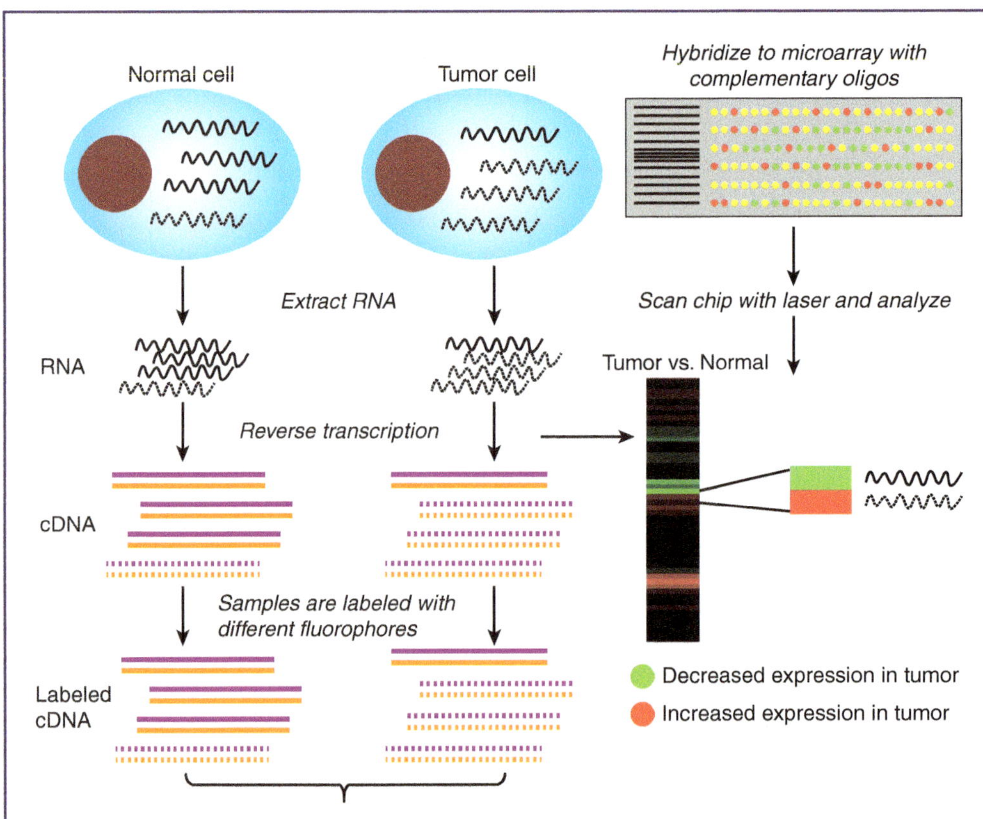

FIGURE 2-43: **Gene expression array. Illustration shows a dual-channel gene expression array. RNA is extracted from tumor and normal tissue and converted to cDNA. The cDNAs from tumor and normal cells are labeled with two different fluorophores. The cDNAs are then mixed and hybridized to an array of complementary oligonucleotides. The chip array is scanned with a laser to measure the intensity of both fluorescent signals at each spot on the array, which is proportional to the relative amounts of hybridized cDNAs. The tumor signal is normalized to create a profile of expression presented as a heat-map. Two different types of RNA molecules are shown; RNA-1 (solid line) with decreased expression in tumor relative to normal and RNA-2 (dotted line) with increased expression in tumor. The heat-map image is shown in intensities of green and red, designating a relative decrease or increase of that RNA type in the tumor. Many hundreds of genes may be represented in the stripe; genes with tumor expression equal to normal expression are black.**

Modification: Gene expression array may be done using single-channel or dual-channel fluorescence. In single-channel, the tumor and normal RNA are labeled with the same fluorophore but analyzed sequentially; in the dual-channel method (shown in the figure), tumor and normal RNA are labeled with different fluorophores and hybridized to the chip simultaneously.

Limitations: RNA, which is used as a starting material, can degrade over time. Also, cell expression can change quickly when subjected to different stresses that are not pertinent to the pathology. It is technically challenging to interpret.

The molecular methods discussed in this section are summarized in Table 2-8. It shows the types of mutations that are generally detected by each method. Limit of detection designates the minimum mutant allele frequency that can be detected by each method in a heterogeneous sample (mixture of WT and tumor DNA). For example, Sanger sequencing has a limit of detection of 20%. Therefore, this method can detect a mutation only if the mutant molecule accounts for at least 20% of all molecules. Because mutations are generally present on only one allele per diploid tumor cell, the method can detect mutations only if the tumor cellularity of the specimen exceeds 40%.

Table 2-8 Summary of molecular methods

ASSAY	VARIANTS				LIMIT OF DETECTION (APPROXIMATE % OF MUTANT MOLECULES)
	SINGLE NUCLEOTIDE VARIANTS	SMALL INDELS	LARGE INDELS CNVs	TRANSLOCATIONS	
RELP/AS-PCR	+	+	–	–	1%–5%
Sanger sequencing	+	+	–	–	20%
Pyrosequencing	+	+	–	–	5%–10%
SNP-array	–	–	+	–	20%
FISH	–	–	+/–	+	3%–10%
NGS-amplicon based	+	+	–*	–*	1%–5%
NGS-hybrid capture	+	+	+	+	1%–5%
DD-PCR	+	+/–	+/–	+/–	0.01%

*Amplicon-based NGS methods can detect large indels and translocations if specifically designed for it.

DD, droplet digital; FISH, fluorescence in situ hybridization; NGS, next generation sequencing; RELP/AS-PCR, restriction fragment length polymorphism/allele-specific polymerase chain reaction; SNP, single nucleotide polymorphism.

HLA typing

Principle: HLA genotyping may be performed in many ways. The commonly used methods include: (a) sequence-specific priming (SSP), (b) sequence-specific oligonucleotide (SSO), (Figure 2-44) (c) sequence-based typing (SBT), and (d) NGS.

The SSP method is conceptually similar to allele-specific PCR, wherein multiple primer sets are used to amplify across several polymorphic regions of HLA loci in individual reactions. Perfectly complementary primers result in amplification, while mismatched primers result in no amplification. The amplification products are then detected by gel electrophoresis. By choosing primers that interrogate each recognized HLA allele, one can obtain the genotype of the entire HLA locus.

In SSO, the polymorphic regions of the HLA loci are amplified using biotin-labeled primers to conserved flanking regions. Amplicons are hybridized under high stringency conditions to sequence-specific oligonucleotide-bound beads; each oligonucleotide is bound to a specific color-coded bead. Hybridization of the test sample to a bead results in fluorescence of that bead. A flow cytometer is used to detect the fluorescent signal as well as the color of the bound bead. By using hundreds of polymorphic oligonucleotide-bound beads, one can investigate all of the polymorphic regions of the HLA loci.

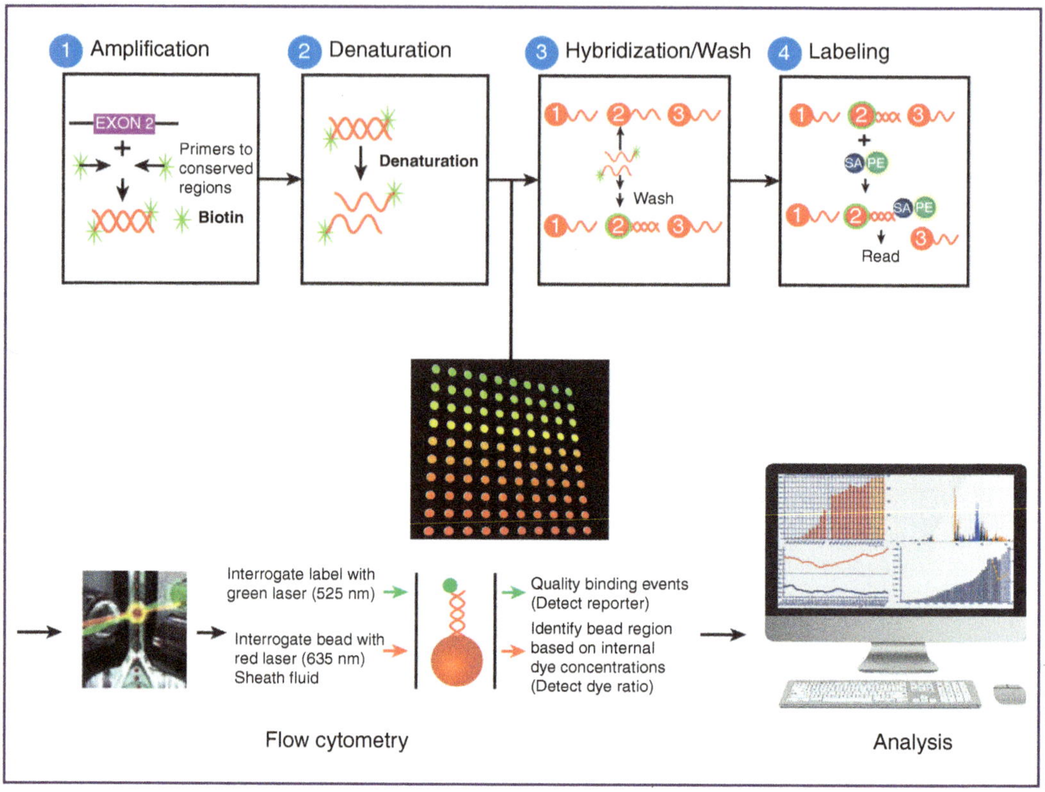

FIGURE 2-44: Sequence-specific oligonucleotide (SSO). Biotinylated primers are used to amplify across the polymorphic exonic HLA regions. The biotinylated amplicons are denatured and hybridized to hundreds of unique oligonucleotide-bound beads. Each oligonucleotide is bound to its respective color-coded bead. Streptavidin (SA)-conjugated phycoerythrin (PE) binds to the biotin in the hybridized DNA molecules. A flow cytometer detects PE and thus hybridization of the DNA molecule to oligonucleotide. Concurrently measuring the color of the bead identifies the bead (and thus the oligonucleotide) that the HLA molecule is bound to. Software analyzes the hybridization signal from each of the polymorphic oligonucleotide-bound beads and reports the HLA genotype of the person.
HLA, human leukocyte antigen.

The SBT method involves amplifying across the polymorphic HLA loci followed by (generally Sanger) sequencing. While conceptually straightforward, the size of the HLA loci makes this method difficult and it is often used as a complement to SSO or SSP to address ambiguities, rather than as a stand-alone method.

With longer sequencing reads and improved bioinformatics pipelines, NGS will likely become the method of choice for high-resolution HLA typing in the near future.

Application: It finds application in bone marrow transplantation.

Limitations: Interpretation of HLA typing can be fairly complex. Rare or unknown alleles may be missed by the SSP and SSO methods.

Selected References

The International Agency for Research on Cancer. In S. Swerdlow, E. Campo, N. Lee Harris, et al, eds, *WHO Classification of Tumours of Haematopoietic and Lymphoid Tissue (IARC WHO Classification of Tumours)*. 4th ed. http://apps.who.int/bookorders/anglais/detart1.jsp?codlan=1&codcol=70&codcch=4002&content=1. Published 2008.

FLT3

Murphy KM, Levis M, Hafez MJ, et al. Detection of FLT3 internal tandem duplication and D835 mutations by a multiplex polymerase chain reaction and capillary electrophoresis assay. *J Mol Diagn*. 2003;5(2):96–102.

STR ANALYSIS

AmpFlSTR Identifiler Plus PCR Amplification Kit User Guide (Pub. no. 4440211 Rev. F). https://www.thermofisher.com/us/en/home/industrial/human-identification/ampflstr-identifiler-plus-pcr-amplification-kit.html

Van Deerlin VM, Leonard DG. Bone marrow engraftment analysis after allogeneic bone marrow transplantation. *Clin Lab Med*. 2000;20(1):197–225.

SNP ARRAY

Affymetrix Genome-Wide Human SNP Array 6.0 data sheet, 2007. http://www.affymetrix.com/catalog/131533/AFFY/Genome-Wide+Human+SNP+Array+6.0#1_1

Wang DG, Fan JB, Siao CJ, et al. Large-scale identification, mapping, and genotyping of single-nucleotide polymorphisms in the human genome. *Science*. 1998;280:1077–1082.

HYBRID CAPTURE

Fisher S, Barry A, Abreu J, et al. A scalable, fully automated process for construction of sequence-ready human exome targeted capture libraries. *Genome Biol*. 2011;12(1):R1.

Gnirke A, Melnikov A, Maguire J, et al. Solution hybrid selection with ultra-long oligonucleotides for massively parallel targeted sequencing. *Nat Biotechnol*. 2009;27(2):182–189.

Shearer AE, Hildebrand MS, Smith RJ. Solution-based targeted genomic enrichment for precious DNA samples. *BMC Biotechnol*. 2012;12:20.

NEXT GENERATION SEQUENCING

Margulies M, Egholm M, Altman WE, et al. Genome sequencing in microfabricated high-density picolitre reactors. *Nature*. 2005;437(7057):376–380.

Metzker ML. Sequencing technologies–the next generation. *Nat Rev Genet*. 2010;11(1):31–46.

Q-RT PCR

Baltimore D. RNA-dependent DNA polymerase in virions of RNA tumour viruses. *Nature*. 1970;226(5252):1209–1211.

Higuchi R, Dollinger G, Walsh PS, Griffith R. Simultaneous amplification and detection of specific DNA sequences. *Biotechnology (NY)*. 1992;10:413–417.

Temin HM, Mizutani S. RNA-dependent DNA polymerase in virions of Rous sarcoma virus. *Nature*. 1970;226(5252):1211–1213.

DD-PCR

Droplet Digital PCR Technology; BIO-RAD. http://www.bio-rad.com/en-us/applications-technologies/droplet-digital-pcr-ddpcr-technology

Hindson BJ, Ness KD, Masquelier DA, et al. High-throughput droplet digital PCR system for absolute quantitation of DNA copy number. *Anal Chem*. 2011;83(22):8604–8610.

RainDrop, RainDance Technologies. http://raindancetech.com/digital-pcr-tech

Sykes PJ, Neoh SH, Brisco MJ, et al. Quantitation of targets for PCR by use of limiting dilution. *Biotechniques*. 1992;13(3):444–449.

GENE EXPRESSION

Schena M, Shalon D, Davis RW, Brown PO. Quantitative monitoring of gene expression patterns with a complementary DNA microarray. *Science*. 1995;270(5235):467–470.

Valk PJ, Verhaak RG, Beijen MA, et al. Prognostically useful gene-expression profiles in acute myeloid leukemia. *N Engl J Med*. 2004;350(16):1617–1628.

SEQUENCE-SPECIFIC OLIGONUCLEOTIDE METHOD FOR HLA TYPING

Erlich HA, Opelz G, Hansen J. HLA DNA typing and transplantation. *Immunity*. 2001;14(4):347–356.

Molecular Mutations in AML

Catherine Lai

FLT3

Mark J. Levis

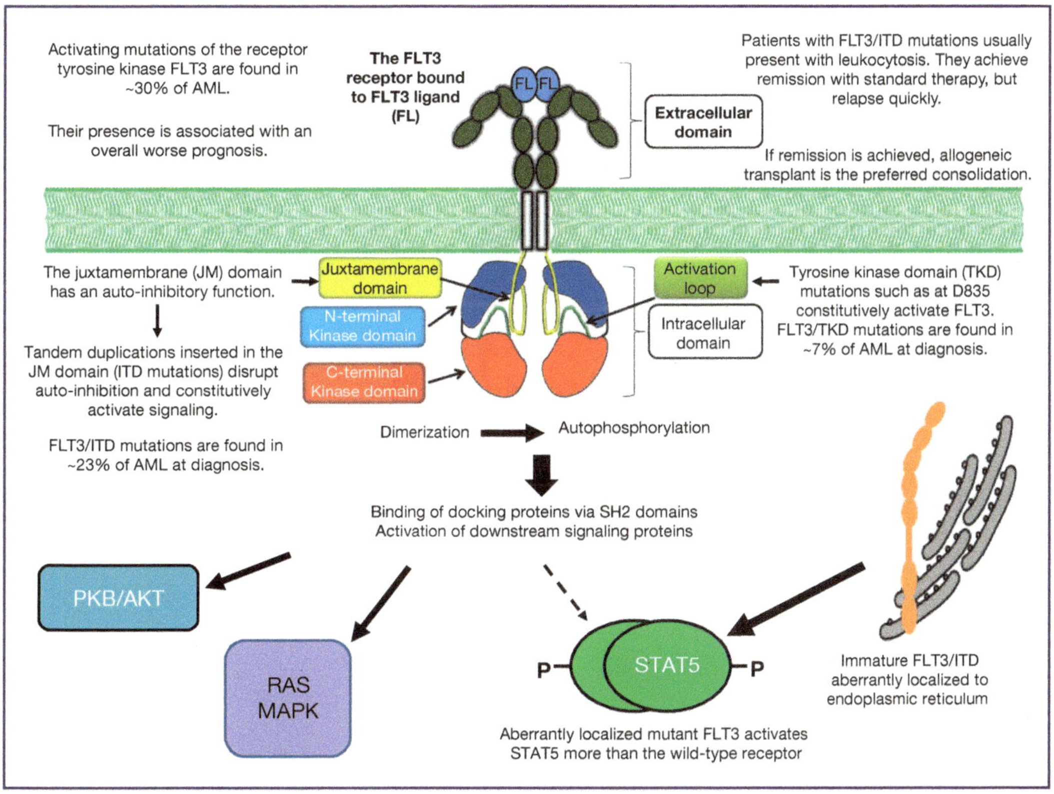

FIGURE 2-45: FLT3 mutation in AML.

AKT, protein kinase B; AML, acute myeloid leukemia; FLT3-ITD, fms-like tyrosine kinase 3 internal tandem duplication; MAPK, mitogen-activated protein kinase; PKB, protein kinase B.

Selected References

Choudhary C, Olsen JV, Brandts C, et al. Mislocalized activation of oncogenic RTKs switches downstream signaling outcomes. *Mol Cell*. 2009;36(2):326–339.

Griffith J, Black J, Faerman C, et al. The structural basis for autoinhibition of FLT3 by the juxtamembrane domain. *Mol Cell*. 2004;13(2):169–178.

Levis M. FLT3 mutations in acute myeloid leukemia: what is the best approach in 2013? *Hematology Am Soc Hematol Educ Program*. 2013;2013:220–226.

Levis M, Small D. FLT3: ITDoes matter in leukemia. *Leukemia*. 2003;17(9):1738–1752.

Mizuki M, Fenski R, Halfter H, et al. FLT3 mutations from patients with acute myeloid leukemia induce transformation of 32D cells mediated by the Ras and STAT5 pathways. *Blood*. 2000;96(12):3907–3914.

Verstraete K, Vandriessche G, Januar M, et al. Structural insights into the extracellular assembly of the hematopoietic FLT3 signaling complex. *Blood*. 2011;118(1):60–68.

C-KIT

Joshua F. Zeidner

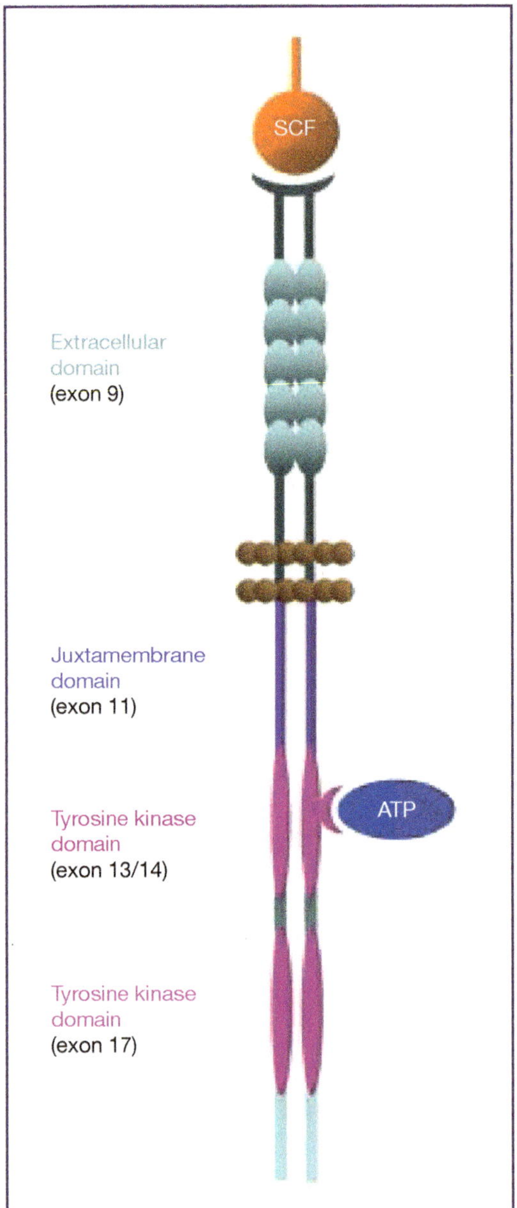

FIGURE 2-46: C-KIT function. A schematic of the structure of the C-KIT receptor. C-KIT, also known as CD117, is a tyrosine kinase receptor in the PDGFR (platelet-derived growth factor receptor) family. The ligand for the C-KIT receptor is stem cell factor (SCF), also known as KIT ligand. When the KIT receptor is activated, downstream signaling pathways are activated, including Ras/ERK, PI3K, Src kinases, and JAK/STAT pathways. KIT is highly expressed in hematopoietic stem cells and the activation of the KIT receptor is critical for the maintenance of normal hematopoiesis.

Source: From Pittoni P, Piconese S, Tripodo C, Colombo MP. Tumor-intrinsic and -extrinsic roles of c-KIT: mast cells as the primary off-target of tyrosine kinase inhibitors. *Oncogene.* 2011;30(7):757–769.

ATP, adenosine triphosphate; C-KIT, c-kit receptor tyrosine kinase.

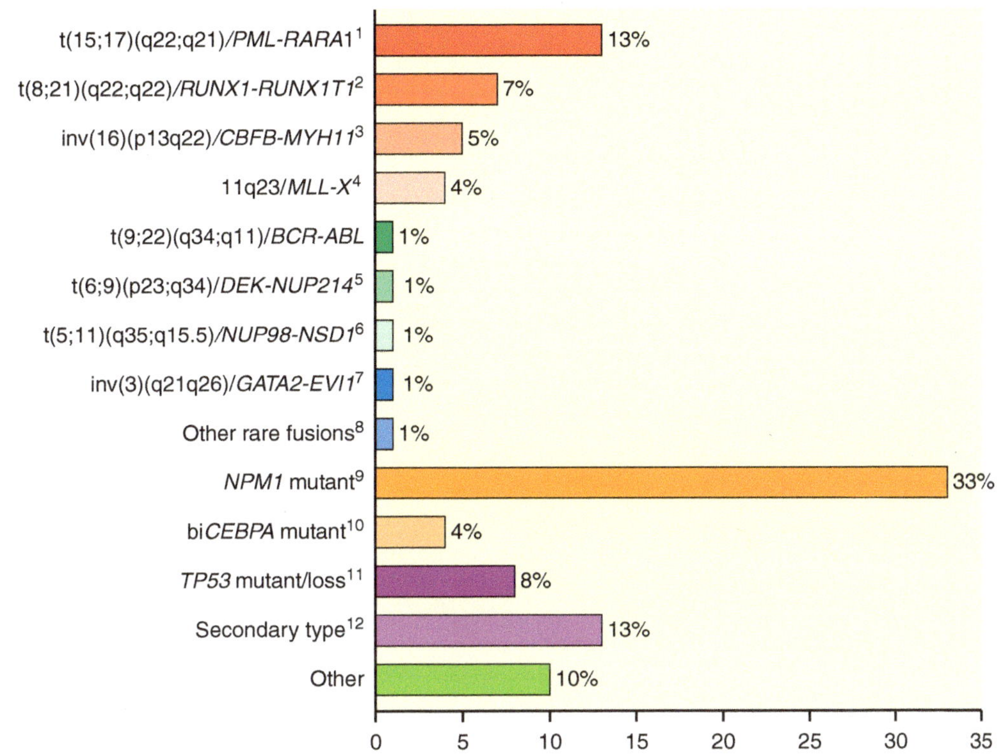

[1]**t(15;17)(q22;q21)/*PML-RARA***
FLT3-ITD ~35%
FLT3-TKD ~20%
WT1 ~10%

[2]**t(8;21)(q22;q22)/*RUNX1-RUNX1T1***
KIT ~25%
ASXL2 ~20%
ASXL1 ~10%

[3]**inv(16)(p13q22)/*CBFB-MYH11***
NRAS ~40%
KIT ~35%
FLT3-TKD ~20%
KRAS ~10%

[4]**1q23/*MLL-X***
KRAS ~20%
NRAS ~20%

[5]**t(6;9)(p23;q34)/*DEK-NUP214***
FLT3-ITD ~70%

[6]**t(5;11)(q35;q15.5)/*NUP98-NSD1***
FLT3-ITD ~85%

[7]**inv(3)(q21q26)/*GATA2-EVI1***
NRAS ~40%
SF3B1 ~20%
ASXL1 ~15%
BCOR1 ~15%
GATA2 ~15%
RUNX1 ~15%

[8]**Other rare fusions**
t(3;5)(q21~25;q31-35)/*NPM1-MLF1*
t(8;16)(p11;p13)/*MYST3-CREBBP*
t(16;21)(p11;q22)/*FUS-ERG*
t(10;11)(p13;q21)/*PICALM-MLLT10*
t(7;11)(p15;p15)/*NUP98-HOXA9*
t(3;21)(p26;q22)/*RUNX1-MECOM*

[9]***NPM1* mutant**
DNMT3A ~50%
FLT3-ITD ~40%
Cohesin ~20%
IDH1 ~15%
IDH2-R140 ~15%
PTPN11 ~15%

[10]**bi*CEBPA* mutant**
GATA2 ~30%

[11]***TP53* mutant/loss**
Complex and Monosomal Karyotype ~90%

[12]**Secondary type**
RUNX1 ~40%
MLL-PTD ~30%
ASXL1 ~30%
SRSF2 ~20%
U2AF1 ~15%
STAG2 ~15%
BCOR ~10%
SF3B1 ~10%
EZH2 ~5%
ZRSR2 ~5%

FIGURE 2-47: KIT mutations in AML. The most common cytogenetic abnormalities (in color) and their co-occurrence with molecular mutations (below the graph) in adults with AML are demonstrated. KIT mutations are seen in approximately 25% of patients with t(8;21)(q22;q22) and approximately 35% of patients with inv(16)(p13.1q22) or t(16;16)(p13.1;q22). KIT mutations are uncommonly seen in patients without CBF AML. Even though KIT mutations are thought to confer a poor prognosis in patients with CBF AML, the type of KIT mutation is important for prognostic implications (see Table 2-9). KIT mutations should be tested for all patients with CBF AML from their diagnostic bone marrow biopsy.

CBF AML, core binding factor acute myeloid leukemia.

Table 2-9 Prognostic significance of C-KIT mutations in CBF AML

TYPE OF CBF AML	EXON 17 MUTATION	EXON 8 MUTATION
t(8;21)	Most studies suggest inferior outcomes	Unclear significance
inv(16)/t(16;16)	Unclear significance	Inconclusive but evidence suggests a possible increased risk of relapse

CBF AML, core binding factor acute myeloid leukemia.

KIT mutations are associated with approximately one-third of patients diagnosed with CBF AML. The majority of the KIT mutations in CBF AML involve either an exon 17 or exon 8 mutation. The prognostic significance of KIT mutations in CBF AML appears to be related to the specific CBF AML abnormality (ie, t(8;21) vs. inv(16)/t(16;16)) and the type of KIT mutation (ie, exon 17 vs. exon 8). In patients with t(8;21) AML, retrospective studies have demonstrated inferior event-free survival (EFS) and overall survival (OS) in patients who harbor exon 17 KIT mutations. Other studies have shown that any KIT mutation (exon 8 or 17) in adults with t(8;21) AML leads to inferior outcomes. In contrast, 197 de novo AML patients were analyzed from the Japan Adult Leukemia Study Group AML201 Study and KIT mutations did not appear to be prognostic for either t(8;21) or inv(16)/t(16;16) patients. In patients with inv(16)/t(16;16) AML, however, the impact of KIT mutations is less clear, with some studies revealing higher relapse rates in patients with KIT exon 8 mutations, and others revealing only higher relapse rates in patients with exon 17 mutations. Analysis from Cancer and Leukemia Group B (CALGB) treatment protocols revealed that any KIT mutation in patients with inv(16)/t(16;16) led to inferior OS, while more recent analyses suggest that KIT mutations have no impact on relapse risk or OS in patients with inv(16)/t(16;16). An analysis of 176 patients with inv(16) from German-Austrian AML Study Group (AMLSG) trials revealed that KIT mutations were most commonly seen in exon 8, and led to inferior relapse-free survival, but did not lead to inferior OS. Given these data, the National Comprehensive Cancer Network (NCCN) classifies patients with t(8;21) or inv(16)/t(16;16) and any KIT mutation as having intermediate-risk disease. In contrast, other groups such as the European LeukemiaNet (ELN) do not incorporate KIT mutations into their respective prognostic risk groups.

Selected References

Grimwade D, Ivey A, Huntly BJP. Molecular landscape of acute myeloid leukemia in younger adults and its clinical relevance. *Blood.* 2016;127(1):29–41.

Kihara R, Nagata Y, Kiyoi T, et al. Comprehensive analysis of genetic alterations and their prognostic impacts in adult acute myeloid leukemia patients. *Leukemia.* 2014;28(8):1586–1595.

O'Donnell MR, Abboud CN, Altman J, et al. Acute myeloid leukemia. *J Natl Compr Canc Netw.* 2012;10(8):984–1021.

Paschka P, Du J, Schlenk RF, et al. Secondary genetic lesions in acute myeloid leukemia with inv(16) or t(16;16): a study of the German-Austrian AML Study Group (AMLSG). *Blood.* 2013;121(1):170–177.

Paschka P, Marcucci G, Ruppert AS, et al. Adverse prognostic significance of KIT mutations in adult acute myeloid leukemia with inv(16) and t(8;21): a Cancer and Leukemia Group B Study. *J Clin Oncol.* 2006;24(24):3904–3911.

Pittoni P, Piconese S, Tripodo C, Colombo MP. Tumor-intrinsic and -extrinsic roles of c-KIT: mast cells as the primary off-target of tyrosine kinase inhibitors. *Oncogene.* 2011;30(7):757–769.

Qin YZ, Zhu HH, Jiang Q, et al. Prevalence and prognostic significance of c-KIT mutations in core binding factor acute myeloid leukemia: a comprehensive large-scale study from a single Chinese center. *Leuk Res.* 2014;38(12):1435–1440.

RAS/RAF/MEK/ERK PATHWAYS

Frank McCormick

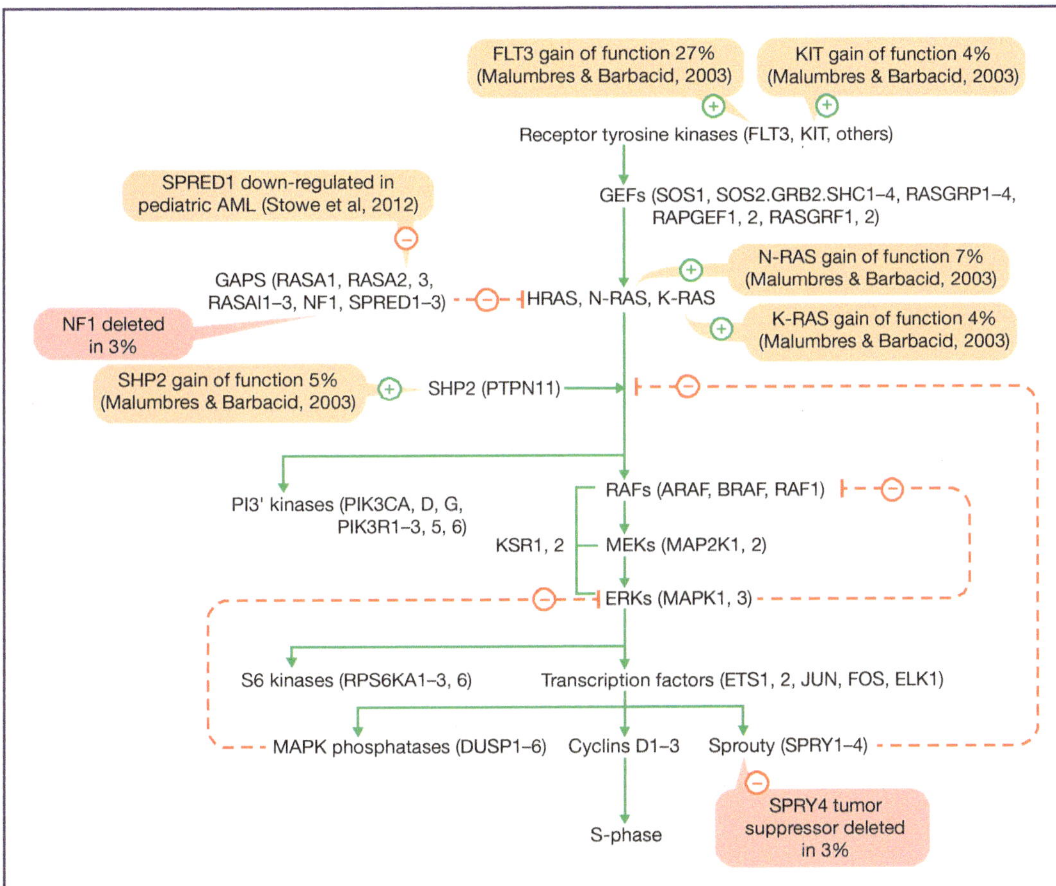

FIGURE 2-48: The Ras–Raf–MEK–ERK pathway. This pathway transduced signals from activated receptor tyrosine kinases in the cell surface to transcription factors in the nucleus, leading to transcription of D-cyclins, and entry in S-phase. Activation of this pathway by mutations results in reduced dependence on growth factors. Frequencies of mutation greater than 1% are shown. Mutation frequencies cited here are in whole or part based upon data generated by the TCGA Research Network (http://cancergenome.nih.gov). Mutations in N-Ras or K-Ras lock these proteins in their active GTP-bound states, making upstream signaling unnecessary. Loss of the tumor suppressor NF1 or its partner SPRED1 also allows Ras proteins to accumulate in their active, GTP-bound state. Gain-of-function mutations in the protein tyrosine phosphates SHP2 and loss of Sprouty proteins contribute to activation of the MAPK pathway downstream of Ras, but the precise mechanisms are not clear. Activation of the pathway is accompanied by induction of feedback pathways, shown here as dotted lines.

AML, acute myeloid leukemia; FLT3, FMS-like tyrosine kinase 3; MAPK, mitogen-activated protein kinase.

Selected References

Malumbres M, Barbacid M. RAS oncogenes: the first 30 years. *Nat Rev Cancer*. 2003;3(6):459–465.

Masoumi-Moghaddam S, Amini A, Morris DL. The developing story of sprouty and cancer. *Cancer Metastasis Rev*. 2014;33(2–3):695–720. doi:10.1007/s10555-014-9497-1

Pasmant E, Gilbert-Dussardier B, Petit A, et al. SPRED1, a RAS MAPK pathway inhibitor that causes Legius syndrome, is a tumour suppressor downregulated in paediatric acute myeloblastic leukaemia. *Oncogene*. 2015;34(5):631–638. doi:10.1038/onc.2013.587

Stowe IB, Mercado EL, Stowe TR, et al. A shared molecular mechanism underlies the human rasopathies Legius syndrome and neurofibromatosis-1. *Genes Dev*. 2012;26(13):1421–1426. doi:10.1101/gad.190876.112

Wang H, Lindsey S, Konieczna I, et al. Constitutively active SHP2 cooperates with HoxA10 overexpression to induce acute myeloid leukemia. *J Biol Chem*. 2009;284(4):2549–2567. doi:10.1074/jbc.M804704200

NPM1

Alexander E. Perl

Leukemogenesis/*NPM1* Normal Function

- Wild-type nucleophosmine 1 (NPM1-WT) normally shuttles between nucleolus and cytoplasm to play key roles in ribosome biogenesis, DNA damage/repair, centrosome duplication during mitosis, and cell cycle progression.
- AML-associated mutations in *NPM1* are small exon 12 insertions that cause frameshifts affecting the protein's C-terminus. *NPM1* mutations all generate a novel nuclear export signal and disrupt a nucleolar localization motif. This leads to exclusively cytoplasmic *NPM1* expression, which is detectable by IHC.
- Functional consequences of mutant *NPM1* may relate to restricted cellular localization and either novel effects of *NPM1mut* or haploinsufficiency of WT-*NPM1* (eg, loss of interaction with ARF or other targets, inability to stabilize WT-p53 to promote cell cycle arrest after DNA damage, inability to transport ribosomal products to cytoplasm).
- The strong association of *NPM1* with mutations affecting signal transduction and DNA methylation suggests additional functions necessary for full leukemic transformation.
- Although *NPM1* is a strongly AML-associated mutation, it frequently occurs in the background of prior *DNMT3A* and/or *IDH* mutation and thus may not strictly be an initiating lesion.

Cooperating Mutations

In patients younger than 60 years of age, striking association exists between *NPM1* and 1) mutations activating signal transduction (82% of cases) including *FLT3-ITD* (41%), *FLT3-TKD* (24%), *N-RAS* (20%), *PTPN11* (17%), and 2) DNA methylation mutations (78%) including *DNMT3A* mutations (50%), *WT1/IDH1/IDH2-R140/TET2* mutations (49%), and 3) cohesin complex (18%).

NPM1 rarely cooperates with splicing mutations (except *SRSF2* (4%)), myeloid transcription factors, (except single *CEBPA* mutation, 4%), chromatin modifier mutations (eg, *ASXL1, EZH2, KDM6A*), and tumor suppressors (eg, *TP53, PHF6, ETV6*)

NPM1 is mutually exclusive with CBF and other transcription factor translocations, *CEBPA* double mutations, *KMT2A* (MLL) translocations.

Clinical Features of Mutant *NPM1*

- Strongly enriched in normal karyotype, de novo AML.
- It is rare in MDS-related AML, though multilineage dysplasia frequently is present at diagnosis of *NPM1* mutant AML and does NOT indicate antecedent MDS.
- Can occur in any non-M3 FAB subtype, but is enriched among myelomonocytic (FAB M4/M5).
- Mutation is enriched among patients with extramedullary disease (eg, leukemia cutis).
- May show "cup-like" morphology, which is associated with *NPM1* and *FLT3-ITD* co-mutation: blasts generally lack CD34 or HLA-DR expression.

Prognostic Effects of *NPM1* Mutation

High response rate of *NPM1* to induction chemotherapy and favorable survival if:

1. No *FLT3-ITD* mutation (favorable risk in European LeukemiaNet, uncertain benefit to CR1 alloHSCT)

2. Minimal residual disease-negative state achieved after induction regardless of *FLT3-ITD* status
3. *DNMT3A*-WT

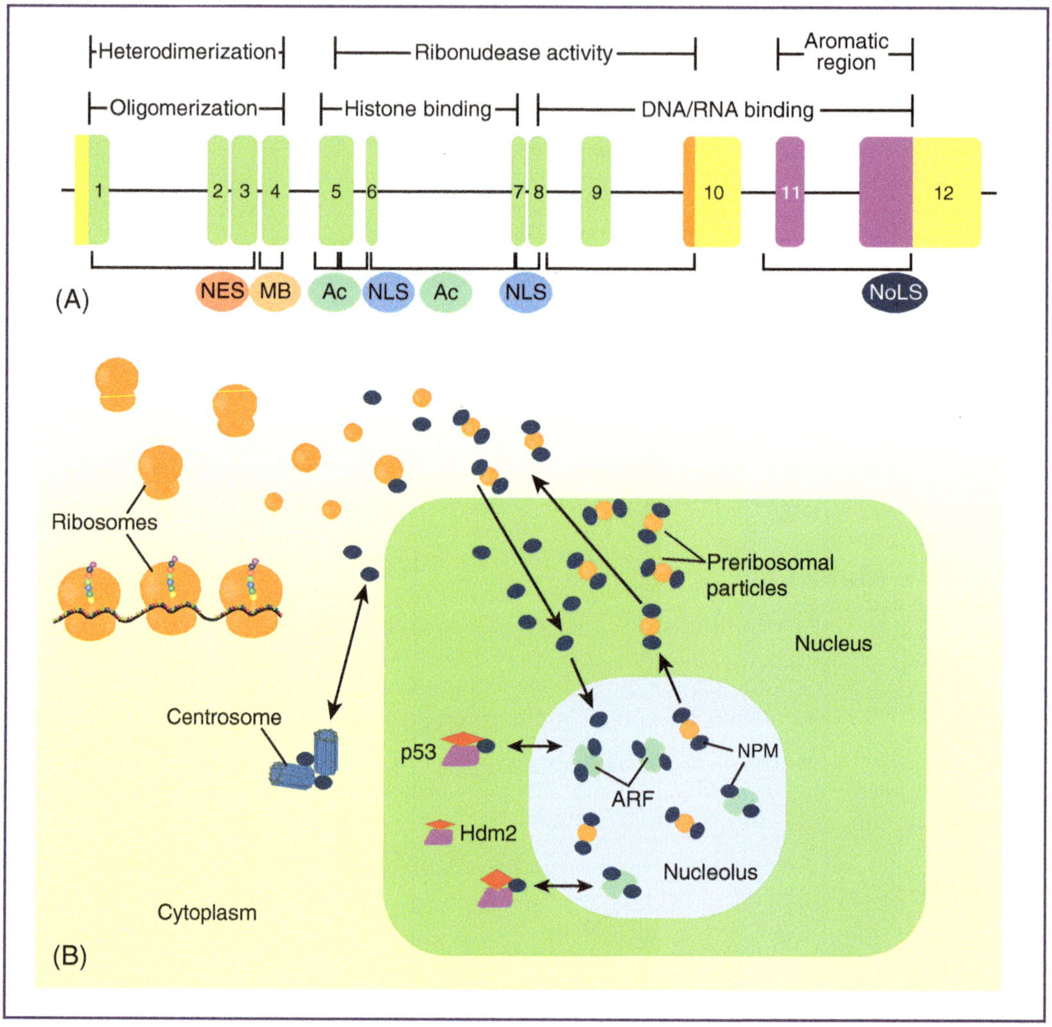

FIGURE 2-49: The *NPM1* gene and protein. (A) Twelve exons of the *NPM1* gene, of which *NPM1* is translated from exons 1 to 9 and 11 to 12. The N-terminus region of *NPM1* protein includes functional nuclear export signal (NES) motifs and a metal-binding (MB) site, which contain a nonpolar domain responsible for oligomerization and heterodimerization. The center of *NPM1* protein confers ribonuclease activity and contains two acidic sites (Ac) for binding to histones, and a two-part nuclear localization signal (NLS). The C-terminus region of *NPM1* protein also confers ribonuclease activity and contains basic regions involved in DNA/RNA binding. The C-terminus region is followed by an aromatic stretch containing two tryptophan residues, which are required for nucleolar localization of the protein (NoLS). (B) NPM is a phosphoprotein located in the nucleolus, which by traveling between the nucleus and cytoplasm and transporting preribosomal particles contribute significantly to the ribosome biogenesis. Other functions of *NPM1* protein include binding to the unduplicated centrosome and regulating its duplication during cell division, interacting with p53 and its regulatory molecules (ARF, Hdm2/Mdm2) manipulating the ARF-Hdm2/Mdm2-p53 suppressive pathway.

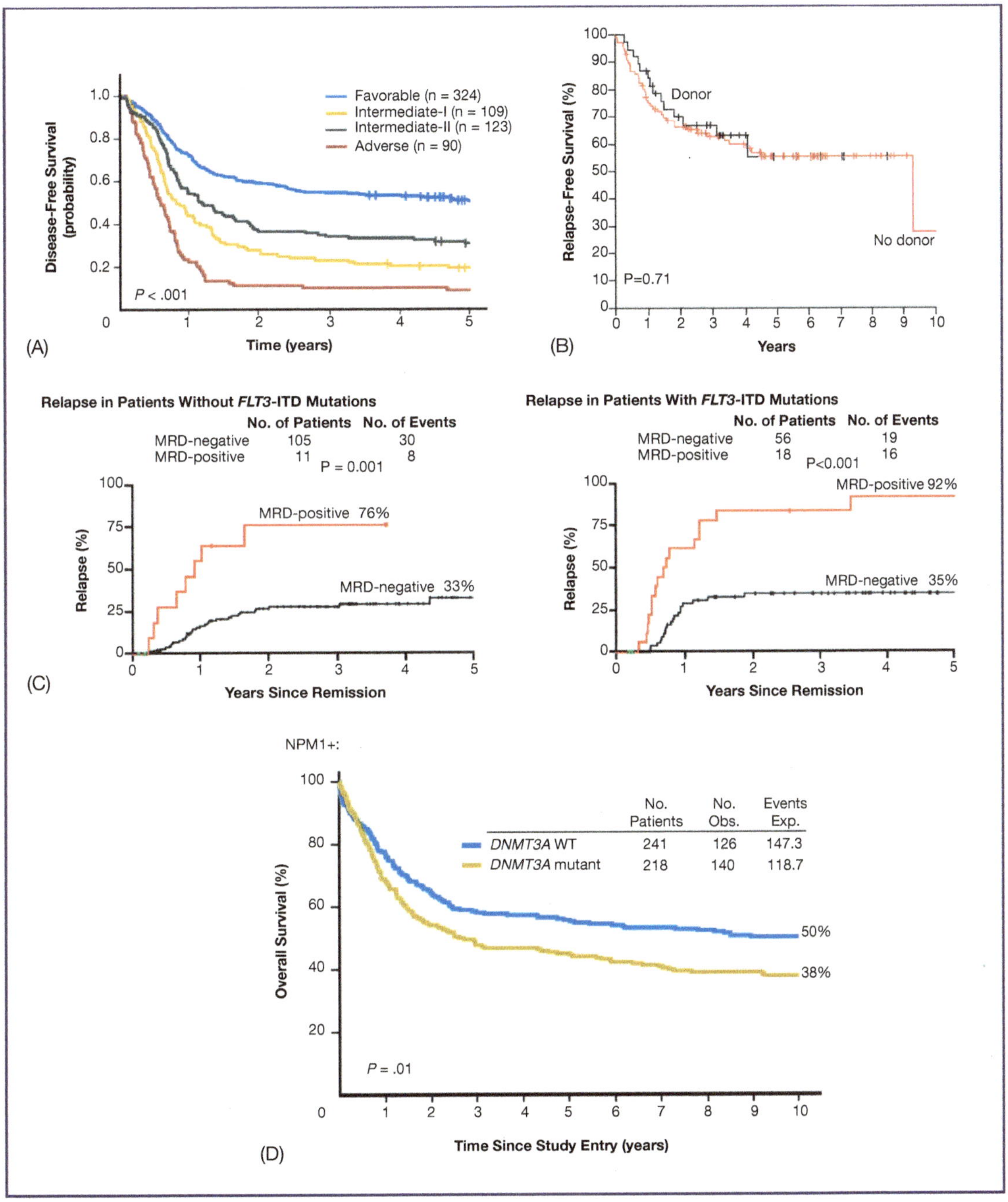

FIGURE 2-50: Survival of patients with AML with *NPM1* mutation in different clinical trials.

Source: (A) From Mrózek K, Marcucci G, Nicolet D, et al. Prognostic significance of the European LeukemiaNet standardized system for reporting cytogenetic and molecular alterations in adults with acute myeloid leukemia. *J Clin Oncol.* 2012;30(36):4515–4523; (B) From Schlenk RF, Dohner K, Krauter J, et al. Mutations and treatment outcome in cytogenetically normal acute myeloid leukemia. *N Engl J Med.* 2008;358(18):1909–1918. (C) From Ivey A, Hills RK, Simpson MA, et al. Assessment of minimal residual disease in standard-risk AML. *N Engl J Med.* 2016;374(5):422–433; (D) From Gale RE, Lamb K, Allen C, et al. Simpson's Paradox and the impact of different *DNMT3A* mutations on outcome in younger adults with acute myeloid leukemia. *J Clin Oncol.* 2015;33(18):2072–2083.

AML, acute myeloid leukemia; ITD, internal tandem duplication; MRD, minimal residual disease; WT, wild-type.

Selected References

Falini B, Nicoletta J, Martelli MF, Mecucci C. Acute myeloid leukemia carrying cytoplasmic/mutated nucleophosmin (NPMc+ AML): biologic and clinical features. *Blood*. 2007;109(3):874–885.

Gale RE, Lamb K, Allen C, et al. Simpson's Paradox and the impact of different *DNMT3A* mutations on outcome in younger adults with acute myeloid leukemia. *J Clin Oncol*. 2015;33(18):2072–2083.

Grimwade D, Ivey A, Huntly BJP. Molecular landscape of acute myeloid leukemia in younger adults and its clinical relevance. *Blood*. 2016;127(1):29–41.

Ivey A, Hills RK, Simpson MA, et al. Assessment of minimal residual disease in standard-risk AML. *N Engl J Med*. 2016;374(5):422–433.

Mrózek K, Marcucci G, Nicolet D, et al. Prognostic significance of the European LeukemiaNet standardized system for reporting cytogenetic and molecular alterations in adults with acute myeloid leukemia. *J Clin Oncol*. 2012;30(36):4515–4523.

Schlenk RF, Dohner K, Krauter J, et al. Mutations and treatment outcome in cytogenetically normal acute myeloid leukemia. *N Engl J Med*. 2008;358(18):1909–1918.

Vidholia A, Menon P. "Cup-like" blasts in acute myeloid leukemia with FLT3 and NPM1 mutations. *Blood*. 2015;15(5):889.

PI3K/AKT/mTOR PATHWAY

Mohamed Rahmani and Steven Grant

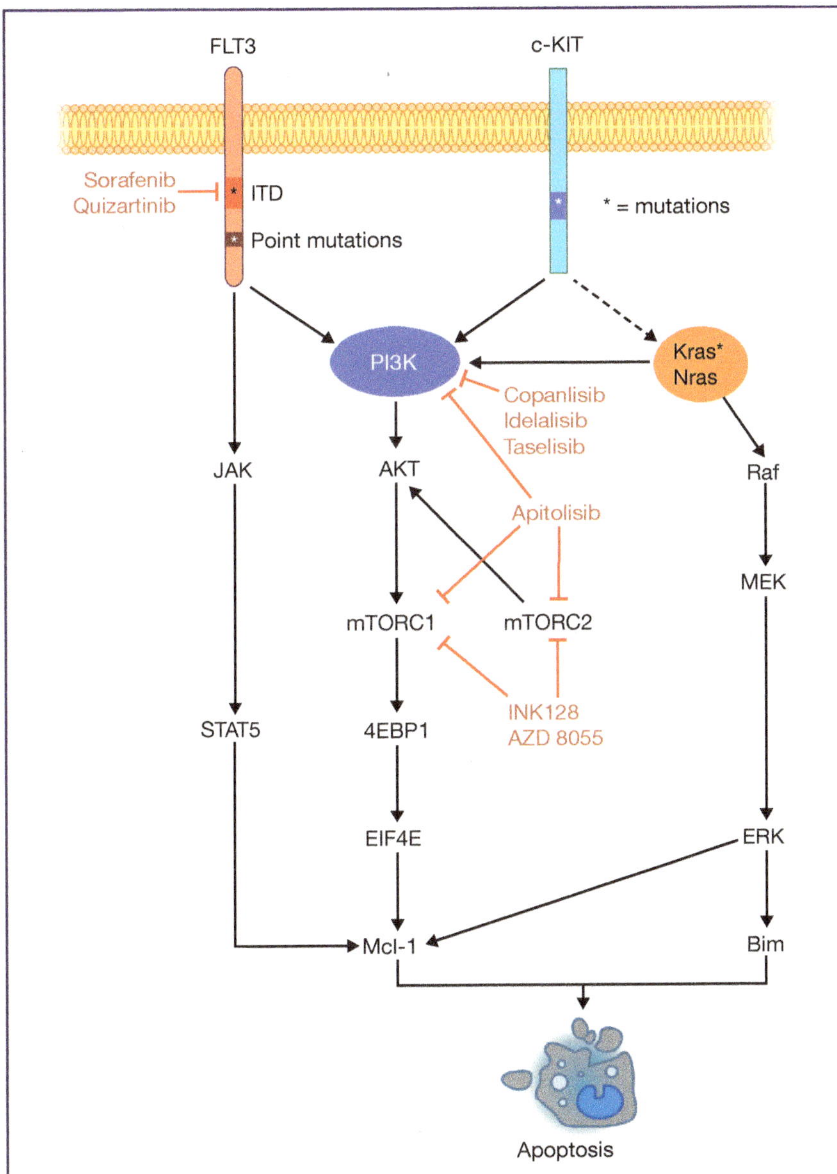

FIGURE 2-51: Activation of the PI3K/AKT pathway in AML. Constitutive activation of the phosphoinositide 3-kinase (PI3K)/Akt signaling pathway is detectable in approximately 50% of AML, cells and potently contributes to proliferation, survival, and chemotherapy resistance of these cells. This activation occurs through a variety of mechanisms including mutations of the FLT3 receptor or Ras or c-Kit. Perturbations of the PI3K/AKT/mTOR pathway by small molecule inhibitors leads to Mcl-1 down-regulation and Bim accumulation, which culminates in apoptotic cell death. Notably, the PI3K/Akt pathway is important for multiple physiological cellular functions including insulin signaling, and its interruption may cause severe systemic adverse events.

AKT, protein kinase B; AML, acute myeloid leukemia; c-KIT, c-kit receptor tyrosine kinase; FLT3, FMS-like tyrosine kinase 3; ITD, internal tandem duplication; mTOR, mechanistic target of rapamycin.

RUNX1

Chandrima Sinha, Lea C. Cunningham, and Paul P. Liu

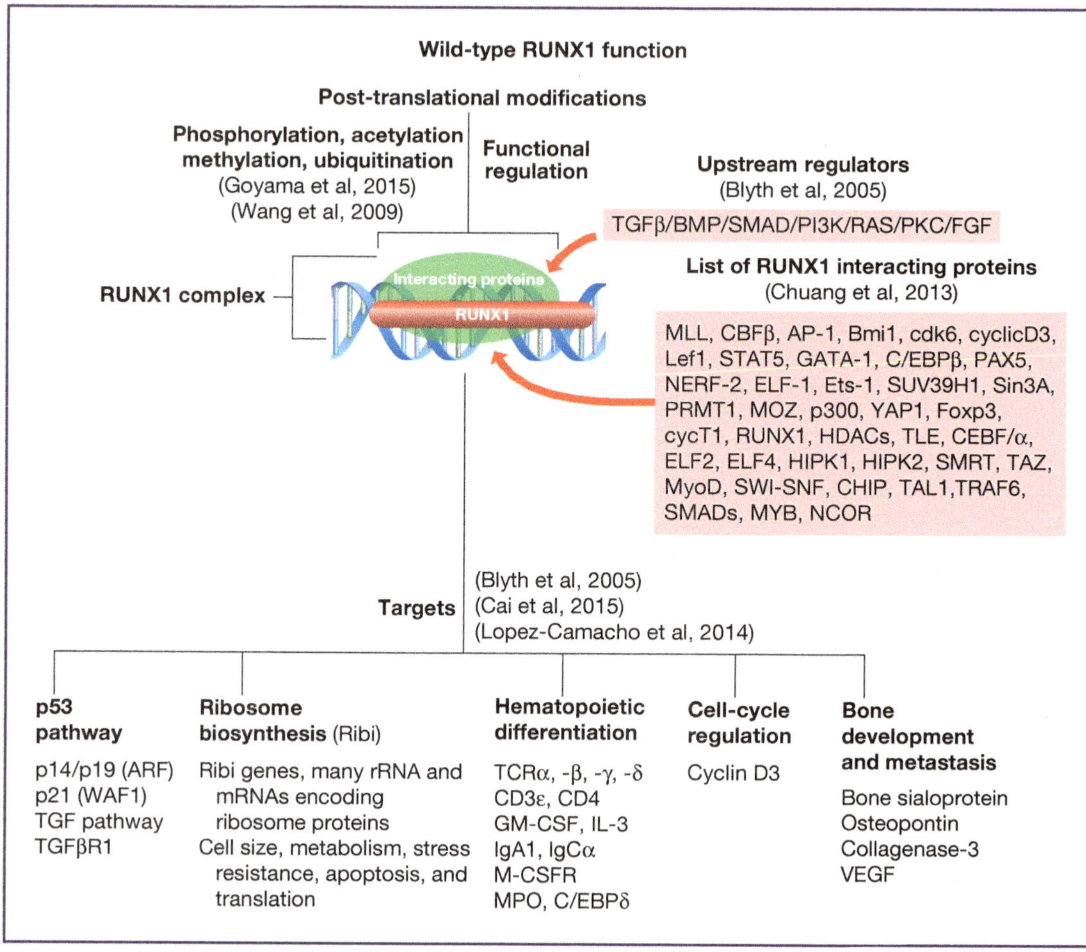

FIGURE 2-52: Upstream regulators and downstream targets of wild-type RUNX1, as well as important binding partners and post-translational modifications.

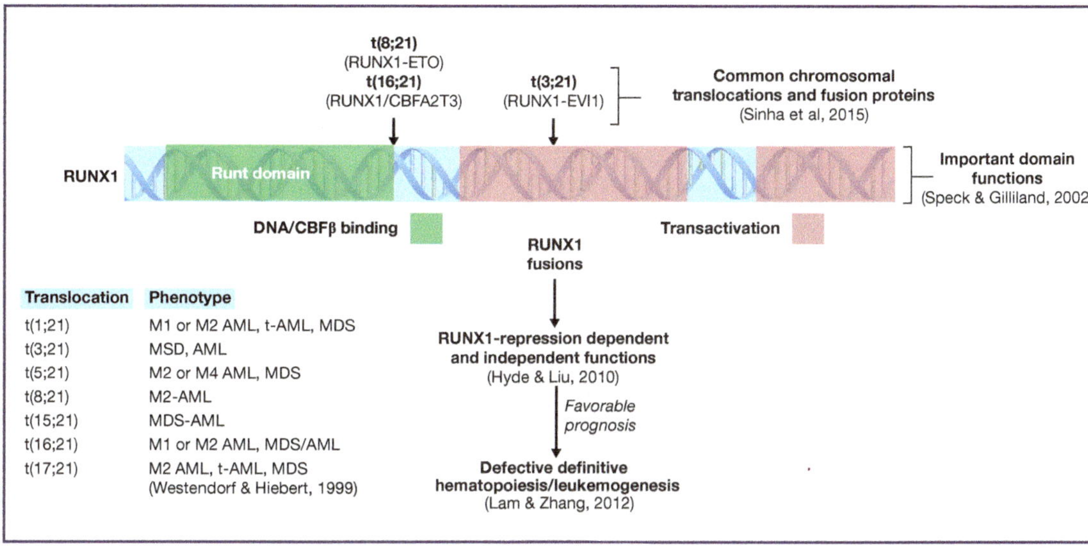

FIGURE 2-53: **RUNX1 translocations and their respective fusion products associated with AML subtypes.**
AML, acute myeloid leukemia; MDS, myelodysplastic syndrome.

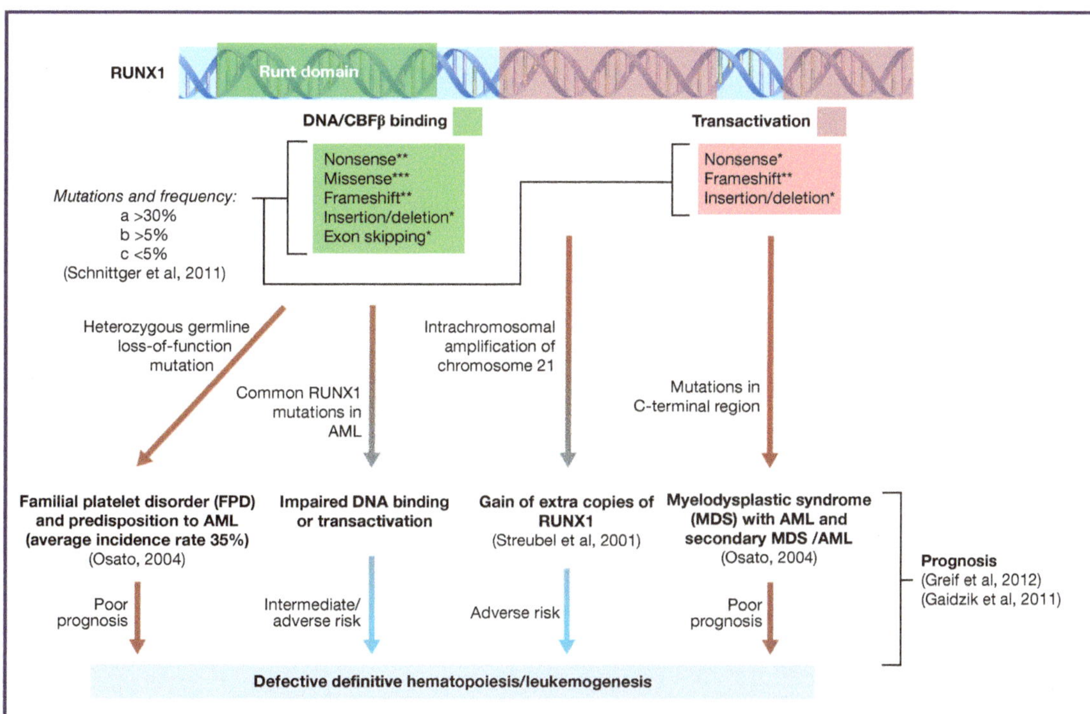

FIGURE 2-54: **Type and frequency of different RUNX1 mutations in AML.**
AML, acute myeloid leukemia.

Selected References

Blyth K, Cameron ER, Neil JC. The RUNX genes: gain or loss of function in cancer. *Nat Rev Cancer*. 2005;5:376–387.

Cai X, Gao L, Teng L, et al. Runx1 Deficiency Decreases Ribosome Biogenesis and Confers Stress Resistance to Hematopoietic Stem and Progenitor Cells. *Cell Stem Cell*. 2015;17:165–177.

Chuang LS, Ito K, Ito Y. RUNX family: regulation and diversification of roles through interacting proteins. *Int J Cancer*. 2013;132:1260–1271.

Gaidzik VI, Bullinger L, Schlenk RF, et al. RUNX1 mutations in acute myeloid leukemia: results from a comprehensive genetic and clinical analysis from the AML study group. *J Clin Oncol*. 2011;29:1364–1372.

Goyama S, Huang G, Kurokawa M, Mulloy JC. Posttranslational modifications of RUNX1 as potential anticancer targets. *Oncogene*. 2015;34:3483–3492.

Greif PA, Konstandin NP, Metzeler KH, et al. RUNX1 mutations in cytogenetically normal acute myeloid leukemia are associated with a poor prognosis and up-regulation of lymphoid genes. *Haematologica*. 2012;97:1909–1915.

Hyde RK, Liu PP. RUNX1 repression-independent mechanisms of leukemogenesis by fusion genes CBFB-MYH11 and AML1-ETO (RUNX1-RUNX1T1). *J Cell Biochem*. 2010;110:1039–1045.

Lam K, Zhang D. RUNX1 and RUNX1-ETO: roles in hematopoiesis and leukemogenesis. *Front Biosci*. 2012;17:1120–1139.

Lopez-Camacho C, van Wijnen AJ, Lian JB, et al. CBFbeta and the leukemogenic fusion protein CBFbeta-SMMHC associate with mitotic chromosomes to epigenetically regulate ribosomal genes. *J Cell Biochem*. 2014;115:2155–2164.

Osato M. Point mutations in the *RUNX1/AML1* gene: another actor in RUNX leukemia. *Oncogene*. 2004;23:4284–4296.

Schnittger S, Dicker F, Kern W, et al. RUNX1 mutations are frequent in de novo AML with noncomplex karyotype and confer an unfavorable prognosis. *Blood*. 2011;117:2348–2357.

Sinha C, Cunningham LC, Liu PP. Core binding factor acute myeloid leukemia: new prognostic categories and therapeutic opportunities. *Semin Hematol*. 2015;52:215–222.

Speck NA, Gilliland DG. Core-binding factors in haematopoiesis and leukaemia. *Nat Rev Cancer*. 2002;2:502–513.

Streubel B, Valent P, Lechner K, Fonatsch C. Amplification of the AML1(CBFA2) gene on ring chromosomes in a patient with acute myeloid leukemia and a constitutional ring chromosome 21. *Cancer Genet Cytogenet*. 2001;124:42–46.

Wang L, Huang G, Zhao X, et al. Post-translational modifications of Runx1 regulate its activity in the cell. *Blood Cells Mol Dis*. 2009;43:30–34.

Westendorf JJ, Hiebert SW. Mammalian runt-domain proteins and their roles in hematopoiesis, osteogenesis, and leukemia. *J Cell Biochem*. 1999;(Suppl. 32–33):51–58.

MLL

Peter D. Aplan

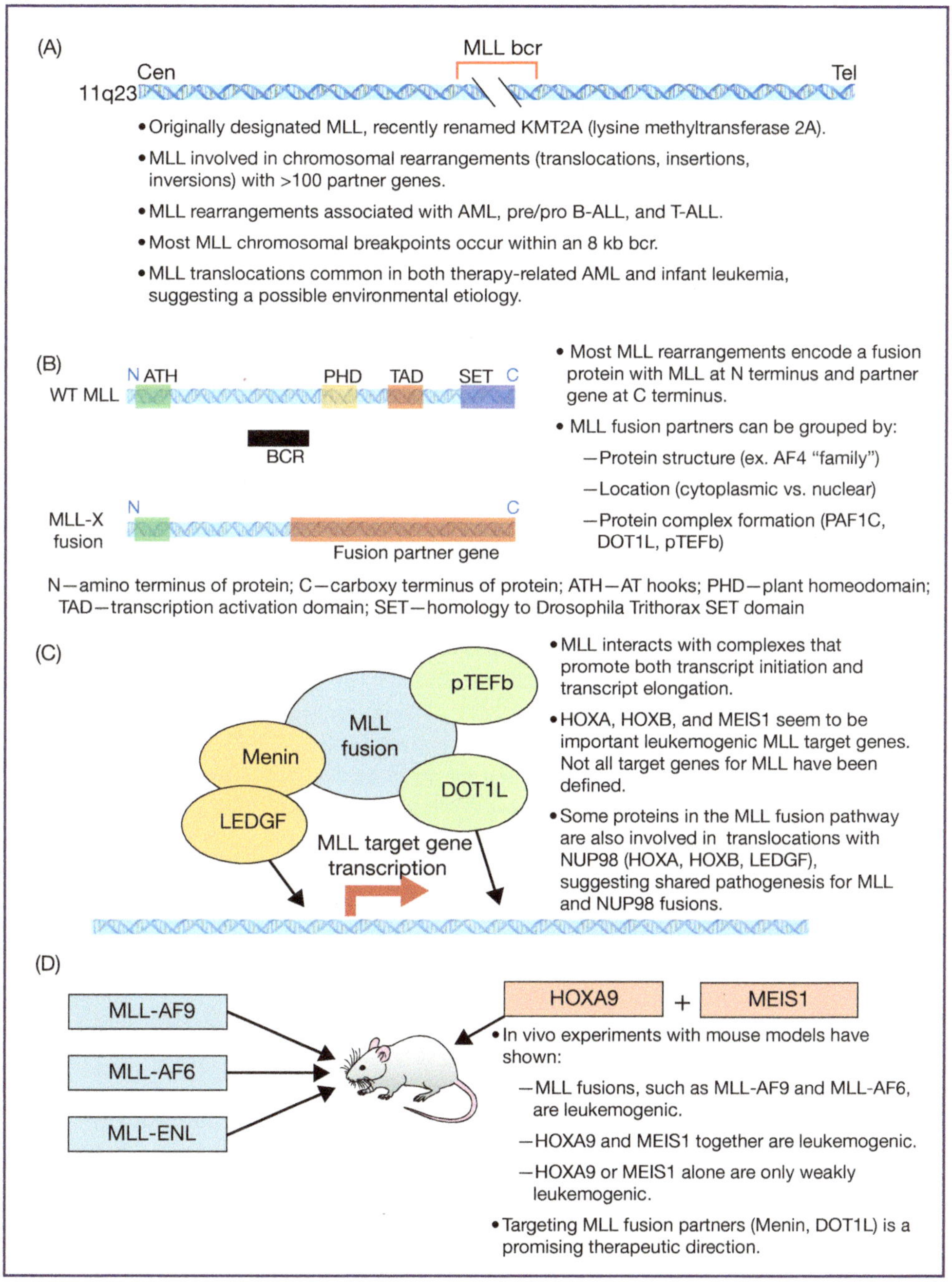

FIGURE 2.55: **MLL fusions in acute leukemia. (A) Location of the MLL bcr on chromosome 11q23. (B) MLL translocations lead to generation of a fusion mRNA, which encodes a fusion protein. (C) MLL fusion proteins function in multi-subunit complexes, and primarily serve to activate transcription of target genes. (D) Mouse models can recapitulate leukemia mediated via MLL fusion proteins in vivo, providing a pre-clinical platform with which to test promising candidate drugs.**

AML, acute myeloid leukemia; B-ALL, B acute lymphoblastic leukemia; bcr, breakpoint cluster region; MLL, mixed lineage leukemia; T-ALL, T acute lymphoblastic leukemia.

CEBPα

Alan D. Friedman

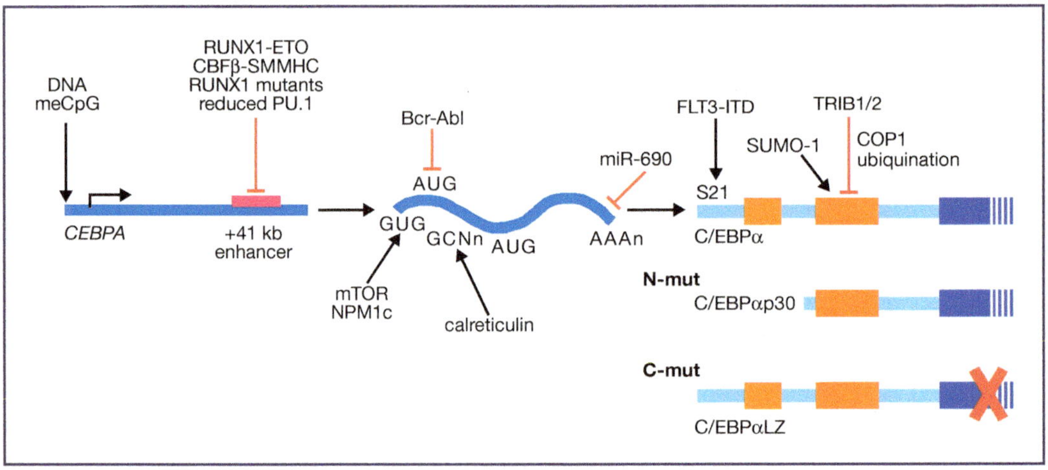

FIGURE 2-56: **CCAAT/enhancer binding protein α (C/EBPα) dimerizes via its C-terminal leucine zipper domain to bind DNA via the adjacent basic region and activate transcription via N-terminal trans-activation domains. C/EBPα is a key mediator of normal myelopoiesis. In the majority of AML cases, multiple pathways likely mediate reduced C/EBPα expression or activity, as diagrammed. Reduced *CEBPA* promoter methylation, dominant inhibition of *RUNX1* by the RUNX1-ETO or CBFβ-SMMHC oncoproteins, *RUNX1* open reading frame point mutations, or reduced PU.1 expression or activity can each reduce *CEBPA* transcription. Expression of Bcr-Abl or NPM1c or increased calreticulin activity can reduce *CEBPA* mRNA translation. FLT3-ITD-mediated phosphorylation of C/EBPα serine 21 or SUMO-1-mediated C/EBPα modification can reduce C/EBPα activity, and Trib1- or Trib2-mediated C/EBPα ubiquitination by COP1 can induce C/EBPα degradation. In addition, approximately 10% of AML cases harbor N- or C-terminal point mutations in one or both *CEBPA* alleles, leading to expression of a truncated C/EBPαp30 protein and C/EBPαLZ variants with leucine zipper in-frame insertions or deletions. Increased mTOR activity can also increase C/EBPαp30 expression, by favoring translational initiation from an internal ATG. Of note, patients whose AML blasts contain both N-terminal and C-terminal *CEBPA* mutants have improved prognosis. Reduction of C/EBPα expression or activity may be a key feature of the majority of AML cases, contributing to transformation by impeding normal myelopoiesis while reducing C/EBPα-mediated cell cycle inhibition.**

AML, acute myeloid leukemia; FLT3-ITD, FMS-like tyrosine kinase 3-internal tandem duplication; mTOR, mechanistic target of rapamycin.

Selected Reference

Friedman AD. C/EBPα in normal and malignant myelopoiesis. *Int J Hematol.* 2015;101:330–342.

GATA2

Dennis D. Hickstein

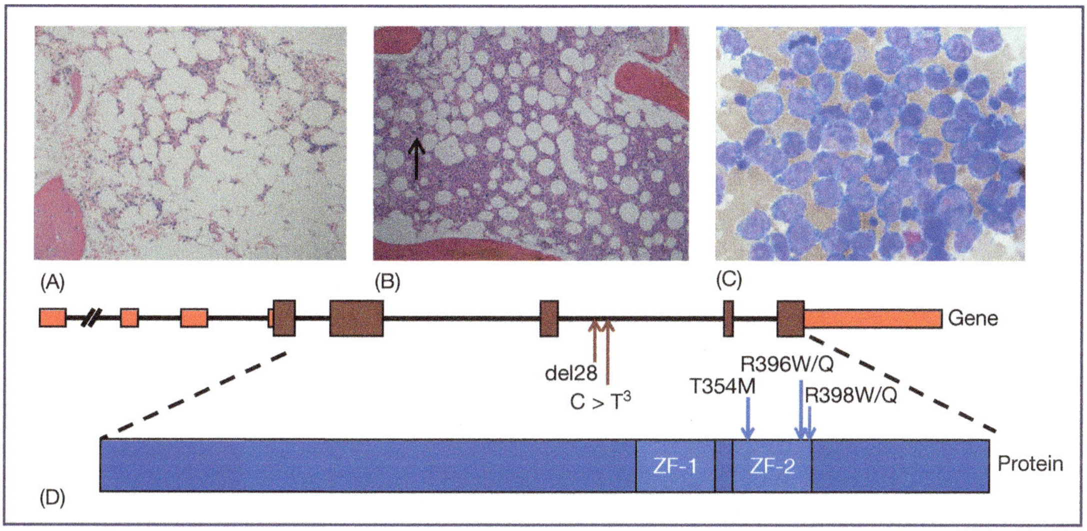

FIGURE 2-57: **Protean bone marrow findings in patients with GATA2 deficiency. (A) Hypocellular marrow with myelodysplastic changes. (B) Bone marrow with micromegakaryocytes (arrow). (C) Acute monocytic leukemia with 85% M5a monoblasts. (D) *GATA2* gene structure and protein domains. The *GATA2* gene (red boxes) has three alternative transcripts (NM_001145661.1, NM_032638.4, NM_00114566.2), with isoforms 1 and 2 having the largest coding region (dark red boxes) (NP_001139133.1). The GATA2 protein (blue boxes) is a transcription factor with two DNA-binding zinc finger domains. Mutations causing hematological disease are heterozygous, somatic, or germline, and appear to function by haploinsufficiency. Missense mutations cluster in the zinc finger domains (ZF-1, ZF-2), while frameshift mutations are more evenly distributed across the protein. Regulatory mutations in intron 5 have also been described. Over 50 mutations are known, with the most common mutations being R396W/Q and R398W/Q.**

Selected References

Dickinson RE, Milne P, Jardine L, et al. The evolution of cellular deficiency in GATA2 mutation. *Blood*. 2014;123(6):863–874.

Spinner MA, Sanchez LA, Hsu AP, et al. GATA2 deficiency: a protean disorder of hematopoiesis, lymphatics, and immunity. *Blood*. 2014;123(6):809–821.

DNMT3A

Timothy J. Ley and David H. Spencer

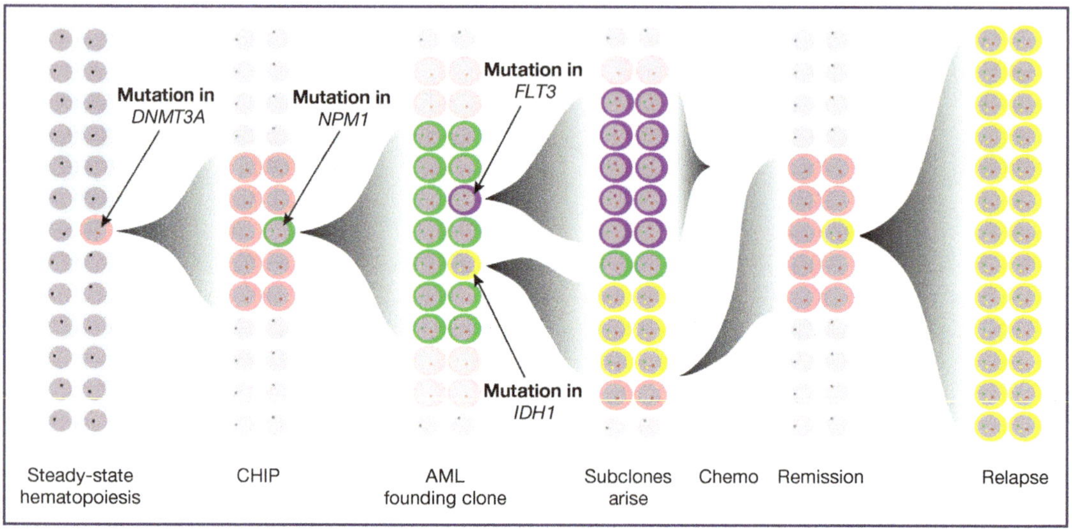

FIGURE 2-58: AML initiated by DNMT3A mutations.

AML, acute myeloid leukemia; CHIP, clonal hematopoiesis of indeterminate potential; DNMT3A, DNA methyltransferase 3A; FLT3, FMS-like tyrosine kinase 3; NPM1, nucleophosmine 1.

Steady-state Hematopoiesis

Early, multipotent hematopoietic stem/progenitor cells (HSPCs) divide infrequently, and accumulate about 1 somatic mutation per cell division (shown as random black dots in the nucleus). Because these cells divide asymmetrically (ie, one daughter cell self-renews to maintain the HSPC pool, and the other contributes to hematopoiesis), these mutations persist in HSPCs and are also present in the mature hematopoietic cells derived from them. Every hematopoietic cell therefore contains a unique set of background mutations.

CHIP (Clonal Hematopoiesis of Indeterminate Potential)

In some individuals, clonal mutations are detected in the blood, which likely reflects the presence of an HSPC with a growth or survival advantage, leading to its clonal expansion. Hematopoiesis is well preserved, however, and blood counts and cellular morphology are normal. Remarkably, the mutations associated with CHIP are the same ones that initiate acute myeloid leukemia (AML); the most common gene to be mutated in people with CHIP is *DNMT3A* (red cells with a red nuclear dot). CHIP appears confer a risk for progression to myelodysplastic syndrome (MDS) or AML, but that risk is thought to relatively small (<5%). The incidence of CHIP increases with age, probably since random mutations in HSPCs increase as a function of age. Current data suggests that more that >10% of people over the age of 80 may have this condition. Since most of the relevant mutations that cause CHIP are in *DNMT3A*, there are probably tens of thousands of people in the US who have clonally skewed hematopoiesis because of *DNMT3A* mutations.

AML Founding Clones

An HSPC with a *DNMT3A* mutation can acquire a second mutation that cooperates with it to contribute to the formation of an AML founding clone. The most common cooperating mutation appears to be one of the canonical frameshifts in the *NPM1* gene (green cells, with red [*DNMT3A*] and green [*NPM1*] mutation dots). At this juncture, it is not at all clear how these two mutant genes cooperate to cause AML. To complicate matters further, there are three distinct classes of *DNMT3A* mutations that all appear to cooperate with progression mutations, but they probably act via different mechanisms.

1. Heterozygous mutations at AA position R882. These are by far the most common, accounting for about 60% of all *DNMT3A* mutations in AML cases. However, they are much less common in people with CHIP. The mutant protein has an 80% reduction in its *de novo* DNA methylase activity. More importantly, it forms a tight heterodimer with the WT protein, preventing it from forming catalytically active homotetramers. It is therefore a strong dominant negative mutation, and it is associated with a focal, canonical hypomethylation phenotype in mutant AML cells.
2. Mutations that cause *DNMT3A* haploinsufficiency. Deletions, nonsense mutations, and frameshifts can abolish the function of mutant alleles, creating a haploinsufficient state. These mutations are certainly associated with AML pathogenesis, but do not have a clear methylation phenotype. They may act by other mechanisms to initiate AML.
3. Other missense mutations. A few of these have been found to be recurrent in AML patients, but they are far less common than the R882 mutations. Their functions are virtually unknown at this time.

Subclones

Subclones can arise when cooperating mutations occur in cells of the AML founding clone. Subclones have been detected at presentation in virtually all AML samples that have been sequenced to date. The most commonly mutated progression gene in *DNMT3A*-initiated AML is *FLT3*, with internal tandem duplication (ITD) mutations being the most common (purple cells with red, green, and purple mutation dots). Several other genes can cooperate, including other well known AML drivers, including mutations in *IDH1/2* (shown, with yellow cells and red, green, and yellow mutation dots), *RAS*, *WT1*, *RUNX1*, and many others. Subclones expand faster than the founding clone, and are often the most prevalent cells in the presenting sample from the bone marrow. Multiple subclones are present in most AML samples, and they have different functional properties, including differential clearance with chemotherapy. Small subclones often contribute to AML relapse.

Clonal Responses to Chemotherapy

About 80% of patients who receive standard induction therapy (3 days of an anthracycline like daunorubicin, and 7 days of cytarabine) go into an initial clinical remission, with clearance of blasts. However, many of these patients still have measurable disease when their leukemia-associated mutations are assessed after they recover from the induction therapy, about 30 days after treatment was started. Despite clearance of blasts, some patients can have founding clones that persist after induction therapy. HSPCs containing initiating mutations in *DNMT3A* are rarely cleared by induction therapy, while cells with *NPM1*, *FLT3*, and *RAS* mutations are usually cleared. In many patients, the most actively dividing subclones (especially those with activating signaling mutations, like *FLT3-ITD*, or *RAS* mutations) are rapidly cleared by induction therapy, perhaps because they are more susceptible to DNA damaging agents that are cell-cycle dependent.

Remission

After induction therapy, many patients with favorable or intermediate risk AML are given high dose cytarabine as consolidation therapy, and usually have a morphologic and cytogenetic remission. However, many of these patients have persistent *DNMT3A* mutations in a small fraction of their marrow cells, suggesting that they have simply returned to a "pre-leukemic" state. This is probably not the same as CHIP, however, since a large fraction of these patients relapse, almost always with the same founding clone variants.

Relapse

A large fraction of patients with *DNMT3A* initiating mutations go on to relapse. Nearly all have persistence of the original *DNMT3A* mutation at relapse, and many have the same founding clone variants. Many relapse with one of the original subclones, which often evolve with new mutations, probably caused at least in part by the chemotherapy itself.

Selected References

STEADY-STATE HEMATOPOIESIS

Welch JS, Ley TJ, Link DC, et al. The origin and evolution of mutations in acute myeloid leukemia. *Cell*. 2012;150(2):264–278.

CHIP

Genovese G, Kähler AK, Handsaker RE, et al. Clonal hematopoiesis and blood-cancer risk inferred from blood DNA sequence. *N Engl J Med*. 2014;371(26):2477–2487.

Jaiswal S, Fontanillas P, Flannick J, et al. Age-related clonal hematopoiesis associated with adverse outcomes. *N Engl J Med*. 2014;371(26):2488–2498.

Steensma DP, Bejar R, Jaiswal S, et al. Clonal hematopoiesis of indeterminate potential and its distinction from myelodysplastic syndromes. *Blood*. 2015;126(1):9–16.

Xie M, Lu C, Wang, J, et al. Age-related cancer mutations associated with clonal hematopoietic expansion. *Nat Med*. 2014;20(12):1472–1478.

AML FOUNDING CLONES

The Cancer Genome Atlas Research Network. Genomic and epigenomic landscapes of adult de novo acute myeloid leukemia. *N Engl J Med*. 2013;368(22):2059–2074.

Ley TJ, Ding L, Walter MJ, et al. DNMT3A mutations in acute myeloid leukemia. *New Engl J Med*. 2010;363(25):2424–2433.

Russler-Germain DA, Spencer DH, Young MA, et al. The R882H DNMT3A mutation associated with AML dominantly inhibits wild-type DNMT3A by blocking its ability to form active tetramers. *Cancer Cell*, 2014;25(4):442–452.

SUBCLONES

Klco JM, Spencer DH, Miller CA, et al. Functional heterogeneity of genetically defined subclones in acute myeloid leukemia. *Cancer Cell*. 2014;25(2):379–392.

CLONAL RESPONSE TO CHEMOTHERAPY

Klco JM, Miller CA, Griffith M, et al. Association between mutation clearance after induction therapy and outcomes in acute myeloid leukemia. *JAMA*. 2015;314(8);811–822.

REMISSION

Corces-Zimmerman MR, Hong WJ, Weissman IL, et al. Preleukemic mutations in human acute myeloid leukemia affect epigenetic regulators and persist in remission. *Proc Natl Acad Sci USA*. 2014;111(7):2548–2553.

Shlush LI, Zandi S, Mitchell A, et al. Identification of pre-leukaemic haematopoietic stem cells in acute leukaemia. *Nature*. 2014;506(7488):328–333.

RELAPSE

Ding L, Ley TJ, Larson DE, et al. Clonal evolution in relapsed acute myeloid leukemia revealed by whole genome sequencing. *Nature*. 2012;481(7382):506–510.

TET AND IDH

Amir T. Fathi

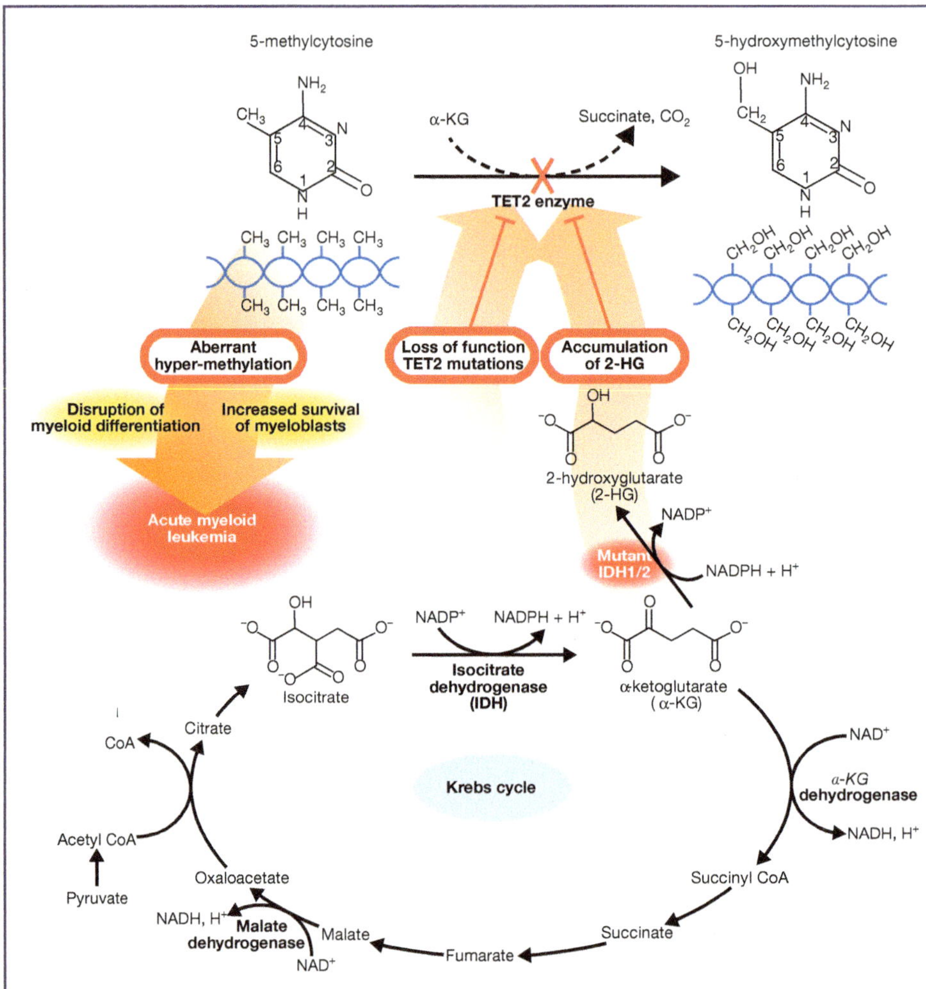

FIGURE 2-59: **Isocitrate dehydrogenase 1 and 2 (IDH1 and IDH2), encoded by their respective genes *IDH1* and *IDH2*, are essential enzyme components of the Krebs cycle and oxidative phosphorylation. They catalyze the decarboxylation of isocitrate to α-keto-glutarate (α-KG) in the cytosol (IDH1) and in mitochondria (IDH2), leading to the production of reduced nicotinamide adenine dinucleotide phosphate (NADPH). Heterozygous and missense mutations of *IDH1* and *IDH2* have been discovered in AML and other myeloid malignancies, and act as "gain of function" alterations. The resultant altered forms of the IDH1/2 enzymes cannot catalyze the conversion of isocitrate to α-KG, and instead, catalyze NADPH-dependent reduction of α-KG to 2-hydroxyglutarate (2-HG). As a result, 2-HG, a metabolite normally present at very low levels in cells, accumulates to high levels. The depletion of α-KG and accumulation of 2-HG in *IDH1/2*-mutant AML both suppress the function of the TET2 enzyme, a key regulator of epigenetic signature. TET2 modifies the conversion of 5-methylcytosine to 5-hydroxymethylcytosine on DNA, and in this fashion triggers the process of demethylation, gene activation, and resultant cell differentiation. TET2 function can also be suppressed in a different manner through loss-of-function mutations involving the *TET2* gene. The resulting abnormal hypermethylation leads to block in myeloid differentiation, enhanced survival of aberrant progenitors, and the phenotype of AML. Therefore, *TET2* and *IDH1/2* mutations appear to form a distinct mutational class in AML, and likely have overlapping roles in leukemogenesis through effects on DNA methylation and epigenetic regulation.**

AML, acute myeloid leukemia; CoA, coenzyme A; TET2, ten-eleven translocation 2.

Epidemiology

- *IDH1* mutations typically impact amino acid R132, and are found in 5% to 10% of cases of AML, whereas *IDH2* mutations, involving either amino acids R172 or R140, are more prevalent and seen in approximately 15% of this population.
- *IDH1/2* mutations are enriched in cytogenetically normal AML, occurring in up to a third of these patients. These mutations also frequently co-occur with *NPM1* gene alterations.
- *TET2* mutations have been reported in 7% to 19% of cases of de novo AML, and typically are mutually exclusive of *IDH1/2* mutations, likely explained by their overlapping impact on suppressing TET2 enzyme function and triggering leukemogenesis.

Prognosis

- The prognostic significance of IDH1/2 remains unclear, with some retrospective studies suggesting a deleterious impact on survival outcomes while others report improved short- and long-term outcomes.
- Similarly, the prognostic impact of *TET2* mutations in AML is controversial, with a few studies suggesting no influence on outcomes, while others suggest a deleterious impact.

Therapeutic Considerations

- IDH1/2 inhibitors are currently under investigation in clinical trials, with early suggestion of tolerability and efficacy.
- Levels of the oncometabolite, 2-hydroxyglutarate (2-HG) can be measured in blood, marrow, and urine of *IDH1/2* mutant AML patients, decrease with therapeutic response, and may have utility as biomarkers in the future.
- *TET2* and *IDH1/2* mutations may render myeloid malignancies more sensitive to hypomethylating therapy, although data are conflicting and prospective studies are necessary for further elucidation.

Selected References

EPIDEMIOLOGY

Abbas S, Lugthart S, Kavelaars FG, et al. Acquired mutations in the genes encoding IDH1 and IDH2 both are recurrent aberrations in acute myeloid leukemia (AML): prevalence and prognostic value. *Blood*. 2010;166(12);2122–2126.

Delhommeau F, Dupont S, Della Valle V, et al. Mutation in TET2 in myeloid cancers. *N Engl J Med*. 2009;360:2289–2301.

Figueroa ME, Abdel-Wahab O, Lu C, et al. Leukemic IDH1 and IDH2 mutations result in a hypermethylation phenotype, disrupt TET2 function, and impair hematopoietic differentiation. *Cancer Cell*. 2010;18:553–567.

Gaidzik VI, Paschka P, Spath D, et al. TET2 mutations in acute myeloid leukemia (AML): results from a comprehensive genetic and clinical analysis of the AML study group. *J Clin Oncol*. 2012;30:1350–1357.

Marcucci G, Maharry K, Wu YZ, et al. IDH1 and IDH2 gene mutations identify novel molecular subsets within de novo cytogenetically normal acute myeloid leukemia: a cancer and leukemia group B study. *J Clin Oncol*. 2010;28:2348–2355.

Ward PS, Patel J, Wise DR, et al. The common feature of leukemia-associated IDH1 and IDH2 mutations is a neomorphic enzyme activity converting alpha-ketoglutarate to 2-hydroxyglutarate. *Cancer Cell*. 2010;17:225–234.

PROGNOSIS

Boissel N, Nibourel O, Renneville A, et al. Prognostic impact of isocitrate dehydrogenase enzyme isoforms 1 and 2 mutations in acute myeloid leukemia: a study by the acute leukemia French Association Group. *J Clin Oncol*. 2010;28:3717–3723.

Green CL, Evans CM, Hills RK, et al. The prognostic significance of IDH1 mutations in younger adult patients with acute myeloid leukemia is dependent on FLT3/ITD status. *Blood*. 2010;116:2779–2782.

Patel JP, Gonen M, Figueroa ME, et al. Prognostic relevance of integrated genetic profiling in acute myeloid leukemia. *N Engl J Med*. 2012;366:1079–1089.

THERAPEUTIC CONSIDERATIONS

Bejar R, Lord A, Stevenson K, et al. TET2 mutations predict response to hypomethylating agents in myelodysplastic syndrome patients. *Blood*. 2014;125:2705–2712.

Emadi A, Faramand R, Carter-Copper B, et al. Presence of isocitrate dehydrogenase mutations may predict clinical response to hypomethylating agents in patients with acute myeloid leukemia. *Am J Hematol*. 2015;90:E77–E79.

Fathi AT, Sadrzadeh H, Borger DR, et al. Prospective serial evaluation of 2-hydroxyglutarate, during treatment of newly diagnosed acute myeloid leukemia, to assess disease activity and therapeutic response. *Blood*. 2012;120:4649–4652.

Itzykson R, Kosmider O, Cluzeau T, et al. Impact of TET2 mutations on response rate to azacitidine in myelodysplastic syndromes and low blast count acute myeloid leukemias. *Leukemia*. 2011;25:1147–1152.

WT1

Sheenu Sheela, John Barrett, and Catherine Lai

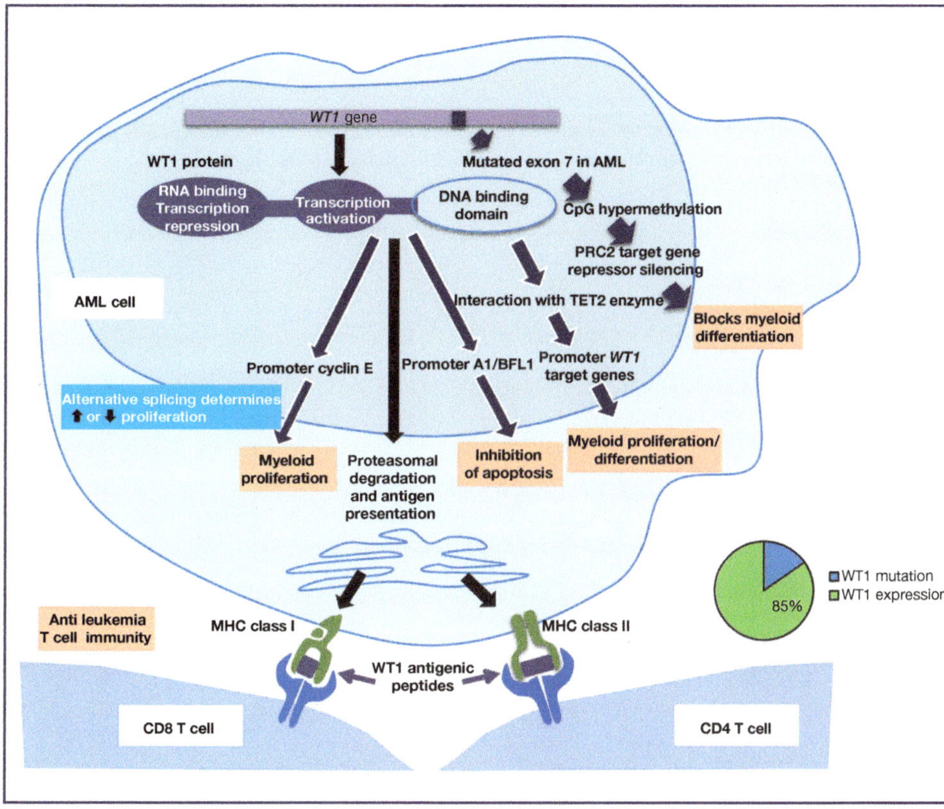

FIGURE 2-60: Wilms' tumor gene (WT1), a zinc finger transcription factor located on chromosome 11p13 activates or represses target genes which participate in cell cycle, proliferation, differentiation, apoptosis and plays a role in post-transcriptional mRNA processing. There are 36 isoforms of WT1 protein. At least one isoform of WT1 is expressed in 80% to 85% of AML patients. Four major isoforms are produced by alternative splicing at exon 5 (17AA insert) and exon 9 (3AA-KTS insert) which are as follows: EX5+/KTS+, EX5-/KTS-, EX5+/KTS-/EX5-/KTS+. The EX5-/KTS- isoform of WT1 up-regulates the antiapoptotic gene *A1/BFL1* (Bcl2 family), thus resisting apoptosis. The EX5+/KTS+ isoform of WT1 inhibits the suppression of cyclin E promoter and allows proliferation. The functions of other isoforms have not been elucidated. WT1 mutations occur in 5% to 7% of AML patients. The *WT1* methylated genes are overrepresented in multiple gene sets of polycomb repressor complex 2 (PRC2). *WT1* exon 7 mutation results in silencing of PRC2 target gene repression and inhibition of myeloid differentiation. The *TET2* and *WT1* genes are mutated in a mutually exclusive manner. The catalytic domain (CD) part of TET2 enzyme binds to the zinc finger or DNA-binding domain of WT1 protein, activating the promoter regions of *WT1* target genes. Any loss-of-function mutations affecting the *WT1* could prevent this sequence of events leading to cell proliferation/lack of differentiation.

WT1 is commonly overexpressed in the majority of AML across a wide diversity of favorable and unfavorable genetic profiles, and it has been extensively studied as a target for the diagnosis and treatment of AML. WT1 expression has been used to stratify the risk of relapse after induction chemotherapy and to monitor minimal residual disease (MRD) before and after allogeneic stem cell transplantation. WT1 also serves as a leukemia associated antigen (LAA) inducing anti-leukemic immunity through WT1-specific cytotoxic T-cells. Clinical trials of WT1 vaccination and adoptive infusion of WT1-specific T-cells have demonstrated clinical responses along with the biological evidence of anti-leukemic immunity. Further studies are necessary to explore the potential of harnessing WT1 as a widely expressed leukemia antigen for immunotherapeutic targeting.

AML, acute myeloid leukemia.

Selected References

The Cancer Genome Atlas Research Network. Genomic and epigenomic landscapes of adult de novo acute myeloid leukemia. *N Engl J Med*. 2013;368(22):2059–2074.

Chapuis AG, Ragnarsson GB, Nguyen HN, et al. Transferred WT1-reactive CD8+ T cells can mediate antileukemic activity and persist in post-transplant patients. *Sci Transl Med*. 2013;5:174ra127.

Cilloni D, Renneville A, Hermitte F, et al. Real-time quantitative polymerase chain reaction detection of minimal residual disease by standardized WT1 assay to enhance risk stratification in acute myeloid leukemia: a European leukemia net study. *J Clin Oncol*. 2009;27:5195–5201.

Di Stasi A, Jimenez AM, Minagawa K, et al. Review of the results of WT1 peptide vaccination strategies for myelodysplastic syndromes and acute myeloid leukemia from nine different studies. *Front Immunol*. 2015;6:36.

Goswami M, Hensel N, Smith BD, et al. Expression of putative targets of immunotherapy in acute myeloid leukemia and healthy tissues. *Leukemia*. 2014;28:1167–1170.

Israyelyan A, Goldstein L, Tsai W, et al. Real-time assessment of relapse risk based on the WT1 marker in acute leukemia and myelodysplastic syndrome patients after hematopoietic cell transplantation. *Bone Marrow Transplant*. 2015;50:26–33.

Kramarzova K, Stuchly J, Willasch A, et al. Real-time PCR quantification of major Wilms' tumor gene 1 (WT1) isoforms in acute myeloid leukemia, their characteristic expression patterns and possible functional consequences. *Leukemia*. 2012;26:2086–2095.

Krauth, MT. Alpermann T, Bacher U, et al. WT1 mutations are secondary events in AML, show varying frequencies and impact on prognosis between genetic subgroups. *Leukemia*. 2015;29:660–667.

Luna I, Such E, Cervera J, et al. WT1 isoform expression pattern in acute myeloid leukemia. *Leuk Res*. 2013;37:1744–1749.

Oka, Y, Udaka K, Tsuboi A, et al. Cancer immunotherapy targeting Wilms' tumor gene WT1 product. *J Immunol*. 2000;164:1873–1880.

Rezvani K, Yong AS, Mielke S, et al. Leukemia-associated antigen-specific T-cell responses following combined PR1 and WT1 peptide vaccination in patients with myeloid malignancies. *Blood*. 2008;111: 236–242.

Simpson LA, Burwell EA, Thompson KA, et al. The antiapoptotic gene *A1/BFL1* is a *WT1* target gene that mediates granulocytic differentiation and resistance to chemotherapy. *Blood*. 2006;107:4695–4702.

Sinha S, Thomas D, Yu L, et al. Mutant WT1 is associated with DNA hyper methylation of PRC2 targets in AML and responds to EZH2 inhibition. *Blood*. 2015;125:316–326.

Van Driessche A, Gao L, Stauss HJ, et al. Antigen-specific cellular immunotherapy of leukemia. *Leukemia*. 2005;19:1863–1871.

Van Tendeloo VF, Van de Velde A, Van Driessche A, et al. Induction of complete and molecular remissions in acute myeloid leukemia by Wilms' tumor 1 antigen-targeted dendritic cell vaccination. *Proc Natl Acad Sci USA*. 2010;107:13824–13829.

Wang Y, Xiao M, Chen X, et al. WT1 recruits TET2 to regulate its target gene expression and suppress leukemia cell proliferation. *Mol Cell*. 2015;57:662–673.

ASXL1 AND EZH2

Lizamarie Bachier-Rodriguez and Joseph M. Scandura

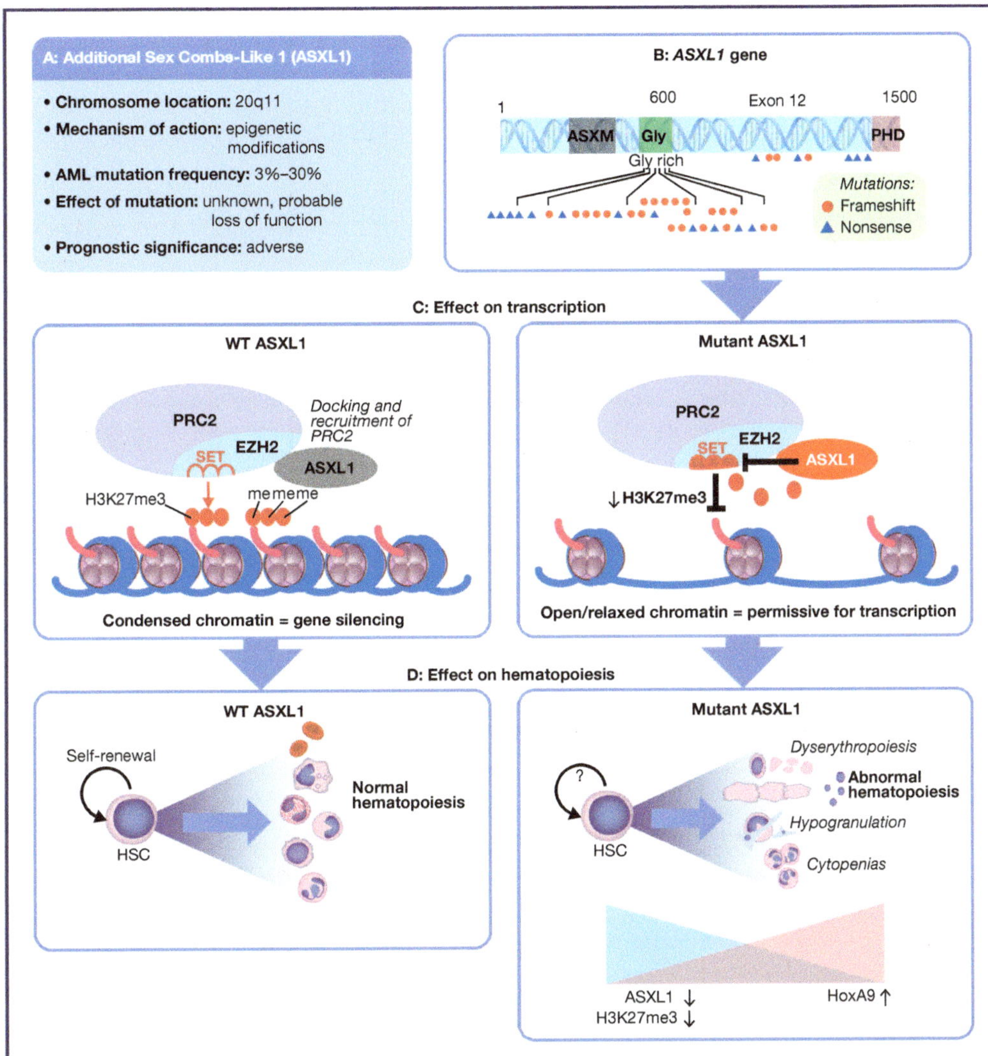

FIGURE 2-61: ASXL1. (A) Additional sex combs-like 1 (ASXL1) is located on chromosome 20q11 and is involved in chromatin modification. ASXL1 mutations are found in 3% to 30% of AML patients and are associated with worse clinical outcomes, including decreased overall survival and progression-free survival. (B) Acquired somatic ASXL1 mutations are frameshift, nonsense, and missense mutations, usually located in exon 12. These result in a truncated protein with loss of the plant-homeodomain (PHD) zinc finger. The PHD domain is found in nuclear proteins involved in chromatin regulation. (C) ASXL1 physically interacts with the Polycomb repressive complex 2 (PRC2). Loss of ASXL1 leads to global reduction of histone H3 lysine 27 (H3K27) tri-methylation (H3K27me3) and de-repression of PRC2 target genes like the posterior *HOXA* cluster genes. (D) Deletion of ASXL1 in mice causes perinatal lethality, defects in lymphopoiesis, and craniofacial and skeletal abnormalities. Conditional deletion of ASXL1 in the hematopoietic compartment results in a phenotype similar to MDS with leukopenia, myeloid dysplasia, impaired erythroid differentiation, and extramedullary hematopoiesis. ASXL1 loss increases the number of immunophenotypic hematopoietic stem and progenitor cells (HSPCs) but reduces the self-renewal capacity of hematopoietic stem cells (HSCs).

AML, acute myeloid leukemia; HSC, hematopoietic stem cells; MDS, myelodysplastic syndrome; WT, wild-type.

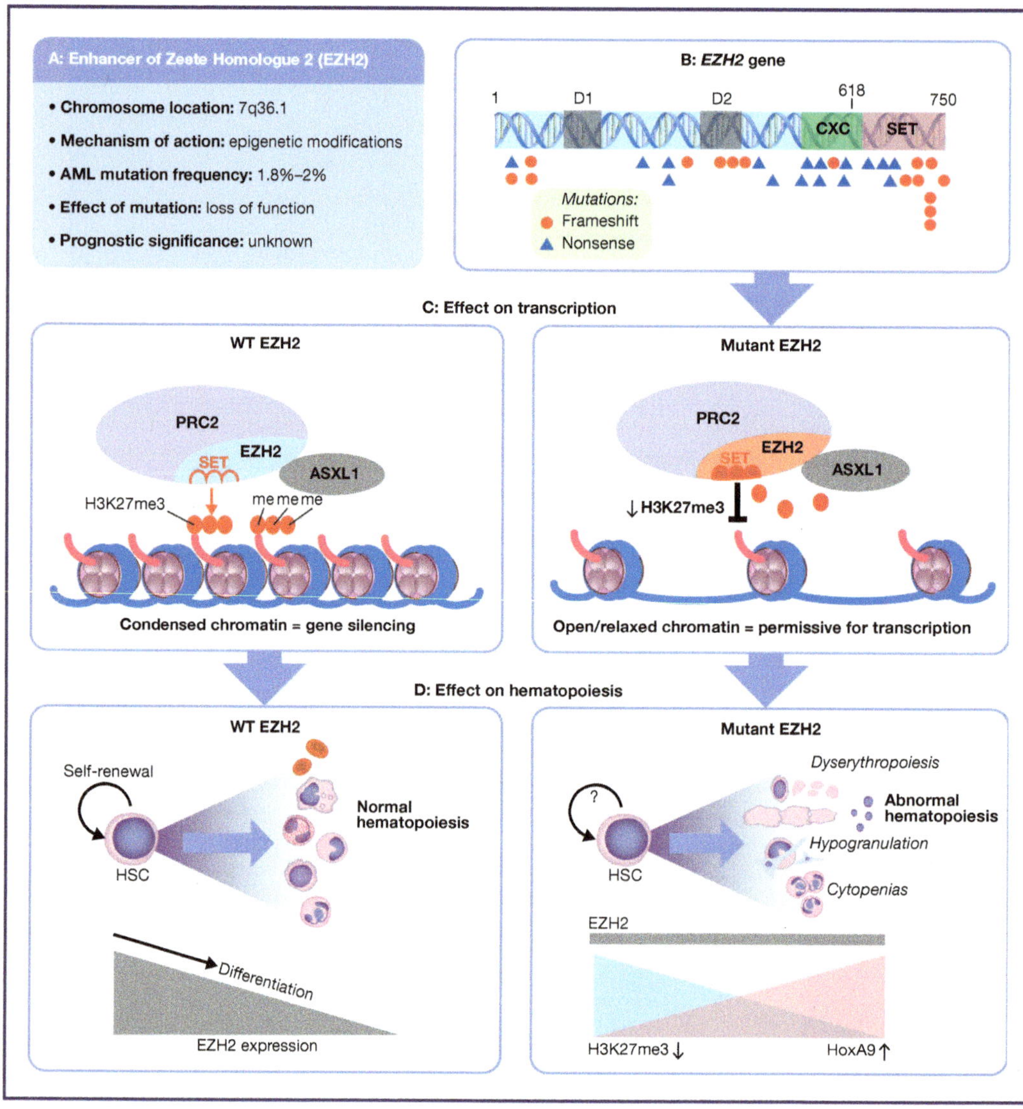

FIGURE 2-62: EZH2. (A) Enhancer of Zeste Homologue 2 (EZH2) is located on chromosome 7q36.1. EZH2 mutations are found in 1.8% to 2% of AML patients. The prognostic significance of EZH2 mutations in AML is unknown. (B) EZH2 mutations in AML cause a loss of function due to missense, frameshift, and nonsense mutations, most commonly in the Su(var), Enhancer of Zeste, Trithorax (SET) domain. The SET domain of EZH2 is required to form the active catalytic unit of the Polycomb repressive complex 2 (PRC2). (C) PRC2 mediates gene silencing via the tri-methylation of Lysine 27 on the N-terminal tail of Histone H3 (H3K27me3). H3K27me3 is a mark of transcriptional repression that leads to chromatin condensation and gene silencing. Similar to ASXL1 mutations, EZH2 loss-of-function mutations lead to global decrease in trimethylation of H3K27 and de-repression of downstream PRC2 target genes like the posterior *HOXA* cluster genes. De-repression or overexpression of *HOXA* genes has been implicated in leukemogenesis and may be one of the mechanisms by which EZH2 loss-of-function mutations contribute to leukemic transformation. (D) EZH2 deletion in mice is developmentally lethal and leads to defects in hematopoiesis, inefficient expansion of hematopoietic stem cells (HSCs), and a global decrease in levels of trimethylation of H3K27. In adult mice, conditional deletion of EZH2 causes myelodysplastic changes and a phenotype similar to human MDS/MPN. EZH2 overexpression prevents HSC exhaustion and stabilizes normal stem cell function. This highlights the importance of EZH2 in regulating gene expression patterns during development via the transcriptional mark H3K27me3.

AML, acute myeloid leukemia; HSC, hematopoietic stem cells; MDS, myelodysplastic syndrome; MPN, myeloproliferative neoplasm; WT, wild-type.

Selected References

ASXL1

Abdel-Wahab O, Adli M, LaFav L, et al. ASXL1 mutations promote myeloid transformation through loss of PRC2-mediated gene repression. *Cancer Cell*. 2012;22(2):180–193.

Abdel-Wahab O, Levine R. Mutations in epigenetic modifiers in the pathogenesis and therapy of acute myeloid leukemia. *Blood*. 2013;121(18):3563–3572.

Abdel-Wahab O, Paradani A, Patel J, et al. Concomitant analysis of EZH2 and ASXL1 mutations in myelofibrosis, chronic myelomonocytic leukemia and blast phase myeloproliferative neoplasms. *Leukemia*. 2011;25(7):1200–1202.

Boultwood J, Perry J, Pellagatti A. Frequent mutation of the polycomb-associated gene *ASXL1* in the myelodysplastic syndromes and in acute myeloid leukemia. *Leukemia*. 2010;24(5):1062–1065.

Schnitter S, Eder C, Jeromin S, et al. ASXL1 exon 12 mutations are frequent in AML with intermediate risk karyotype and are independently associated with an adverse outcome. *Leukemia*. 2013;27(1):82–91.

EZH2

Ernst T, Chase AJ, Score J, et al. Inactivation mutations of the histone methyltransferase gene *EZH2* in myeloid disorders. *Nat Genet*. 2010;42(8):722–727.

Kamminga L, Bystrykh L, de Boer A, et al. The polycomb group gene *EZH2* prevents hematopoietic stem cell exhaustion. *Blood*. 2006;107(5):2170–2179.

Khan SN, Jankowska AM, Mahrouz R, et al. Multiple mechanisms deregulate EZH2 and histone H3 lysine 27 epigenetic changes in myeloid malignancies. *Leukemia*. 2013;27(6):1301–1309.

Konuma T, Oguro H, Iwama A. Role of the polycomb group proteins in hematopoietic stem cells. *Dev Growth Differ*. 2010;52(6):505–516.

Mochizuki-Kashio M, Mishima Y, Miyagi S, et al. Dependency on the polycomb gene *EZH2* distinguishes fetal from adult hematopoietic stem cells. *Blood*. 2011;118(25):6553–6561.

Su H, Dobenecker M, Dickinson E, et al. Polycomb group protein EZH2 controls acting polymerization and cell signaling. *Cell*. 2005;121(3):425–436.

Wang X, Dai H, Wang W, et al. EZH2 mutations are related to low blast percentage in bone marrow and -7/del (7q) in de novo acute myeloid leukemia. *PLoS One*. 2013;8(4).

EVI1

Ling Li and Guido Marcucci

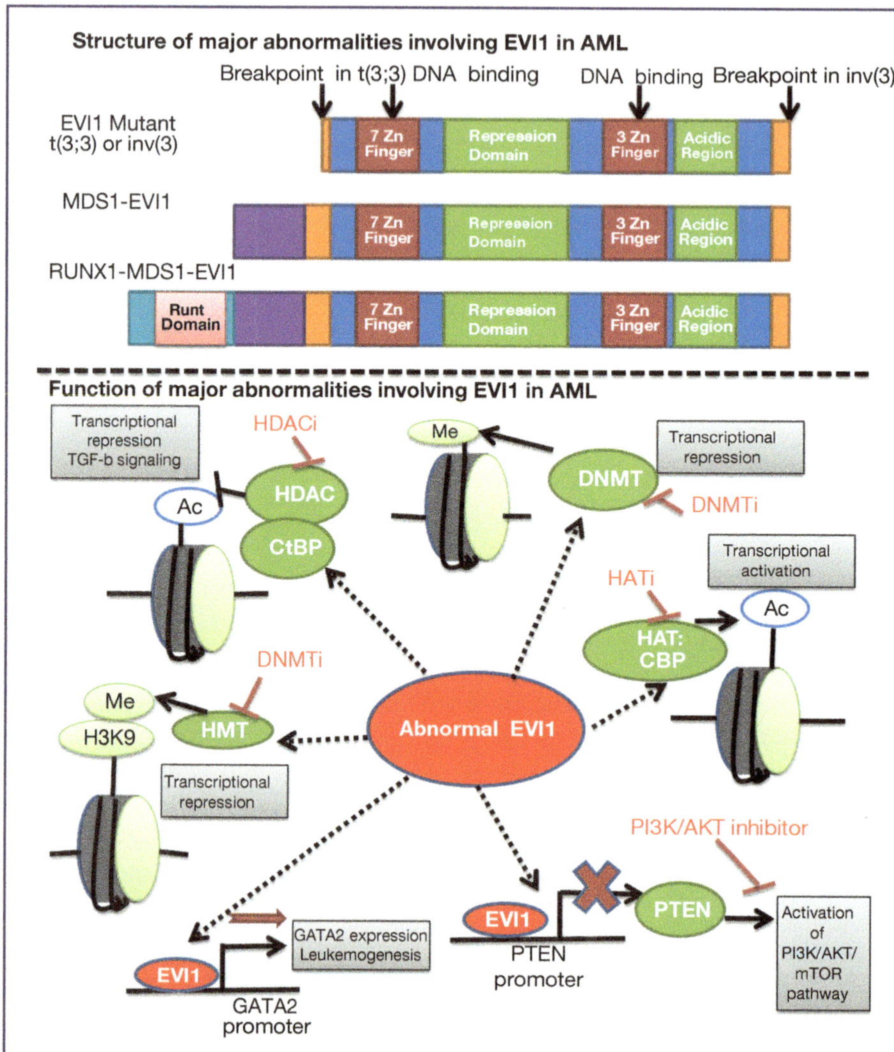

FIGURE 2-63: Top panel: Diagram of the genes and proteins involved in the rearrangements of EVI1. Top: Two forms of EVI1 mutation, the zinc finger domains (RED), the repression domain (GREEN), and the acidic domain (GREEN), are indicated. The breakpoints of the t(3;3) and of the inv(3) are indicated by the arrows. Bottom: Diagram of the proteins MDS1-EVI1 and fusion protein (RUNX1-MDS1-EVI1) are shown. Lower panel: Mechanistic link of epigenetic machinery and EVI1. EVI1 interacts with multiple components of various epigenetic machineries, including histone deacetylases (HDAC), DNA methyltransferases (DNMT), and H3K9-specific histone methyltransferases (HMT), leading to transcriptional repression. EVI1 interacts with histone acetyltransferase (HAT), which mediates transcriptional activation. EVI1 also related to leukemias-associated molecular targets, including the PI3K/AKT/mTOR pathway and GATA2; it can positively promote leukemogenesis.

Source: From Buonamici S, Chakraborty S, Senyuk V, Nucifora G. The role of EVI1 in normal and leukemic cells. *Blood Cells Mol Dis.* 2003;31(2):206–212. Hinai AA, Valk PJ. Aberrant EVI1 expression in acute myeloid leukaemia. *Br J Haematol.* 2016;172(6):870–878. Kataoka K, Kurokawa M. Ecotropic viral integration site 1, stem cell self-renewal and leukemogenesis. *Cancer Sci.* 2012;103(8): 1371–1377.

AKT, protein kinase B; AML, acute myeloid leukemia; MDS, myelodysplastic syndrome; mTOR, mechanistic target of rapamycin.

Selected References

Buonamici S, Chakraborty S, Senyuk V, Nucifora G. The role of EVI1 in normal and leukemic cells. *Blood Cells Mol Dis*. 2003;31(2):206–212.

Hinai AA, Valk PJ. Aberrant EVI1 expression in acute myeloid leukaemia. *Br J Haematol*. 2016; 172(6):870–878.

Kataoka K, Kurokawa M. Ecotropic viral integration site 1, stem cell self-renewal and leukemogenesis. *Cancer Sci*. 2012;103(8):1371–1377.

p53

Sami N. Malek

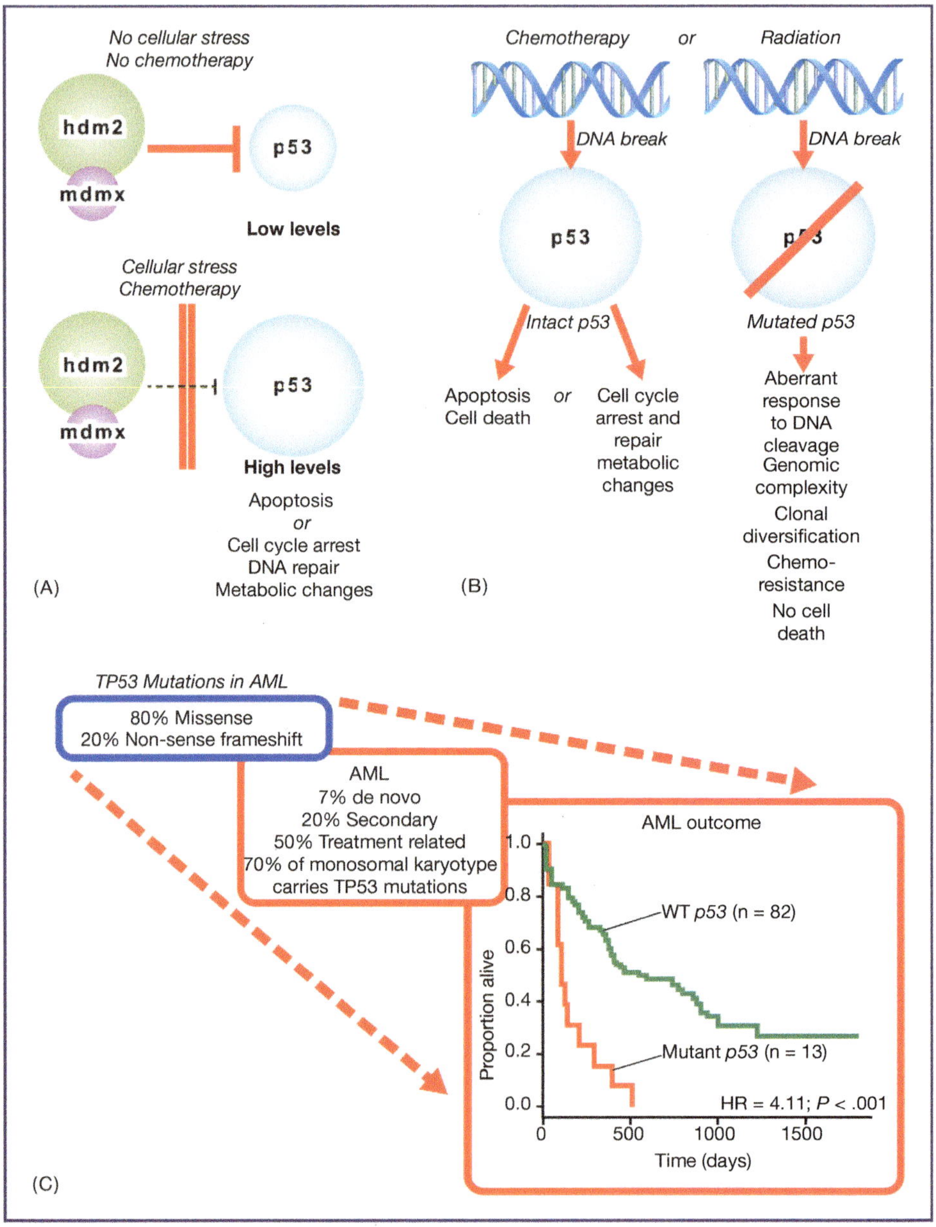

FIGURE 2-64: Inadequate p53 expression in AML. (A) Schema of the regulation of p53 protein levels by the ubiquitin ligase MDM2/MDMX. During stress, MDM2-mediated degradation of p53 is inhibited, resulting in high p53 protein levels. (B) Cellular responses to chemotherapy or radiation therapy, which induces DNA breaks, in cells with intact or mutated *TP53*. (C) Details and incidence of *TP53* mutations detected in human AML.

Source: Adapted from Parkin B, Erba H, Ouillette P, et al. Acquired genomic copy number aberrations and survival in adult acute myelogenous leukemia. *Blood.* 2010;116(23):4958–4967.

AML, acute myeloid leukemia; HR, high risk; WT, wild-type.

Selected Reference

Parkin B, Erba H, Ouillette P, et al. Acquired genomic copy number aberrations and survival in adult acute myelogenous leukemia. *Blood*. 2010;116(23):4958–4967.

SECONDARY AML (s-AML)

R. Coleman Lindsley

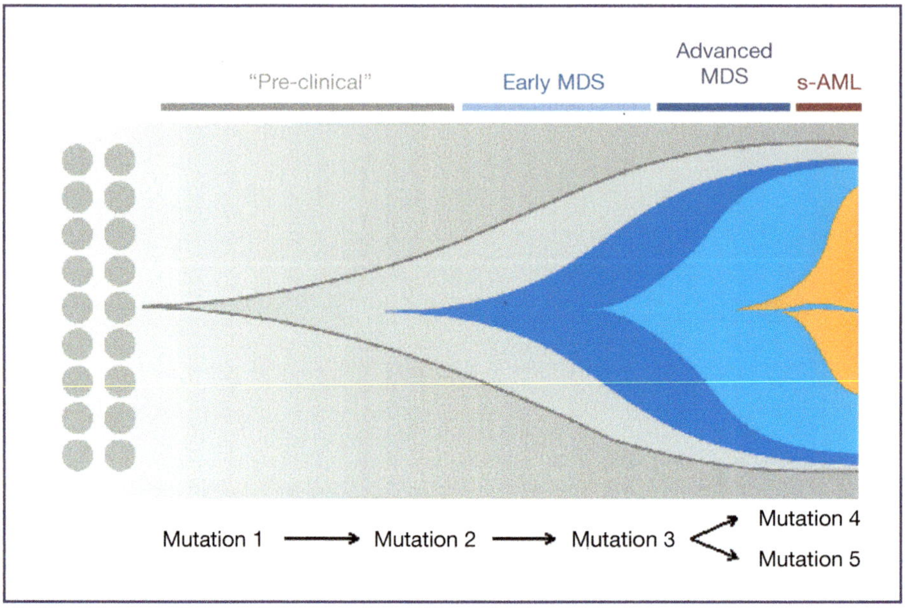

FIGURE 2-65: Secondary AML is the culmination of clonal and clinical evolution. The bone marrow of a healthy individual contains a diverse complement of normal stem cells (shown by the gray circles). Somatic acquisition of a pathogenic mutation drives selective expansion of a single stem cell (mutation 1). Additional mutations (mutations 2, 3, 4), shown by different colors moving through "clonal time," define individual daughter subclones, each with successive competitive advantage over its parent. The specific complement of mutations at any single point in time—and their relative abundance—is the clonal architecture. The dynamic changes in clonal architecture over time define clonal evolution. The earliest, disease-initiating mutations may cause an unrecognized, preclinical condition of variable latency and propensity for progression, called clonal hematopoiesis of indeterminate potential (CHIP), that can evolve further into MDS and, ultimately, secondary AML. Here the *x*-axis is clonal time and y-axis is proportional involvement of the bone marrow.

AML, acute myeloid leukemia; MDS, myelodysplastic syndrome.

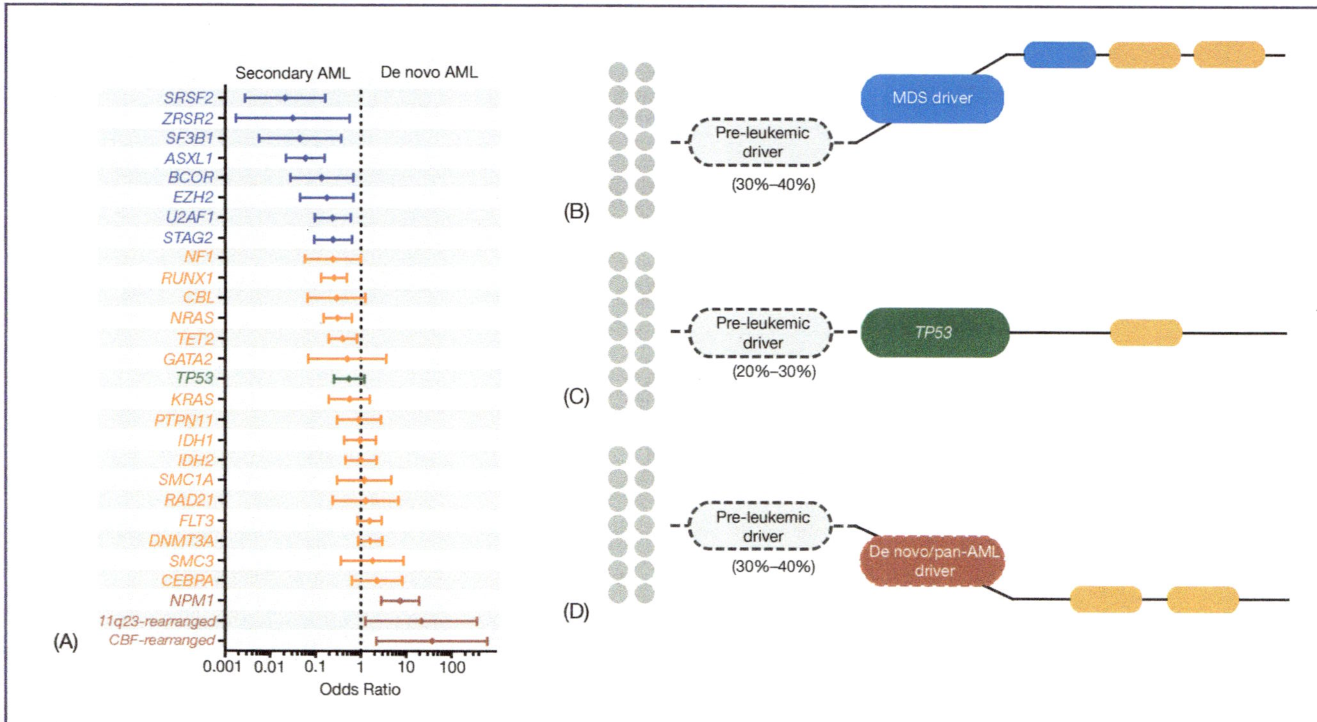

FIGURE 2-66: Objective genetic ontogeny classification in AML. AML ontogeny has historically been classified based on clinical history as secondary AML (arising as transformation of an antecedent myeloid neoplasm, such as MDS or MPN), therapy-related AML (arising after exposure to leukemogenic therapy for a nonmyeloid disease), or de novo AML (arising without identifiable exposure or prodromal myeloid disorder). (A) By comparing the mutational profile of confirmed secondary AML cases (arising after WHO-confirmed MDS) to that of non-M3 de novo AML cases, some mutated genes were found to have high specificity for ontogeny, independent of clinical history. The forest plot shows odds ratios with 95% confidence intervals and demonstrates the strength of association between individual mutated genes and either secondary AML (left) or de novo AML (right). Mutations in eight genes (colored in blue and termed "secondary-type mutations") have greater than 95% specificity for secondary AML. Three alterations (colored in red) with equally high specificity for de novo AML include *NPM1* frameshift mutations and rearrangements of *MLL* and core binding factor genes. The remaining genes (shown in yellow and termed "pan-AML mutations") are commonly mutated in AML but are not ontogeny-restricted. (B–D) A schematized view of three genetic pathways of AML ontogeny, where ontogeny is defined by either "secondary-type" MDS driver mutation (blue), *TP53* mutation (green), or only de novo/pan-AML mutation (red). Preleukemic driver mutations (*TET2* or *DNMT3A*, in gray) or pan-AML mutations (in yellow) are not ontogeny-restricted and do not define clinically consistent groups of patients.

AML, acute myeloid leukemia; MDS, myelodysplastic syndrome; MPN, myeloproliferative neoplasm; WHO, World Health Organization.

Table 2-10 Relationship of genetic ontogeny, clinical ontogeny, and selected mutations. Genetic ontogeny categories define subgroups of AML patients with consistent clinicopathologic features

		CLINICAL ONTOGENY					Pan-AML MUTATIONS (%)			
		DE NOVO (NO EXPOSURE OR PRIOR MYELOID DISEASE)	SECONDARY (POST-MDS OR MPN)	THERAPY-RELATED (POST-EXPOSURE)	AGE	RELATIVE CHEMOSENSITIVITY	RAS/TK*	MYELOID TF**	IDH1/2	COMPLEX/MONOSOMAL KARYOTYPE
Genetic ontogeny	**Secondary-type**	10	70	35	+++	low	40–50	30–40	20	rare
	***TP53* mutated**	10	15	20–30	+/–	low	25	5–10	<2	frequent
	de novo or Pan-AML only	80	25	50	+/–	high	40-50	15	20	rare

*Mutations in Ras or genes encoding tyrosine kinases.

**Mutations or translocations of gene encoding myeloid transcription factors.

AML, acute myeloid leukemia; MDS, myelodysplastic syndrome; MPN, myeloproliferative neoplasm.

Selected References

Cancer Genome Atlas Research Network. Genomic and epigenomic landscapes of adult de novo acute myeloid leukemia. *N Engl J Med*. 2013;368(22):2059–2074.

Lindsley RC, Mar BG, Mazzola E, et al. Acute myeloid leukemia ontogeny is defined by distinct somatic mutations. *Blood*. 2015;125(9):1367–1376.

Pedersen-Bjergaard J, Christiansen DH, Desta F, Andersen MK. Alternative genetic pathways and cooperating genetic abnormalities in the pathogenesis of therapy-related myelodysplasia and acute myeloid leukemia. *Leukemia*. 2006;20(11):1943–1949.

Rücker FG, Schlenk RF, Bullinger L, et al. TP53 alterations in acute myeloid leukemia with complex karyotype correlate with specific copy number alterations, monosomal karyotype, and dismal outcome. *Blood*. 2012;119(9):2114–2121.

Steensma DP, Bejar R, Jaiswal S, et al. Clonal hematopoiesis of indeterminate potential and its distinction from myelodysplastic syndromes. *Blood*. 2015;126(1):9–16.

Walter MJ, Shen D, Ding L, et al. Clonal architecture of secondary acute myeloid leukemia. *N Engl J Med*. 2012;366(12):1090–1098.

MICRORNAs: NETWORKS IN ACUTE LEUKEMIA

Lukasz P. Gondek and Gabriel Ghiaur

Introduction

MicroRNAs (miRNAs) are small noncoding RNAs (about 22 nucleotides) that act as biological regulators via interactions with unique mRNA sequences (Figure 2-67). By specifically targeting multiple mRNAs within a signaling pathway, miRNAs can exert global control of biological processes such as cell cycle, metabolism, or differentiation. More so, the effect is usually quantitative (subtle modulation of the pathway output) rather than a binary on/off switch imposing another layer of post-transcriptional fine-tuning. MicroRNAs play pivotal roles in the hematopoietic system regulating self-renewal, proliferation, and differentiation of both myeloid and lymphoid cells. Dysregulation of miRNA transcriptome leads to disruption of the hematopoiesis and may result in leukemic transformation and/or disease progression. The miRNA transcriptome can be deregulated in cancer either by numerical and structural chromosomal alterations or by somatic mutations in their loci or in genes responsible for their processing (Figure 2-67). In addition to these mechanisms, miRNA loci are also subject to epigenetic modulation. Not only are the miRNA loci under epigenetic control but these molecules can also target the epigenetic machinery to control global cellular fate (Figure 2-69). MicroRNAs can act either as oncogenes or as tumor suppressors (Figure 2-68), and they tend to cluster in unique genomic regions with common transcriptional control. Thus, either single miRNA or miRNA signatures have been shown to serve as prognostic factors in subtypes of acute leukemia (Table 2-11). Not only do these highly stable molecules exert their cellular function intrinsically but they can also be delivered via direct cell-to-cell communication to adjacent cells or via exosomes to distant target cells. Their role in leukemogenesis or as potential pharmacological agents/targets is just starting to be explored (Figures 2-68 and 2-69).

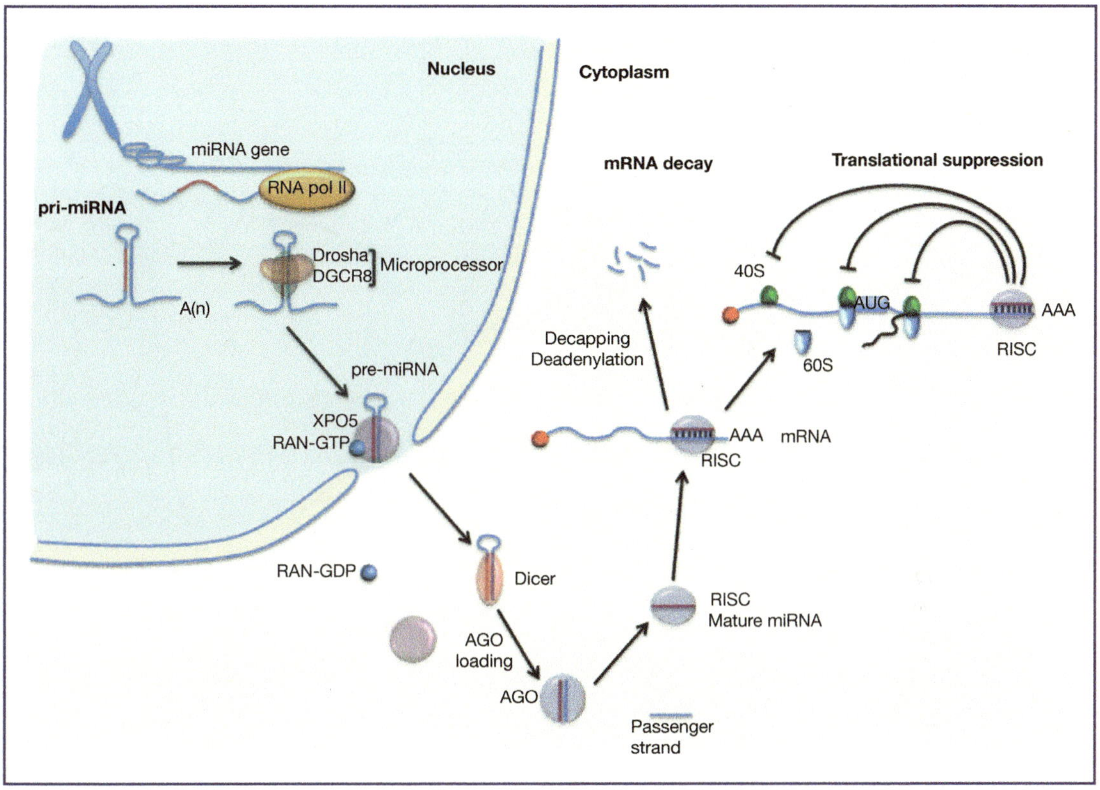

FIGURE 2-67: MicroRNA processing and mechanism of action. MicroRNAs are transcribed from genomic DNA by RNA polymerase II (RNA Pol II). Primary miRNA (pri-miRNA) is then processed in the nucleus by Drosha and DGCR8 (microprocessor complex) to produce pre-miRNA. Pre-miRNA is exported to the cytoplasm via export 5 (XPO5), which forms a transport complex with GTP-binding nuclear protein RAN (RAN-GTP). On cytoplasmic entry, GTP is hydrolyzed and the pre-miRNA is released. Pre-miRNA is then cleaved by RNase III type endonuclease (DICER) and subsequently loaded on Argonaute protein (AGO 1-4) to form the RNA-induced silencing complex (RISC). The passenger strand is then removed and mature RISC is formed. The mature 22-nucleotide strand recognizes a complementary sequence in the 3′ untranslated region (3′-UTR) of the target mRNA. The RISC–mRNA complex promotes mRNA destabilization by recruiting deadenylases onto target mRNA. Deadenylation results in 5′-to-3′ mRNA degradation. Alternatively, RISC can also directly promote mRNA decapping and the subsequent mRNA decay by recruiting decapping factors onto the target mRNAs. Both mechanisms result in miRNA-mediated decay of target mRNA. Additionally, the binding of miRNA to target mRNA could result in translation inhibition by interfering with any of the three steps of the translation process: initiation, elongation, or termination.

GTP, guanosine triphosphate.

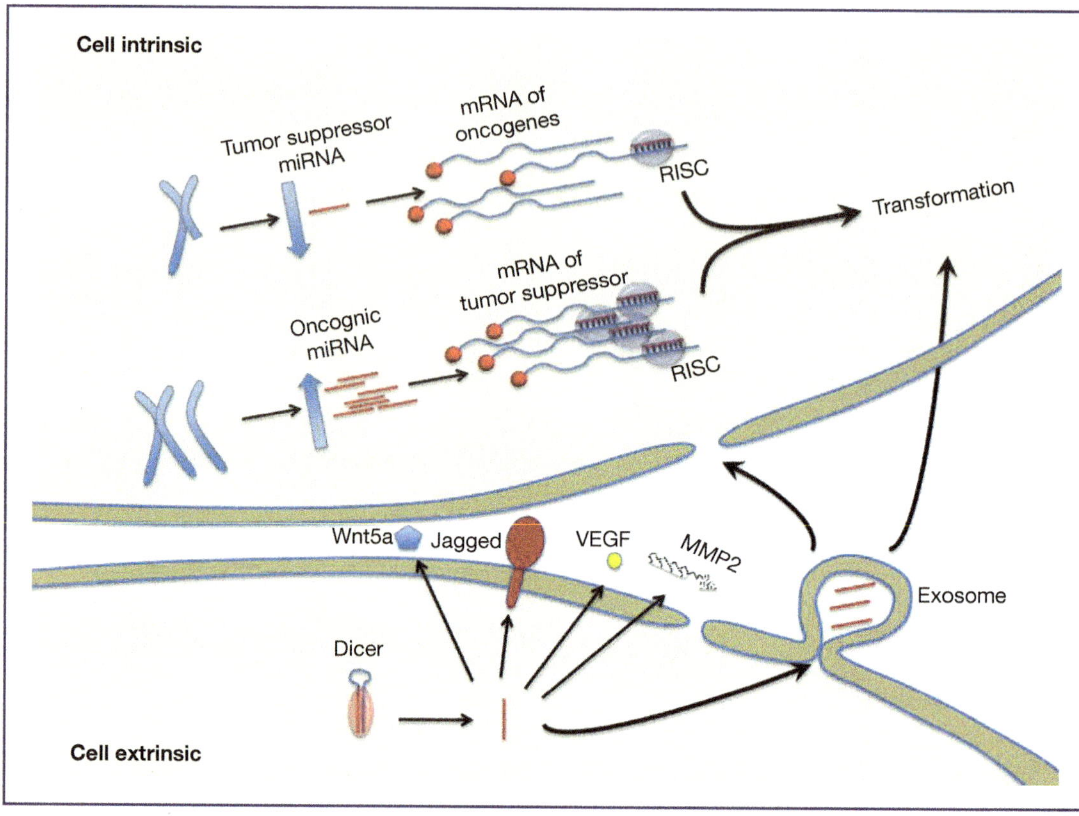

FIGURE 2-68: Biological effects of miRNAs in leukemia homeostasis. Dysregulation of miRNAs (either overexpression and/or silencing) results in changes in transcriptome with subsequent decreased mRNA levels of tumor suppressors and/or increased levels of oncogenes. In addition to these cell-intrinsic mechanisms of leukemogenesis, cell-extrinsic changes in noncoding RNAs, such as those induced by DICER knockout in bone marrow mesenchymal stroma cells, are enough to induce genomic instability in hematopoietic cells with subsequent AML/MDS. While the exact pathway by which the DICER knockout mesenchymal cells dysregulate the neighboring hematopoietic cells remains unknown, some candidates include miRNAs that target Wnt, NOTCH, VEGF, or MMP activity. In addition, extracellular vesicle (for instance, exosomes) and other cell-to-cell communication pathways can be used to transfer abnormal miRNAs between bone marrow microenvironment and the hematopoietic cells and impact leukemia homeostasis. One family of miRNAs that has been extensively studied for its role in cancer homeostasis with an eye toward therapeutic potential is the Let7 family. This is a class of miRNAs highly conserved from *C. elegans* to human and found to be deregulated in a variety of cancers, including leukemia. Let7 is a powerful tumor suppressor miRNA via targeting Ras, Myc, HMGA2 and other oncogenes. Thus, rescuing Let7 activity negatively impacts leukemia and offers another potential therapeutic tool.

AML/MDS, acute myeloid leukemia/myelodysplastic syndrome; MMP, matrix metalloproteinase; RISC, RNA-induced silencing complex; VEGF, vascular endothelial growth factor.

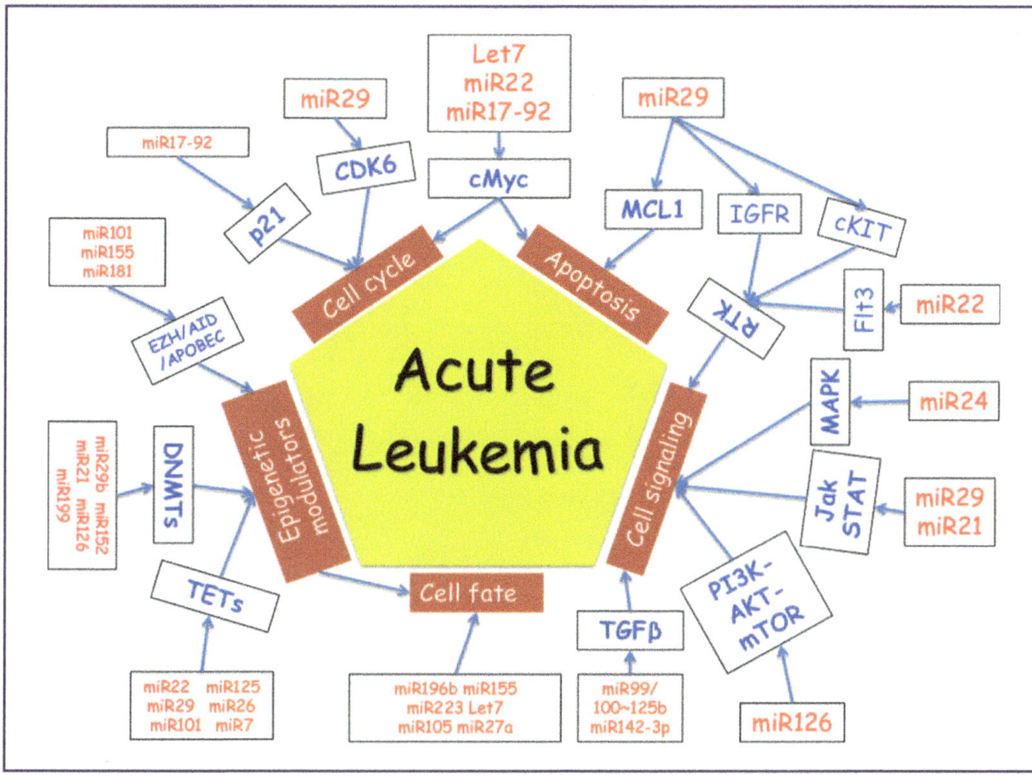

FIGURE 2-69: Cell-intrinsic mechanisms of leukemogenesis of miRNA. A variety of cellular processes are impacted by miRNAs, with the end result being cellular transformation. While this map is ever expanding and does not capture the entire complexity of miRNA signatures, some mechanisms have been better defined than others. For instance, miRNAs can target and dysregulate epigenetic modulators such as TET2 and DNMTs and act as true oncogenes. To this end, miR22 overexpression, for instance (as seen in MDS), targets TET2, resulting in increased HSC activity and MDS, and the phenotype is rescued by overexpression of TET2. On the other hand, the miR29 family can target all three TET isoforms and DNMTs with resultant myeloproliferation. This phenotype is also rescued by the overexpression of TET2. More so, miRNAs have been shown to target a variety of cell signaling programs, from RTKs such as c-Kit and FLT3 to downstream signaling pathways such as MAPK, JAK/STAT, or PI3K. To this end, miR126, for instance, negatively regulates the PI3K/AKT pathway in leukemia stem cells and promotes their self-renewal. More often than not, the effects of miRNAs are pleiotropic and at times divergent with impacts on multiple pathways that can lead to cellular transformation. A prime example in this sense is the miR29 family, composed of miR29a, miR29b, and miR29c. These miRNAs, down-regulated in AML with 11q23 or del7, can act as oncogenes via their effects on epigenetic modulators (see earlier) or as tumor suppressor via their effects on cell cycling/apoptosis as well as differentiation downstream of JAK/STAT. Interestingly, forced up-regulation of miR29b in AML as seen with either ectopic overexpression or treatment with pharmacologic agents (for instance, bortezomib) disrupts the protein–miRNA network, decreases c-Kit levels, and carries therapeutic potential.

DNMT, DNA methyltransferase; HSC, hematopoietic stem cell; MAPK, mitogen-activated protein kinases; RTK, receptor tyrosine kinase; TET2, ten-eleven translocation 2.

Table 2-11 MicroRNAs deregulated in most common subtypes of AML

	microRNAs	
CHROMOSOME ABERRATION	**UP-REGULATED**	**DOWN-REGULATED**
t(15;17)	miR127	miR17
	miR299	miR126
	miR323	
	miR368	
	miR382	
t(8;21)	miR126	miR133
	miR24a, -b	Let7b, Let7c
inv(16)	miR126	Let7b, Let7c
t(11q23)/MLL	miR326	miR29
	miR219	miR34
	miR17-92	miR16
	miR196a	
Trisomy 8	miR124a	
	miR30d	
del7		miR29
Normal Karyotype		
Molecular lesions		
NPM1 mutations	miR10a/miR10b	miR204
	miR196a/miR196b	miR128
	Let7a/Let7c	miR126
		miR130a
		miR451
FLT3-ITD	miR155	
IDH mutations	miR1	
	miR125b	
	miR133a	
CEBPα mutations	miR181a	miR34a
	miR335	

Source: Adapted and updated from Marcucci G, Mrozek K, Radmacher MD, et al. The prognostic and functional role of microRNAs in acute myeloid leukemia. *Blood.* 2011;117(4):1121–1129.

AML, acute myeloid leukemia; FLT3-ITD, FMS-like tyrosine kinase 3 internal tandem duplication; NPM1, nucleophosmine 1.

Selected References

Bussing I, Slack FJ, Grosshans H. *let-7* microRNAs in development, stem cells, and cancer. *Trends Mol Med.* 2008;14(9):400–409.

Cheng J, Guo S, Chen S, et al. An extensive network of Tet2-targeting microRNAs regulates malignant hematopoiesis. *Cell Rep.* 2013;5(2):471–481.

Fabian MR, Sonenberg N. The mechanics of miRNA-mediated gene silencing: a look under the hood of miRISC. *Nat Struct Mol Biol.* 2012;19(6):586–593.

Garzon R, Heaphy CE, Havelange V, et al. MicroRNA 29b functions in acute myeloid leukemia. *Blood.* 2009;114(26):5331–5341.

Ha M, Kim VN. Regulation of microRNA biogenesis. *Nat Rev Mol Cell Biol.* 2014;15(8):509–524.

Kats LM, Reschke M, Tauli R, et al. Proto-oncogene role of mutant *IDH-2* in leukemia initiation and maintenance. *Cell Stem Cell.* 2014;14(3):329–341.

Lechman ER, Gentner B, Ng SWK, et al. miR-126 regulates distinct self-renewal outcomes in normal and malignant hematopoietic stem cells. *Cancer Cell.* 2016;29(2):214–228.

Marcucci G, Mrozek K, Radmacher MD, et al. The prognostic and functional role of microRNAs in acute myeloid leukemia. *Blood.* 2011;117(4):1121–1129.

Raaijmakers MHGP, Mukherjee S, Guo S, et al. Bone progentior dysfunction induces myelodysplasia and secondary leukaemia. *Nature.* 2010;464(7290):852–857.

Winter J, Jung S, Keller S, et al. Many roads to maturity: microRNA biogenesis pathways and their regulation. *Nat Cell Biol.* 2009;11(3):228–234.

Zipeto MA, Court AC, Sadarangani A, et al. ADAR1 activation drives leukemia stem cell renewal by impairing Let-7 biogenesis. *Cell Stem Cell.* 2016;19(2):177–191.

PROGNOSTIC IMPLICATION OF MUTATIONAL INTERPLAY

Ashkan Emadi and Judith E. Karp

Based on the patterns of co-mutation found in 1,540 patients with AML in three prospective multicenter clinical trials of the German-Austrian AML Study Group, Papaemmanuil et al developed a Bayesian statistical model to classify AML into subtypes that are mutually exclusive, and proposed the subgroups or classes of AML described in Table 2-12.

Table 2-12 Frequency (%) of specific gene mutations or genetic abnormalities in addition to the main genomic feature

GENOMICALLY DETERMINED AMLs	ACCOMPANIED GENE MUTATIONS OR GENETIC ABNORMALITIES (% CO-OCCURRENCE)
Favorable	
AML with t(15;17)(q22;q12); *PML-RARA*	*FLT3*-ITD (35%), *WT1* (17%)
AML with inv(16)(p13.1q22) or t(16;16)(p13.1;q22); *CBFB-MYH11*	*NRAS* (53%), +8/8q (16%), +22 (16%), *KIT* (15%), *FLT3*-TKD (15%)
AML with t(8;21)(q22;q22); *RUNX1-RUNX1T1*	*KIT* (38%), −Y (33%), −9q (18%)
AML with biallelic *CEBPA* mutations	*NRAS* (30%), *WT1* (21%), *GATA2* (20%)
AML with *NPM1* mutation	*DNMT3A* (54%), *FLT3*-ITD (39%), *NRAS* (19%), *TET2* (16%), *PTPN11* (15%)
AML with *IDH2*-R172 mutations and no other class-defining lesions	*DNMT3A* (67%), +8/8q (17%)
Unfavorable	
AML with *TP53* mutations, chromosomal aneuploidy, or both	Complex karyotype (68%), −5/5q (47%), −7/7q (44%), *TP53* (44%), −17/17p (31%), −12/12p (17%), +8/8q (16%)
AML with mutated chromatin, RNA-splicing genes, or both	*RUNX1* (39%), *MLL*-PTD (25%), *SRSF2* (22%), *DNMT3A* (20%), *ASXL1* (17%), *STAG2* (16%), *NRAS* (16%), *TET2* (15%), *FLT3*-ITD (15%)
AML with *MLL* fusion genes; t(x;11)(x;q23)	*NRAS* (23%)
AML with inv(3)(q21q26.2) or t(3;3)(q21;q26.2); *GATA2, MECOM(EVI1)*	−7 (85%), *KRAS* (30%), *NRAS* (30%), *PTPN11* (30%), *ETV6* (15%), *PHF6* (15%), *SF3B1* (15%)
AML with t(6;9)(p23;q34); *DEK-NUP214*	*FLT3*-ITD (80%), *KRAS* (20%)
AML with driver mutations but no detected class-defining lesions	*FLT3*-ITD (39%), *DNMT3A* (16%)

AML, acute myeloid leukemia.

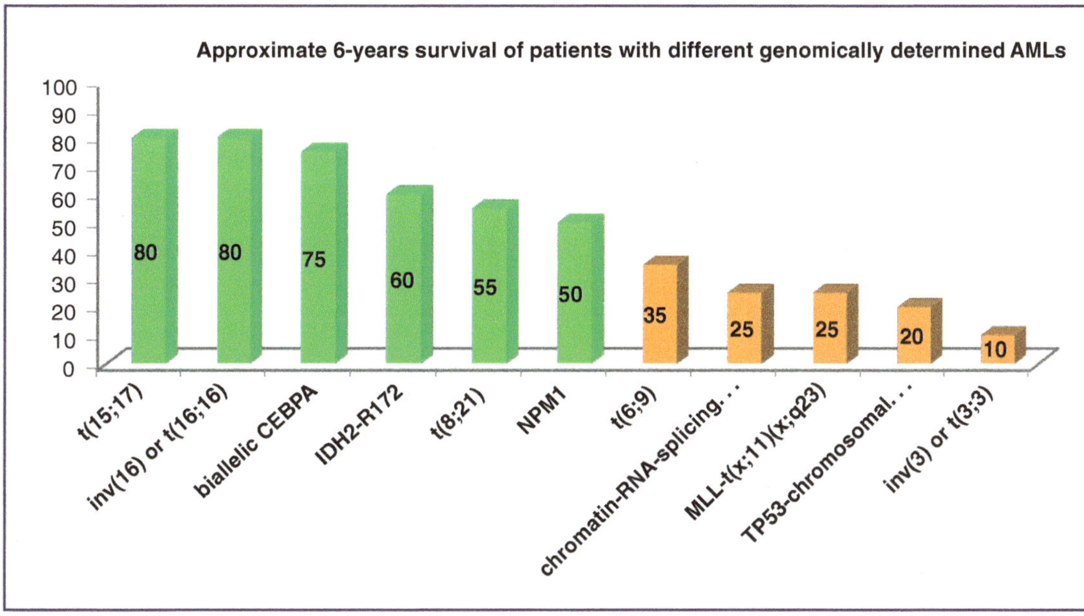

FIGURE 2-70: Probability of 6-year overall survival of patients with AML on the basis of the specific genomically determined subgroups.
AML, acute myeloid leukemia.

Table 2-13 The effect of presence or absence of *FLT3-ITD* or *NRAS* codon 12/13 mutations on approximate 6-year overall survival (%) of patients with AMLs with wild-type (WT) or mutant (mut) *NPM1* or *DNMT3A*

		NPM1			
		WT		mut	
		DNMT3A			
		WT	mut	WT	mut
FLT3-ITD	Present	No effect (P = .1) (40%)	No effect (P = .9) (25%)	40%	20%
	Absent			55% (P = .2)	60% (P = .009)
NRAS-G12/13	Present	No effect (P = .8) (40%)	No effect (P = 1.0) (30%)	60% (P = .5)	75% (P = .0007)
	Absent			50%	40%

Yellow, no effect; green, positive effect on survival; orange, negative effect on survival; dark orange and dark green represent more negative and positive impact on survival, respectively.
AML, acute myeloid leukemia.

Selected Reference

Papaemmanuil E, Gerstung M, Bullinger L, et al. Genomic classification and prognosis in acute myeloid leukemia. *N Engl J Med*. 2016;374:2209–2221.

Molecular Mutations in ALL

Kristen O'Dwyer and Anjali Advani

Table 2-14 Distinct genetic subtypes of ALL. Recurrent chromosome translocations occur frequently in ALL. These genetic events are important for leukemia initiation, but alone are insufficient for transformation to a full leukemia phenotype. The prevalence of each of the genetic subtypes varies among children and adults. The prognosis varies with subtype.

GENETIC SUBTYPE	GENE	COOPERATING GENOMIC ALTERATIONS	PREVALENCE IN ADULTS	PREVALENCE IN CHILDREN	PROGNOSIS
B-lineage ALL					
Hyperdiploidy (>50 chromosomes)	Extra copies of chromosomes 21, X, 14, 4 are the most common	Genomic gains	5%	25%	Favorable
Hypodiploidy (<44 chromosomes)		*PAX5*	2%	2%–3%	Poor
t(12;21)(p13;q22)	*TEL-AML1* *(ETV6-RUNX1)*	Deletion *12p13.2, PAX5, EBF1, ETV6, CDKN2A, RAGI, RAG2, BTLA, CD200, TOX, TBL1XR1, NR3C1, BTG1*	2%	25%	Favorable
t(1;19)(q23;p13)	*E2A-PBX1 (TCF3-PBX1)*	Deletion of *CDKN2A, PAX5,* chromosome 6q, 13q, and formation of isochromosome 9q	1%–3%	5%	Favorable
t(9;22)(q34;q11.2)	*BCR-ABL1*	Deletions of *IKZF1 (IKAROS), CDKN2A, PAX5*	25%	2%–5%	Improved with TKI therapy
t(v;11q23); MLL rearranged	*MLL*-many fusion partners including *AF4, ENL, AF9*	Activating mutations in PI3 kinase, *RAS, FLT3, NF1, PTPN11, PIK3R1*	2%	1%	Poor
t(5;14)(q35;q32)	*IL3-IGH*		1%	1%	Poor
Ph-like	No common chromosome rearrangement or translocation	Multiple mutations, including IKZF1	10%–30%	10%–15%	Poor

(*continued*)

Table 2-14 Distinct genetic subtypes of ALL. Recurrent chromosome translocations occur frequently in ALL. These genetic events are important for leukemia initiation, but alone are insufficient for transformation to a full leukemia phenotype. The prevalence of each of the genetic subtypes varies among children and adults. The prognosis varies with subtype. (*continued*)

GENETIC SUBTYPE	GENE	COOPERATING GENOMIC ALTERATIONS	PREVALENCE IN ADULTS	PREVALENCE IN CHILDREN	PROGNOSIS
T-lineage ALL					
t(7;9)(q34;q34.3)	*TCRB-NOTCH1*		<1%	<1%	Poor
t(10;14)(q24;q11)	*HOX 11*		30%	7%	Favorable
t(5;14)(q35;q32)	*BCL11B-TLX3*		1%	20%	Poor
t(11;14)(p15;q11)	*TRA/D-LMO1*		20%–25%	10%	Favorable with intensive chemotherapy
t(1;14)(p32;q11)	*TRA-TAL1*		12%	7%	Favorable
Early T-cell precursor ALL	No common chromosome rearrangement or translocation; characterized by a distinct immunophenotype: cytoplasmic $CD3^{+}$, $CD8^{-}$, $CD1a^{-}$, CD5 weak, and express one or more myeloid or stem cell marker (CD13, CD33, CD34, CD117, and HLA-DR)	Gene regulators of hematopoiesis and lymphoid development (*RUNX1, IKZF1, ETV6, GATA3, EP300*). Activating mutations in signaling pathways (*N-RAS, K-RAS, FLT3, IL7R, JAK3, JAK1, SH2B3*). Mutations in epigenetic regulators (*PRC2, SETD2*)	Unknown	15%	Historically poor, but improved with risk-adapted therapy

ALL, acute lymphoblastic leukemia; MLL, mixed lineage leukemia; TKI, tyrosine kinase inhibitor.

Table 2-15 Distinct genetic alterations in ALL. Key genes from commonly altered pathways in B-ALL and T-ALL are listed. In B-lineage ALL, the genes most frequently mutated are transcription factors that control early lymphoid development. In T-lineage ALL, NOTCH1 is mutated in more than 50% of cases.

GENE	FUNCTION	MECHANISM OF GENETIC ALTERATION	CLINICAL SIGNIFICANCE
B-lineage			
PAX5	The *PAX5* gene is a member of the paired box (PAX) family of transcription factors. It is essential for B-lineage commitment and B-lineage differentiation.	Mono-allelic deletions, chromosomal translocations, point mutations that initiate loss of PAX5 function and arrest B-cell differentiation.	Incidence is 32% of B-ALL. Implicated in development of B-ALL. Not associated with prognosis.
IKZF1	The *IKZF1* gene encodes the transcription factor, Ikaros, which is a member of the zinc-finger nuclear proteins. It is essential for development of all lymphoid lineages.	Point mutations, copy number deletions lead to disturbed lymphoid maturation.	Incidence is 15% of all pediatric B-ALL. Increased incidence in poor-risk subtypes: Ph-positive ALL (80%) and high-risk Ph-negative ALL (33%).
EBF1	The *EBF1* gene encodes transcription factors required for specification to B-lineage and for B-lineage differentiation.	Mono-allelic deletions. Loss of function arrests B-cell differentiation.	Implicated in development of B-ALL. Associated with poor prognosis.
CDKN2A/B	Cell cycle gene, controls two important tumor suppressor genes, *p16INK4A* and *p14ARF*. Deletions of this gene lead to defects in the normal control of the cell cycle.	Copy number alterations (most commonly deletions) identified in 40% of patients.	Prognostic significance is unclear; some studies show poor prognosis, while others have no impact.
T-lineage			
NOTCH1	This transcription factor is required for commitment of bone marrow stem cells to becoming T-lymphocytes. Also leads to proliferation of T-cells in the thymus (thymocytes).	– Identified in >50% of T-ALL cases – Activating mutations cause constitutive activation of NOTCH1 signaling – Single amino acid substitutions or short in-frame mutations or deletions in exons 26 and 27	Activating mutations are associated with improved early response and increased sensitivity to steroids. Some studies have demonstrated improved overall survival.
FBXW7	A tumor suppressor gene; when mutated, it impairs proteasomal degradation of activated *NOTCH1*.	Found in approximately 20% of cases, commonly with an associated *NOTCH1* mutation.	Improved overall survival, especially with associated *NOTCH1* mutations.
CDKN2A/B	Cell cycle gene, which controls two important tumor suppressor genes, *p16INK4A* and *p14ARF*. Deletions of this gene lead to defects in the normal control of the cell cycle.	Copy number deletions identified >70% of T-ALL cases.	Favorable prognosis
IL7R	This receptor activates the JAK/STAT signal transduction pathway and is required for the growth, proliferation, and survival of developing T-cells. This gain of function mutation results in ligand-independent activation of JAK/STAT signaling.	Identified in 10% of cases, notably found in ETP ALL.	Unknown

ALL, acute lymphoblastic leukemia, B-ALL, B acute lymphoblastic leukemia, ETP, early T-cell precursor; T-ALL, T acute lymphoblastic leukemia.

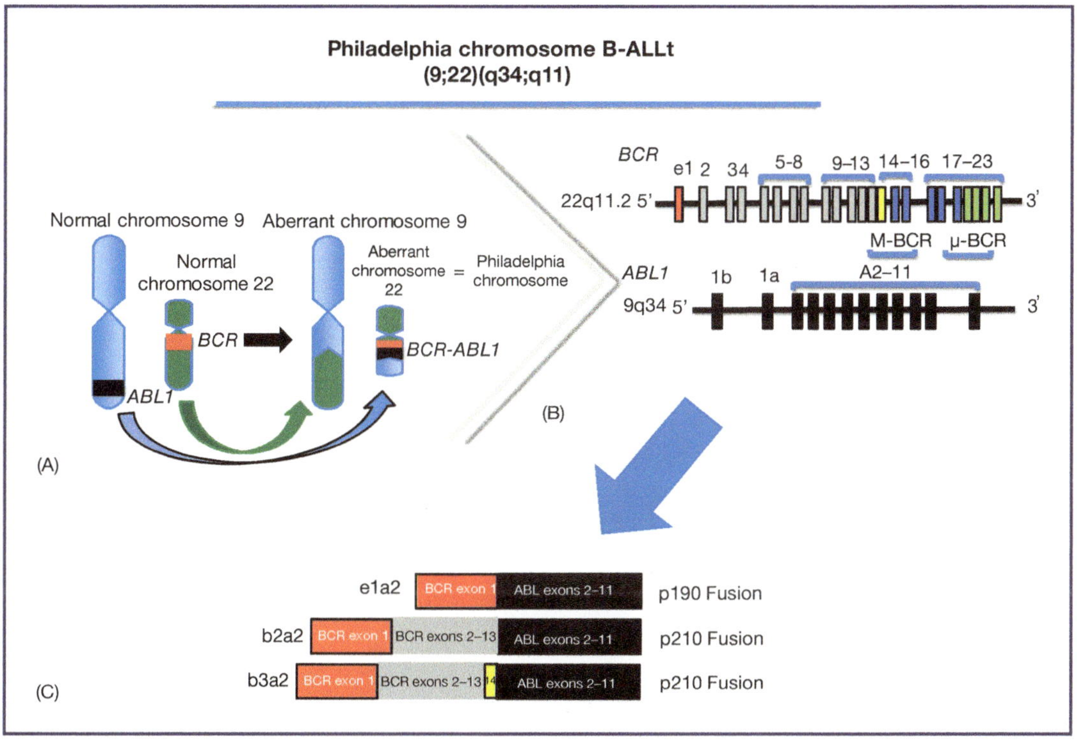

FIGURE 2-71: **Philadelphia chromosome in ALL: The Philadelphia chromosome (Ph) is the most common translocation in adult ALL, accounting for 25% to 30% of patients with ALL. It is rare in pediatric ALL. It is defined by a reciprocal translocation between chromosomes 9 and 22, and produces the oncogenic fusion gene *BCR/ABL1* (panel A). Specific exons of the 5′ *BCR* on chromosome band 22q11.2 fuse with exon 2 of the *ABL1* gene located on chromosome band 9q34. Two main fusion proteins, $p190^{BCR/ABL}$ and $p210^{BCR/ABL}$, are produced depending on the location of the breakpoint within the *BCR* gene (panel B and C). The p190 product contains the first exon of *BCR* and occurs in the majority of patients with Ph^{+}-ALL (approximately 66%). The p210 product contains either exon 13 or exon 14 of BCR and is less frequent in ALL (approximately 33% of patients), but is found universally in patients with chronic myeloid leukemia (CML).**

ALL, acute lymphoblastic leukemia; B-ALL, B acute lymphoblastic leukemia.

BCR-ABL1 Mutations Reported for Ph(+) B-ALL

(A)

Mutation/Frequency	Amino Acid Exchange	Clinical Management
T315I (37%)	Threonine 315-Isoleucine	Ponatinib and HSCT
E255K (18%)	Glutamic acid 255-Lysine	Consider Dasatinib
Y253H (18%)	Tyrosine 253-Histadine	Consider Dasatinib
F359V (4.6%)	Phenylalanine 359-Valine	Consider Dasatinib
G250E (4.6%)	Glysine 250-Glutamic acid	Consider Nilotinib
L387M (3.8%)	Leucine 387-Methionine	Consider Dasatinib or Nilotinib
M244V (3.8%)	Methionine 244-Valine	Consider Dasatinib or Nilotinib
M351T (3.8%)	Methionine 351-Threonine	Consider Dasatinib or Nilotinib
F317L (3.8%)	Phenylalanine 317-Leucine	Consider Nilotinib
Q252H (3.1%)	Glutamine 252-Histidine	Consider Nilotinib
D276G (2.3%)	Aspartic acid 276-Glycine	Consider Dasatinib or Nilotinib
F311I (1.5%)	Phenylalanine 311-Isoleucine	Consider Dasatinib or Nilotinib
F359I (1.5%)	Phenylalanine 359-Isoleucine	Unknown
E279K (0.8%)	Glutamic acid 279-Lysine	Consider Dasatinib
E255V (0.8%)	Glutamic acid 255-Valine	Consider Dasatinib or Nilotinib
L248R (0.8%)	Leucine 248-Arginine	Unknown
V299L (1%)	Valine 299-Leucine	Consider Nilotinib

(B)

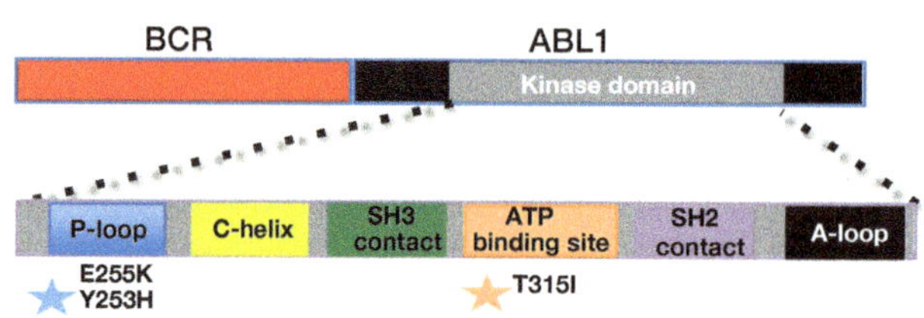

FIGURE 2-72: ***BCR-ABL1*** **mutations: Incorporating tyrosine kinase inhibitors into the cytotoxic chemotherapy regimens of patients with Ph+ ALL is the standard of care for newly diagnosed patients. Most patients with Ph+ chromosome are highly susceptible to develop TKI-resistant mutations, and therefore treatment responses are not sustained. Resistance is frequently caused by point mutations in the ABL kinase domain of BCR-ABL. The specific mutations that have been reported in ALL are listed in Panel A, with the most common mutations identified in bold. These three mutations account for approximtely 70% of cases. Panel B is a representation of the BCR/ABL1 fusion that depicts key structural motifs within the kinase domain and the location of mutations within the key motifs: P-loop indicates phosphate binding loop; C-helix participates in the active and inhibited state of the kinase domain; ATP-binding site is where ATP is captured and hydrolyzed to ADP; SH2 contact and SH3 contact indicates contact regions with SH2 and SH3 domain-containing proteins; A-loop indicates the activation loop.**

ADP, adenosine diphosphate; ATP, adenosine triphosphate; B-ALL, B acute lymphoblastic leukemia.

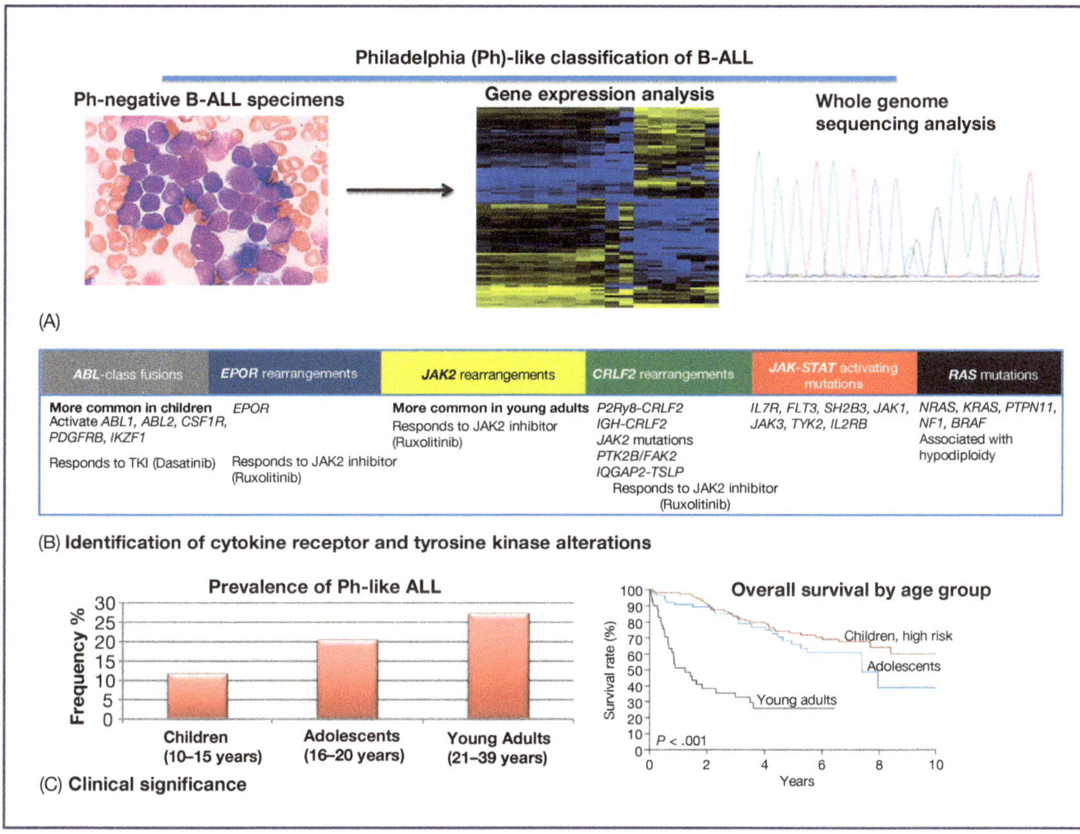

FIGURE 2-73: Philadelphia-like B-ALL. This important biologic subtype of precursor B-ALL is characterized by a gene expression profile that is similar to that of patients with Ph-positive ALL, but it does not contain the BCR-ABL1 fusion protein expressed from the t(9;22)(q34;q11.2). The so-called Ph-like or *BCR-ABL1*-like cases have been identified in both children and young adults. (A) B-lymphoblasts from patients with precursor B-ALL were analyzed by gene expression profiling and next-generation sequencing. A hierarchical clustering dendogram identified a gene expression pattern that was similar to Ph-positive ALL and dissimilar from other subtypes of B-ALL. Detailed genome sequencing was performed on a subset of cases to identify recurrent genetic abnormalities in the Ph-like cases. (B) 91% of the patient specimens had genomic mutations that altered distinct kinase signaling pathways. The signaling pathways included ABL-class fusions, the erythropoietin receptor (EPOR) or Janus kinase 2 (JAK2) rearrangements, cytokine receptor-like 2 (CRLF2) rearrangements, other JAK-STAT activating mutations, and other alterations in the Ras pathway. (C) The identification of Ph-like ALL has significant clinical relevance. The prevalence of the Ph-like ALL increases with age, and the overall survival rates are inferior in all age groups, as compared to patients without the Ph-like ALL. Utilizing tyrosine kinase inhibitors in these cases may improve the outcome for these patients.

ALL, acute lymphoblastic leukemia; B-ALL, B acute lymphoblastic leukemia.

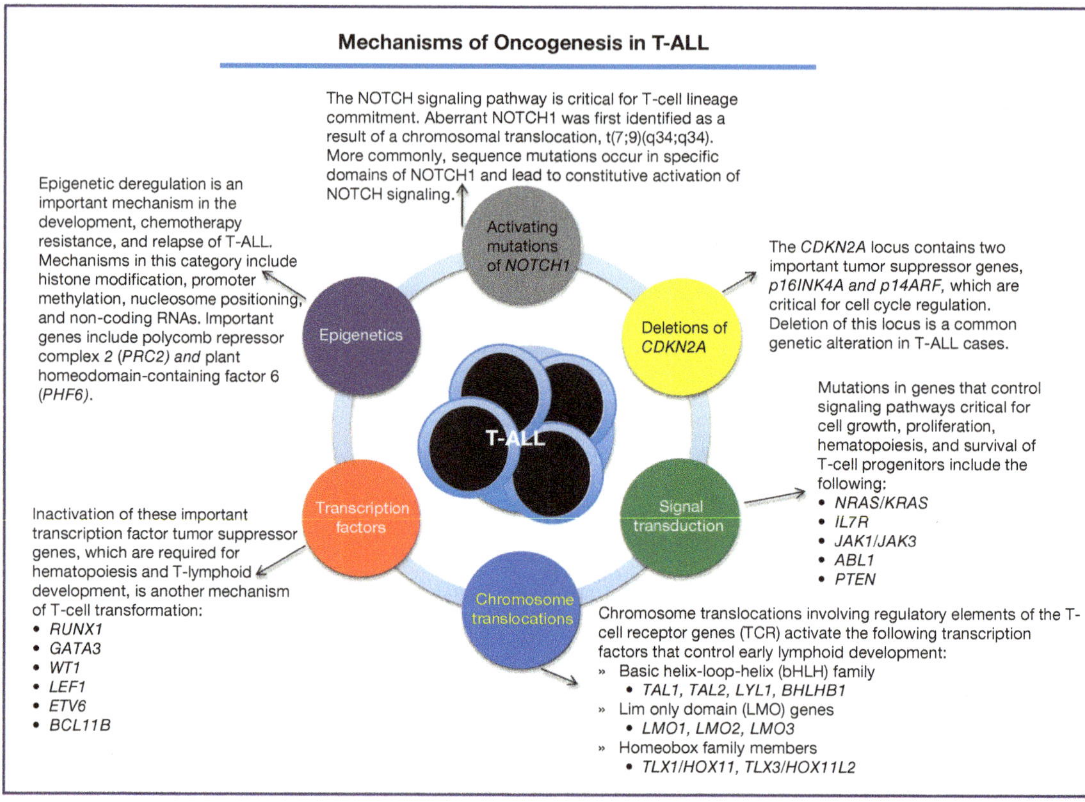

FIGURE 2-74: Mechanisms of oncogenesis in T-ALL: The genetic changes that contribute to the development of T-ALL are complex and include chromosome rearrangements, sequence mutations that target critical cellular growth pathways, and deletions and/or mutations of transcription factor tumor suppressor pathways, as well as epigentic deregulation. Activating mutations in *NOTCH1* have been identified in more than 50% of T-ALL cases, and deletions of the *CDKN2A* locus are present in more than 70% of T-ALL cases. Thus, these two genes account for the majority of the genetic alterations in T-ALL cases.

T-ALL, T acute lymphoblastic leukemia.

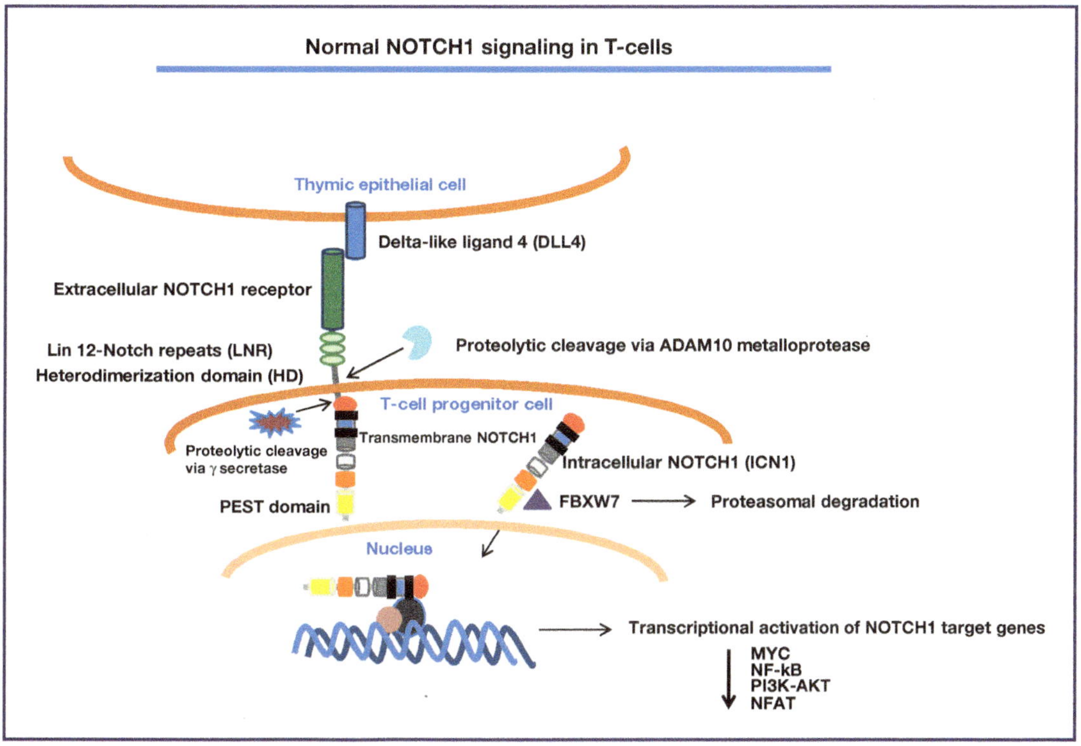

FIGURE 2-75: Physiologic notch signaling. The NOTCH1 receptor is a ligand-activated transcription factor that transmits extracellular signals at the cell membrane to the nucleus and causes changes in gene expression of multiple cell growth processes. In T-lymphocytes, the NOTCH1 signal is essential for T-cell lineage commitment. Thymic epithelial cells express Delta-like ligand 4 (DLL4) (blue) and activate the NOTCH1 receptor in T-lineage progenitor cells. The extracellular segment of NOTCH1 (green) contains the ligand–receptor interaction, a region of three Lin 12-Notch repeats (LNRs), and a heterodimerization (HD) domain. The intracellular segment of NOTCH1 (ICN1) contains several different domains: Recombination-signal-sequence binding protein for Jk genes (RBP-Jk)-associated molecule (RAM) (red), two nuclear localization sequences (NSL)(black bars), an ankyrin repeat region (blue), the repression/activation domain (RE/AC)(gray), C-terminal domain with a glutamine-rich region (OPA) (white), C-terminal transactivation domain (TAD)(orange), and a proline-, glutamate-serine-, and threonine-rich region (PEST) (yellow). The LNR-HD domain connects the extracellular NOTCH1 receptor with the intracellular segment. DLL4 ligand binding induces a conformational change in the NOTCH1 receptor, and results in two key proteolytic cleavage events: 1) cleavage of the HD domain by the metalloprotease ADAM10; and 2) cleavage of ICN1 by gamma secretase. These cleavages free the intracellular NOTCH1 from the membrane, and translocate it to the nucleus and form a transcription complex to activate NOTCH1 target genes. The NOTCH1 signal is terminated by degradation in the proteasome. This event is coordinated by the F-box protein (FBXW7-SCF ubiquitin ligase complex), which recognizes the PEST domain and targets ICN1 for proteasomal degradation in the nucleus.

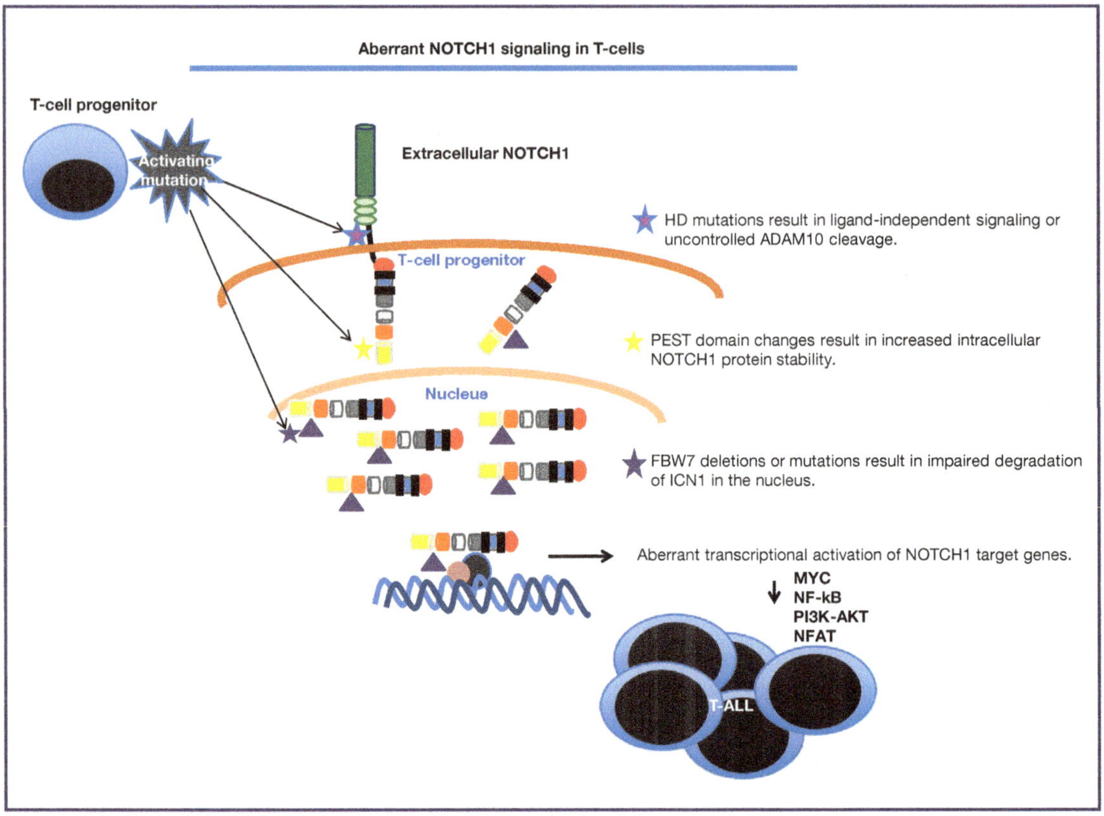

FIGURE 2-76: **Aberrant notch signaling. Activating mutations of *NOTCH1* have been identified in more than 50% of human T-ALL specimens. The most common class of *NOTCH1* mutations occurs in the HD domain and results in either ligand-independent activation of the *NOTCH1* receptor or increased ADAM10 or γ secretase cleavage. Other *NOTCH1* mutations result in truncation of the PEST domain, which results in increased ICN1 protein stability and impaired proteasomal degradation in the nucleus. Additionally, mutations or deletions in FBXW7 also result in increased ICN1 stability and impaired degradation in the nucleus, and thus aberrant *NOTCH1* signaling.**

T-ALL, T acute lymphoblastic leukemia.

Selected References

Aplan PD, Lombardi DP, Ginsberg AM, et al. Disruption of the human SCL locus by "illegitimate" V-(D)-J recombinase activity. *Science*. 1990;250:1426–1429.

Coustan-Smith E, Mullighan CG, Onciu M, et al. Early T-cell precursor leukaemia: a subtype of very high-risk acute lymphoblastic leukaemia. *Lancet Oncol*. 2009;10(2):147–156.

Dastugue N, Suciu S, Plat G, et al. Hyperdiploidy with 58-66 chromosomes in childhood B-acute lymphoblastic leukemia is highly curable: 58951 CLG-EORTC results. *Blood*. 2013;121:2415–2423.

Den Boer ML, van Slegtenhorst M, De Menezes RX, et al. A subtype of childhood acute lymphoblastic leukaemia with poor treatment outcome: a genome-wide classification study. *Lancet Oncol*. 2009;10: 125–134.

Hatano M, Roberts CW, Minden M, et al. Deregulation of a homeobox gene, HOX11, by the t(10;14) in T cell leukemia. *Science*. 1991;253:79–82.

Holmfeldt L, Wei L, Diaz-Flores E, et al. The genomic landscape of hypodiploid acute lymphoblastic leukemia. *Nat Genet*. 2013;45:242–252.

Joshi I, Yoshida T, Jena N, et al. Loss of Ikaros DNA-binding function confers integrin-dependent survival on pre-B cells and progression to acute lymphoblastic leukemia. *Nat Immunol.* 2014:15;294–304.

Kennedy MA, Gonzalez-Sarmiento R, Kees UR, et al. *HOX11*, a homeobox-containing T-cell oncogene on human chromosome 10q24. *Proc Natl Acad Sci USA.* 1991;88:8900–8904.

Martinelli G, Iacobucci I, Storlazzi CT, et al. IKZF1 (Ikaros) deletions in *BCR-ABL1*-positive acute lymphoblastic leukemia are associated with short disease-free survival and high rate of cumulative incidence of relapse: a GIMEMA AL WP report. *J Clin Oncol.* 2009;27:5202–5207.

Moorman AV, Harrison CJ, Buck GA, et al. Karyotype is an independent prognostic factor in adult acute lymphoblastic leukemia (ALL): analysis of cytogenetic data from patients treated on the Medical Research Council (MRC) UKALLXII/Eastern Cooperative Oncology Group (ECOG) 2993 trial. *Blood.* 2007;109:3189–3197.

Mullighan CG, Goorha S, Radtke I, et al. Genome-wide analysis of genetic alterations in acute lymphoblastic leukemia. *Nature.* 2007;446:758–764.

Mullighan CG, Su X, Zhang J, et al. Deletion of IKZF1 and prognosis in acute lymphoblastic leukemia. *N Eng J Med.* 2009;360:470–480.

Nutt SL, Heavey B, Rolink A, et al. Commitment to the B-lymphoid lineage depends on the transcription factor Pax5. *Nature.* 1999;401:556–562.

Pui CH, Raimondi SC, Hancock ML, et al. Immunologic, cytogenetic, and clinical characterization of childhood acute lymphoblastic leukemia with the t(1;19) (q23; p13) or its derivative. *J Clin Oncol.* 1994;12:2601–2606.

Ribeiro RC, Abromowitch M, Raimondi SC, et al. Clinical and biologic hallmarks of the Philadelphia chromosome in childhood acute lymphoblastic leukemia. *Blood.* 1987;70:948–953.

Roberts KG, Li Y, Payne-Turner D, et al. Targetable kinase-activating lesions in Ph-like acute lymphoblastic leukemia. *N Engl J Med.* 2014;371:1005–1015.

Roberts KG, Pei D, Campana D, et al. Outcomes of children with *BCR-ABL1*-like acute lymphoblastic leukemia treated with risk-directed therapy based on the levels of minimal residual disease. *J Clin Oncol.* 2014;32:3012–3020.

Romana SP, Poirel H, Leconiat M, et al. High frequency of t(12;21) in childhood B-lineage acute lymphoblastic leukemia. *Blood.* 1995;86:4263–4269.

Schwickert TA, Tagoh H, Gultekin S, et al. Stage-specific control of early B cell development by the transcription factor Ikaros. *Nat Immunol.* 2014;15:283–293.

Trinquand A, Tanguy-Schmidt A, Ben Abdelali R, et al. Toward a NOTCH/FBXW7/RAS/PTEN-based oncogenetic risk classification of adult T-cell acute lymphoblastic leukemia: a group for research on adult acute lymphoblastic leukemia study. *J Clin Oncol.* 2013;31:4333–4342.

Van Vlierberghe P, Ambesi-Implombato A, De Keersmaecker K, et al. Prognostic relevance of integrated genetic profiling in adult T-cell acute lymphoblastic leukemia. *Blood.* 2013;122(1):74–82.

Weng AP, Ferrando AA, Lee W, et al. Activating mutations of NOTCH1 in human T cell acute lymphoblastic leukemia. *Science.* 2004;306:269–271.

Zhang J, Ding L, Holmfeldt L, et al. The genetic basis of early T-cell precursor acute lymphoblastic leukemia. *Nature.* 2012;481:157–163.

3

Therapy

Management of Early Crisis

Initial diagnostic workup includes obtaining complete blood counts (CBCs), peripheral blood smear to be reviewed by an expert, peripheral blood flow cytometry, bone marrow aspiration and biopsy, and evaluation for disseminated intravascular coagulation (DIC) and tumor lysis syndrome (TLS).

HYPERLEUKOCYTOSIS

Heather J. Male and Tara Lin

Management of Early Crisis

Hyperleukocytosis is present upon presentation in

- up to 20% of acute myeloid leukemias (AMLs)
- up to 30% of acute lymphoblastic leukemias (ALLs)

Hyperleukocytosis is most commonly seen in myeloid leukemias due to reduced pliability of the myeloid blast cells in the microcirculation. In AML, leukostasis appears to be mediated in large part by increased vascular adhesion by blasts through up-regulation of adhesion molecules such as NCAM and CD11c on the surface of blasts and E-selectin, ICAM, and VCAM on the surface of endothelial cells in the setting of AML.

Within the first 7 days, the risk of mortality for patients with leukostasis is up to 20%. The following scoring system identifies patients with symptoms attributable to leukostasis and at risk for early mortality.

Table 3-1 Symptoms of probable and highly probable leukostasis

PROBABLE LEUKOSTASIS	HIGHLY PROBABLE LEUKOSTASIS
• Symptoms with activity, limited function • Dyspnea with exertion but not at rest • Fatigue limiting normal activity • Mild vision changes, headache, dizziness • Severe tinnitus	• Marked reduction of normal function due to symptoms • Pulmonary symptoms at rest, oxygen required • Impaired neurologic function including CNS hemorrhage, somnolence, confusion, vision impairment, ischemia

Source: From Novotny JR, Müller-Beißenhirtz H, Herget-Rosenthal S, et al. Grading of symptoms in hyperleukocytic leukaemia: a clinical model for the role of different blast types and promyelocytes in the development of leukostasis syndrome. *Eur J Haematol.* 2005;74:501–510.
CNS, central nervous system.

Given the association of high mortality with leukostasis, it is recommended that patients with hyperleukocytosis with symptoms of leukostasis be managed in an intensive care unit (ICU) until definitive treatment is initiated and the leukemic blast burden has been lowered.

Transfusion with packed red blood cells should be avoided as this increases blood viscosity, but liberal use of platelets is recommended due to the risk of intracranial hemorrhage, coagulopathy, and falsely elevated platelet count due to blast fragments mistaken for platelets on automated

CBCs. Assessment of hypoxemia is best done by peripheral pulse oximetry, as pO_2 is often falsely low in arterial blood gas sampling due to blasts consuming the oxygen in vitro, though this can be minimized by placing samples on ice and performing the test immediately.

Treatment of Hyperleukocytosis

In patients identified as having symptomatic leukostasis, options for treatment include cytoreduction with chemotherapy, hydroxyurea, and/or leukapheresis. Chemotherapy is the most effective and beneficial treatment modality. However, this requires the patient to have a definitive diagnosis, and this is not immediately available at presentation for most patients. Hydroxyurea and/or leukapheresis are used as a bridge until definitive diagnosis can be made and induction chemotherapy started.

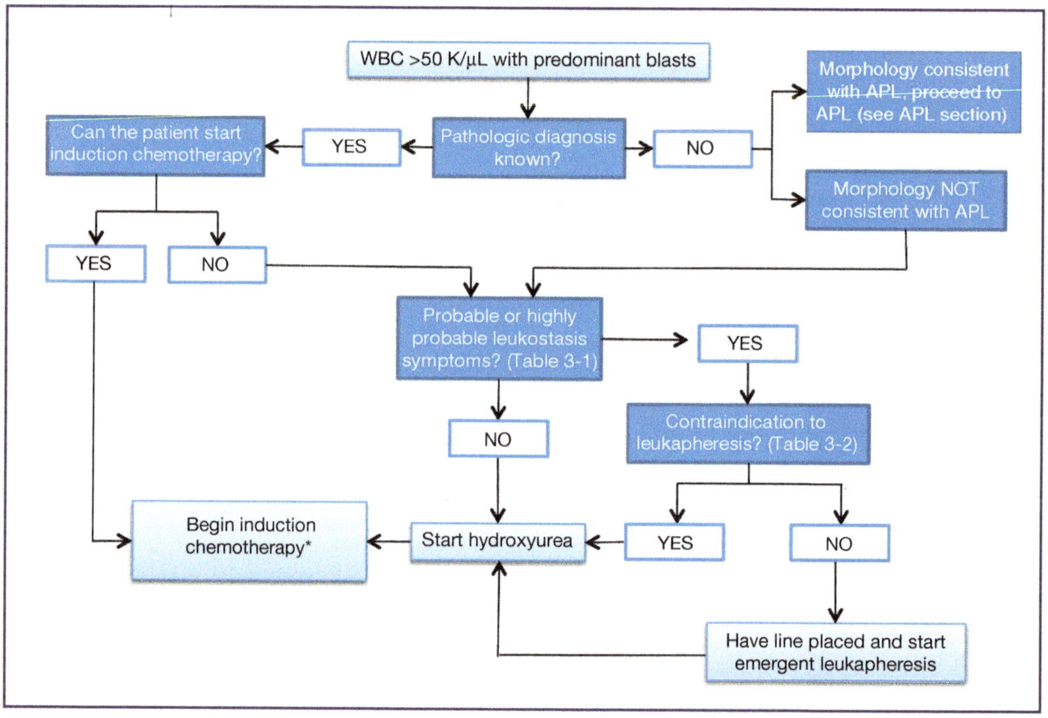

FIGURE 3-1: Algorithm for hyperleukocytosis with predominant blasts.

*If >12 hour delay to start chemotherapy, reassess for leukostasis symptoms and consider additional hydrea and/or leukapheresis until chemotherapy initiated.

APL, acute promyelocytic leukemia; WBC, white blood cell.

Hydroxyurea is the recommended bridging agent if symptoms of leukostasis are mild, and the use of leukapheresis is limited to those with probable or highly probable leukostasis symptoms. Although there is no literature to support the survival benefit of leukapheresis, most experts believe it to be an effective modality to rapidly reduce leukemic blast burden in patients having leukostasis symptoms. Use of leukapheresis is not available at all institutions, and it requires placement of a large catheter able to rapidly pull and return blood to the patient, such as the ones usually used for hemodialysis. Contraindications for leukapheresis include diagnosis of acute promyelocytic leukemia, severe coagulopathy, and hemodynamic/cardiovascular instability.

Table 3-2	Contraindications to leukapheresis
Cardiovascular comorbidities	
Hemodynamic instability	
Coagulation disturbances	
Acute promyelocytic leukemia	

Source: From Röllig C, Ehninger G. How I treat hyperleukocytosis in acute myeloid leukemia. *Blood.* 2015;125(21):3246–3252.

Selected References

Novotny JR, Müller-Beißenhirtz H, Herget-Rosenthal S, et al. Grading of symptoms in hyperleukocytic leukaemia: a clinical model for the role of different blast types and promyelocytes in the development of leukostasis syndrome. *Eur J Haematol.* 2005;74:501–510.

Porcu P, Cripe LD, Ng EW, et al. Hyperleukocytic leukemias and leukostasis: a review of pathophysiology, clinical presentation and management. *Leuk Lymphoma.* 2000;39(1–2):1.

Röllig C, Ehninger G. How I treat hyperleukocytosis in acute myeloid leukemia. *Blood.* 2015; 125(21):3246–3252.

TUMOR LYSIS AND CYTOKINE RELEASE SYNDROMES

Ashkan Emadi and Judith E. Karp

Tumor Lysis Syndrome (TLS)

Patients at high risk for development of TLS include those with:

- Burkitt's leukemia/lymphoma
- Acute myeloid leukemia (AML) and acute lymphoblastic leukemia (ALL), particularly with white blood count (WBC) >50K/mcL
- T-cell ALL
- Extramedullary leukemia
- Small cell lung cancer
- Testicular cancers

Etiologic factors

Pretreatment	**Cytotoxic treatment**
Massive tumor burden	Rapid cell kill
Enzyme-rich cells	Cell necrosis
High cell turnover	

Clinical and laboratory manifestations

Hyperuricemia (uric acid >8 mg/dL)

Hyperphosphatemia (phosphorus >4.5 mg/dL)

Hyperkalemia (potassium >6 mmol/L)

Hypocalcemia (corrected calcium <7 mg/dL, ionized Ca <1.1)

Marked elevation of lactate dehydrogenase (LDH)

Acute kidney injury

Cardiac arrhythmias

Seizure/neuromuscular irritability

Management of TLS

- Expect tumor lysis with initiation of cytotoxic therapy, and be prepared for it.
- Start aggressive intravenous hydration with normal saline.
- Start allopurinol, a xanthine oxidase inhibitor, to decrease production of uric acid.
- Start rasburicase if uric acid is more than 8 mg/dL.
    - Rasburicase is a recombinant uricase (urate oxidase) enzyme that has been approved for the prevention and treatment of tumor lysis syndrome in patients receiving chemotherapy for hematologic and solid neoplasms.
    - Rasburicase can cause severe hypersensitivity reactions including anaphylaxis.
    - Due to production of reactive oxygen species, rasburicase should not be administered to patients with glucose-6-phosphate dehydrogenase (G6PD) deficiency. Rasburicase should be immediately and permanently discontinued in patients developing hemolysis.
    - Rasburicase can result in methemoglobinemia in some patients.

- Rasburicase can enzymatically degrade uric acid in blood samples left at room temperature. Blood samples should be collected in prechilled tubes containing heparin and immediately be immersed and maintained in an ice water bath. Assay plasma samples within 4 hours of collection.

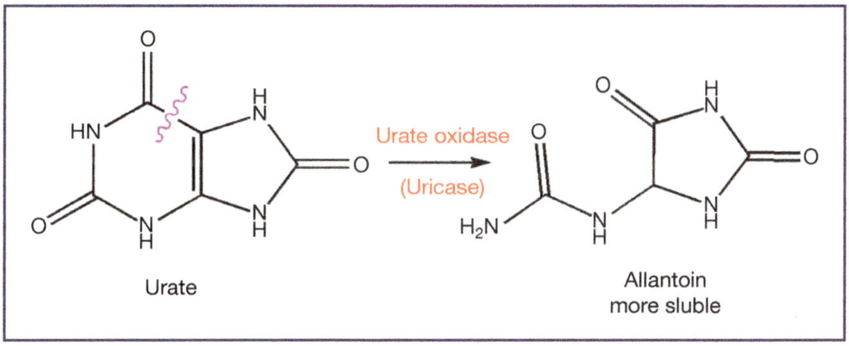

FIGURE 3-2: **Conversion of uric acid to allantoin catalyzed by rasburicase. In a randomized study of the use of allopurinol versus rasburicase for patients at risk for TLS, the mean serum uric acid levels decreased by 86%, to 1 mg/dL, at 4 hours in the rasburicase arm compared with 10.3 mg/dL in the allopurinol group.**

TLS, tumor lysis syndrome.

- Start phosphate binding drugs such as sevelamer to treat hyperphosphatemia.
- Monitor electrolytes, uric acid, and LDH every 6 to 8 hours in the first few days of initiation of chemotherapy.

Inflammatory/Cytokine Release Syndrome (CRS)

Cytokine release syndrome (CRS) can be a life-threatening condition that can occur after administration of chemotherapeutic antibodies, including:

- naked antibodies such as anti-CD20 rituximab, anti-CD52 alemtuzumab, and anti-CD3 OKT3,
- bispecific antibodies such as blinatumomab,
- adoptive T-cell therapies such as T-cells engineered to express chimeric receptor antigens (CARs) for neoplastic conditions, and
- infusion of haploidentical mononuclear cells to patients with refractory leukemia.

CRS is associated with elevated cytokines including IL-6, IFNγ, TNFα, IL-2, granulocyte macrophage–colony-stimulating factor (GM-CSF), IL-10, IL-8, and IL-5. Interleukin 6 (IL-6) is the key mediator in the pathophysiology of CRS.

Table 3-3 Clinical manifestation of CRS

ORGAN SYSTEM	SYMPTOMS
Constitutional	Fever, chills, fatigue, anorexia, myalgias, arthalgias
Neurologic	Headache, altered mental status, delirium, difficulty finding words, aphasia, hallucinations, tremor, abnormal gait, seizures
Skin	Rash
Gastrointestinal	Nausea, vomiting, diarrhea
Lung	Tachypnea, hypoxemia, ARDS
Cardiovascular	Tachycardia, hypotension, widened pulse pressure, cardiomyopathy
Kidney	Azotemia, elevated creatinin
Liver	Transaminitis, hyperbilirubinemia

ARDS, acute respiratory distress syndrome; CRS, cytokine release syndrome.

Table 3-4	Grading system for CRS
GRADE	**TOXICITY**
Grade 1	Symptoms are not life-threatening and require symptomatic treatment only, such as fever, nausea, fatigue, headache, myalgias, and malaise
Grade 2	Symptoms require and respond to moderate intervention Oxygen requirement <40% or Hypotension responsive to fluids or low-dose of one vasopressor or Grade 2 organ toxicity
Grade 3	Symptoms require and respond to aggressive intervention Oxygen requirement ≥40% or Hypotension requiring high-dose or multiple vasopressors or Grade 3 organ toxicity or Grade 4 transaminitis
Grade 4	Life-threatening symptoms Requirement for ventilator support or Grade 4 organ toxicity (excluding transaminitis)
Grade 5	Death

CRS, cytokine release syndrome.

Management of CRS

Grade 1 and Grade 2 in the absence of comorbidities: Supportive care including treatment of febrile neutropenia, monitor fluid balance, antipyretic, and close monitoring of cardiac, renal, and hepatic function

Grade 2 with comorbidities and in older patients, Grade 3, and Grade 4: Aggressive supportive care plus tocilizumab ± corticosteroids

Anti-IL-6 antibodies

- Tocilizumab: Anti-IL6-receptor humanized IgG1κ monoclonal antibody blocks IL6 binding to soluble and membrance receptor
    - Approved for treatment of rheumatoid arthritis, juvenile idiopathic arthritis, and polyarticular juvenile rheumatoid arthritis.
    - It is an effective treatment for severe or life-threatening CRS at a dose of 4 mg/kg in adults and 8 mg/kg in children over 1 hour; repeat the dose if clinical improvement does not occur within 24 to 48 hours.
- Siltuximab: anti-IL6 (not used frequently)

Selected References

Coiffer B, Altman A, Pui CH, et al. Guidelines for the management of pediatric and adult tumor lysis syndrome: an evidence-based review. *J Clin Oncol.* 2008;26(16):2767–2778.

DeConti RC, Calabrese P. Use of allopurinol for prevention and control of hyperuricemia in patients with neoplastic disease. *N Engl J Med.* 1966;274:481–486.

Howard SC, Jones DP, Pui CH. The tumor lysis syndrome. *N Engl J Med.* 2011;364(19):1844–1854.

Jeha S, Kantarjian H, Irwin D, et al. Efficacy and safety of rasburicase, a recombinant urate oxidase (Elitek), in the management of malignancy-associated hyperuricemia in pediatric and adult patients: final results of a multicenter compassionate use trial. *Leukemia.* 2005;19:34–48.

Lee DW, Gardner R, Porter DL, et al. Current concepts in the diagnosis and management of cytokine release syndrome. *Blood*. 2014;124(2):188–195.

Zusman J, Brown DM, Nesbit ME, et al. Hyperphosphatemia, hyperphosphaturia and hypocalcemia in acute lymphoblastic leukemia. *N Engl J Med*. 1972;289:1335–1340.

FEBRILE NEUTROPENIA

Judith E. Karp

Principles of Antibiotic Therapy During Leukemia or Chemotherapy-Induced Neutropenia

- Recognition of:
  - commonly occurring pathogens
  - commonly infected sites
  - links between specific pathogens and specific sites
  - drug- and/or leukemia-related barrier breakdown (eg, oraUGI mucosa)
- Prompt initiation of broad-spectrum antibiotic coverage directed against the most common pathogenic organisms arising in the specific clinical setting and at the specific time during intensive chemotherapy (ie, Gram-negative bacteria, especially *Pseudomonas aeruginosa*, causing first posttherapy fever)
- Prevention of the development of multiple resistant organisms
- Continued antimicrobial coverage until the underlying lesion is corrected (ie, by the return of functional neutrophils and monocytes)

Guidelines for Prevention and Management of Infections in Neutropenic Hosts

Prophylaxis: Start day 0 or when neutrophils <500 × 10^9/L, maintain throughout neutropenia

Quinolone (prevent Gram-negative sepsis)

Antiviral (prevent herpes simplex virus reactivation)

Echinocandin or azole (prevent yeast or filamentous fungal infection)

Bactrim, dapsone, atovaquone, or pentamidine (anti-*Pneumocystis carinii*, PCP) for lymphoid disease or immunosuppressive therapies

First infectious fever: Gram-negative, anaerobe, some Gram-positive bacteria

Carbapenem (imipenem–cilastin, meropenem) or antipseudomonal penicillin (piperacillin–tazobactam)

Add vancomycin for oral mucositis or other sites of potential Gram-positive infection

Reasons for Increased Incidence of Gram-Positive and Fungal Infectious Complications During Induced Neutropenia

- Effective empiric antibacterial coverage of early infections due to serious Gram-negative infections (eg, *Pseudomonas aeruginosa*)
- Heightened ability to deliver dose-intensive chemotherapy with resultant increase in skin, oropharyngeal, and gastrointestinal mucosal cytotoxicity
- Increased use of indwelling catheters
- Increased use of parenteral nutrition
- Development of resistance to vancomycin and β-lactam antibiotics by Gram-positive organisms

- Concurrent immunosuppression (particularly important with fungal infections)
- Graft vs. host disease (GVHD) in bone marrow transplant recipients

Management of Refractory or Recurrent Fever

Progressive disease (no response in 48 to 72 hours of starting coverage for first fever)

Add vancomycin if not already started or linezolid for vancomycin-resistant enterococci (VRE)

Add metronidazole or oral vancomycin for *Clostridium dificile*

If there is rapid clinical deterioration, add aminoglycoside to augment Gram-negative coverage

If there is suspicion of fungal infection (5%–10% of first fevers), change to liposomal Amphotericin or increase dose of azole or echinocandin

Recrudescent fever (more than 72 hours after starting coverage for first fever)

Assess serum galactomannan, chest CT (without contrast)

Augment antifungal coverage (liposomal Amphotericin, increase dose of echinocandin or azole)

Add Bactrim for suspicion of *Stenotrophomonas* or aminoglycoside for rapid clinical deterioration

Carry out bronchoscopy if progressive symptoms of fungal pneumonia ensue

Add metronidazole or oral vancomycin for *Clostridium difficile*

Invasive Fungal Infections Among Patients With Newly Diagnosed Acute Myeloid Leukemia Postinduction Chemotherapy

Risk Factors for Development of Fungal Infections

Invasive Fungus (Mold)	Invasive Candidiasis
Female	Mucositis
Creatinine ≥1.5 mg/dL	Baseline organ dysfunction

MORTALITY PREDICTORS

	UNIVARIATE ANALYSIS	MULTIVARIATE ANALYSIS
Age ≥50 years	<0.0001	<0.001
Female	0.03	0.005
Secondary AML (MDS/AML)	0.03	
Creatinine ≥1.5 mg/dL	0.01	
AST and/or ALT >3X normal	0.05	
Total bilirubin ≥2.0 mg/dL	0.007	
Baseline organ dysfunction	<0.001	<0.001

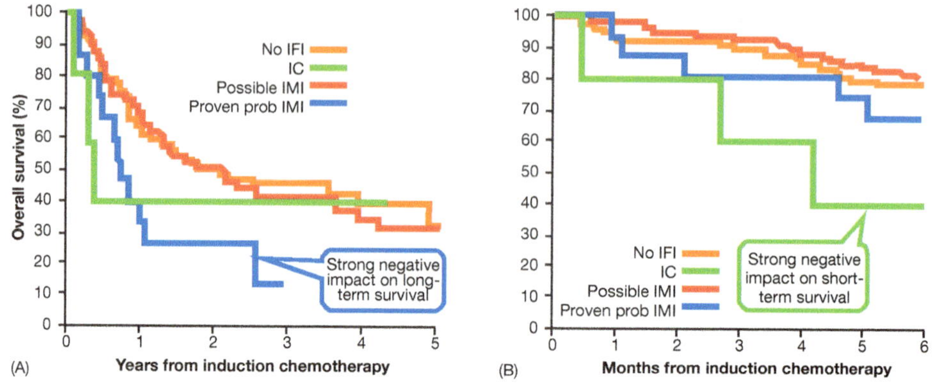

Number at risk

	(A)							(B)						
No IFI	131	81	48	27	21	12	6	131	129	121	118	112	104	95
IC	15	6	4	1	0	0	0	15	14	13	12	12	11	10
Possible IMI	103	56	36	28	15	10	4	103	97	92	89	85	78	74
Proven possible IMI	5	1	1	1	1	1	0	5	4	4	3	3	2	2

FIGURE 3-3: Impact of invasive fungal infections on overall survival.

Source: **From Neofytos D, Lu K, Hatfield-Seung A, et al. Epidemiology, outcomes, and risk factors of invasive fungal infections in adult patients with acute myelogenous leukemia after induction chemotherapy. *Diag Microbial Infect Dis*. 2013;75:144–149.**

IC, invasive candidiasis; IFI, invasive fungal infection; IMI, invasive mold infection.

Selected References

Baden LR, Bensinger B, Angarone M, et al. NCCN clinical practice guidelines in oncology: prevention and treatment of cancer-related infections. Version 1. *J Natl Comp Canc Netw*. 2012;10:1412–1445.

Karp JE, Merz WG, Hendricksen C, et al. Orla norfloxacin for prevention of Gram-negative bacterial infections in patients with acute leukemia and granulocytopenia. *Ann Int Med*. 1987;106:1–7.

Neofytos D, Lu K, Hatfield-Seung A, et al. Epidemiology, outcomes, and risk factors of invasive fungal infections in adult patients with acute myelogenous leukemia after induction chemotherapy. *Diag Microbial Infect Dis*. 2013;75:144–149.

Pizzo PH, Robichaud KJ, Gill FA, et al. Empiric antibiotics for cancer patients with prolonged fever and granulocytopenia. *Am J Med*. 1982;72:101–112.

Schimpff S, Satterlee W, Young VM, et al. Empiric therapy with carbenicillin and gentamicin for febrile patients with cancer and granulocytopenia. *N Engl J Med*. 1971;284:1061–1064.

Treatment of AML in Adults

AML TREATMENT IN YOUNGER PATIENTS

Joshua F. Zeidner and Matthew C. Foster

Table 3-5 European LeukemiaNet (ELN) risk groups for AML

RISK GROUP	CYTOGENETIC/MOLECULAR FEATURES
Favorable	t(8;21); RUNX1-RUNX1T1*
	inv(16) or t(16;16); CBFB-MYH11*
	Normal karyotype + NPM1 mutation without FLT3-ITD
	Normal karyotype + CEBPA double mutation
Intermediate-1	Normal karyotype + NPM1 mutation + FLT3-ITD mutation
	Normal karyotype + NPM1 wild-type + FLT3-ITD mutation
	Normal karyotype + NPM1 wild-type + FLT3-ITD wild-type
Intermediate-2	t(9;11); MLLT3-mixed lineage leukemia (MLL)
	Cytogenetic abnormalities not classified as favorable or adverse
Adverse	inv(3); RPN1-EVI1
	t(6;9); DEK-NUP214
	t(v;11); MLL rearranged other than t(9;11)
	–5 or del(5q)
	–7
	Abnormal(17p)- signifying TP53 abnormality
	Complex karyotype[+]

*C-Kit mutations have been shown to confer a worse prognosis in patients with core-binding factor AML [t(8;21); inv(16); t(16;16)]. Although these patients are still classified as favorable-risk as per ELN criteria, other scores such as the NCCN Guidelines classify these patients as intermediate risk.
[+]Complex karyotype = 3 or more chromosomal abnormalities in absence of one of WHO-designated recurring translocations or inversions such as t(15;17); t(8;21); inv(16); t(16;16); t(9;11); t(v;11); t(6;9); inv(3); t(3;3).
Source: Adapted from Dohner H, Estey EH, Amadori S, et al. Diagnosis and management of acute myeloid leukemia in adults: recommendations from an international expert panel, on behalf of the European LeukemiaNet. *Blood.* 2010;115(3):453–474.
AML, acute myeloid leukemia; FLT3-ITD, FMS-like tyrosine kinase 3 internal tandem duplication; MLL, mixed lineage leukemia; NPM1, nucleophosmine 1.

- Clinical trials are imperative for front-line induction therapy in all newly diagnosed AML patients (Figure 3-4). Newly diagnosed AML patients should be promptly referred to tertiary care cancer centers with expertise in the management of acute leukemia, and careful consideration of clinical trials should be made.
- In the absence of clinical trials, 7 + 3 (cytarabine 100 mg/m^2 daily continuous infusion IV days 1–7, daunorubicin 45–90 mg/m^2 daily IV days 1–3 or idarubicin 12 mg/m^2 daily IV days 1–3) remains the standard and most commonly used regimen in the United States.
- Patients with favorable and intermediate-risk cytogenetics have improved outcomes with high doses of daunorubicin (ie, 90 mg/m^2). A recent update of the original E1900 Eastern Cooperative Oncology Group randomized clinical trial of 7 + 3 with high dose daunorubicin versus low dose (45 mg/m^2) suggests that patients with adverse-risk cytogenetics may also confer benefit from high dose daunorubicin on adjusted analyses. Complete remission (CR; see Table 3-6) rates with 7 + 3 depend on many factors such as age, performance status, ELN risk, and secondary versus de novo AML. In general, CR rates with 7 + 3 are approximately 80% to 90%, 60% to 75%, and 40% to 50% in favorable, intermediate, and poor-risk patients, respectively.
- Unfortunately, the majority of patients who achieve a CR with 7 + 3 (and other conventional chemotherapy induction regimens) will ultimately relapse.

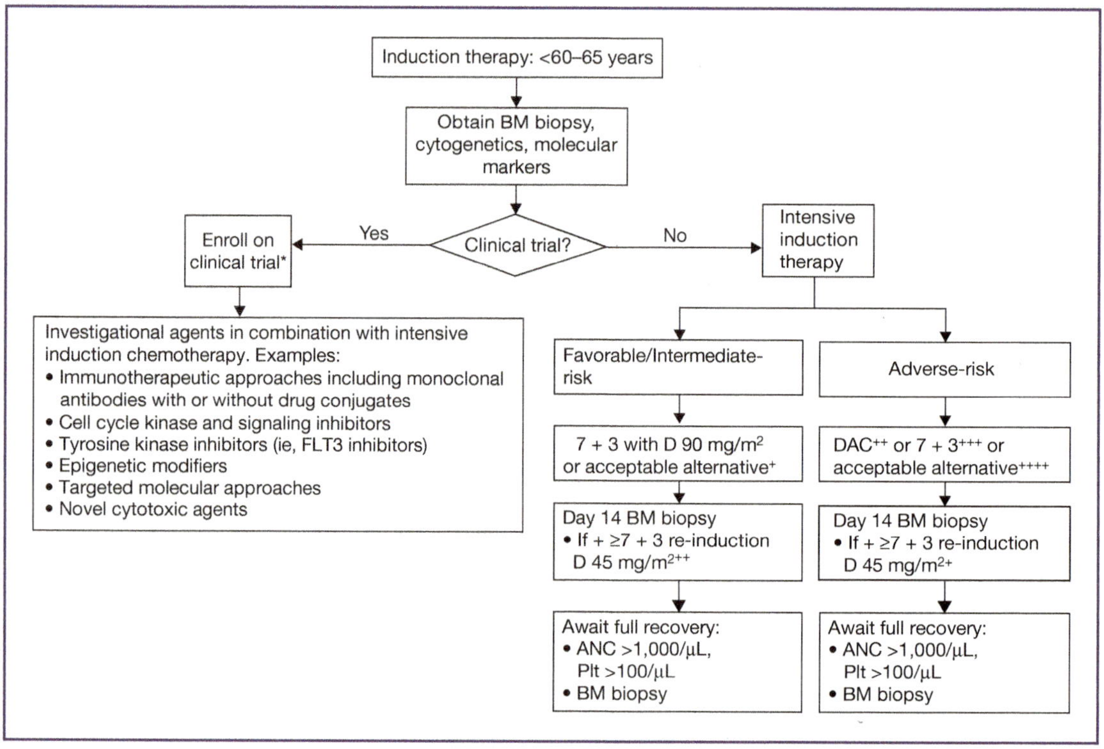

FIGURE 3-4: Treatment diagram for newly diagnosed adult patients with AML.

*All newly diagnosed younger (ie, <60–65 years) AML patients should be considered for clinical trials evaluating novel agents. In particular, patients with nonfavorable risk cytogenetics (ie, intermediate and adverse risk) should be highly prioritized for clinical trials. Examples of promising classes of agents being investigated in AML include immunotherapeutic approaches such as IMiDs (Thalidomide derivatives), checkpoint receptor inhibitors, monoclonal antibody-drug conjugates, and chimeric antigen receptor (CAR) T-cell therapies.

+Acceptable alternatives for 7 + 3 in favorable/intermediate-risk patients include DAC++ (daunorubicin 60 mg/m^2 IV days 1–3, cytarabine 200 mg/m^2 continuous infusion IV days 1–7, cladribine 5 mg/m^2 IV days 1–5), high-dose cytarabine-containing regimens such as IA (cytarabine 1.5 gm/m^2/day IV continuous infusion IV days 1 to 4, idarubicin 12 mg/m^2 IV days 4–6), and timed-sequential therapy regimens such as AcDVP16 (cytarabine 667 mg/m^2/day continuous infusion IV days 1–3, daunorubicin 45 mg/m^2 IV days 1–3, etoposide 400 mg/m^2 IV days 8–10).

++Although there is a lack of grade 1 evidence that reinduction in patients with residual leukemia on day 14 improves overall outcomes, standard recommendations include reinduction with either 7 + 3 (cytarabine 100 mg/m^2/day IV continuous infusion days 1–7, daunorubicin 45 mg/m^2 IV days 1–3) or 5 + 2 (cytarabine 100 mg/m^2/day IV continuous infusion days 1–5, daunorubicin 45 mg/m^2 IV days 1–2) or high-dose cytarabine (in patients with cardiomyopathy) for patients with residual leukemia (variably defined as BM blasts ≥5% with or without cellularity ≥10%–20%) on day 14 BM biopsy. Patients receiving DAC or other alternative regimens do not receive reinduction based on a day 14 BM biopsy.

+++These patients should be treated with standard-dose anthracyclines such as daunorubicin 45 to 60 mg/m^2 or idarubicin 12 mg/m^2 in conjunction with cytarabine 100 mg/m^2/day continuous infusion (ie, 7 + 3) with or without cladribine (ie, DAC). These patients do poorly with conventional chemotherapy regimens and should be highly prioritized for investigational agents. A recent adjusted analysis suggests that patients with adverse-risk cytogenetics may confer benefit from high dose daunorubicin (90 mg/m^2).

++++Acceptable alternatives to DAC or 7 + 3 in adverse-risk AML patients include IA, AcDVP16, and other similar intensive induction regimens.

AML, acute myeloid leukemia; ANC, absolute neutrophil count; BM, bone marrow; D, daunorubicin; FLT3, FMS-like tyrosine kinase 3; Plt, platelet.

Table 3-6 AML response criteria

RESPONSE CATEGORY	BONE MARROW FINDINGS	PERIPHERAL BLOOD FINDINGS	CLINICAL OR RADIOGRAPHIC FINDINGS	GENETIC OR MOLECULAR FINDINGS
Complete Remission (CR)	Blasts <5%; no blasts with Auer rods	ANC >1,000/μL, platelets >100,000/μL	Independent of RBC transfusions; no extramedullary leukemia	n.a.
CR With Incomplete Recovery (CRi)	Blasts <5%; no blasts with Auer rods	Either residual neutropenia (<1,000/μL) or thrombocytopenia (<100,000/μL)	Independent of RBC transfusions; no extramedullary leukemia	n.a.
Partial Remission (PR)	Both absolute bone marrow blast percentage 5%–25% AND decrease of blast percentage 50% relative to pretreatment bone marrow	ANC >1,000/μL, platelets >100,000/μL	Independent of RBC transfusions; no extramedullary leukemia	n.a.
Cytogenetic CR (CRc)	Blasts <5%; no blasts with Auer rods	Criteria for CR or CRi	Independent of RBC transfusions; no extramedullary leukemia	Reversion to normal karyotype in at least 20 metaphase bone marrow cells (if pretreatment karyotype abnormal)
Treatment Failure–Resistant Disease (RD)	Failure to achieve CR or CRi, with evidence of persistent leukemia in peripheral blood or bone marrow		Patient survived ≥7 days following completion of initial treatment	n.a.
Treatment Failure–Death in Aplasia	Aplastic or hypocellular marrow (examined within 7 days of death) without evidence of leukemia	Persistent cytopenias (RBC transfusion dependence, neutropenia, or thrombocytopenia)	Death ≥7 days following completion of initial treatment	n.a.
Treatment Failure–Death From Indeterminate Cause	Marrow examination unavailable	No blasts	Death during or within 7 days of completion of therapy (or ≥7 days following completion of initial therapy but without available bone marrow examination)	n.a.
Relapse	Blasts ≥5%	Reappearance of circulating blasts	Development of extramedullary leukemia	n.a.

Note that Molecular CR (CRm) has been proposed though no standard definition exists. Certain criteria are most applicable to particular clinical trials: CRi is relevant in clinical trials of double induction strategies and novel agents that are continued regardless of recovery; PR is most relevant in phase 1 and 2 trials.

Source: Adapted from Dohner H, Estey EH, Amadori S, et al. Diagnosis and management of acute myeloid leukemia in adults: recommendations from an international expert panel, on behalf of the European LeukemiaNet. *Blood.* 2010;115(3):453–474.

AML, acute myeloid leukemia; RBC, red blood cell.

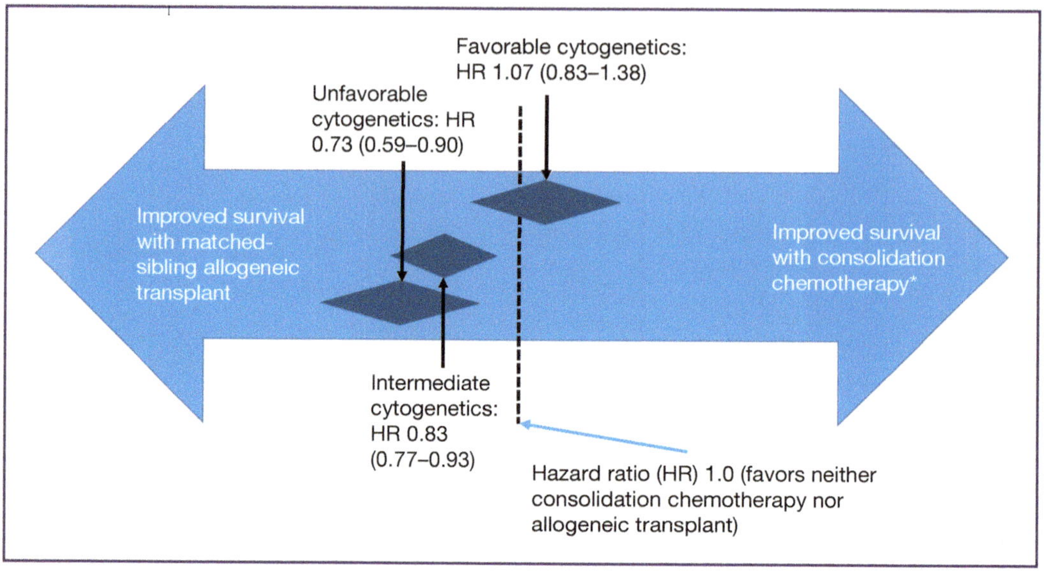

FIGURE 3-5: **Postremission treatment for younger patients with AML in first CR. Hazard ratios in this figure are derived from a meta-analysis of studies assigning AML patients to myeloablative conditioning allogeneic stem cell transplant if an HLA-matched sibling donor was available. Subjects in these studies without sibling donors were assigned to consolidation chemotherapy. Though these data are generalizable to patients eligible for myeloablative conditioning matched-sibling transplants, there is increasing evidence that outcomes from alternative donor sources such as matched unrelated and haploidentical donors confer similar benefits.**

In general, patients diagnosed with intermediate- or adverse-risk cytogenetics/genetics have improved outcomes with an allogeneic stem cell transplant in first CR. There are many factors that are considered when discussing an allogeneic stem cell transplant with patients including disease biology, minimal residual disease indices, donor availability, patient preference, patient resources, age, performance status, and comorbidities. It takes approximately 4 weeks to prepare for a matched-sibling or haploidentical stem cell transplant, and can take 8 to 12 weeks to prepare for a matched unrelated stem cell transplant. Therefore, the general recommendations are to proceed with standard consolidation chemotherapy consisting of high-dose cytarabine (3 gm/m² IV every 12 hours on days 1, 3, and 5) for as many as 3 to 4 cycles while awaiting definitive stem cell transplantation.

***Consolidation chemotherapy regimens were variable in the studies included in the meta-analysis. The most widely used consolidation chemotherapy for patients with favorable-risk ELN criteria is 3 to 4 cycles of high-dose cytarabine—3 gm/m² IV every 12 hours on days 1, 3, and 5 of approximately 28-day cycles.**

AML, acute myeloid leukemia; CR, complete remission.

Selected References

Byrd JC, Mrozek K, Dodge RK, et al. Pretreatment cytogenetic abnormalities are predictive of induction success, cumulative incidence of relapse, and overall survival in adult patients with de novo acute myeloid leukemia: results from Cancer and Leukemia Group B (CALGB 8461). *Blood.* 2002;100(13):4325–4336.

Ciurea SO, Zhang MJ, Bacigalupo AA, et al. Haploidentical transplant with posttransplant cyclophosphamide vs matched unrelated donor transplant for acute myeloid leukemia. *Blood.* 2015;126(8), 1033–1040.

Dohner H, Estey EH, Amadori S, et al. Diagnosis and management of acute myeloid leukemia in adults: recommendations from an international expert panel, on behalf of the European LeukemiaNet. *Blood.* 2010;115(3):453–474.

Fernandez HF, Sun Z, Yao X, et al. Anthracycline dose intensification in acute myeloid leukemia. *N Engl J Med.* 2009;361(13):1249–1259.

Garcia-Manero G, Tambaro FP, Bekele NB, et al. Phase II trial of vorinostat with idarubicin and cytarabine for patients with newly diagnosed acute myelogenous leukemia or myelodysplastic syndrome. *J Clin Oncol.* 2012;30(18):2204–2210.

Geller RB, Burke PJ, Karp JE, et al. A two-step timed sequential treatment for acute myelocytic leukemia. *Blood.* 1989;74(5):1499–1506.

Holowiecki J, Grosicki S, Giebel S, et al. Cladribine, but not fludarabine, added to daunorubicin and cytarabine during induction prolongs survival of patients with acute myeloid leukemia: a multicenter, randomized phase III study. *J Clin Oncol.* 2012;30(20):2441–2448.

Koreth J, Schlenk R, Kopecky KJ, et al. Allogeneic stem cell transplantation for acute myeloid leukemia in first complete remission: systematic review and meta-analysis of prospective clinical trials. *JAMA.* 2009;301(22), 2349–2361.

Luskin MR, Lee JW, Fernandez HF, et al. Benefit of high-dose daunorubicin in AML induction extends across cytogenetic and molecular groups. *Blood.* 2016;127:1551–1558.

Mayer RJ, Davis RB, Schiffer CA, et al. Intensive postremission chemotherapy in adults with acute myeloid leukemia. Cancer and Leukemia Group B. *N Engl J Med.* 1994;331(14):896–903.

Mrozek K, Marcucci G, Nicolet D, et al. Prognostic significance of the European LeukemiaNet standardized system for reporting cytogenetic and molecular alterations in adults with acute myeloid leukemia. *J Clin Oncol.* 2012;30(36):4515–4523.

Saber W, Opie S, Rizzo JD, et al. Outcomes after matched unrelated donor versus identical sibling hematopoietic cell transplantation in adults with acute myelogenous leukemia. *Blood.* 2012;119(17):3908–3916.

AML TREATMENT IN OLDER PATIENTS

Houman Nourkeyhani and Eunice S. Wang

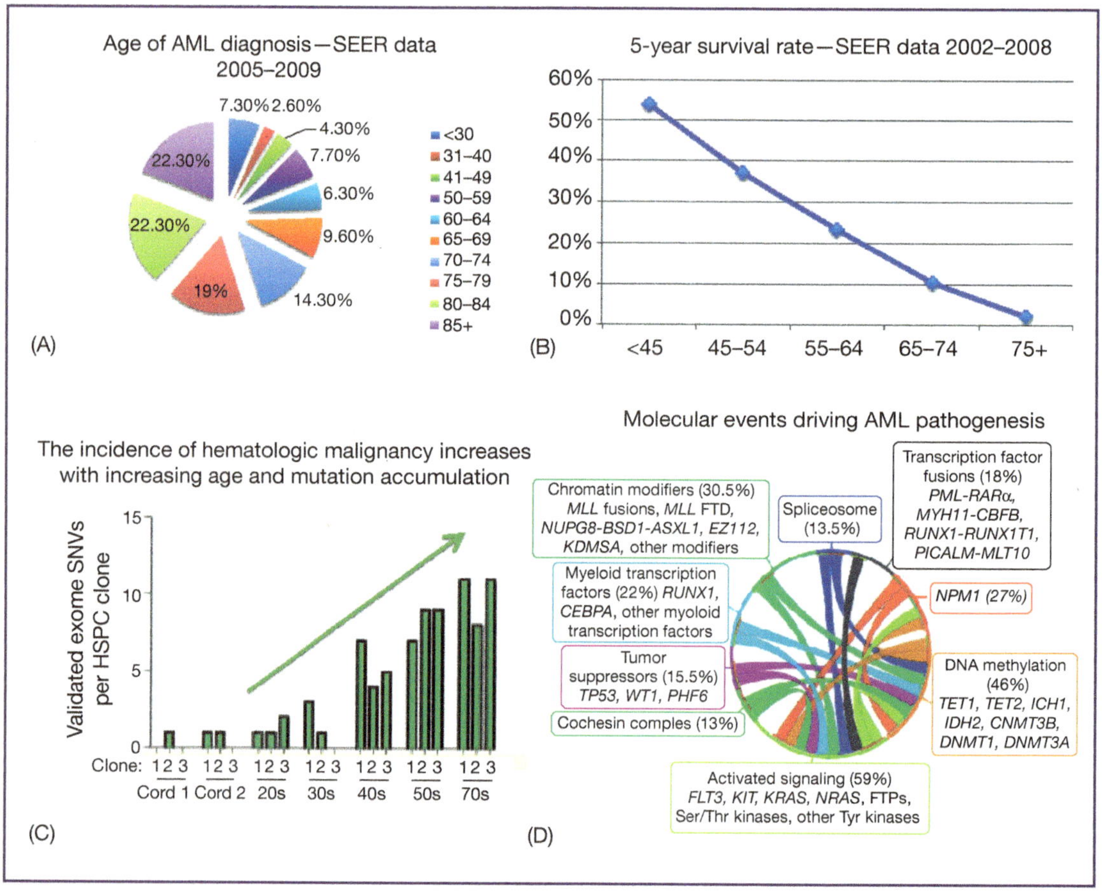

FIGURE 3-6: **Incidence, survival, and biology of AML in older individuals. (A) The incidence of AML increases with increasing age. The average age at diagnosis is 66 years. (B) The 5-year survival rate for AML decreases with increasing age. The 5-year survival for patients younger than 65 years is 40.6%, while it is only 5.4% for patients older than 65 years. (C) One of the reasons why AML occurs largely in older individuals is the fact that as a human ages, the number of mutations occurring in one's HSC increases. It is reported that the number of coding mutations in HSC in normal individuals increase with age with much higher numbers occurring in the 50s to 70s (average 8–10 and above) as compared with HSC taken from cord blood cells or adults in their 20s to 30s (only one mutation on average). (D) This diagram highlights our current understanding of the biology of AML in human patients. The interplay of these gene mutations shows both complex patterns of cooperation as well as mutual exclusivity. Each AML case may have several gene mutations in different functional categories. The presence of such extreme biological heterogeneity within AML disease confers significant therapeutic challenges.**

Source: (C) Adapted from Welch JS, Ley TJ, Link DC, et al. The origin and evolution of mutations in acute myeloid leukemia. *Cell.* 2012;150:264–278; (D) Reprinted by permission from Macmillan Publishers Ltd: Adapted from: Chen SJ, Shen Y, Chen Z. A panoramic view of acute myeloid leukemia. *Nat Genet.* 2013;45:586–587.

AML, acute myeloid leukemia; HSC, hematopoietic stem cell; HSPC, hematopoietic stem/progenitor cell; SEER, surveillance, epidemiology, and end results; SNVs, single nucleotide variants.

	Population	Comparison	Age	CRrate	Survival	Early death rates
Juliusson et al (2009)	Sweden/Swedish Acute Leukemia Registry	Swedish regions with low rates of intensive therapy vs. regions with high rates of intensive therapy	70–79	41% vs. 49%	2-year survival: 24% vs. 50% 5-year survival: 1% vs. 13%	All ages combined, 30-day mortality: Intensive therapy: 10% Palliative treatment 34%. Increased with declining performance status
Oran and Weisdorf (2012)	US SEER database 2000–2007	Treated (all treatments included) vs. untreated patients	All patients aged 65 and over	–	OS: 2 months (untreated) vs. 6 months (treated) (*P* <.01)	Mortality within 2 months: Untreated 52.7%; receiving intensive chemotherapy: 36%; receiving hypomethylating therapy: 18.7%
Lowenburg et al (2009)	Phase III trial consisting of 813 elderly patients with previously untreated AML	Induction cytarabine 200 mg/m^2/day and daunorubicin doses of 45 mg/m^2 or 90 mg/m^2	60–83	64% for patients receiving daunorubicin at 90 mg/m^2 vs. 54% in 45 mg/m^2 group		11% for patients receiving daunorubicin at 90 mg/m^2 vs. 12% in 45 mg/m^2 group

(A)

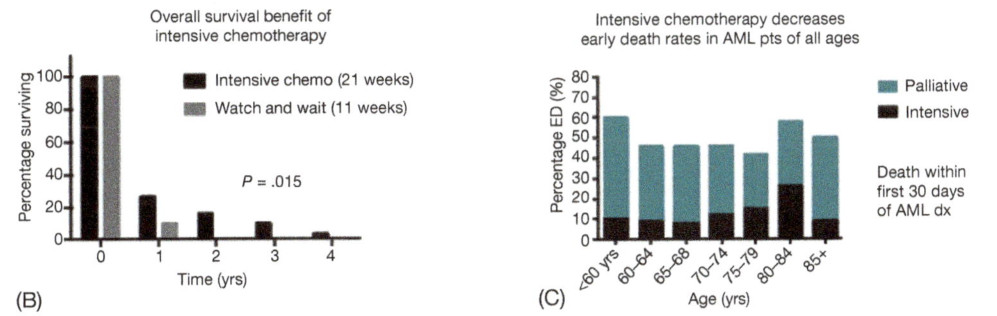

FIGURE 3-7: Benefit of chemotherapy over supportive care for upfront therapy of older adults. (A) In the past, a majority of elderly patients were not offered intensive chemotherapy as a treatment option solely based on their age. However, as summarized here, multiple clinical studies have consistently shown that individuals up to 80 years of age clearly benefited from intensive treatment over supportive care as reflected in improved complete remission (CR) and overall survival rates. Achieving CR also has been shown to improve quality of life by reducing the number of hospitalizations, infections, and transfusion requirements. (B) In their seminal study, Lowenberg and colleagues randomized 60 adults aged 65 years and over to receive either intensive chemotherapy or a "watch and wait" supportive approach after AML diagnosis. Their results demonstrated a clear survival benefit for intensive therapy with a doubling of overall survival over the control arm. (C) Juliusson et al demonstrated using Swedish Acute Leukemia Registry that early death rates were lower in patients treated with intensive chemotherapy as opposed to palliative or supportive therapy.

AML, acute myeloid leukemia; OS, overall survival; SEER, surveillance, epidemiology, and end results.

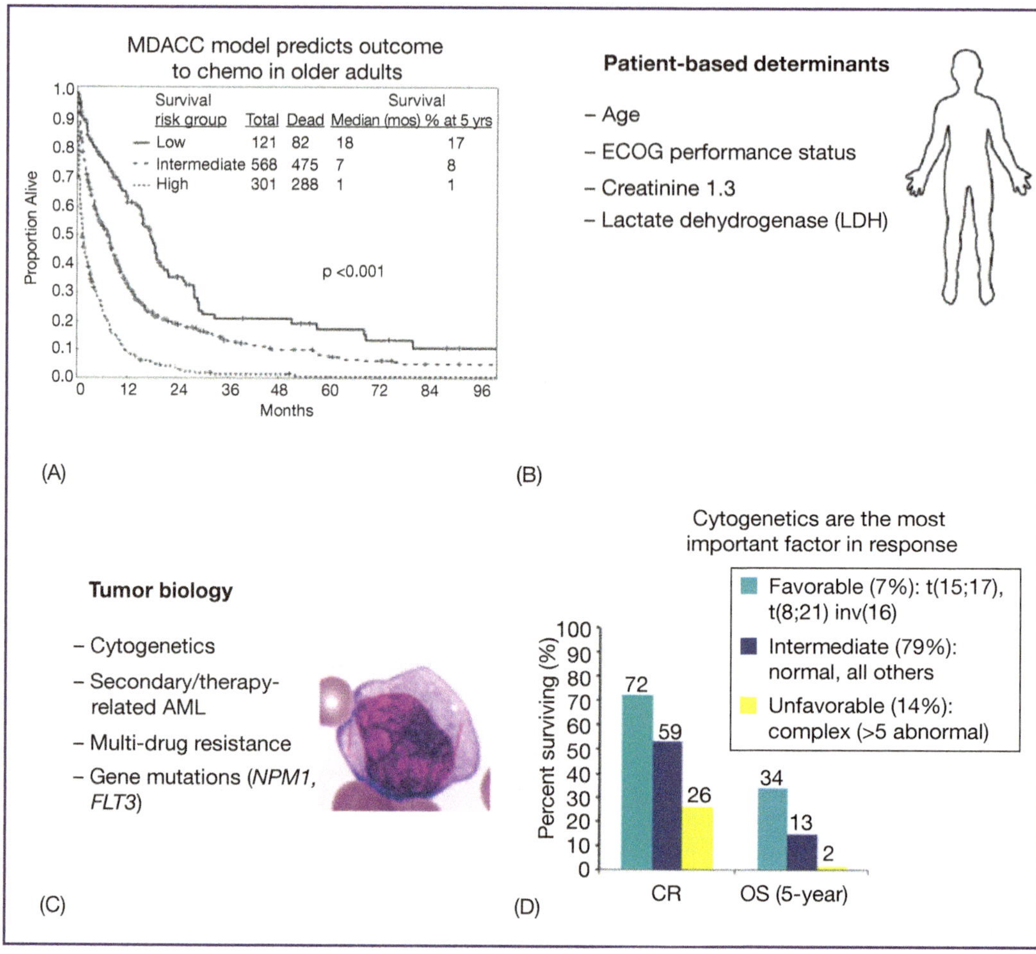

FIGURE 3-8: Predictors of clinical outcome in older patients receiving intensive chemotherapy for AML. (A) Treatment mortality scores have been developed to predict the risk of toxicity and poor outcomes of intensive cytarabine- and anthracycline-based chemotherapy for older patients with AML, recognizing the fact that chronological age may not be the sole measure of treatment outcome. For example, MD Anderson developed a model to predict outcomes in 998 older patients with AML and MDS. (B) Patient-based determinants: Elderly patients are more likely than their younger counterparts to present with multiple comorbidities, limiting their therapeutic options. Moreover, frail elderly patients with an ECOG performance status greater than or equal to 2 generally tend to have a worse clinical outcome. (C) Tumor biology: Elderly patients are much more likely than younger patients to have AML harbor high-risk cytogenetic abnormalities. They may also have disease arising from prior chemotherapy or radiation or secondary AML following a prior hematological diagnosis (MDS, MPN). AML cells expressing multidrug resistance due to drug efflux pumps or whose disease is refractory to initial therapy also have poorer prognoses. Older patients whose AML cells contain *NPM1* mutations in the absence of *FLT3* mutations are the molecularly identified group thus far to clearly benefit from intensive chemotherapy. (D) AML cytogenetics remains the strongest prognostic factor for response to chemotherapy. Patients with favorable or intermediate-risk karyotype have higher rates of complete remission, as high as 60% to 70%, following standard 7 + 3 induction chemotherapy compared to those patients with unfavorable karyotype. Survival decreases drastically with worsening cytogenetic features, despite aggressive chemotherapy.

Source: From Kantarjian H, O'Brien S, Cortes J et al. Results of intensive chemotherapy in 998 patients age 65 years or older with acute myeloid leukemia or high-risk myelodysplastic syndrome. *Cancer.* 2006;106(5):1090–1098.

AML, acute myeloid leukemia; CR, complete remission; ECOG, Eastern Cooperative Oncology Group; FLT3, FMS-like tyrosine kinase 3; MDS, myelodysplastic syndrome; MPN, myeloproliferative neoplasm; NPM1, nucleophosmine 1; OS, overall survival.

Authors	Patient population	Intervention	Overall survival
Dombret et al (2015)	488 patients ages 65 and above (median 75, with newly diagnosed AML with 30% of greater bone marrow blasts)	Azacitidine (Aza) 75 mg/m^2 subcutaneous, daily for 7 days, on a 28-day cycle versus conventional care regimen low-dose cytarabine (LDAC) or best supportive or induction chemotherapy	Median overall survival 10.4 months in aza arm vs. 6.5 months in CCR
Fenaux et al (2009) AZA-001	358 patients, median age 69, with high-risk MDS by French-American-British criteria. Of these, 113 patients (median age 70) fulfilled AML criteria based on WHO classification	Azacitidine (Aza) 75 mg/m^2 subcutaneous, daily for 7 days, on a 28-day cycle versus conventional care regimen (low-dose cytarabine (LDAC) or best supportive or induction chemotherapy)	Median overall survival 24.5 months in aza arm vs. 15 months in CCR. 2-year OS 50% in aza group vs. 16% in CCR group
Kantarjian et al (2012)	485 new diagnosed de novo or secondary AML, ages 65 or above,	Decitabine (Dec) 20 mg/m^2 daily intravenous infusion for 5 days, on a 28-day cycle versus best supportive care of LDAC	Trend toward improved OS (7.7 months vs. 5.0 months) but did not reach statistical significance
Quintas-Cardama et al (2012)	Retrospective review of 671 patients with newly diagnosed AML treated at MD Anderson cancer center between 2000 and 2010	Intensive chemotherapy versus epigenetic therapy (decitabine or azacitidine)	Median OS 6.7 months (intensive chemotherapy group) vs. 6.5 months (hypomethylating therapy group)

(A)

	Intensive chemotherapy	10-day decitabine	*P* value
Number of pateints	84	63	–
CR	43%	19%	<.01
ORR	50%	28%	.01
Median OS (mos)	10.7	8.0	.026
30 day mortality	11%	13%	.80
60 day mortality	18%	24%	.41

(B)

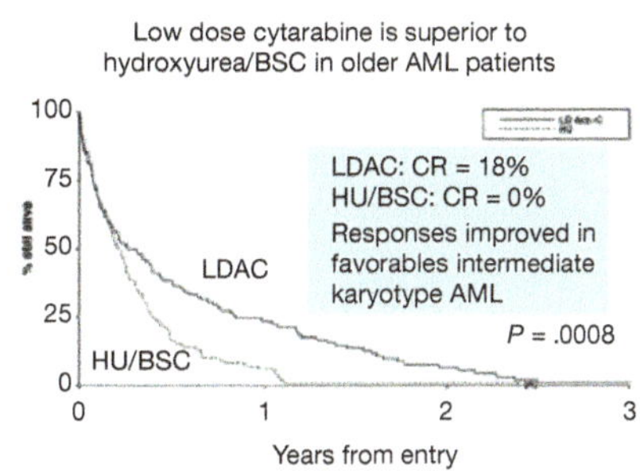

(C)

FIGURE 3-9: Clinical outcomes of lower-dose chemotherapy approaches for older adults with AML. (A) Summary of clinical trials utilizing hypomethylating agents in older individuals with AML. DNA hypermethylation leading to gene silencing has been linked to leukemogenesis. Reversal of this process using the hypomethylating pyrimidine nucleoside analogs, decitabine (Dec) and azacitidine (Aza), has demonstrated clinical benefit in older individuals with de novo AML in multiple trials. Dombret et al compared Aza 75 mg/m^2 for 7 days of each 28-day cycle with conventional care regimens (CCR, consisting of induction chemotherapy, low-dose cytarabine (LDAC) or best supportive care) in 488 older patients with newly diagnosed AML. Subgroup analysis revealed azacitidine to be superior in patients with unfavorable cytogenetics, as demonstrated by a twofold higher median overall survival (OS) over CCR (6.4 vs. 2–3 months). Kantarjian et al conducted a phase III, multicenter trial comparing a 5-day regimen of Dec versus CCR in older patients with AML. While the results trended toward survival advantage with Dec, the results failed to reach statistical significance. In a retrospective study comparing the outcomes of 671 older patients with AML treated at MD Anderson Cancer Center, Quintas-Cardama et al demonstrated similar OS rates following either intensive or hypomethylating therapy despite lower CR rates following epigenetic therapy. Based on all of these results, decitabine or azacitidine have increasingly become the preferred first-line treatment for many older patients with AML, particularly those individuals with compromised functional/performance status, organ dysfunction, and tumor biology (ie, karyotype and molecular aberrations) predicting poor response to intensive chemotherapy. (B) Data from Roswell Park Cancer Institute on the outcomes of intensive chemotherapy versus a 10-day decitabine regimen for upfront treatment of older patients with AML showed higher CR rates following intensive treatment but similar OS and treatment-related mortality. Of note, nearly half of these patients had secondary AML and a poor-risk karyotype. (C) For older patients considered unfit for other treatment, another option is low-dose cytarabine (LDAC), which is associated with minimal but real benefit over best supportive care. While inferior to hypomethylating and induction therapy, LDAC induces CR in up to 18% of patients and results in prolonged OS.

Source: **(C) From Burnett AK, Milligan D, Prentice AG, et al. A comparison of low-dose cytarabine and hydroxyurea with or without all-trans retinoic acid for acute myeloid leukemia and high-risk myelodysplastic syndrome in patients not considered fit for intensive treatment. *Cancer*. 2007;109:1114–1124.**

AML, acute myeloid leukemia; CCR, conventional care regimen; CR, complete remission; ORR, overall response rate; OS, overall survival.

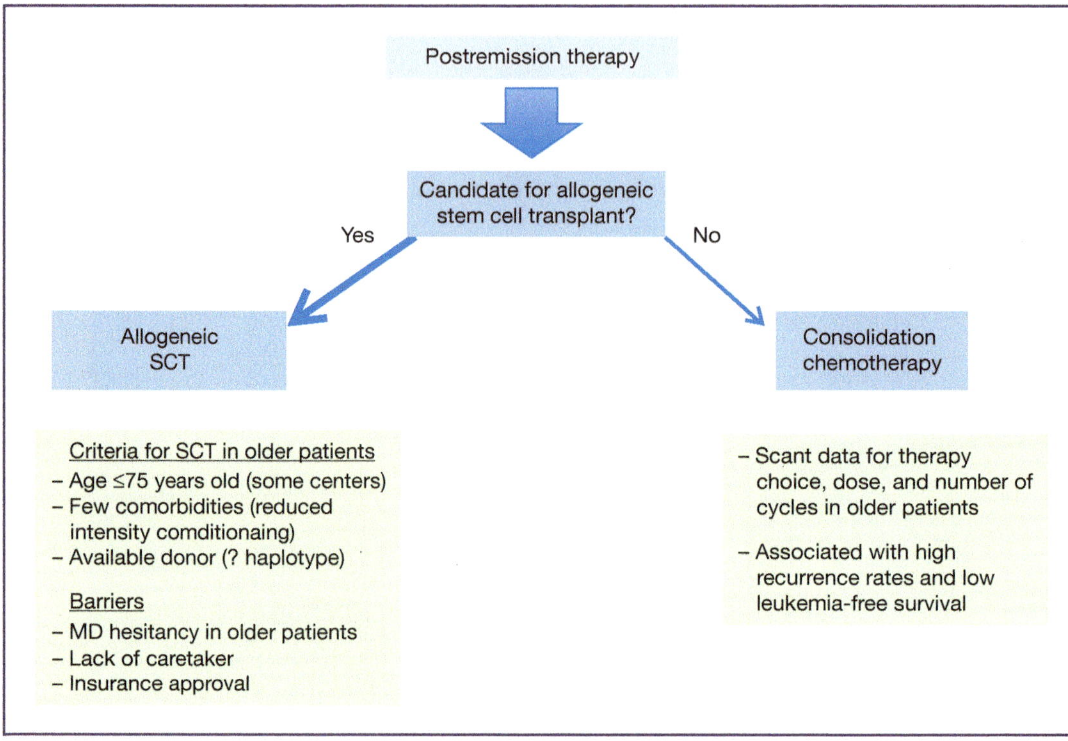

FIGURE 3-10: Considerations for consolidation/postremission therapy of older patients with AML. (LEFT SIDE) Following upfront therapy, the choice of subsequent therapy is dictated by the patient's ability and willingness to undergo allogeneic hematopoietic stem cell transplant (alloSCT). Older patients with AML who underwent alloSCT consistently lived longer than their counterparts. Reported 2-year survival rates are 50% for patients aged 65 to 69 years and 30.5% for patients aged 70 to 74 years. Though age alone is not a disqualifying factor, other comorbid conditions must be taken into consideration as well as the availability of a matched donor. Reduced-intensity (nonmyeloablative) conditioning regimens for older individuals is also associated with similar leukemia-free and overall survival as younger patients based on the Center for International Blood and Marrow Transplant Research (CIBMTR). Although consolidation chemotherapy has never been prospectively compared against alloSCT, a retrospective study comparing the results of alloSCT versus maintenance chemotherapy in patients with AML aged 60 to 70 years found a significantly longer leukemia-free survival (32% vs. 15% at 3 years; $P = .001$), a lower risk of relapse (32% vs. 81%; $P < .001$), and a higher treatment-related mortality (36% vs. 4% at 3 years; $P < .001$) in patients undergoing alloSCT. Though OS trended toward favoring the alloSCT group, this did not reach statistical significance (37% vs. 25% at 3 years; $P = .08$), leaving the question of which treatment was superior still unanswered. (RIGHT SIDE) Older patients with AML who are not transplant candidates and/or are unwilling to undergo an alloSCT for any reason typically proceed onto consolidation chemotherapy. Consolidation chemotherapy typically consists of either high-dose cytarabine or cytarabine combined with anthracycline at lower doses than during induction. To date, due to a lack of randomized prospective data, a consensus regarding the optimal number of agents, their dosages, and the optimal number of consolidation cycles has not yet been reached. The Medical Research Council AML 11 trial examined 1,314 patients in CR, who were randomized to receive either 1 or 3 additional cycles of consolidation chemotherapy after standard induction therapy. No benefit was observed in those receiving the longer course of consolidation therapy. In patients with favorable or intermediate-risk AML who achieve CR after standard 7 + 3 induction therapy, two to four additional cycles of consolidation chemotherapy with intermediate- or high-dose cytarabine has been shown to be beneficial. Patients with poor-risk disease tend to have a worse outcome, regardless of postinduction therapy, and would be best managed on a clinical trial.

AML, acute myeloid leukemia; CR, complete remission; SCT, stem cell transplantation.

Selected novel agent	Mechanism of action	Current phase trail	Projected enrollment
KX2-391	Src kinase and tubulin polymerization inhibitor	Phase Ib	N = 20
Pracinostat	Histone deacetylase (HDAC) inhibitor	Phase II	N = 50
Dasatinib and all-trans-retinoic acid (ATRA)	BCR-ABL tyrosine kinase inhibitor	Phase I	N = 24
BIBF 1120 (Nintedanib)	Multi-tyrosine kinase inhibitor	Phase I/II	N = 140
Temsirolimus	mTOR inhibitor	Phase II	N = 224
Plerixafor and clofarabine	CXCR4 antagonist	Phase I/II	N = 66
Sapacitabine	Nucleoside analog	Phase III	N = 486
OCV-501	Wilms tumor gene 1-derived peptide vaccine	Phase I	Not available

FIGURE 3-11: Overview of current investigational agents for the treatment of older patients+ with AML. Numerous clinical trials are investigating novel agents targeting biological pathways, receptors, or signaling pathways relevant to myeloid leukemogenesis for AML therapy. Several agents are known to be active in other malignancies.
AML, acute myeloid leukemia.

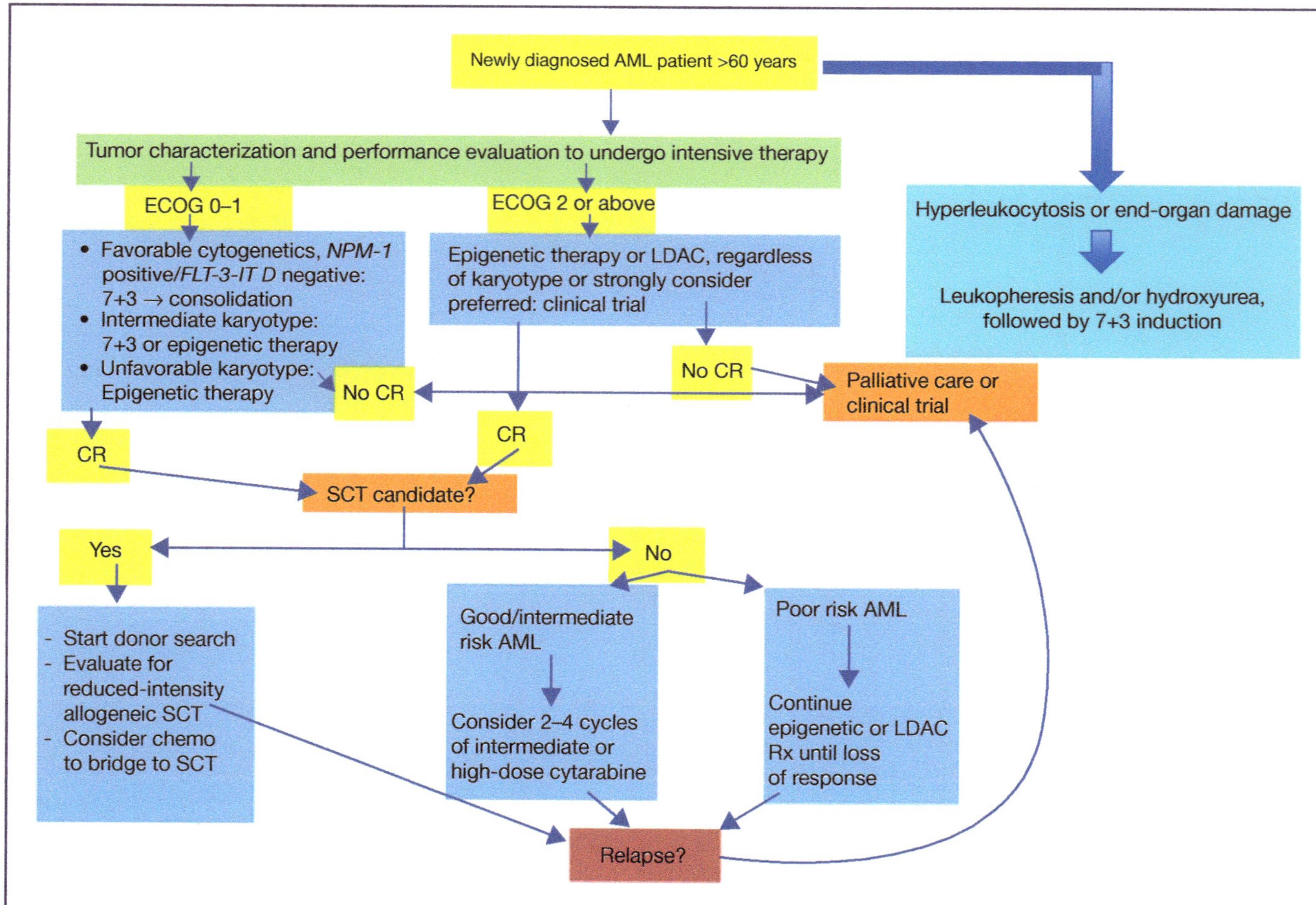

FIGURE 3-12: Proposed treatment algorithm for older patients with acute myeloid leukemia.

AML, acute myeloid leukemia; CR, complete remission; ECOG, Eastern Cooperative Oncology Group; LDAC, low-dose cytosine arabinoside; SCT, stem cell transplantation.

Selected References

Brandts C. Study with temsirolimus added to standard chemotherapy for patients over 60 years with acute myeloblastic leukemia (TOR-AML); 2017. https://ClinicalTrials.gov/show/NCT01611116

Burnett AK, Milligan D, Prentice AG, et al. A comparison of low-dose cytarabine and hydroxyurea with or without all-trans retinoic acid for acute myeloid leukemia and high-risk myelodysplastic syndrome in patients not considered fit for intensive treatment. *Cancer*. 2007;109:1114–1124.

Chen SJ, Shen Y, Chen Z. A panoramic view of acute myeloid leukemia. *Nat Genet*. 2013;45:586–587.

Cyclacel Pharmaceuticals, Inc. A study of oral sapacitabine in elderly patients with newly diagnosed acute myeloid leukemia (SEAMLESS); 2015. https://ClinicalTrials.gov/show/NCT01303796

Dombret H, Seymour JF, Butrym A, et al. International phase 3 study of azacitidine vs conventional care regimens in older patients with newly diagnosed AML with >30% blasts. *Blood*. 2015;126:291–299.

Doria-Rose VP, Harlan LC, Stevens J, Little RF. Treatment of de novo acute myeloid leukemia in the United States: a report from the Patterns of Care program. *Leuk Lymphoma*. 2014;55:2549–2655.

Farag SS, Maharry K, Zhang MJ, et al. Comparison of reduced-intensity hematopoietic cell transplantation with chemotherapy in patients age 60–70 years with acute myelogenous leukemia in first remission. *Biol Blood Marrow Transplant*. 2011;17:1796–1803.

Fenaux P, Mufti G, Hellstrom-Lindberg E, et al. Efficacy of azacytidine compared with that of conventional care regimens in the treatment of higher-risk myelodysplastic syndromes: a randomized, open-label phase III study. *Lancet Oncol*. 2009;10:223–232.

Gupta N, Miller A, Gandhi S, et al. Comparison of epigenetic versus standard induction chemotherapy for newly diagnosed acute myeloid leukemia patients ≥60 years old. *Am J Hematol*. 2015;90: 639–646.

Helsinn Healthcare SA. Safety and efficacy study of pracinostat with azacitadine in elderly patients with newly diagnosed acute myeloid leukemia (AML); 2015. https://ClinicalTrials.gov/show/NCT01912274

Howlader N, Noone AM, Krapcho M, et al. SEER cancer statistics review, 1975–2012, National Cancer Institute. Bethesda, MD. http://seer.cancer.gov/csr/1975_2012

Juliusson G, Antunovic P, Derolf A, et al. Age and acute myeloid leukemia: real world data on decision to treat and outcomes from the Swedish Acute Leukemia Registry. *Blood*. 2009;113:4179–4187.

Kantarjian H, O'Brien S, Cortes J et al. Results of intensive chemotherapy in 998 patients age 65 years or older with acute myeloid leukemia or high-risk myelodysplastic syndrome. *Cancer*. 2006;106(5):1090–1098

Kantarjian H, Ravandi F, O'Brien S, et al. Intensive chemotherapy does not benefit most older patients (age 70 years or older) with acute myeloid leukemia. *Blood*. 2010;116:4422–4429.

Kantarjian HM, Thomas XG, Dmoszynska A, et al. Multicenter, randomized, open-label, phase III trial of decitabine versus patient choice, with physician advice, of either supportive care or low-dose cytarabine for the treatment of older patients with newly diagnosed acute myeloid leukemia. *J Clin Oncol*. 2012;30:2670–2677.

Kinex Pharmaceuticals Inc. Evaluation of KX2-391 in elderly subjects with acute myeloid leukemia (AML); 2015. https://clinicaltrials.gov/ct2/show/NCT01397799?term=kx2-391&rank=2

Krug U, Rollig C, Koschmieder A, et al. Complete remission and early death after intensive chemotherapy in patients aged 60 years or older with acute myeloid leukaemia: a web-based application for prediction of outcomes. *Lancet*. 2010;376:2000–2008.

Lowenberg B, Ossenkoppele GJ, van Putten W, et al. High-dose daunorubicin in older patients with acute myeloid leukemia. *N Engl J Med*. 2009;361:1235–1248.

Malfuson JV, Etienne A, Turlure P, et al. Risk factors and decision criteria for intensive chemotherapy in older patients with acute myeloid leukemia. *Haematologica*. 2008;93:1806–1813.

M.D. Anderson Cancer Center, Genzyme, a Sanofi Company. Plerixafor and clofarabine in frontline treatment of elderly patients with acute myelogenous leukemia (AML); 2017. https://ClinicalTrials.gov/show/NCT01160354

Naing A, Cohen R, Dy GK, et al. A phase I trial of KX2-391, a novel non-ATP competitive substrate-pocket-directed SRC inhibitor, in patients with advanced malignancies. *Invest New Drugs*. 2013;31:967–973.

Oran B, Weisdorf DJ. Survival for older patients with acute myeloid leukemia: a population-based study. *Haematologica*. 2012;97:1916–1924.

Otsuka Pharmaceutical Co., Ltd, Korea Otsuka Pharmaceutical Co., Ltd. A Phase 2 trial to evaluate the efficacy and safety of OCV-501 in elderly patients with acute myeloid leukemia; 2017. https://ClinicalTrials.gov/show/NCT01961882

Quintas-Cardama A, Ravandi F, Liu-Dumlao T, et al. Epigenetic therapy is associated with similar survival compared with intensive chemotherapy in older patients with newly diagnosed acute myeloid leukemia. *Blood*. 2012;120:4840–4845.

Sorror ML, Estey E. Allogeneic hematopoietic cell transplantation for acute myeloid leukemia in older adults. *Hematology Am Soc Hematol Educ Program*. 2014;2014:21–33.

University Hospital Muenster, Boehringer Ingelheim. Phase I/II Trial: BIBF 1120 added to low-dose cytarabine in elderly patients with acute myeloid leukemia (AML); 2014. https://ClinicalTrials.gov/show/NCT01488344

University of Pittsburgh. Study of dasatinib and all-trans retinoic acid for relapsed/refractory and/or elderly patients with acute myelogenous leukemia (AML) or myelodysplastic syndrome; 2016. https://ClinicalTrials.gov/show/NCT00892190

Welch JS, Ley TJ, Link DC, et al. The origin and evolution of mutations in acute myeloid leukemia. *Cell*. 2012;150:264–278.

TREATMENT OF RELAPSED/REFRACTORY AML

Mark R. Litzow and Selina M. Luger

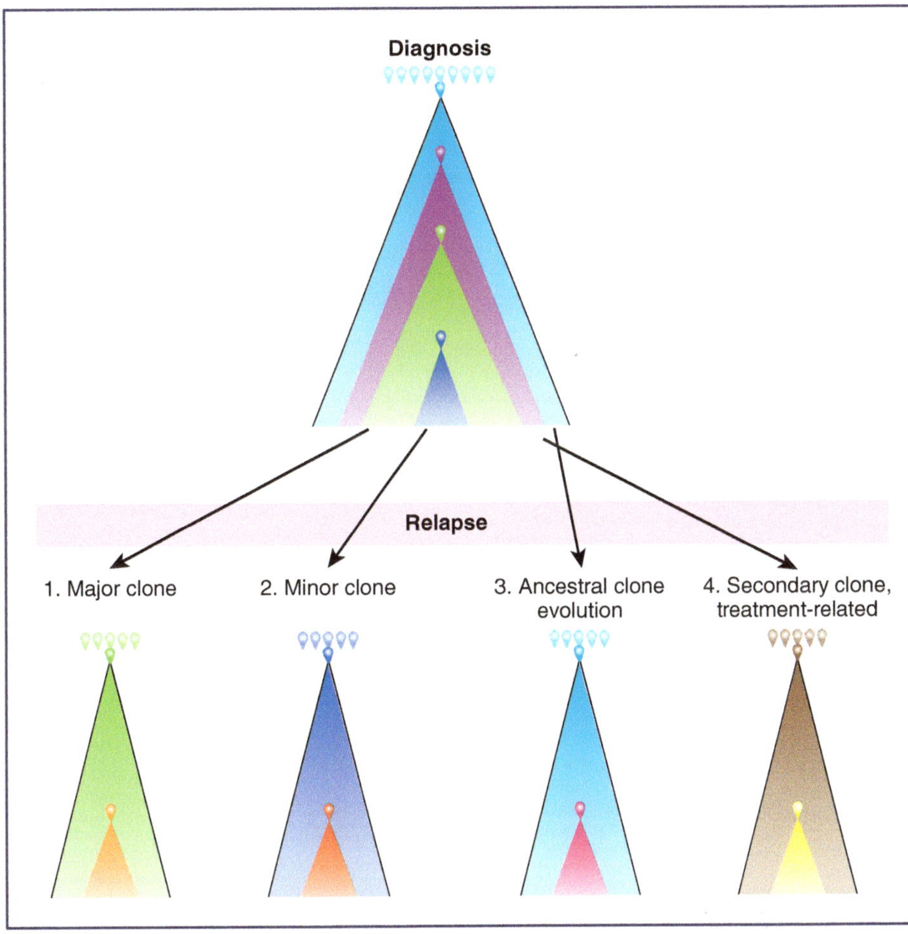

FIGURE 3-13: AML at the time of relapse carries a heterogeneous clonal pattern. AML, acute myeloid leukemia.

There are many established patient- and disease-related factors at presentation predictive of primary refractory disease (PRD). Karyotype has historically been demonstrated to be a significant predictor, while the importance of recurrent molecular mutations and epigenetic changes in AML have been more

Table 3-7 Predictive factors of achieving complete remission with induction therapy

PREDICTIVE FACTORS	COMMENTS
Disease Related	
Cytogenetics	One of the strongest factors determining chance of complete remission
Molecular mutations	Most prognostic when intermediate karyotype present • Numerous studies and reviews looking at impact of both isolated and multiple mutations with significant heterogeneity in findings
Epigenetic changes	Global and specific gene methylation patterns affect complete remission rates

(*continued*)

Table 3-7 Predictive factors of achieving complete remission with induction therapy (*continued*)

PREDICTIVE FACTORS	COMMENTS
Cell counts	Elevated white blood cell count, thrombocytopenia
AML type	Secondary after cytotoxic therapy or antecedent hematological disorder decreases rate of complete remission in some studies
Patient Related	
Performance status	>1 is negative prognostic factor
Age	Age >65 is adverse prognostic factor Even higher risk if age >75
Comorbidities	Predictive of early death during induction
Treatment Response	
Nadir bone marrow biopsy	>5% and especially >15% blasts are negative prognostic marker
Peripheral blast clearance	Rapid decrease in peripheral blasts highly predictive of complete remission

AML, acute myeloid leukemia.

Table 3-8 Prognostic scoring systems for patients with refractory/relapsed AML

A. GOELAMS SCORE

FACTOR	POINTS
CR1 Duration	
≥12 mo	0
≤12 mo (refractory/early relapse)	1
FLT3-ITD Status	
Negative	0
Positive	1
Cytogenetics*	
Favorable/intermediate	0
High risk	1

Prognostic groups: good (0 points; OS 58%, event-free survival [EFS] 45% at 7 years); intermediate (1 point; OS 37%, EFS 31% at 2 years); poor (2–3 points; OS 12%, EFS 12% at 2 years).

B. EUROPEAN PROGNOSTIC INDEX SCORE

FACTOR	POINTS
CR1 Duration	
≥18 mo	0
7–18 mo	3
≤6 mo	5
Cytogenetics at Diagnosis	
t(16;21) or inv(16)	0
t(8;21)	3
Other	5
Age at Relapse	
≤35 y	0
36–45 y	1
>45 y	2
SCT Before First Relapse	
No	0
Yes	2

Prognostic groups: favorable (1–6 points; OS of 70% at 1 year and 46% at 5 years); intermediate (7–9 points; OS of 49% at 1 year and 18% at 5 years); poor (10–14 points; OS of 16% at 1 year and 4% at 5 years).

AML, acute myeloid leukemia; FLT3-ITD, FMS-like tyrosine kinase 3 internal tandem duplication; SCT, stem cell transplantation.

Table 3-9 Conventional and novel cytotoxic salvage chemotherapy regimens utilized in patients with relapsed/refractory acute myeloid leukemia (AML)

REGIMEN	AGENTS	CR	TRM OR 30-DAY MORTALITY
HiDAC	Cytarabine 3 g/m^3 every 12 hours days 1–6	32%–47%	12%–15%
FLAG/FLAG-IDA	Fludarabine 30 mg/m^2 days 1–5 Cytarabine 2 g/m^2 days 1–5 G-CSF 5 mcg/kg day 0 until ANC recovery	48%–55%	10%–11%
	Fludarabine 30 mg/m^2 days 1–5 Cytarabine 2 g/m^2 days 1–5 G-CSF 300 mcg day 0 until ANC recovery Idarubicin 8 mg/m^2 days 1–3	63%	17%
FLA	Fludarabine 30 mg/m^2 days 1–5 Cytarabine 2 g/m^2 days 1–5	61%	7%
CLAG/CLAG-M	Cladribine 5 mg/m^2 days 2–6 Cytarabine 2 g/m^2 days 2–6 G-CSF 300 mcg days 1–6	38%–50%	0%–17%
	Cladribine 5 mg/m^2 days 1–5 Cytarabine 2 g/m^2 days 1–5 G-CSF 300 mcg days 0–5 Mitoxantrone 10 mg/m^2 days 1–3	50%–58% (53% after first course)	0%–7%
MEC	Mitoxantrone 6 mg/m^2 days 1–6 Etoposide 80 mg/m^2 days 1–6 Cytarabine 1 g/m^2 days 1–6	59%–66%	3%–6%
	Mitoxantrone 8 mg/m^2 days 1–5 Etoposide 100 mg/m^2 days 1–5 Cytarabine 1 mg/m^2 days 1–5	18%–24%	7%–11%
MEC/Decitabine	Decitabine 20 mg/m^2 days 1–10 Mitoxantrone 8 mg/m^2 days 16–20 Etoposide 100 mg/m^2 days 16–20 Cytarabine 1 mg/m^2 days 16–20	30% (CR + CRp + Cri = 50%)	20%
EMA-86	Mitoxantrone 12 mg/m^2 days 1–3 Cytarabine 500 mg/m^2 CI days 1–3 & 8–10 Etoposide 200 mg/m^2 CI days 8–10	60%	11%
MAV	Mitoxantrone 10 mg/m^2 days 4–8 Cytarabine 100 mg/m^2 CI days 1–8 Etoposide 100-120 mg/m^2 days 4–8	58%	11%
FLAD	Fludarabine 30 mg/m^2 days 1–3 Cytarabine 2 g/m^2 days 1–3 Liposomal daunorubicin 100 mg/m^2 days 1–3	53%	7.5%
FLAM	Flavopiridol 50 mg/m^2 days 1–3 Cytarabine 2 g/m^2/72 h starting day 6 Mitoxantrone 40 mg/m^2 day 9	28%–43%	5%–28%
Hybrid FLAM	Flavopiridol 30 mg/m^2 bolus, 60 mg/m^2 over 4 h days 1–3 Cytarabine 2 g/m^2/72 h starting day 6 Mitoxantrone 40 mg/m^2 day 9	40%	9%

(*continued*)

Table 3-9 Conventional and novel cytotoxic salvage chemotherapy regimens utilized in patients with relapsed/refractory acute myeloid leukemia (AML) (*continued*)

REGIMEN	AGENTS	CR	TRM OR 30-DAY MORTALITY
Clofarabine Cytarabine	Clofarabine 40 mg/m² days 2–6 Cytarabine 1 g/m² days 1–5 Clofarabine 40 mg/m² days 1–5; Cytarabine 1 g/m² days 1–5 Clofarabine 22.5 mg/m² days 1–5; Cytarabine 1 g/m² days 1–5	28%–51%	6.2%–13%
GCLAC	Clofarabine 25 mg/m² days 1–5; Cytarabine 2 g/m² days 1–5; G-CSF 5 mcg/kg day 0 until ANC recovery	46% (CR+CRp 61%)	13%
HAA	Homoharringtonine 4 mg/m² days 1–3 Cytarabine 150 mg/m² days 1–7 Aclarubicin 12 mg/m² days 1–7	76%–80%	0%
CPX 351	CPX 351 101 units/m² days 1, 3, and 5 CPX 351 100 units/m² days 1, 3, 5 (first induction) and days 1 and 3 (second induction and consolidation)	23%–37% (CR + CRi = 49%)	7%–13%

CDK, cyclin-dependent kinase; CI, continuous infusion; CR, complete remission; CRi, complete remission with incomplete blood count recovery; CRp, complete remission with incomplete platelet recovery; G-CSF, granulocyte colony-stimulating factor; HiDAC, high-dose arabinoside cytarabine; TRM, treatment-related mortality.

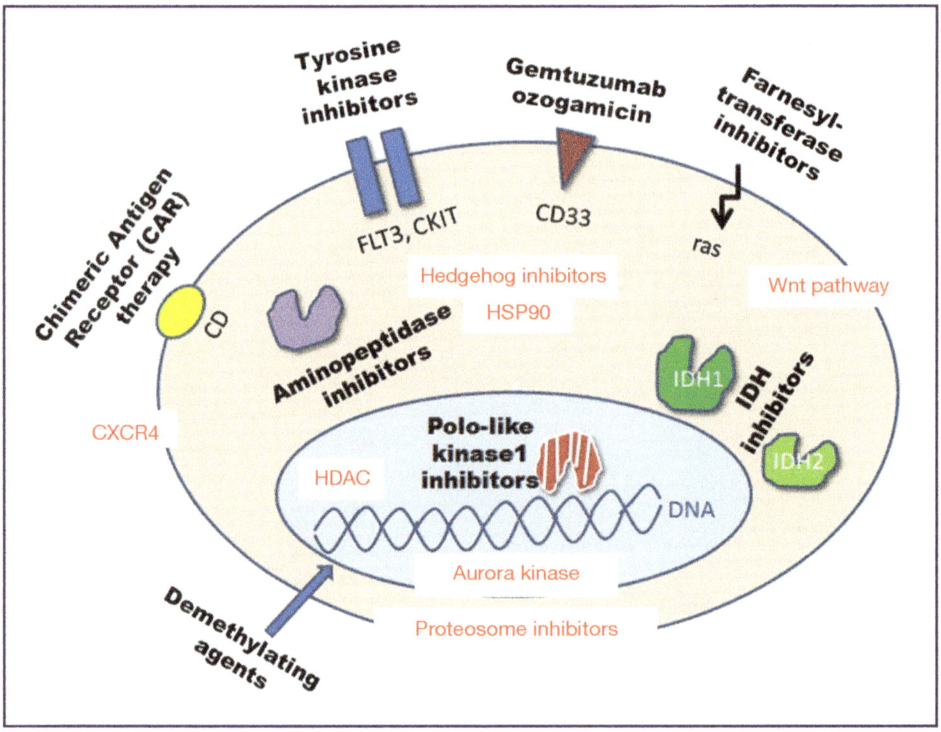

FIGURE 3-14: The candidate gene targets in AML.

AML, acute myeloid leukemia; FLT3, FMS-like tyrosine kinase 3; HDAC, histone deacetylase; HSP90, heat shock protein 90; IDH, isocitrate dehydrogenase; ras, rat sarcoma; Wnt, wingless-type MMTV (mouse mammary tumor virus) integration site.

Table 3-10 Targeted agents under active evaluation for treatment of patients with relapsed/refractory AML (RR-AML)

AGENT	MECHANISM OF ACTION	ONGOING CLINICAL TRIAL
Ruxolitinib	JAK1 and JAK2 inhibitor	NCT02257138, NCT00674479, NCT01251965
Rapamycin	mTOR inhibitor	NCT01184898, NCT01869114, NCT00634244, NCT02109744
Everolimus	mTOR inhibitor	NCT00819546
Tosedostat	Aminopeptidase activity inhibitor	NCT01636609
Vorinostat	Histone deacetylase inhibitor	NCT01130506, NCT01534260, NCT01550224, NCT01617226, NCT02083250
AG-120	IDH1 inhibitor	NCT02074839
AG-221	IDH2 inhibitor	NCT01915498
Elacytarabine	Elaidic acid ester of cytarabine	No active studies found
Vosaroxin	Anticancer quinolone derivative	NCT01191801
Pravastatin	HMG-CoA reductase inhibitor	NCT00840177
Bortezomib	Proteasome inhibitor	NCT01174888, NCT01127009, NCT01736943, NCT01861314, NCT01534260, NCT01075425, NCT00410423
Lenalidomide	Immunomodulatory agent	NCT01681537, NCT01904643, NCT01629082, NCT01132586, NCT01246622, NCT01743859, NCT01016600, NCT00466895, NCT01615042
CPI-613	Lipoate derivative	NCT01768897
ABT-199	BCL-2 inhibitor	NCT01994837
Erismodegib	Hedgehog inhibitor	NCT02129101
PF-04449913	Hedgehog inhibitor	NCT02038777

AML, acute myeloid leukemia.

Table 3-11 Immunotherapeutic agents under evaluation for treatment of patients with relapsed/refractory AML (see also immunology in Chapter 8)

AGENT	MECHANISM OF ACTION	ONGOING CLINICAL TRIAL
Gemtuzumab ozogamicin	Conjugated antibody targeting CD33	NCT01869803, NCT00766116, NCT02221310
SGN-CD33A	Conjugated antibody targeting CD33	NCT01902329
Lintuzumab	Unconjugated antibody targeting CD33	No active studies found
CSL362	Unconjugated antibody targeting CD123	No active studies found
AMG330	Bispecific T-cell engaging antibody targeting CD33 and CD3	No active studies found
MGD006	Dual affinity re-targeting antibody targeting CD123 and CD3	NCT02152956
CD16x33 BiKE	Bispecific killer cell engager antibody against CD16 and CD33	No active studies found
CART33	Chimeric antigen receptor-transduced T-cells targeting CD33	NCT01864902
CART123	Chimeric antigen receptor-transduced T-cells targeting CD123	NCT02159495
WT1 peptide vaccine	Vaccine targeting WT1	NCT00965224

(*continued*)

Table 3-11 Immunotherapeutic agents under evaluation for treatment of patients with relapsed/refractory AML (see also immunology in Chapter 8) (*continued*)

AGENT	MECHANISM OF ACTION	ONGOING CLINICAL TRIAL
WT1-specific CD8(+) T-cell infusion	Adoptive cell transfer	NCT01640301
Haploidentical NK cell infusion	Adoptive cell transfer	NCT01947322, NCT01385423, NCT01370213, NCT00303667, NCT01621477, NCT00526292, NCT00789776, NCT02259348, NCT01795378, NCT01898793, NCT01386619
Allo-HSCT	Adoptive cell transfer	More than 40 active clinical trials identified
Donor lymphocyte infusion (post-allo-HSCT)	Adoptive cell transfer	NCT01758367, NCT01390311, NCT00068718, NCT01523223, NCT01760655, NCT00534118, NCT00005799, NCT00448357

Source: www.clinicaltrials.gov

Allo-HSCT, allogeneic hematopoietic stem cell transplant; AML, acute myeloid leukemia; NK, natural killer; WT, wild-type.

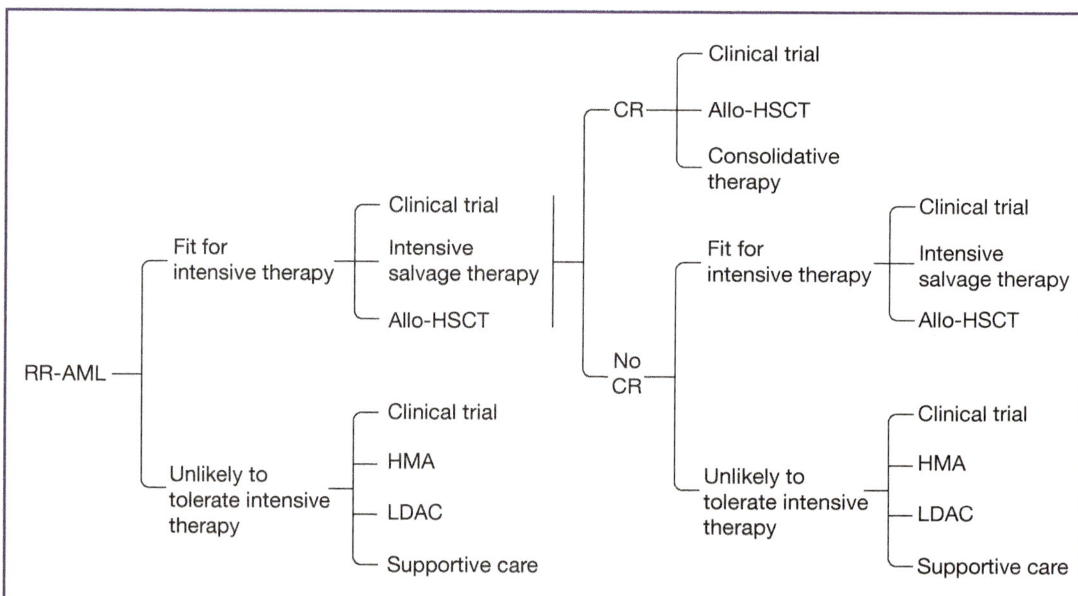

FIGURE 3-15: Treatment algorithm for patients with RR-AML in 2016. The management of relapsed and refractory AML has not been standardized, but the algorithm presented here represents an accepted approach. A clinical trial, if available, is often preferred given the poor outcomes with standard therapy. Hopefully, many of the immunotherapeutic and targeted approaches outlined in Tables 3-10 and 3-11 will find utility in the treatment of AML either as initial therapy, salvage therapy as a bridge to allo-HSCT, or as part of consolidation therapy. Prior to allo-HSCT, it is desirable to achieve a complete remission to maximize the chances of survival as patients with residual disease who undergo an allo-HSCT have poorer outcomes in general.

Allo-HSCT, allogeneic hematopoietic stem cell transplant; AML, acute myeloid leukemia; CR, complete remission; HMA, hypomethylating agent; LDAC, low-dose cytosine arabinoside; RR, relapsed/refractory.

recent findings. Integration of cytogenetics and molecular mutations can help predict PRD, especially in the largest category of intermediate-risk karyotype. Older age (>60) has repeatedly been an independent poor prognostic factor for any given cytogenetic or mutational change. In addition to presenting features, kinetics of peripheral and marrow blast clearance have some predictive value. A negative nadir bone marrow biopsy is defined as less than 10% to 20% cellularity with less than 5% to 10% residual blasts Patients, however, can have a morphologically negative nadir bone marrow and not achieve complete remission, while other patients with residual disease at nadir can achieve complete remission without further treatment. The percentage of blasts present, though, is still meaningful, with increasing percentage worsening the prognosis, as 5% to 15% seems to represent a different prognostic group than more than 15%. The less invasive technique of flow cytometry on peripheral blood has also been utilized early during induction therapy to evaluate the kinetics of blast clearance. At this time, it is useful to evaluate these factors, but no compilation of prognostic factors or tests is completely satisfactory in determining who will or will not achieve the important milestone of complete remission with induction therapy.

Please see Chapter 4 (Allogeneic Transplant in Adults and Children for AML and ALL) for issues related to allogeneic transplantation in adults and children.

Selected References

GENERAL

Breems DA, Van Putten WL, Huijgens PC, et al. Prognostic index for adult patients with acute myeloid leukemia in first relapse. *J Clin Oncol*. 2005;23:1969–1978.

Bryan JC, Jabbour EJ. Management of relapsed/refractory acute myeloid leukemia in the elderly: current strategies and developments. *Drugs Aging*. 2015;32:623–637.

Chevallier P, Labopin M, Turlure P, et al. A new leukemia prognostic scoring system for refractory/relapsed adult acute myelogeneous leukaemia patients: a GOELAMS study. *Leukemia*. 2011;25:939–944.

Grimwade D, Ivey A, Huntly BJ. Molecular landscape of acute myeloid leukemia in younger adults and its clinical relevance. *Blood*. 2016;127:29–41.

Litzow MR. Progress and strategies for patients with relapsed and refractory acute myeloid leukemia. *Curr Opin Hematol*. 2007;14:130–137.

Mangan JK, Luger SM. Salvage therapy for relapsed or refractory acute myeloid leukemia. *Ther Adv Hematol*. 2011;2:73–82.

National Comprehensive Cancer Network. NCCN clinical practice guidelines in oncology: acute myeloid leukemia version 2. http://www.nccn.org/professionals/physician_gls/f_guidelines.asp

Orlowski RJ, Mangan JK, Luger SM. Approach to patients with primary refractory acute myeloid leukemia. *Curr Opin Hematol*. 2015;22:97–107.

Price SL, Lancet JE, George TJ, et al. Salvage chemotherapy regimens for acute myeloid leukemia: Is one better? Efficacy comparison between CLAG and MEC regimens. *Leuk Res*. 2011;35:301–304.

Ramos NR, Mo CC, Karp JE, Hourigan CS. Current approaches in the treatment of relapsed and refractory acute myeloid leukemia. *J Clin Med*. 2015;4:665–695.

Thol F, Schlenk RF, Heuser M, Ganser A. How I treat refractory and early relapsed acute myeloid leukemia. *Blood*. 2015;126:319–327.

Walter RB, Othus M, Burnett AK, et al. Resistance prediction in AML: analysis of 4601 patients from MRC/NCRI, HOVON/SAKK, SWOG and MD Anderson cancer center. *Leukemia*. 2015;29:312–320.

CHEMOTHERAPY-BASED REGIMENS

Archimbaud E, Thomas X, Leblond V, et al. Timed sequential chemotherapy for previously treated patients with acute myeloid leukemia: long-term follow-up of the etoposide, mitoxantrone, and cytarabine-86 trial. *J Clin Oncol*. 1995;13:11–18.

Becker PS, Kantarjian HM, Appelbaum FR, et al. Retrospective comparison of clofarabine versus fludarabine in combination with high-dose cytarabine with or without granulocyte colony-stimulating factor as salvage therapies for acute myeloid leukemia. *Haematologica*. 2013;98:114–118.

Feldman EJ, Lancet JE, Kolitz JE, et al. First-in-man study of CPX-351: a liposomal carrier containing cytarabine and daunorubicin in a fixed 5:1 molar ratio for the treatment of relapsed and refractory acute myeloid leukemia. *J Clin Oncol*. 2011;29:979–985.

Herzig RH, Lazarus HM, Wolff SN, et al. High-dose cytosine arabinoside therapy with and without anthracycline antibiotics for remission reinduction of acute nonlymphoblastic leukemia. *J Clin Oncol*. 1985;3:992–997.

Karanes C, Kopecky KJ, Head DR, et al. A phase III comparison of high dose ARA-C (HIDAC) versus HIDAC plus mitoxantrone in the treatment of first relapsed or refractory acute myeloid leukemia. Southwest Oncology Group Study. *Leuk Res*. 1999;23:787–794.

Karp JE, Smith BD, Resar LS, et al. Phase 1 and pharmacokinetic study of bolus-infusion flavopiridol followed by cytosine arabinoside and mitoxantrone for acute leukemias. *Blood*. 2011;117:3302–3310.

Lancet JE, Ravandi F, Ricklis RM, et al. A phase Ib study of vosaroxin, an anticancer quinolone derivative, in patients with relapsed or refractory acute leukemia. *Leukemia*. 2011;25:1808–1814.

Ravandi F, Cortes J, Faderl S, et al. Characteristics and outcome of patients with acute myeloid leukemia refractory to 1 cycle of high-dose cytarabine-based induction chemotherapy. *Blood*. 2010;116:5818–5823;quiz 6153.

Roboz GJ, Rosenblat T, Arellano M, et al. International randomized phase III study of elacytarabine versus investigator choice in patients with relapsed/refractory acute myeloid leukemia. *J Clin Oncol*. 2014;32:1919–1926.

IMMUNE-BASED REGIMENS

Chapuis AG, Ragnarsson GB, Nguyen HN, et al. Transferred WT1-reactive CD8+ T cells can mediate antileukemic activity and persist in post-transplant patients. *Sci Transl Med*. 2013;5:174ra127.

Cilloni D, Renneville A, Hermitte F, et al. Real-time quantitative polymerase chain reaction detection of minimal residual disease by standardized WT1 assay to enhance risk stratification in acute myeloid leukemia: a European LeukemiaNet study. *J Clin Oncol*. 2009;27:5195–5201.

Feldman EJ, Brandwein J, Stone R, et al. Phase III randomized multicenter study of a humanized anti-CD33 monoclonal antibody, lintuzumab, in combination with chemotherapy, versus chemotherapy alone in patients with refractory or first-relapsed acute myeloid leukemia. *J Clin Oncol*. 2005;23:4110–4116.

Goswami M, Hensel N, Smith BD, et al. Expression of putative targets of immunotherapy in acute myeloid leukemia and healthy tissues. *Leukemia*. 2014;28:1167–1170.

Thol F, Schlenk RF. Gemtuzumab ozogamicin in acute myeloid leukemia revisited. *Expert Opin Biol Ther*. 2014;14:1185–1195.

ACUTE PROMYELOCYTIC LEUKEMIA (APL)

Aziz Nazha, Steven D. Gore, and Amer Methqal Zeidan

Acute promyelocytic leukemia (APL) or AML with t(15;17)(q22;q12)/*PML-RARα* has a predominant population of abnormal promyelocytes (considered as blast equivalents). The genetic abnormality confers high sensitivity of the leukemic promyelocytes to all-trans-retinoic acid (ATRA) treatment. The abnormal promyelocytes may have oval, folded, or bilobed nuclei, and typically have numerous cytoplasmic granules and multiple Auer rods (Figure 3-16A). The hypo or microgranular variant of APL has blasts with bilobed, "apple core," or "sliding plates" nuclei, and usually has a high leukocyte

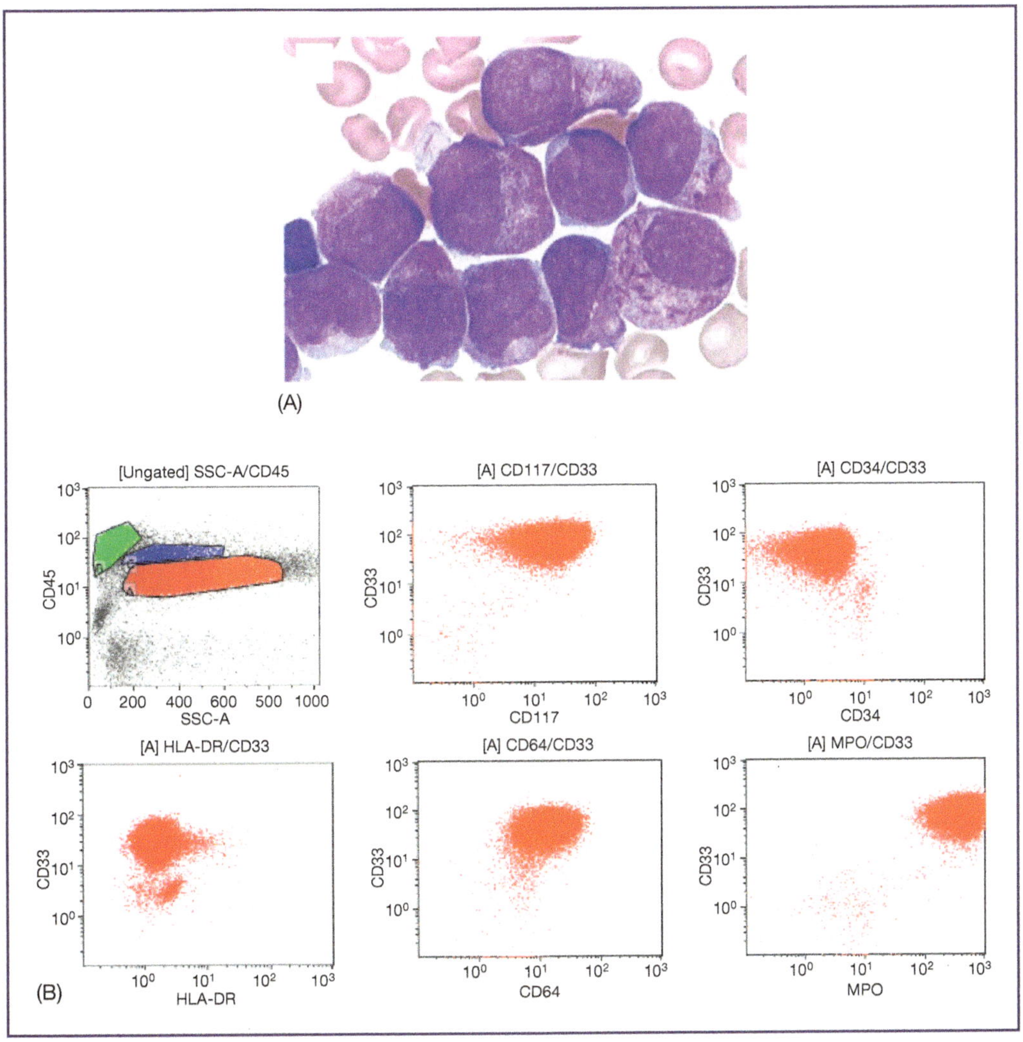

FIGURE 3-16: (A) AML with t(15;17), also known as acute promyelocytic leukemia (APL). Bone marrow aspirate showing abnormal promyelocytes with bilobed or folded nuclei, prominent nucleoli, and numerous azurophil granules in the cytoplasm. Note the multiple Auer rods in the cells. Wright stain X50. (B) Flow cytometric analysis of a case of AML with t(15;17). The abnormal promyelocytes (red) exhibit a high SSC and express bright CD33 and MPO, but lack CD34 and HLA-DR expression. CD64 is also characteristically expressed on promyelocytes.

Source: **Courtesy of Dr. Zeba Singh.**

AML, acute myeloid leukemia; HLA-DR, human leukocyte antigen-D related; MPO, myeloperoxidase; SSC-A, side scatter-A.

count at presentation (Figure 3-16B). Both the typical and microgranular variant are frequently complicated by development of disseminated intravascular coagulation (DIC). Presence of schistocytes on the peripheral blood (PB) film is an indicator for accompanying DIC and warrants assessment of coagulation parameters, importantly fibrinogen and D-dimer level. The immunophenotype is characteristic, but not diagnostic of, APL—the blasts have high side scatter, are negative for CD34 and HLA-DR, and have bright CD33 expression (Figure 3-16B). Of note, the microgranular variant may have a partial expression of CD34, and is difficult to distinguish morphologically from acute monocytic leukemia. Confirmation requires demonstration of the t(15;17)/*PML-RARα* or the chimeric gene product. In a minority of cases, the *RARα* gene may have variant translocation partners—*ZBTB1* (11q23), *NUMA1* (11q13), *NPM1* (5q35), and *STAT5* (17q11.2). The variant translocations are not picked up by the usual FISH probe set for the t(15;17), but a *RARα* breakapart probe indicates involvement of the *RARα* gene in a translocation. Variant translocations involving the *ZBTB1* (11q23) and *STAT5* (17q11.2) genes do not respond to ATRA.

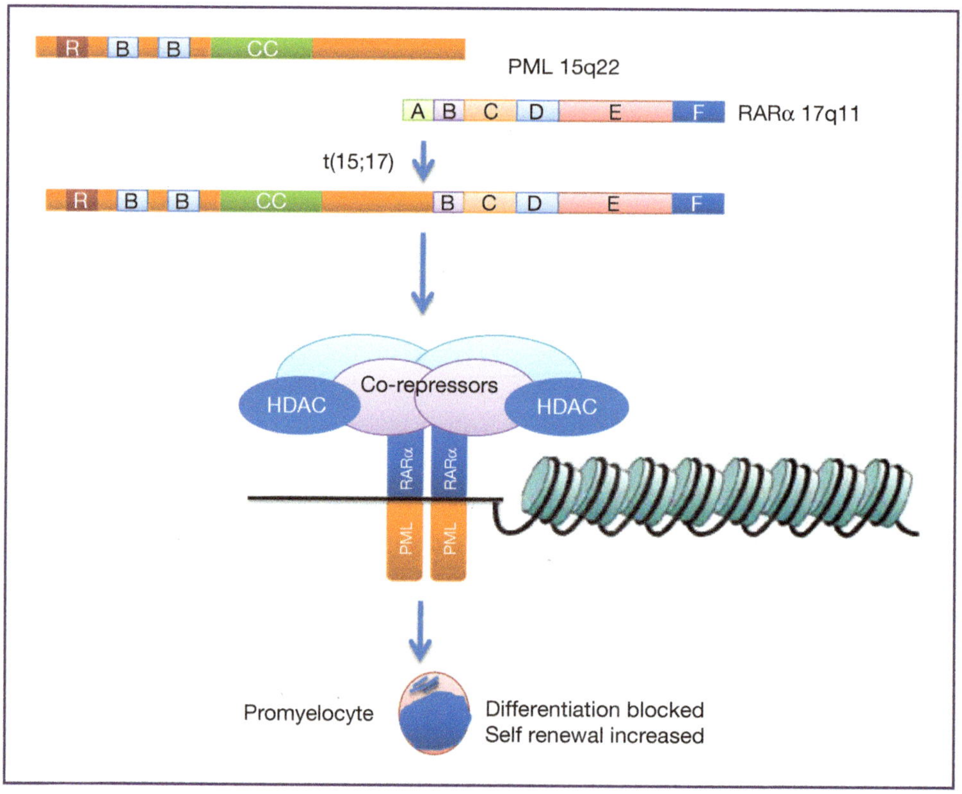

FIGURE 3-17: Model of APL pathogenesis and pathophysiology. Structures of PML (promyelocytic leukemia), RARα (retinoic acid receptor-alpha), and the fusion PML-RARα proteins that result from the t(15:17) translocation. Boxes with R, B, CC, C, E, and F indicate regulatory domains in each protein. PML induces dimerization and represses RARα targets through recruitment of co-repressors and HDAC, in turn leading to blockade of differentiation in myeloid precursors. APL, acute promyelocytic leukemia; HDAC, histone deacetylase.

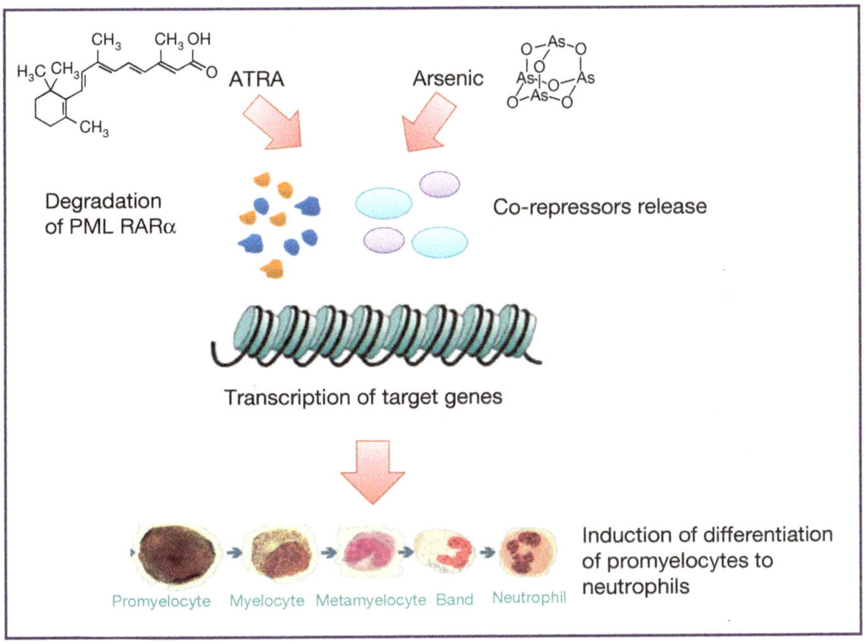

FIGURE 3-18: ATRA and ATO degrade the PML-RARα protein. **Treatment with all-trans-retinoic acid (ATRA) and arsenic trioxide (ATO) induces degradation of the PML-RARα protein and the release of co-repressors, thereby inducing histone acetylation and transcription of *RARα* target genes, which in turn induces differentiation in myeloid progenitors. APL is a medical emergency often presenting with DIC, bleeding, and thrombosis. At first suspicion for APL, *even without confirmed diagnosis*, ATRA must be initiated along with aggressive transfusion support. The patients who are receiving ATRA should be monitored for signs and symptoms of *differentiation syndrome* and be treated with steroids.**

APL, acute promyelocytic leukemia; PML, promyelocytic leukemia; RARα, retinoic acid receptor alpha.

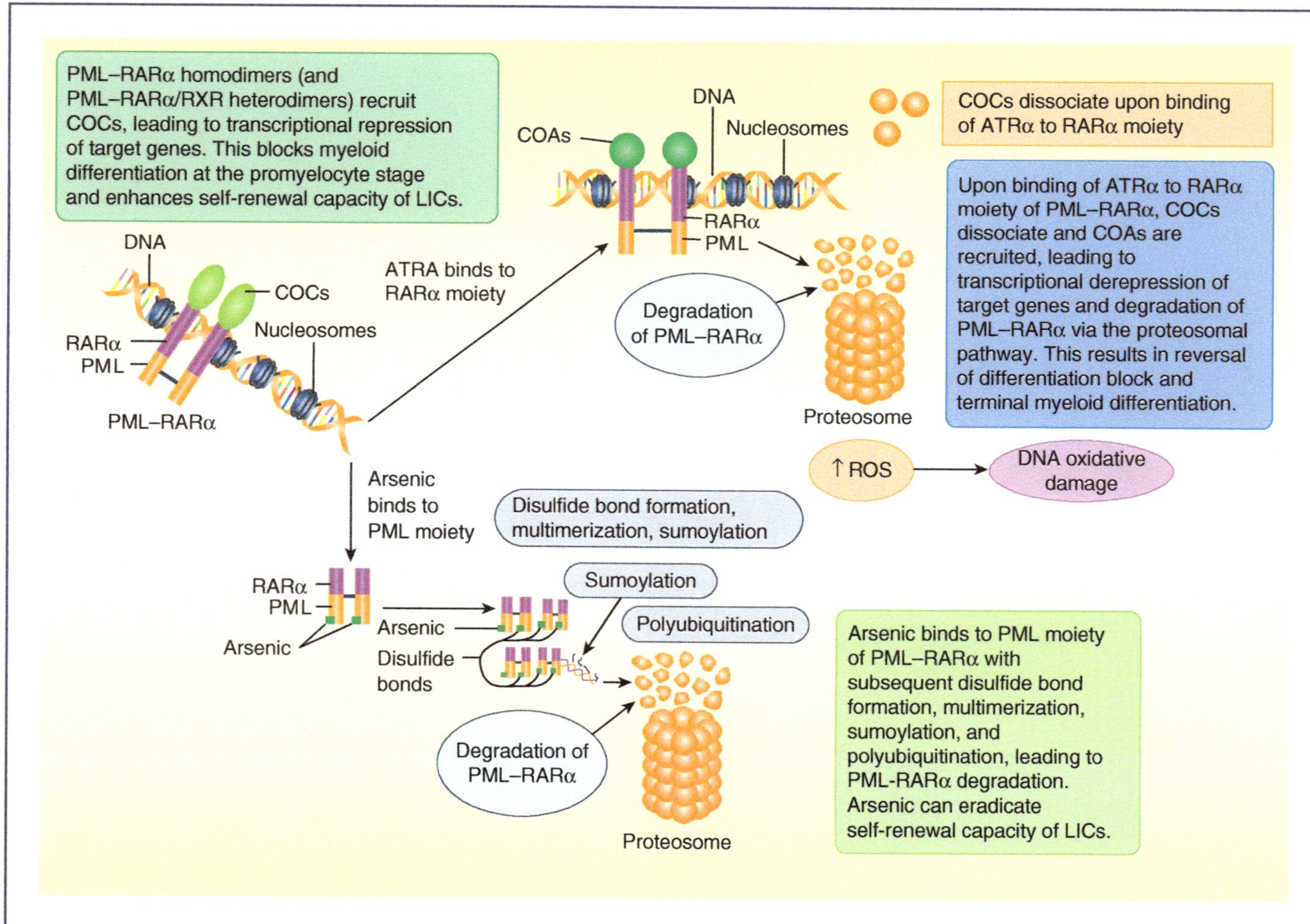

FIGURE 3-19: **Mechanisms of action of ATRA and arsenic trioxide in APL.**

Source: Adapted from Zeidan AM, Gore SD. New strategies in acute promyelocytic leukemia: moving to an entirely oral, chemotherapy-free upfront management approach. *Clin Cancer Res.* 2014;20(19):4985–4993. doi:10.1158/1078-0432.CCR-13-2725

APL, acute promyelocytic leukemia; ATRA, all-trans retinoic acid; COA, coactivator complex; LIC, leukemia-initiating cells; PML, promyelocytic leukemia; RARα, retinoic acid receptor alpha; ROS, reactive oxygen species.

Study, year of publication, type of study, # of patients (reference)	Follow-up, median (range) in months	Age, median (range) in years	Risk group (# patients)		Induction (complete remission %)	Consolidation	Maintenance	Survival
			High	Non-high				
Induction ± consolidation ± maintenance in combination with other agents								
Shen et al (2004), randomized, 61	18 (8–30)	30.5–39.5 (14–74)	14	47	Randomized to: • ATRA (95%) • ATO (90%) • ATRA + ATO (95.2%)	Three courses of sequential DA-cytarabine "pulse" regimen-HA	Five cycles of either: • ATRA + 6-MP + MTX • ATO + 6-MP + MTX • ATRA + ATO+ -MP + MTX	Median DFS (months): ATRA: 13 ATO: 16 ATRA + ATO: 20
Estey et al (2006), single-arm, 44	16 (N/A)	45	19	25	ATRA + ATO (+GO for high-risk) (89%)	Four courses of ATRA-ATO (28 weeks)	No additional therapy	Two-year OS: 86% Two-year DFS: 86%
Ravandi et al (2009), single-arm, 82	23 (0.47–65.6)	47 (14–81)	26	56	ATRA + ATO (+GO for high-risk) (92%)	Four courses of ATRA-ATO (28 weeks)	No additional therapy	Three-year OS: 85% Three-year DFS: 81%
Hu et al (2009), single-arm, 85	70 (21–88)	N/A (<15 – >55)	19	66	ATRA + ATO (+hydroxyurea for high-risk)(94.1%)	Three courses of sequential DA-cytarabine "pulse" regimen-HA	Five cycles of either: -ATRA + 6-MP + MTX -ATO + 6-MP + MTX -ATRA + ATO+-MP + MTX	Five-year OS: 91.7% Five-year EFS: 89.2% Five-year DFS: 94.8%
Dai et al (2009), non-randomized, two-arm, 162	30–32 (1–59)	32–34 (14–69)	39	123	Group A (72 patients): ATRA (90.3%) Group B (90 patients): ATRA + ATO (93.3%, $P = .57$)	Group A: A2: Five cycles of ATRA + DA + HA; A1: Four cycles of ATRA + DA + HA + one cycle of ATO Group B: Four cycles of ATRA + DA + HA + one cycle of ATO	Group A: A2: Two years of ATRA + DA + HA; A1: Two years of ATRA + ATO + DA Group B: Two years of ATRA + ATO + DA	Three-year DFS: Group A2 (no ATO): 72.4%, Group A1 (ATO in consolidation and maintenance): 93.8% Group B (ATO in induction, consolidation, and maintenance): 92.6%
Iland et al (2012), single-arm, 124	24 (2–61)	44 (3–78)	24	99	ATRA + ATO + Ida (95%)	Two courses of ATO + ATRA	Two years (8 cycles) of ATRA, 6-MP, and MTX	Two-year OS: 93.2% Two-year EFS: 88.1% Two-year DFS: 98%

FIGURE 3-20: Selected clinical trials that used ATO along with other agents (not as a single agent) in upfront induction +/– consolidation of APL. (*continued*)

Study, year of publication, type of study, # of patients (reference)	Follow-up, median (range) in months	Age, median (range) in years	Risk group (# patients)		Induction (complete remission %)	Consolidation	Maintenance	Survival
			High	Non-high				
Lo-Coco et al (2013), randomized non-inferiority, 156	34.4 (0.5–55.8)	44.6–46.6 (18.7–70.2)	0	156	Randomized (1:1) to: - ATRA-ATO (100%) - ATRA-Ida (95%), *P*-value = (.12)	- For ATRA-ATO group: Four courses of ATRA-ATO (28 weeks) - For ATRA-Ida group: Three sequential cycles of ATRA-Ida, ATRA-MA, ATRA-Ida	- For ATRA-ATO: No additional therapy - For ATRA-Ida group: Two years of ATRA, 6-MP, and MTX	Two-year EFS:ATRA-ATO: 97% ATRA-Ida: 86% (non-inferiority *P*-value <.001, superiority *P*-value = .02). Two-year OS:ATRA-ATO: 99% ATRA-Ida: 91% (*P*-value = .02)
Consolidation								
Gore et al (2010), single arm, 45	32.4 (18–66)	50 (19–70)	14	31	ATRA + daunorubicin	One course of cytarabine + daunorubicin + ATO	High-risk: Two years of ATRA, 6-MP, and MTX Low-risk: Two-year [ATRA]	Three-year OS: 88% Three-year DFS: 88.7% Three-year EFS: 76%
Powell et al (2010), randomized, 481	28.8 (N/A)	N/A (15–79)	113	368	ATRA + cytarabine + daunorubicin (90%)	Randomized (1:1) to: - Two courses of ATRA + daunorubicin - Two courses of ATO followed by two courses of ATRA + daunorubicin	Randomized to 1 year of: - ATRA - ATRA + 6-MP + MTX	-Three-year EFS:ATO arm: 80% Non-ATO arm: 63% (*P*-value <.0001), 3-year OS: ATO arm: 86% Non-ATO arm: 81% (*P*-value = .059), 3-year DFS: ATO arm: 90% Non-ATO arm: 70% (*P*-value <.0001).

FIGURE 3-20: (*continued*) **Selected clinical trials that used ATO along with other agents (not as a single agent) in upfront induction +/– consolidation of APL.**

#All patients were required to be in CR after induction and consolidation at registration for the trial.

Risk grouping according to Sanz et al (2000).

Source: From Zeidan AM, Gore SD. New strategies in acute promyelocytic leukemia: moving to an entirely oral, chemotherapy-free upfront management approach. *Clin Cancer Res.* 2014;20(19):4985–4993. doi:10.1158/1078-0432.CCR-13-2725

6-MP, 6-mercaptopurine; AS_4S_4, tetra-arsenic tetra-sulfide; ATO, arsenic trioxide; ATRA, all-trans retinoic acid; DA, daunorubicin + cytarabine; DFS, disease-free survival; EFS, event-free survival; GO, gemtuzumab ozogamicin; HA, homoharringtonine + cytarabine; Ida, idarubicin; MA, mitoxantrone + cytarabine; MTX, methotrexate; N/A, not available; OS, overall survival; RIF, realgar-indigo naturalis (an AS_4S_4-containing formulation).

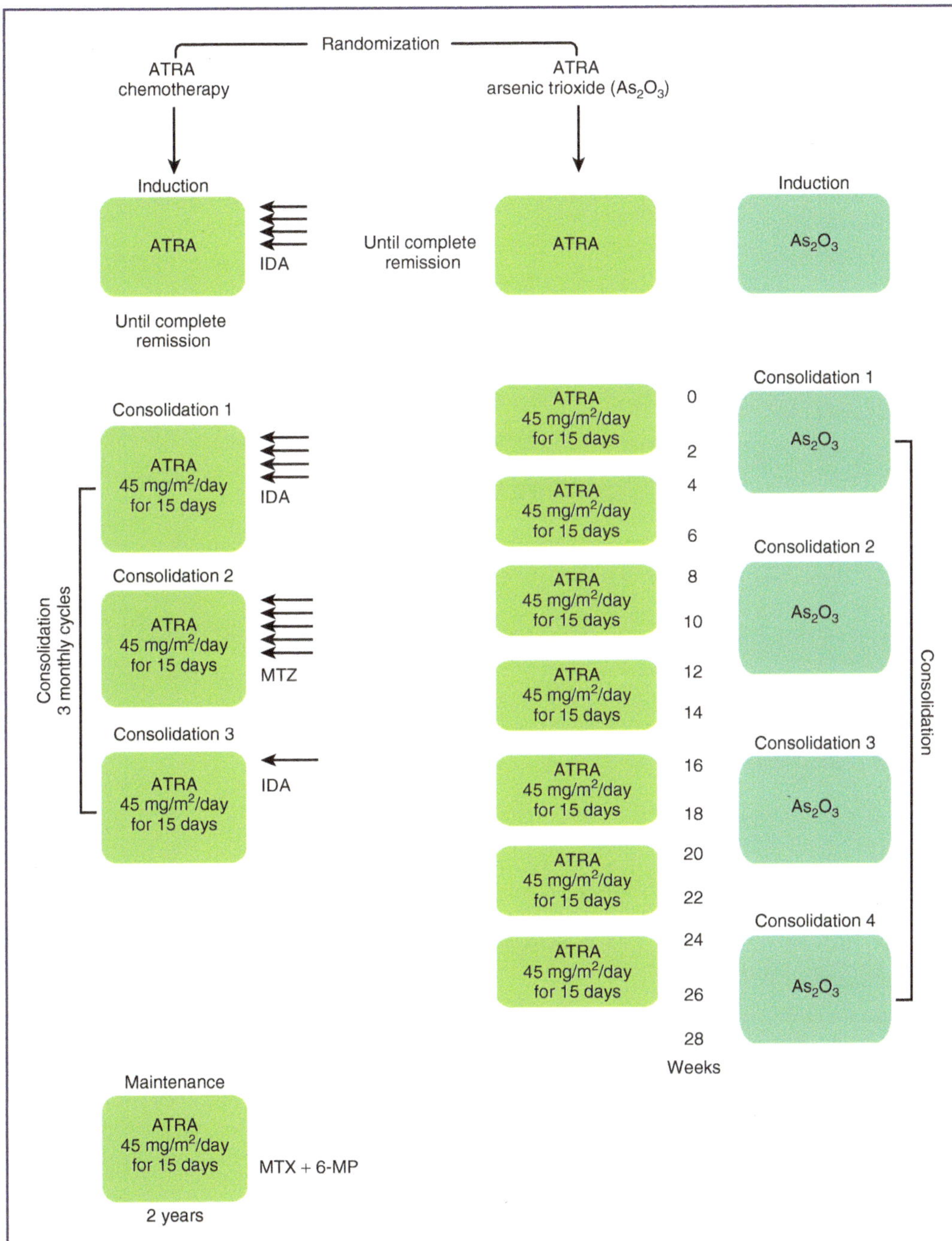

FIGURE 3-21: Chemotherapy-free regimen for low- and intermediate-risk APL (WBC <10K/mcL) at presentation.

Dose of ATRA 45 mg/m²/day in two divided doses orally. Dose of As_2O_3 0.15 mg/kg intravenously (given daily during induction, and 5 days per week [Monday through Friday] during consolidations).

Source: Adapted from Lo-Coco F, Avvisati G, Vignetti M, et al. Retinoic acid and arsenic trioxide for acute promyleocytic leukemia. *N Engl J Med.* 2013;369(2):111–121.

6-MP, 6-mercaptopurine; As_2O_3, arsenic trioxide; ATRA, all-trans retinoic acid; IDA, idarubicin; MTX, methotrexate; MTZ, mitoxantrone.

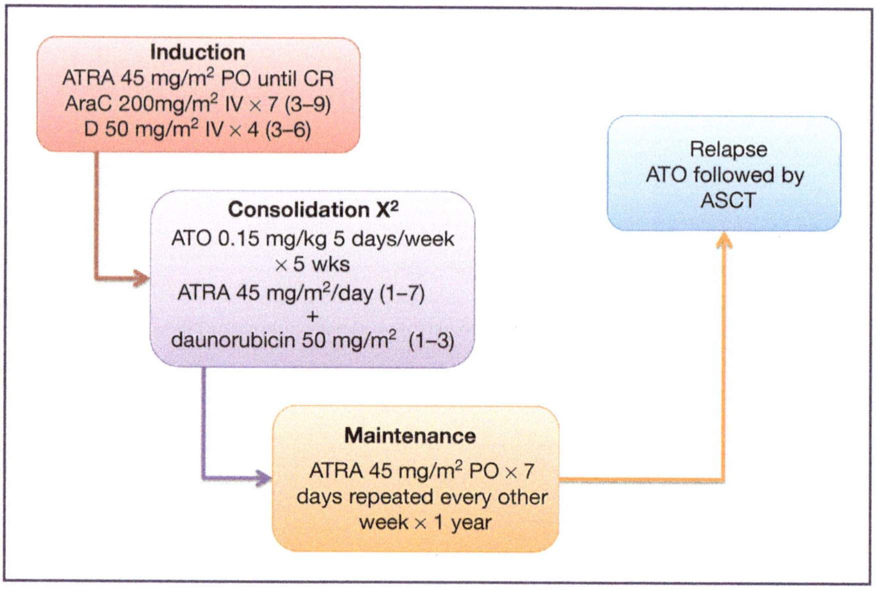

FIGURE 3-22: Suggested treatment schema for high-risk APL at presentation: North American Leukemia Intergroup Study.

APL, acute promyelocytic leukemia; AraC, cytarabine; ASCT, autologous stem cell transplantation; ATO, arsenic trioxide; ATRA, all-trans retinoic acid; D, daunorubicin.

Selected References

Collins SJ. Acute promyelocytic leukemia: relieveing repression induces remission. *Blood*. 1998; 91(8):2631–2633.

Dai CW, Zhang GS, Shen JK, et al. Use of all-trans retinoic acid in combination with arsenic trioxide for remission induction in patients with newly diagnosed acute promyelocytic leukemia and for consolidation/maintenance in CR patients. *Acta Haematol*. 2009;121(1):1–8.

de The H, Chomienne C, Lanotte M, et al. The t(15;17) translocation of acute promyelocytic leukaemia fuses the retinoic acid receptor alpha gene to a novel transcribed locus. *Nature*. 1990;347(6239):558–561.

Estey E, Garcia-Manero G, Ferrajoli A, et al. Use of all-trans retinoic acid plus arsenic trioxide as an alternative to chemotherapy in untreated acute promyelocytic leukemia. *Blood*. 2006;107(9):3469–3473.

Gore SD, Gojo I, Sekeres MA, et al. Single cycle of arsenic trioxide-based consolidation chemotherapy spares anthracycline exposure in the primary management of acute promyelocytic leukemia. *J Clin Oncol*. 2010;28(6):1047–1053.

Hu J, Liu YF, Wu CF, et al. Long-term efficacy and safety of all-trans retinoic acid/arsenic trioxide-based therapy in newly diagnosed acute promyelocytic leukemia. *Proc Natl Acad Sci USA*. 2009;106(9):3342–3347.

Iland HJ, Bradstock K, Supple SG, et al. All-trans-retinoic acid, idarubicin, and IV arsenic trioxide as initial therapy in acute promyelocytic leukemia (APML4). *Blood*. 2012;120(8):1570–1580.

Lo-Coco F, Avvisati G, Vignetti M, et al. Retinoic acid and arsenic trioxide for acute promyleocytic leukemia. *N Engl J Med*. 2013;369(2):111–121.

Melnick A, Licht JD. Deconstructing a disease: RARalpha, its fusion partners, and their roles in the pathogenesis of acute promyelocytic leukemia. *Blood*. 1999;93(10):3167–3215.

Powell BL, Moser B, Stock W, et al. Arsenic trioxide improves event-free and overall survival for adults with acute promyelocytic leukemia. North American Leukemia Intergroup Study C9710. *Blood.* 2010;116(19):3751–3757.

Ravandi F, Estey E, Jones D, et al. Effective treatment of acute promyelocytic leukemia with all-trans-retinoic acid, arsenic trioxide, and gemtuzumab ozogamicin. *J Clin Oncol.* 2009;27(4):504–510.

Sanz MA, Lo Coco F, Martín G, et al. Definition of relapse risk and role of nonanthracycline drugs for consolidation in patients with acute promyelocytic leukemia: a joint study of the PETHEMA and GIMEMA cooperative groups. *Blood.* 2000;96:1247.

Shen ZX, Shi ZZ, Fang J, et al. All-trans retinoic acid/As2O3 combination yields a high quality remission and survival in newly diagnosed acute promyelocytic leukemia. *Proc Natl Acad Sci USA.* 2004;101(15):5328–5335.

Zeidan AM, Gore SD. New strategies in acute promyelocytic leukemia: moving to an entirely oral, chemotherapy-free upfront management approach. *Clin Cancer Res.* 2014;20(19):4985–4993. doi:10.1158/1078-0432.CCR-13-2725

MDS/AML

FUNDAMENTALS OF EPIGENETICS

Monica Reddy Muppidi, Priyank P. Patel, Adam R. Karpf, and Elizabeth A. Griffiths

Introduction

Epigenetics (*epi* meaning *"above" genes*) refers to the heritable changes in gene expression that are not associated with changes in nucleic acid sequence in DNA–a change in phenotype without a change in genotype. It is these naturally occurring epigenetic changes that lead to the differentiation of the embryo into specialized cells with specific functions such as skin, liver, and brain. Epigenetic changes are also known to play critical roles in X chromosome inactivation and genomic imprinting. Epigenetic alterations to gene expression are known to be influenced by a myriad of factors including age, environmental/lifestyle exposures, and disease states and are changeable across an organism's lifetime. In addition, there is increasing recognition for the transgenerational inheritance of epigenetic marks that can profoundly alter phenotype for a wide variety of different disease states. Dysregulated epigenetic signaling is linked to the pathogenesis of various cancers and has been extensively studied in myelodysplastic syndromes and acute myeloid leukemia.

Structure of Chromatin

Every cellular nucleus contains genetic information in the form of DNA, which is packed by protein complexes composed of histone proteins to form chromatin. Approximately 147 base pairs of DNA wrap around a histone protein complex known as the nucleosome. The nucleosome core particle consists of DNA wrapped around a histone octamer that contains two copies each of four major types of histone proteins: H2A, H2B, H3, and H4. Histone protein H1 provides structural stability to the complex by acting as a linker between two nucleosomes. Chromatin in a tightly wound, compact state is called heterochromatin and is generally inaccessible for transcription, whereas chromatin in a relaxed configuration, generally accessible for transcription, is called euchromatin (Figure 3-23).

DNA consists of four primary nucleotides (adenine, thiamine, guanine, and cytosine). Two additional bases, formed through modifications to cytosine with the addition of either a methyl group (CH_3) or a hydroxymethyl group (CH_2OH) to the carbon 5 (C5) of the cytosine ring, have also been identified, and it is these modified bases that form the skeleton for epigenetic changes at the DNA level. Modified cytosine is generally restricted to cytosines found adjacent and 5′ to guanine. This sequence, cytosine-phosphate-guanine (CpG), or C followed by G within the nucleotide sequence, occurs less frequently in the genome than would be expected by random chance. This deficiency of CpG dinucleotides within the genome likely results from the tendency of methylcytosine to spontaneously deaminate to uracil, a base that is then copied forward as thymidine, converting CpG to TpG. Despite the relative deficiency of CpGs across the genome, the promoters of many critical genes are relatively CpG rich (containing >50% G-C content and enriched for CpG sites); such regions are referred to as CpG islands. The presence of such C-G–rich regions within the genome is the result of evolutionary conservation in order to impart the important information related to gene expression conferred by epigenetic modifications. Chemical modifications to CpG sites and adjacent histone proteins, without alteration of the DNA structure, resulting in silencing (inactivation) or expression (activation) of CpG-rich genes, is the basis of epigenetic regulation.

Epigenetic Modifications

Epigenetic modifications include direct DNA modifications (methylation, hydroxymethylation), histone modifications, and RNA interference with noncoding RNAs. All these epigenetic mechanisms are interlinked. Epigenetic modifications are made, interpreted, and removed by several classes of conserved proteins called writers, readers, and erasers. Such genes interact to form one large regulatory

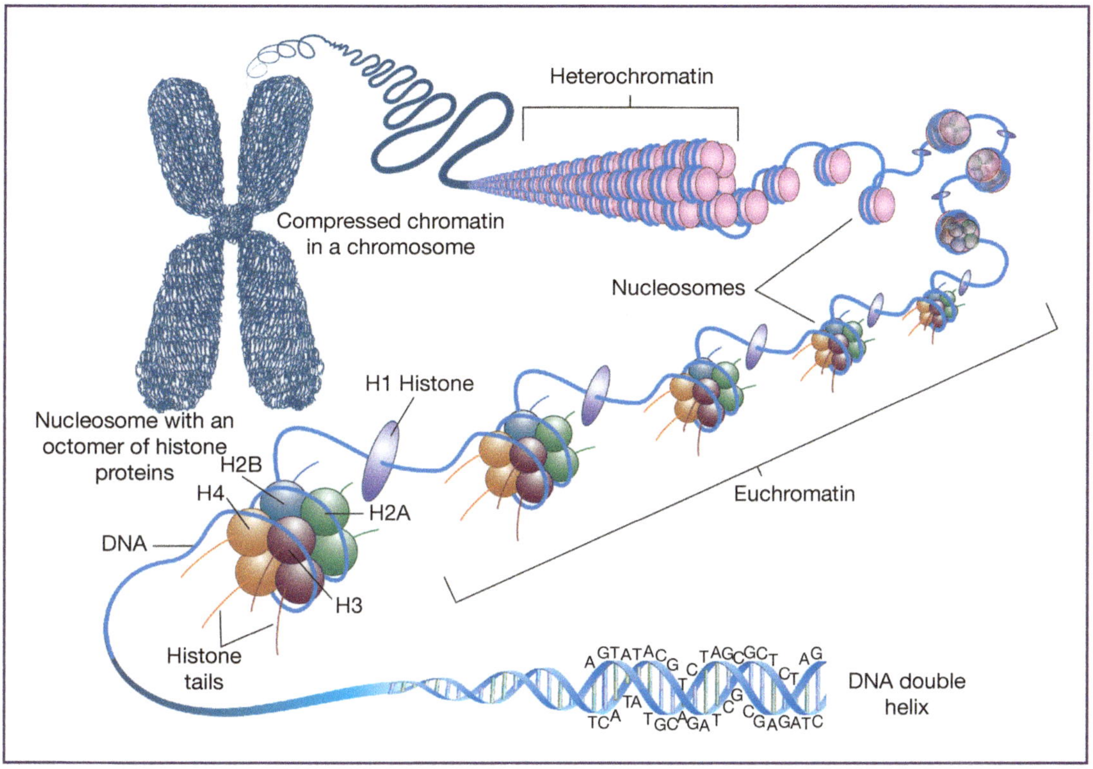

FIGURE 3-23: **Structure of chromatin in a mitotic chromosome, heterochromatin, euchromatin, and nucleosome. Heterochromatin is tightly packed and transcriptionally inactive. DNA in euchromatin is in a relaxed state accessible for transcription. A nucleosome containing 147bp DNA wrapped around a histone octamer. The octomer consists of two each of histone proteins H2A, H2B, H3, and H4. Histone H1 acts as a linker between two nucleosomes.**

network. The two most common and well-studied epigenetic modifications are DNA methylation and histone modifications.

1. **DNA methylation**

   DNA methylation occurs via the addition of a methyl group at the C5 position of the cytosine ring. 5-Methyl-cytosine occurs in the genome mostly in the context of the cytosine phosphate-guanine dinucleotide (CpG islands). This process of DNA methylation is catalyzed by a group of enzymes called DNA methyltransferases (DNMTs). During DNA replication, the parent DNA methylation pattern acts as a template for the addition of methyl groups to newly synthesized DNA. Promoter regions rich in CpG islands can become heavily methylated, resulting in the recruitment of DNA-binding proteins and histone deacetylase inhibitors, which produce transcriptional repression. Demethylation/hypomethylation of such regions will permit reexpression of such genes. In cancer cells, genes related to cell cycle regulation, DNA repair, and tumor suppression can become aberrantly hypermethylated, leading to their silencing.

   Genome-wide methylation is regulated by a variety of different mechanisms. Recently, recurrent nonoverlapping mutational events within an important set of epigenetic regulatory genes including DNA methyltransferase 3A (*DNMT3A)* (see DNMT3A in Chapter 2), isocitrate dehydrogenase 1 and 2 (*IDH1/2*), and the ten-eleven translocation *(Tet methylcytosine dioxygenase, TET)* enzymes (see TET and IDH in Chapter 2) have been identified as among the most common events in hematological malignancies. Inactivating mutations in *WT1* have also been shown to impact the function of TET enzymes and have been identified as yet another gene in

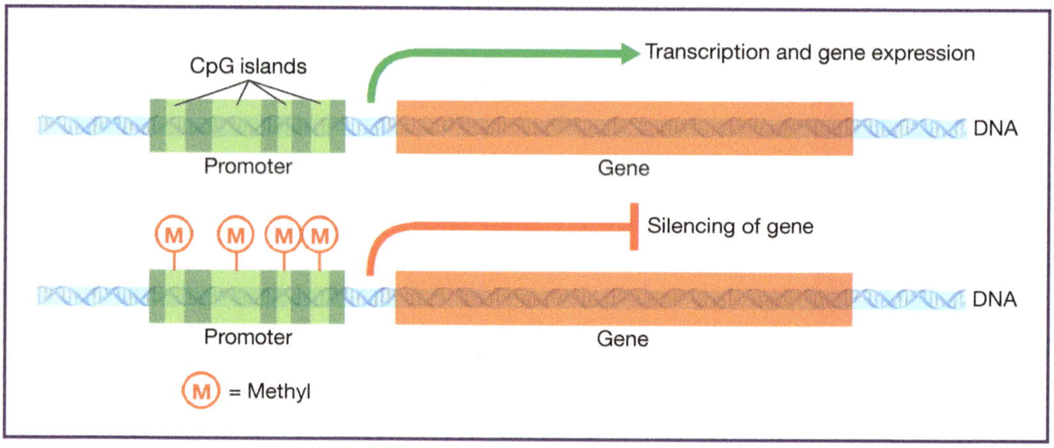

FIGURE 3-24: **The gene promotor regions are often rich in cytosine phosphate-guanine dinucleotides (CpGs) called CpG islands. Addition of methyl groups form 5-methylcytosine (methylation), leading to silencing of gene expression.**

the family of epigenetic modifiers frequently mutated in AML (see WT1 in Chapter 2). Extensive evaluation of these epigenetic driver mutational events has demonstrated them to be founder mutations in several myeloid malignancies. Importantly, we now recognize that mutations in these genes are present in older adults without identified hematological malignancy where clonal hematopoiesis appears to develop in association with aging. Furthermore, mouse models of *DNMT3A/B*, *IDH*, and *TET* mutant hematopoiesis have demonstrated enhanced stem cell self-renewal and leukemic transformation, validating the role of epigenetic mutational events as drivers of hematologic malignancies.

2. **Histone Modifications**

Histone modifications occur mostly on the flexible NH_2-terminal region of histone proteins called the histone tail. These post-translational modifications serve to allocate the genome into active regions (euchromatin) and inactive regions (heterochromatin) leading to gene expression or silencing, respectively. Amino acids such as lysine, arginine, glutamic acid, serine, threonine, and proline, which are present in histone proteins, are subject to specific chemical modifications such as acetylation, ubiquitination, phosphorylation, or methylation, among others.

Histone modification is regulated by writer enzymes including acetylases, methylases, and phosphorylases. Eraser enzymes including deacetylases, demethylases, and phosphatases catalyze the hydrolytic removal of respective chemical groups from histone tails. Readers are proteins that bind to modified histones and interpret the histone code laid down by writers and erasers. Disruption of the normal patterns of these modifications can contribute to cancer. The nomenclature for these modifications includes the histone protein involved (eg, H3), a single-letter code for the altered amino acid (eg, lysine, K), and the specific modification (eg, acetyl, ac or methyl, Me); H3K9ac denotes monoacetylation of the 9th lysine residue on histone H3. The well-characterized modifications to histones are acetylation and methylation.

- **Histone acetylation:** Acetylation of histone tails leads to relaxation of the local chromatin structure and allows access for transcriptional machinery, increasing gene expression. The enzymes responsible for regulation of this process are histone acetyltransferases (HAT; the writer) and deacetylases (HDAC, the eraser).
- **Histone methylation:** Histone methylation can either repress or activate transcription depending on the amino acid being methylated and the site of methylation. Arginine methylation of histones H3 and H4 result in transcriptional activation, whereas lysine methylation of the same histones leads to either activation or repression depending on the site of methylation. Tri-methylation of lysine 4 (K4) leads to transcriptional activation, while tri-methylation of lysine 9 (K9) is associated with transcriptional repression.

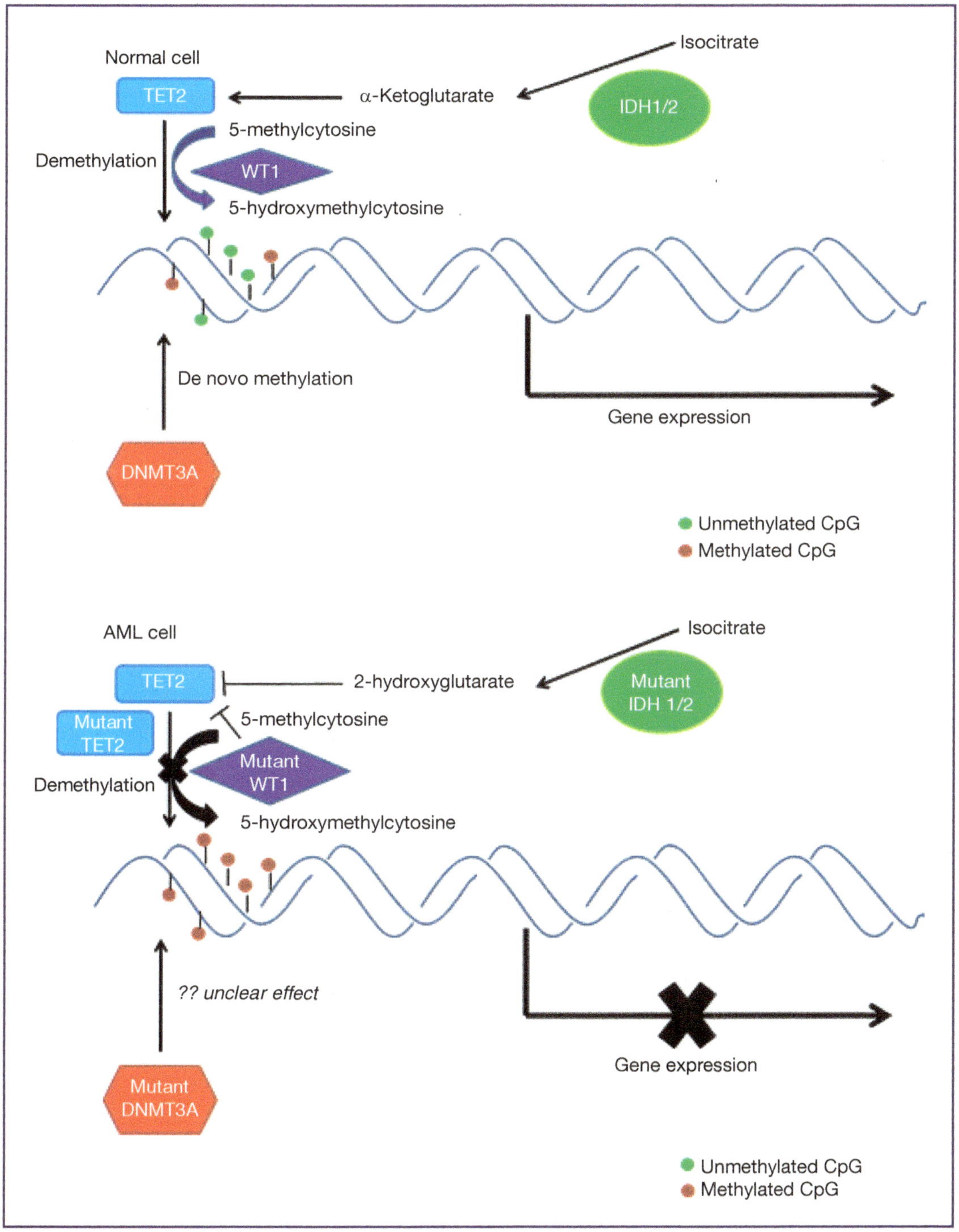

FIGURE 3-25: In a normal cell, isocitrate dehydrogenase (IDH) catalyzes the conversion of isocitrate to α-ketoglutarate (α-KG) in the Krebs cycle. α-KG along with iron and oxygen enhance TET2 catalytic activity for conversion of 5-methylcytosine to 5-hydroxymethylcytosine, which leads to demethylation. DNMT3A is an enzyme that catalyzes de novo methylation of CpG dinucleotides. In an AML cell, the mutant IDH converts isocitrate to α-KG and further to 2-hydroxyglutarate (2-HG). The lack of availability of α-KG leads to loss of function of TET2, which cannot perform demethylation. The effects of mutant DNMT3A are unclear as of now.

AML, acute myeloid leukemia; TET2, ten-eleven translocation 2; WT1, Wilms' tumor.

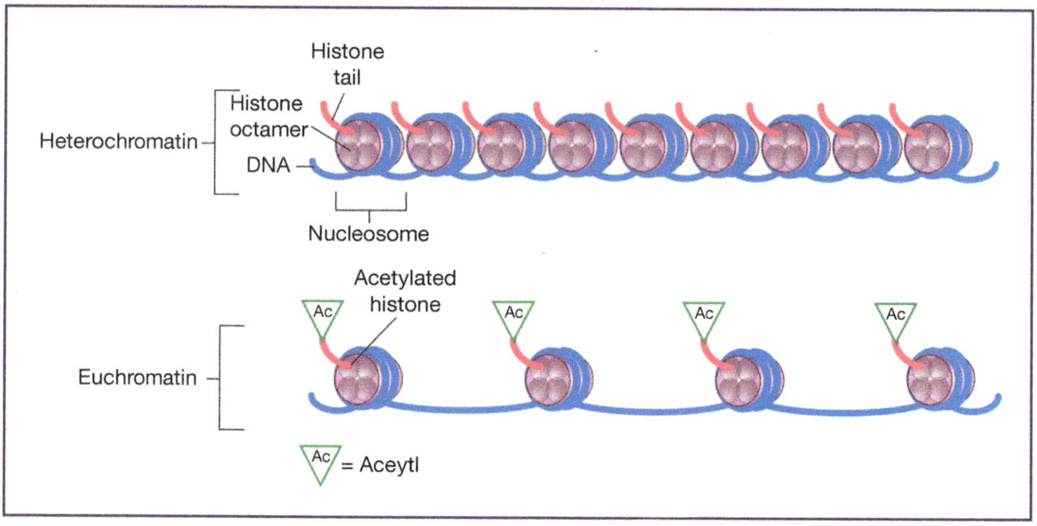

FIGURE 3-26: Acetylation of histone proteins causes more open chromatin configuration (euchromatin) leading to transcription and gene expression.

Table 3-12 Common mutations in epigenetic genes

GENE	MUTATION EFFECT	FREQUENCY OF MUTATION IN AML
DNMT3A	Reduced binding affinity and catalytic activity of DNMT3A during de novo methylation Loss of function	15%–25%
TET2	Truncated protein and consequent reduction in demethylation (reduction in hydroxymethylation) Loss of function	7%–23%
IDH1/2	Neomorphic enzyme by production of 2-hydroxyglutarate and inhibition of TET2 function Gain of function	15%–30%
ASXL1	Reduced expression, which results in reduced histone methylation and overexpression of leukemia-promoting genes	10%–15%
EZH2	Truncated SET domain leads to reduced catalytic activity of protein during histone modifications Loss of function	Occasional
WT1	Alterations in 5-hydroxymethylation (leads to site-specific effects on DNA methylation) and reduced function of TET2-loss of function	~10%

AML, acute myeloid leukemia; TET2, ten-eleven translocation 2.

3. Noncoding RNAs

Approximately 70% of the genome is transcribed but only 1% to 2% of it encodes protein. The transcribed RNAs that do not encode protein are called noncoding RNAs (ncRNAs). They include microRNA (miR), small nucleolar RNA (snoRNAs), Piwi-interacting RNAs (PiRNA), small interfering RNAs (siRNAs), and others. These ncRNAs regulate gene expression by recognizing target nucleotide sequences through complementarity. The well-studied ncRNAs are the miRs. MiRs are produced in the nucleus by transcription of the micro RNA gene to form a hairpin loop structure called pre-micro RNA. The pre-micro RNA undergoes cropping in the nucleus and dicing in the cytoplasm with the help of enzymes Drosha and Dicer, respectively, to form a mature miR. The mature miR is a double-stranded RNA with both sense and antisense strands, which is then incorporated into a larger complex known as the RNA-induced silencing complex (RISC). Once the miR is transferred to RISC, it is unwound by helicase forming single-stranded RNAs. Complementary base pairing between miR and mRNA signals RISC to either degrade the mRNA in case of complementary match or cause translational halt if there is a partial match, ultimately leading to regulation of gene expression. This process of silencing is called RNA interference. Dysregulation or mutations in ncRNA have been linked to cancer and other diseases, and can also determine response to chemotherapy agents.

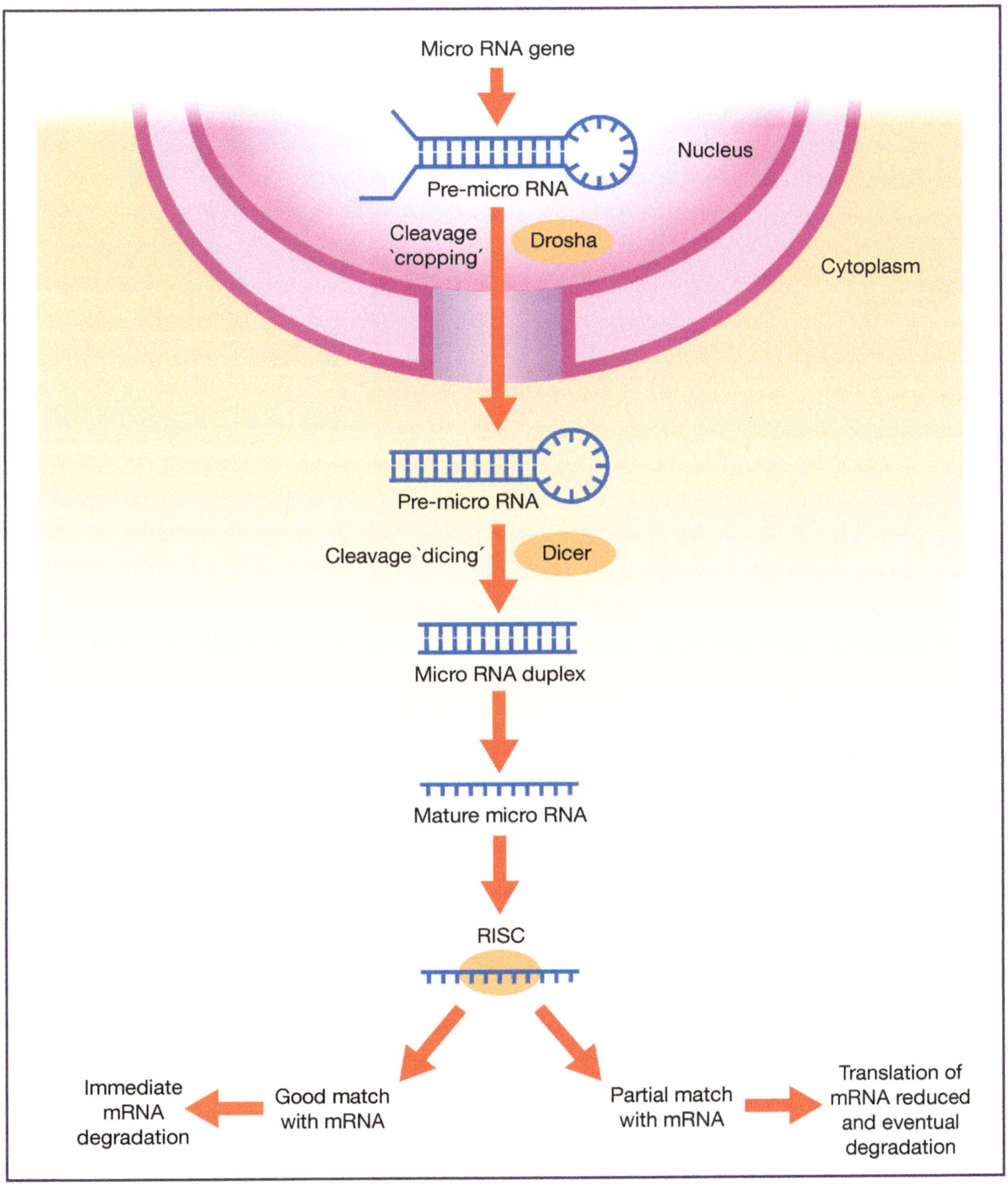

FIGURE 3-27: miRNA genes encode pre-miRNA, which is cleaved by cropping and dicing, leading to formation of mature miRNA. miRNA is incorporated into a larger complex called RNA-induced silencing complex (RISC). A good complementary match of miRNA with messenger RNA (mRNA) leads to immediate mRNA degradation. A partial match will reduce mRNA translation.

Epigenetics as Therapeutic Targets in Leukemia

Epigenetic modifications to the genome play a critical role in normal development and are among the most frequently disrupted marks in cancer. Deep sequencing studies, both of cancer genomes and those of younger and older adults, have now identified mutations within epigenetic driver genes as among the most frequently observed events associated with malignant transformation. Dysfunction of epigenetic mechanisms leads to lasting changes in gene expression that can confer cancer cells with survival advantage due to uninhibited growth, invasiveness, and delayed apoptosis. Global hypomethylation, down-regulation of miRNAs, promotor-specific hypermethylation, and histone deacetylation are some of the epigenetic dysregulations seen in malignancy.

Increased understanding of epigenetic mechanisms and their pathological implications in myelodysplastic syndromes and acute myeloid leukemia has opened a new treatment landscape. There are several arenas in epigenetics in which drugs can be designed to target and activate the suppressed genes, for example, demethylating the DNA, promoting acetylation of histone residues, or modifying the genes altering the epigenetic signatures (*DNMT3A*, *TET*, etc.).

Selected References

Bohacek J, Mansuy IM. Molecular insights into transgenerational non-genetic inheritance of acquired behaviours. *Nat Rev Genet*. 2015;16(11):641–652.

Djebali S, Davis CA, Merkel A, et al. Landscape of transcription in human cells. *Nature*. 2012;489:101–108.

Egger G, Liang G, Aparicio A, Jones PA. Epigenetics in human disease and prospects for epigenetic therapy. *Nature*. 2004;429:457–463.

Greer EL, Shi Y. Histone methylation: a dynamic mark in health, disease and inheritance. *Nat Rev Genet*. 2012;13:343–357.

Jaenisch R, Bird A. Epigenetic regulation of gene expression: how the genome integrates intrinsic and environmental signals. *Nat Genet*. 2003;33(Suppl):245–254.

Kats LM, Reschke M, Taulli R, et al. Proto-oncogenic role of mutant IDH2 in leukemia initiation and maintenance. *Cell Stem Cell*. 2014;14(3):329–341.

Mayle A, Yang L, Rodriguez B, et al. DNMT3A loss predisposes murine hematopoietic stem cells to malignant transformation. *Blood*. 2015;125(4):629–638.

McKerrell T, Park N, Moreno T, et al. Leukemia-associated somatic mutations drive distinct patterns of age-related clonal hemopoiesis. *Cell Rep*. 2015;10(8):1239–1245.

Rana TM. Illuminating the silence: understanding the structure and function of small RNAs. *Nat Rev Mol Cell Biol*. 2007;8:23–36.

Shih AH, Jiang Y, Meydan C, et al. Mutational cooperativity linked to combinatorial epigenetic gain of function in acute myeloid leukemia. *Cancer Cell*. 2015;27(4):502–515.

Stresemann C, Lyko F. Modes of action of the DNA methyltransferase inhibitors azacitidine and decitabine. *Int J Cancer*. 2008;123(1):8–13.

Walter MJ, Shen D, Ding L, et al. Clonal architecture of secondary acute myeloid leukemia. *N Engl J Med*. 2012;366(12):1090–1098.

CLONAL EVOLUTION AND TREATMENT OF SECONDARY AML AND MDS/AML

Vu H. Duong and Amer Methqal Zeidan

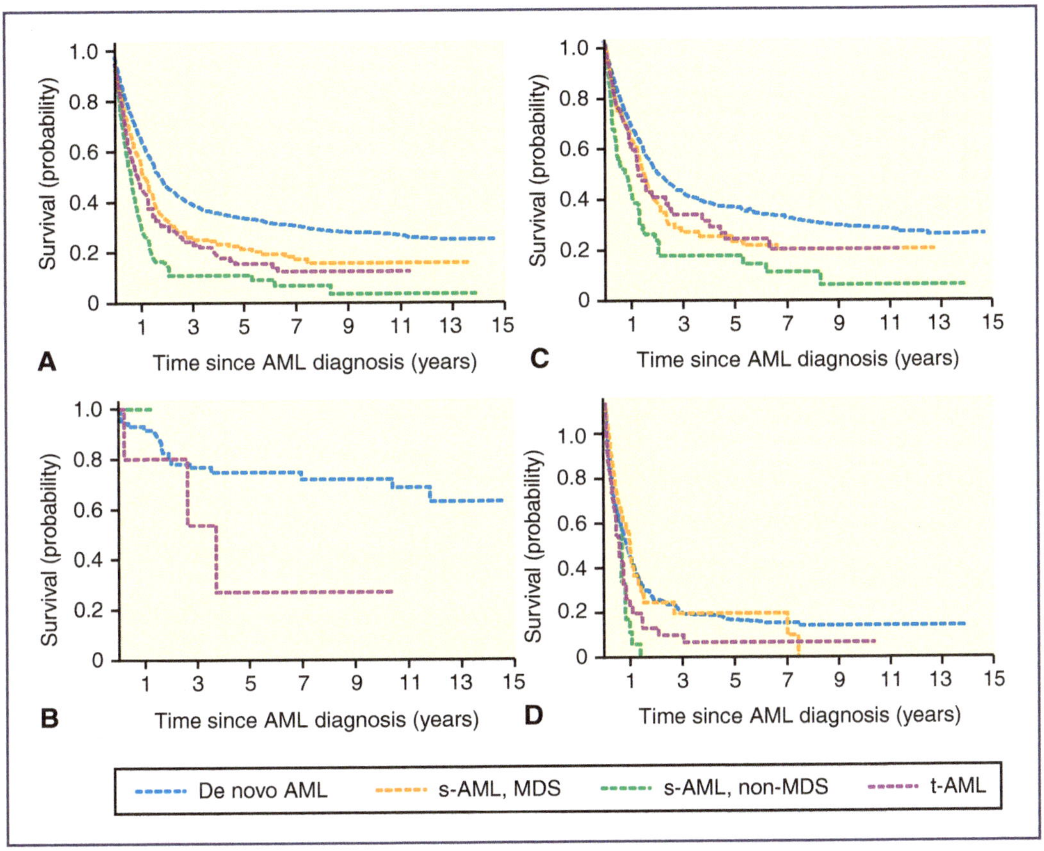

FIGURE 3-28: **Natural history of secondary AML (s-AML). Kaplan–Meier curves of survival for 1,567 adults with AML. (A) Overall survival, AML with (B) favorable cytogenetics (C) intermediate cytogenetic risk (D) adverse cytogenetic risk.**

Source: **Adapted from Granfeldt Østgård LS, Medeiros BC, Sengeløv H, et al. Epidemiology and clinical significance of secondary and therapy-related acute myeloid leukemia: a national population-based cohort study. *J Clin Oncol.* 2015;33(31):3641–3649.**

AML, acute myeloid leukemia; MDS, myelodysplastic syndrome; s-AML, secondary AML; t-AML, therapy-related AML.

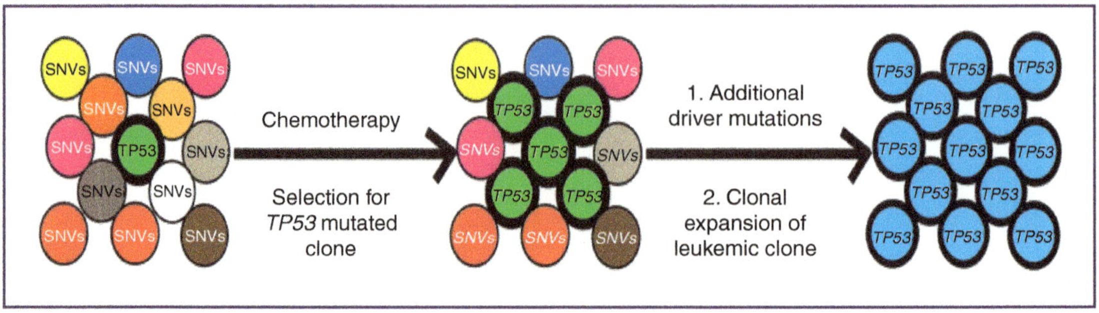

FIGURE 3-29: Age-related mutations in hematopoietic stem/progenitor cells (HSPCs) result in the production of a genetically heterogeneous population of HSPCs, including rare HSPCs with heterozygous *TP53* mutations in some individuals. During chemotherapy and/or radiotherapy for the primary cancer, HSPC clones harboring a *TP53* mutation have a competitive advantage, resulting in expansion of that clone. Subsequent acquisition of additional driver mutations results in transformation to t-AML/t-MDS. Of note, the presence of *TP53* mutations probably accounts for the high incidence of cytogenetic abnormalities in t-AML/t-MDS and poor response to chemotherapy.

Source: Reprinted by permission from Macmillan Publishers Ltd: Wong TN, Ramsingh G, Young AL, et al. Role of *TP53* mutations in the origin and evolution of therapy-related acute myeloid leukaemia. *Nature*. 2015;518:552–555. doi:10.1038/nature13968

SNVs, single nucleotide variants; t-AML/t-MDS, therapy-related acute myeloid leukemia/myelodysplastic syndrome.

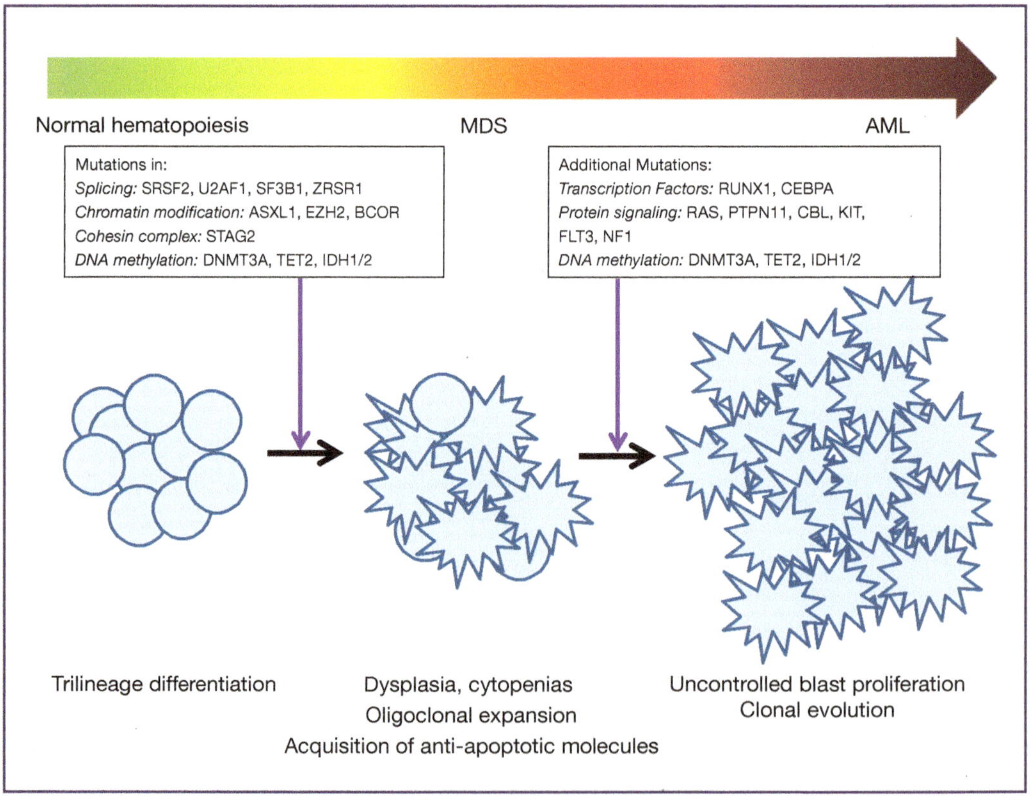

FIGURE 3-30: Progression from MDS to secondary AML.

AML, acute myeloid leukemia; FLT3, FMS-like tyrosine kinase 3; MDS, myelodysplastic syndrome.

TABLE 3-13 Mutually exclusive patterns of specific somatic gene mutations in secondary AML vs. de novo AML

SECONDARY (ANTECEDENT MDS, CMML)	DE NOVO AML
RNA Splicing: SRF2, SF3B1, U2AF, ZRSR2	NPM1
DNA Methylation: EZH	MLL/11q23 Translocations
Chromatin Modification/Co-repressors: ASXL, BCOR	Core Binding Factor Rearrangements
Cohesin Complex: STAG2	

AML, acute myeloid leukemia; CMML, chronic myelomonocytic leukemia; MDS, myelodysplastic syndrome; MLL, mixed lineage leukemia; NPM1, nucleophosmine 1.

The 8 genes that are mutated preferentially in secondary AML ("secondary-type mutations") are characteristic of MDS-associated dysplasia and aberrant differentiation. For both secondary and de novo AMLs, the presence of *TP53* mutations is associated with complex karyotypes and the clinical phenotype of intrinsic drug resistance. Roughly 15% of secondary AMLs carry *TP53* mutations and are linked to cytogenetic complexity (10 alterations vs 1) and shortened overall survival (4 vs. 8.5 months) relative to those secondary AMLs without *TP53* mutations.

Table 3-14 Results of cytotoxic induction chemotherapy for patients with secondary AML evolved from MDS

REFERENCE AND POPULATION	NO. OF PATIENTS	CHEMOTHERAPY REGIMEN	CR RATE	OVERALL SURVIVAL
Stone R, 2015 Therapy-related or prior MDS	111 104	Daunorubicin 45 mg/m² d1-3 Cytarabine 200 mg/m² d1-7 vs. Amonafide 600 mg/m² d1-5 Cytarabine 200 mg/m² d1-7	41% 40%	Median: 7.0 months 1 year: 31% Median: 7.0 months 1 year: 36%
Gajewski, 1989 Prior MDS or >2 months of cytopenias	44	Cytarabine 100–200 mg/m² x 7d Daunorubicin 60 mg/m² x 3d Thioguanine 100 mg/m² BID x 7d	41%	At 3 years: 8%
Bello, 2011 Prior MDS or MPN	61	Cytarabine 100–200 mg/m² x 7d with daunorubicin or idarubicin x 3d or high-dose cytarabine-based regimen	59% (48% CR, 11% CRp)	Median: 6.5 months
Knipp, 2007 Age ≥60, high-risk karyotype AML from prior MDS	42	Cytarabine 200 mg/m² x 5d Idarubicin 12 mg/m² x 3d +/– Thioguanine 100 mg/m² x 6d or Etoposide 100 mg/m² x 3d	62%	Median: 12 months
Jabbour, 2014 Prior MDS with failure of hypomethylating agents	63	Various	23% (10% CR, 13% CRp)	Median: 5 months At 1 year: 19% At 2 years: 8%

(continued)

Table 3-14 Results of cytotoxic induction chemotherapy for patients with secondary AML evolved from MDS (*continued*)

REFERENCE AND POPULATION	NO. OF PATIENTS	CHEMOTHERAPY REGIMEN	CR RATE	OVERALL SURVIVAL
Löwenberg, 2009 Age ≥60, prior MDS	119	Cytarabine 200 mg/m² x 7d Daunorubicin 60 mg/m² x 3d or Cytarabine 200 mg/m² x 7d Daunorubicin 90 mg/m² x 3d	45%	At 2 years: 22%
Rizzieri, 2009 Prior MDS or MPN	51	Various	62%	Median: 12 months At 1 year: 48%
Holowiecki, 2004 Prior MDS	57	Cytarabine 200 mg/m² x 7d Daunorubicin 60 mg/m² x 3d vs. Cytarabine 200 mg/m² x 7d Daunorubicin 60 mg/m² x 3 Cladribine 5 mg/m² x 5d	48% 60%	LFS at 3 years: 35% 42%

AML, acute myeloid leukemia; CR, complete remission; LFS, leukemia-free survival; MDS, myelodysplastic syndrome; MPN, myeloproliferative neoplasm.

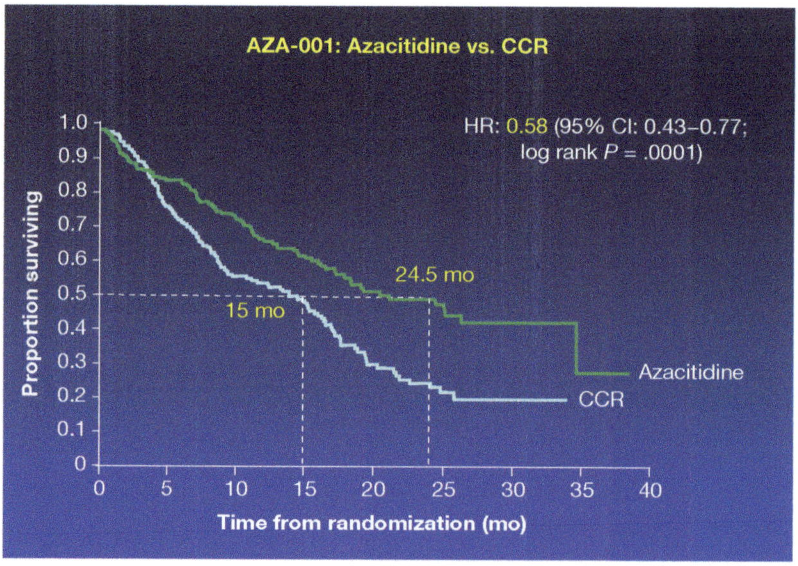

FIGURE 3-31: **Azacitidine prolongs overall survival in patients with MDS compared to conventional care regimens (CCR). Hazard ratio 0.58 (95% confidence intervals 0.43–0.77; log rank *P* = .0001).**

Source: From Fenaux P, Mufti G, Hellstrom-Lindberg E, et al. Efficacy of azacytidine compared with that of conventional care regimens in the treatment of higher-risk myelodysplastic syndromes: a randomized, open-label phase III study. *Lancet Oncol.* 2009;10:223–232.

CCR, conventional care regimen; CI, continuous infusion; HR, high risk; MDS, myelodysplastic syndrome.

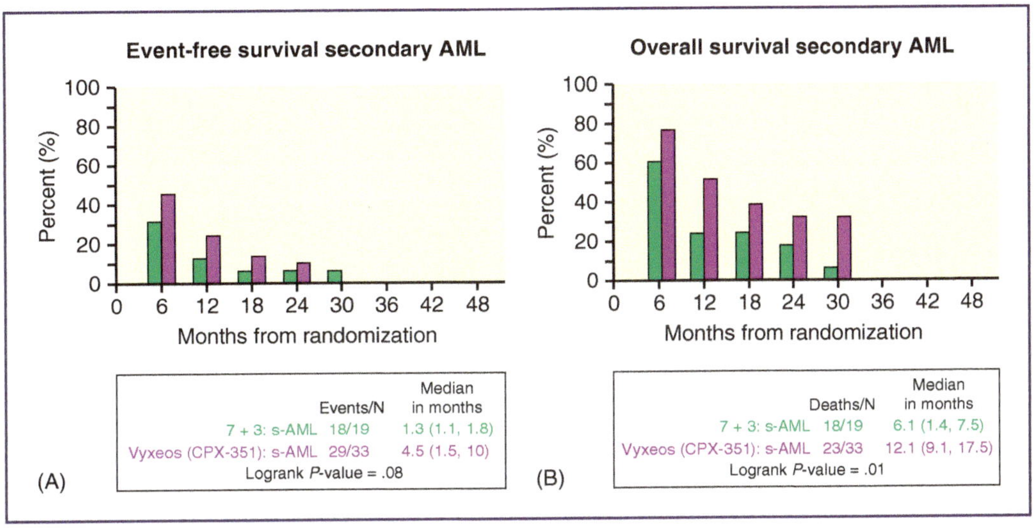

FIGURE 3-32: Vyxeos (CPX-351) (cytarabine:daunorubicin) liposome injection vs. "7 + 3"; CPX-351 improves event-free survival (A) and overall survival (B) in older adults with secondary AML.

Source: **Adapted from Lancet JE, Cortes JE, Hogge DE, et al. Phase 2 trial of CPX-351, a fixed 5:1 molar ratio of cytarabine/daunorubicin, vs cytarabine/daunorubicin in older adults with untreated AML. *Blood.* 2014;123(21):3239–3246.**

AML, acute myeloid leukemia; s-AML, secondary AML.

Selected References

Bello C, Yu D, Komrokji RS, et al. Outcomes after induction chemotherapy in patients with acute myeloid leukemia arising from myelodysplastic syndrome. *Cancer.* 2011;117(7):1463–1469.

Fenaux P, Mufti G, Hellstrom-Lindberg E, et al. Efficacy of azacytidine compared with that of conventional care regimens in the treatment of higher-risk myelodysplastic syndromes: a randomized, open-label phase III study. *Lancet Oncol.* 2009;10:223–232.

Gajewski JL, Ho WG, Nimer SD, et al. Efficacy of intensive chemotherapy for acute myelogenous leukemia associated with a preleukemic syndrome. *J Clin Oncol.* 1989;7(11):1637–1645.

Granfeldt Østgård LS, Medeiros BC, Sengeløv H, et al. Epidemiology and clinical significance of secondary and therapy-related acute myeloid leukemia: a national population-based cohort study. *J Clin Oncol.* 2015;33(31):3641–3649.

Holowiecki J, Grosicki S, Robak T, et al; Polish Adult Leukemia Group (PALG). Addition of cladribine to daunorubicin and cytarabine increases complete remission rate after a single course of induction treatment in acute myeloid leukemia. Multicenter, phase III study. *Leukemia.* 2004;18(5):989–997.

Jabbour E, Ghanem H, Huang X, et al. Acute myeloid leukemia after myelodysplastic syndrome and failure of therapy with hypomethylating agents: an emerging entity with a poor prognosis. *Clin Lymphoma Myeloma Leuk.* 2014;14(2):93–97.

Knipp S, Hildebrand B, Kündgen A, et al. Intensive chemotherapy is not recommended for patients aged >60 years who have myelodysplastic syndromes or acute myeloid leukemia with high-risk karyotypes. *Cancer.* 2007;110(2):345–352.

Lancet JE, Cortes JE, Hogge DE, et al. Phase 2 trial of CPX-351, a fixed 5:1 molar ratio of cytarabine/daunorubicin, vs cytarabine/daunorubicin in older adults with untreated AML. *Blood.* 2014;123(21):3239–3246.

Lindsey RC, Mar BG, Mazzola E, et al. Acute myeloid leukemia ontogeny is defined by distinct somatic mutations. *Blood*. 2015;125(9):1367–1376.

Löwenberg B, Ossenkoppele GJ, van Putten W, et al; Dutch-Belgian Cooperative Trial Group for Hemato-Oncology (HOVON); German AML Study Group (AMLSG); Swiss Group for Clinical Cancer Research (SAKK) Collaborative Group. High-dose daunorubicin in older patients with acute myeloid leukemia. *N Engl J Med*. 2009;361(13):1235–1248.

Ossenkoppele G, Lowenberg B. How I treat the older patient with acute myeloid leukemia. *Blood*. 2015;125(5):767–774.

Ostergard LSG, Medeiros BC, Sengelov H, et al. Epidemiology and clinical significance of secondary and therapy-related acute myeloid leukemia: a national population-based cohort study. *J Clin Oncol*. 2015;33(31):3641–3649.

Rizzieri DA, O'Brien JA, Broadwater G, et al. Outcomes of patients who undergo aggressive induction therapy for secondary acute myeloid leukemia. *Cancer*. 2009;115(13):2922–2929.

Stone RM, Mazzola E, Neuberg D, et al. Phase III open-label randomized study of cytarabine in combination with amonafide L-malate or daunorubicin as induction therapy for patients with secondary acute myeloid leukemia. *J Clin Oncol*. 2015;33(11):1252–1257.

Wong TN, Ramsingh G, Young AL, et al. Role of *TP53* mutations in the origin and evolution of therapy-related acute myeloid leukaemia. *Nature*. 2015;518:552–555. doi:10.1038/nature13968

Treatment of ALL in Adults

Matthew J. Wieduwilt

- Approximately 6,000 new cases of ALL are diagnosed yearly in the United States with roughly half of these cases occurring in patients over the age of 18 years.
- Hispanic populations have a higher incidence of ALL than other racial/ethnic populations due in part to polymorphisms in the *ARID5B* gene.
- Compared to children, ALL in adults has a poorer prognosis. Inferior outcomes in adult ALL may result from fewer randomized trials, lack of standard treatment approaches, lack of routine national and international cooperation on clinical trials, higher-risk ALL genetics conferring chemotherapy resistance, reduced tolerability of intensive chemotherapy, more frequent and severe comorbidities, and poorer compliance with the rigors of therapy for ALL.

RISK STRATIFICATION

- Consistent high-risk features include poor-risk cytogenetics, such as t(9;22), t(4;11), t(1;19), or complex karyotype (≥4–5 abnormalities), WBC ≥30,000/mcL with B-cell immunophenotype or WBC ≥50,000/mcL with T-cell immunophenotype, requiring more than 4 weeks to achieve a complete remission (CR), and age 35 years or older.
- The Ph-like phenotype, which is associated with targetable kinase mutations and gene fusions, is being recognized as a high-risk feature as well.
- Positive minimal residual disease (MRD), generally defined as greater than 0.1% (10^{-3}) or greater than 0.01% (10^{-4}) lymphoblasts in the bone marrow at the end of induction, has also been associated with poor relapse-free survival. Bassan et al measured molecular MRD at 10, 16, and 22 weeks of therapy in 236 remission patients treated on study NILG-ALL 09/00. Using an MRD positivity cut-off of 10^{-4}, 5-year overall survival (OS) and disease-free survival (DFS) were 75% and 72%, respectively, for MRD-negative patients versus 33% and 14% for MRD-positive patients ($P = .001$). Notably, OS and DFS were not different between MRD-negative patients with very high risk, high risk, or standard risk characteristics at diagnosis. In multivariate analysis, MRD negativity was the most significant risk factor for disease relapse.

GENERAL THERAPEUTIC PRINCIPLES

Initial Evaluation and Management

- The diagnosis of ALL requires 20% or more lymphoblasts in the bone marrow by morphology and/or flow cytometry. Comprehensive assessment of the leukemia immunophenotype and genetic assessment at diagnosis are essential for determining prognosis and guiding the choice of treatment, especially decision making regarding treatment of Ph/BCR-ABL1-positive disease with tyrosine kinase inhibitors (TKIs).
- Comprehensive cytogenetics should include standard karyotyping and FISH for t(9;22)(q34;q11.2)/BCR-ABL1, t(v;11q23)/MLL rearranged, t(12;21)(p13;q22)/ETV6-RUNX1, and t(1;19)(q23;p13.3)/TCF3-PBX1 translocations.
- ALL is a very aggressive hematologic malignancy generally requiring urgent inpatient evaluation, management, and treatment. A complete physical examination is warranted with special focus for detection of lymphadenopathy, signs of superior vena cava syndrome, hepatomegaly, splenomegaly, testicular masses, cranial nerve deficits, and other neurologic abnormalities.

- Initial laboratory evaluation of a newly diagnosed or suspected ALL includes a complete blood count; chemistry panel; AST; ALT; total bilirubin; alkaline phosphatase; tumor lysis assessment with LDH, uric acid, potassium, magnesium, phosphorous, and calcium; and disseminated intravascular coagulation (DIC) assessment with prothrombin time, partial thromboplastin time, fibrinogen, and d-dimer. Additional workup should include CT scans of the chest to assess for mediastinal masses in patients with T-cell ALL. Patients with evidence of extramedullary disease at diagnosis should be considered for CT scans of the chest, abdomen, and pelvis to fully assess the extent of disease prior to starting chemotherapy for response assessment during and after therapy.
- For patients with concerning testicular examination findings, further evaluation with scrotal content ultrasound is useful.
- Diagnostic lumbar puncture is generally performed per chosen treatment protocol with intrathecal chemotherapy administered at the time of the first lumbar puncture.
- Patients with neurologic symptoms at diagnosis should have brain imaging with CT or MRI to assess for parenchymal brain masses prior to a lumbar puncture.
- Assessment of cardiac function for patients receiving anthracycline chemotherapy should be considered, especially in patients with a history of or risk factors for cardiac disease.
- Unless allogeneic HCT is contraindicated or not possible for the patient, human leukocyte antigen (HLA)-typing of the patient and potentially siblings should be performed to expedite allogeneic HCT if ultimately indicated for the patient.
- See Management of Early Crisis in Chapter 3.
- Organ failure may be evident at the time of diagnosis, frequently manifesting as liver test abnormalities or acute kidney injury. Generally, these are from organ infiltration by lymphoblasts or, in the case of acute kidney injury, as a consequence of hyperuricemia from tumor lysis. Early institution of induction chemotherapy may stop and reverse organ malfunction from tissue infiltration by lymphoblasts.

Overview of Adult ALL Chemotherapy

- B-cell and T-cell ALLs are typically treated with the same regimen, although ongoing studies are evaluating targeted therapies directed against B-cell-specific antigens in the front-line. Nelarabine has been added to front-line therapy for T-cell ALL.
- Therapy for newly diagnosed ALL generally consists of three or more unique chemotherapy blocks of non-cross-resistant chemotherapy that are often repeated during the intensive portion of chemotherapy.
- Induction therapy utilizes a backbone of an anthracycline (eg, daunorubicin), vincristine, and a high-dose corticosteroid, with some regimens using a corticosteroid prephase to reduce disease burden prior to intensive induction. Specific regimens may add asparaginase and/or cyclophosphamide to induction in an attempt to improve response rates and MRD-negativity rates accepting the risk of greater induction toxicity.
- For patients not achieving a CR after induction, some regimens integrate a second induction course to try to get more patients to CR prior to consolidation.
- Consolidation therapy follows successful induction and contains regimen-specific courses of non-cross-resistant chemotherapy.
- Many regimens repeat the induction course or a similar anthracycline-containing course later in therapy, called delayed or late intensification.
- Interim maintenance has been rarely used in adults.
- For patients with Ph/BCR-ABL1-positive ALL, a tyrosine kinase inhibitor against BCR-ABL1 (eg, dasatinib) is typically added given improved outcomes, especially with second-generation TKIs (Figure 3-33).

- All regimens employ CNS prophylaxis with intrathecal chemotherapy with or without prophylactic cranial irradiation. Regimens employing high-dose methotrexate, high-dose cytarabine, and/or etoposide provide additional CNS prophylaxis with these CNS-penetrating chemotherapy agents.
- Given the rarity of adult ALL, the complexity of treatment, the unique complications of treatment, and the frequent need for allogeneic HCT, it is generally recommended that adult ALL patients be treated at a center specialized in the treatment of ALL as survival appears superior if ALL patients are treated at academic/research centers.

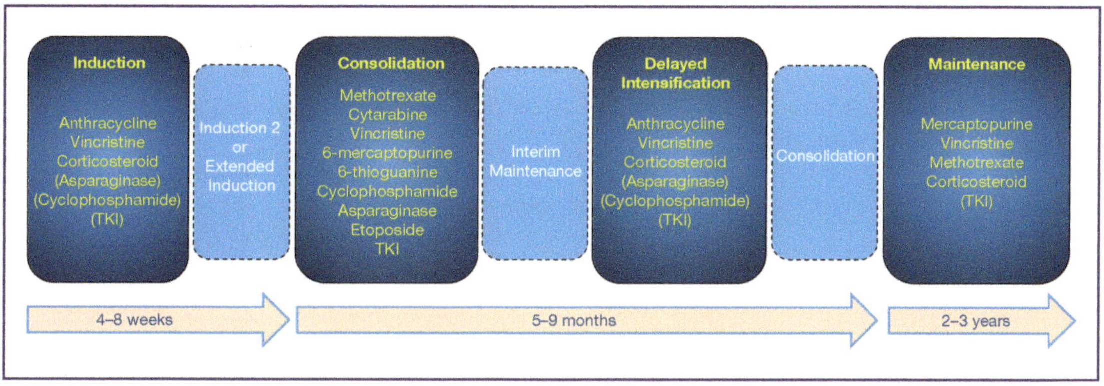

FIGURE 3-33: Treatment overview of pediatric-inspired regimens for adults with ALL. Design of front-line adult acute lymphoblastic leukemia regimens. Common courses of therapy (large dark blue rectangles) include induction, consolidation, delayed intensification, and 2 to 3 years of maintenance. Some regimens add additional courses (small light blue rectangles) including extended induction or second induction, interim maintenance, and/or additional consolidation.
ALL, acute lymphoblastic leukemia; TKI, tyrosine kinase inhibitor.

- See Chapter 3 for Treatment of ALL in the adolescent and young adult population.
- Consolidation of response to initial therapy with myeloablative allogeneic HCT yields 5-year overall survival rates of approximately 50%, higher than traditional moderate-intensity adult ALL regimens. Given the toxicity of myeloablative conditioning, it is generally reserved for those younger than age 60 to 65 years although a large meta-analysis suggested benefit is restricted to patients younger than age 35 years.

CNS Evaluation and Management

- Active CNS involvement by lymphoblasts is uncommon at the time of diagnosis (about 5%–10% of cases) but approximately 50% of patients will relapse in the CNS without administration of adequate CNS prophylaxis.
- CNS involvement is characterized as CNS-1 (no lymphoblasts in CSF), CNS-2 (WBC <5/mcL with lymphoblasts present), or CNS-3 (WBC ≥5/mcL with lymphoblasts present).
- For patients with a "traumatic" tap with peripheral blood contamination and a WBC ≥5/mcL with blasts in the CSF, the CSF WBC/RBC ratio and peripheral blood WBC/RBC ratio should be calculated. If the CSF ratio is greater than twice the peripheral blood ratio, then the patient is characterized as CNS-3; otherwise, the patient is classified as CNS-2.
- Patients presenting with cranial nerve abnormalities are presumed to have CNS involvement regardless of the presence of blasts in the CSF and should be treated as CNS-3 disease.
- Numerous approaches may be used to prevent CNS relapse, including intrathecal chemotherapy (eg, methotrexate, cytarabine, or triple therapy with methotrexate, cytarabine, and

corticosteroid), high-dose systemic but CNS-penetrating chemotherapy (eg, high-dose cytarabine and high-dose methotrexate), and prophylactic cranial irradiation. The schedule of treatment depends on the regimen administered and the use of cranial irradiation in adults is limited in some protocols to those with T-cell ALL, CNS-3 CSF disease, CNS masses at diagnosis, and/or persistent testicular involvement. For patients presenting with CNS-3 CSF involvement or cranial nerve abnormalities at diagnosis, intensified treatment with intrathecal chemotherapy given 2 to 3 times a week until CSF clearance and/or improvement in cranial nerve deficits followed by weekly intrathecal treatments is a common approach.

Evaluation and Management of Extramedullary Disease

- Extramedullary involvement is frequently present at diagnosis of ALL. Hepatomegaly and splenomegaly may be present and liver infiltration by ALL may lead to abnormalities including hyperbilrubinemia, transaminitis, and elevation of alkaline phosphatase that can limit safe delivery of full-dose induction chemotherapy.
- Significant palpable lymphadenopathy at diagnosis should prompt staging computed tomography scans of the chest, abdomen, and pelvis to aid in response assessment to therapy.
- The testicles may act as a sanctuary site for ALL and a testicular examination is essential for the evaluation of all male patients with newly diagnosed ALL.
- Patients with lymphoblastic lymphoma manifest only extramedullary disease. Patients typically not only have T-cell lineage disease and mediastinal masses, but also may have lymphadenopathy and extranodal masses. Although often excluded from studies of ALL, they are frequently treated with the same regimens with good outcomes.

Management and Prophylaxis of Infectious Complications

- Patients undergoing therapy for ALL have compromised cellular immunity due to destruction of normal T- and B-lymphocytes that are sensitive to ALL chemotherapy. As such, patients are at risk for opportunistic infections. Of greatest concern are reactivation of herpes viruses and pneumonia caused by *Pneumocystis jiroveci*.
- Herpes virus reactivation, especially herpes simplex virus (HSV)-1, HSV-2, and varicella zoster virus, can complicate immunosuppressive therapy and may cause significant morbidity. Prophylaxis with acyclovir is typically used until the patient completes all therapy.
- Symptomatic or invasive disease with cytomegalovirus, adenovirus, and Epstein-Barr virus is rare and routine prophylaxis or monitoring for these viruses is not recommended.
- The risk of *Pneumocystis jiroveci* pneumonia due to extended immunosuppressive chemotherapy is generally ameliorated through the use of trimethoprim-sulfamethoxazole (TMP-SMX) prophylaxis. For those intolerant of TMP-SMX, alternative prophylactic agents include dapsone, atovaquone, and pentamidine.
- In the setting of neutropenia, the risk of bacterial and fungal infections increases and prophylaxis against bacterial infections with an agent active against *Pseudomonas* spp. (eg, ciprofloxacin) and an antifungal such as fluconazole is generally indicated. For those with prolonged neutropenia (greater than 7 days), especially if receiving concomitant corticosteroids, consideration should be given to starting an antifungal active against mold species (eg, voriconazole or posaconazole).

Response Assessment

- Response assessment is typically performed at the end of induction, ideally at count recovery, and includes evaluation of peripheral blood, bone marrow, and any sites of extramedullary disease identified at diagnosis.

- A complete remission (CR) is defined as
  - <5% lymphoblasts in the bone marrow with no circulating lymphoblasts,
  - no evidence of extramedullary disease, including absence of CNS involvement, testicular involvement, lymphadenopathy, or organomegaly related to ALL,
  - marrow that must show trilineage hematopoiesis,
  - an absolute neutrophil count greater than 1,000/mcL, and
  - platelet count greater than 100,000/mcL.
- CR with incomplete count recovery (CRi) is defined as per CR but without recovery of platelets or neutrophils.
- Those who fail to achieve a CR or CRi at the end of protocol-defined induction are considered to have refractory ALL.
- CNS remission is defined as achievement of CNS-1 status in a patient with CNS-2 or CNS-3 disease at diagnosis.
- For patients with documented extramedullary disease at diagnosis, repeat imaging is necessary to confirm remission status. For patients with mediastinal masses, complete resolution of mediastinal mass is required for CR with PR defined as greater than 50% reduction in the sum of the perpendicular diameters (SPDs) of measurable lesions.
- Given its prognostic implications, MRD monitoring has now become part of the standard response assessment for ALL. MRD may be assessed by multiparameter flow cytometry, quantitative PCR for diagnostic immunoglobulin heavy chain and T-cell receptor rearrangements, or both. For Ph/BCR-ABL1-positive ALL, quantitative RT-PCR is typically used to monitor for minimal residual disease. Minimal residual disease levels greater than 0.1% (10^{-3} lymphoblasts) or 0.01% (10^{-4} lymphoblasts), depending on the regimen administered, are generally considered "positive" as they are associated with a higher relapse risk and are an indication for allogeneic HCT or therapy on a clinical trial.

Therapeutic Approaches to Adult Philadelphia Chromosome Negative (Ph-) ACUTE Lymphoblastic Leukemia

Conventional Adult Regimens

- Relative to pediatric regimens, conventional adult regimens are typically less intense in the administration of non-myelosuppresive agents, especially corticosteroids, vincristine, and asparaginase, although overall intensity is difficult to ascertain.
- The Cancer and Leukemia Group B (CALGB) 8811 utilized a five-drug induction containing asparaginase followed by standard-dose postremission chemotherapy for adults aged 16 to 80 years with newly diagnosed Ph- and Ph+ ALL. For the entire cohort, CR rate was 85% with 3-year DFS and OS of 46% and 50%, respectively. For those under the age of 30, CR rate was 94% with 3-year DFS and OS of 51% and 69%, respectively. For those 60 years of age and older, the CR rate was only 39%, with an induction mortality of 50%, and a 3-year OS of only 17%.
- The UKALLXII/E2993 trial studied newly diagnosed adult ALL patients aged 15–59 years. A four-drug induction containing asparaginase was followed by postremission therapy that included three cycles of high-dose methotrexate in addition to standard-dose chemotherapy courses. Patients were allocated to allogeneic HCT if they had a matched-sibling donor and randomized between chemotherapy alone or autologous HCT if they did not have a donor. For the Ph- cohort, the CR rate was 90% with a 5-year overall survival of 43% (44% for chemotherapy alone vs. 54% allogeneic HCT, *P* = .007).

- The hyper-CVAD regimen deserves special attention as an intense adult regimen that differs significantly from other regimens in its basic design and notable lack of asparaginase. Treatment consists of alternating courses of hyperfractionated cyclophosphamide given twice daily for 3 days, doxorubicin, vincristine, and dexamethasone (hyper-CVAD) alternating with high-dose methotrexate/high-dose cytarabine for a total of eight courses followed by POMP maintenance in standard hyper-CVAD and adding two late intensification blocks of hyper-CVAD followed by MTX/asparaginase during maintenance in modified hyper-CVAD. With standard hyper-CVAD, the CR rate was 91% with a 5-year OS of 39% in the entire cohort and 54% in patients under the age of 30. Relative to standard hyper-CVAD historical controls, modified hyper-CVAD improved CR duration without improvement in 3-year OS. For the CD20-positive subgroup younger than 60 years, modified hyper-CVAD with rituximab improved 3-year OS (75% vs. 47%, $P = .03$) for CD20+ ALL. Attempts to intensify this regimen with the addition of asparaginase in the front-line have been difficult due to high treatment-related mortality, principally from infection.
- The GRAALL investigators recently reported results of 209 patients treated on GRAALL-2005, a Phase III randomized study of rituximab vs. no rituximab in combination with the pediatric-inspired GRAALL regimen for adults ages 18 to 59 with newly diagnosed CD20+ B-cell ALL. Similar to the experience with rituximab added to modified hyper-CVAD, complete response rates and minimal residual disease negativity rates were not different between the two groups, although 2-year EFS, but not OS, was significantly improved with the addition of rituximab (65% rituximab vs. 52% control, HR = 0.66 [0.45–0.98], $P = .038$). When patients undergoing allogeneic HCT were censored, 2-year OS was superior in the rituximab arm (2-year OS, 74% vs. 63%; HR = 0.55 [0.34–0.91], $P = .018$). Notably, significantly more patients in the rituximab cohort proceeded to allogeneic HCT (35% vs. 20%, $P = .029$).
- Current clinical trials studying the addition of the anti-CD20 antibody rituximab, the anti-CD3/CD19 bifunctional T-cell engager blinatumomab, and the antibody-drug conjugate targeting CD22 inotuzumab-ozagamicin in the front-line are planned or ongoing.

Pediatric and Pediatric-Inspired Regimens

- Improvement in the treatment of pediatric ALL and 5-year survival rates of greater than 80% have been realized through the integration of new and effective agents, intensification of therapy, institution of CNS prophylaxis, and improvements in risk stratification. Although adult ALL has integrated similar approaches, outcomes have been disappointing with 5-year survival rates of 30% to 50% in most studies.
- Numerous country-specific retrospective studies have compared outcomes of adolescent and young adult ALL patients ages 15–21 years receiving therapy on pediatric or adult regimens on national trials. Superior 5-year event-free survival of 60% to 70% was observed for those treated on pediatric protocols relative to 30% to 50% for those treated on conventional adult chemotherapy trials.
- The intensity of therapy, especially with nonmyelosuppressive agents such as corticosteroids, vincristine, and asparaginase, is higher in the pediatric regimens with roughly equivalent levels of myelosuppressive agents such as anthracyclines. Patient compliance with therapy may also differ between adolescent and young adult (AYA) patients treated on pediatric versus adult protocols as those treated on pediatric regimens by pediatricians may have a more extensive support system including both family and social support services available through pediatric centers. Nonetheless, intensive conventional adult regimens may give similar outcomes to pediatric or pediatric-inspired regimens outside of the 15- to 20-year age group. Notably, intensive adult regimens have yielded 3- to 5-year survival of greater than 60% in patients under the age of 30.

Table 3-15 Conventional adult and pediatric/pediatric-inspired ALL regimens

STUDY	N	AGENTS	PH+, %	AGE	CR	EFS	DFS	OS
"Conventional" Adult								
CALGB 8811	197	D, V, P, A, C (D, P, C ≥60)/C, 6MP, AraC, V, A/6MP, M/Dox, V, Dex, C, TG, AraC/POMP	Yes, est. 27%	16–80	85%	–	46% (3-year)	50% (3-year)
				<30	94%		51%	69%
				30–59	85%		43%	39%
				>59	39%		43%	17%
UKALLXII/E2993	1646	D, V, P, A/C, AraC, 6MP/HD-MTX, A/AraC, E, V, Dex/AraC, E/D, C, AraC, TG/POMP	No	15–59	90%	–	–	43% (5-year) Chemo 44% AlloHCT 54%
UCSF 8707	84	D, V, P, A/E, HD-AraC/HD-MTX, 6MP/POMP	Yes, 16%	16–59	93%	48% (5-year)	54% (5-year)	47% (5 yr)
				<30		63% (5-year)		
JALG ALL93	263	V, Dox, Psl, A, C/Mit, E, AraC/MTX, A/ACR, AraC, Psl/6MP, M	Yes, 22%	15–59	78%	33% (6-year)	30% (6-year)	33% (6-year)
				<30	84%		33.5%	47.5%
				<40	83%		30.2%	43.4%
Hyper-CVAD	204	C, Dox, V, Dex/HD-MTX, HD-Ara-C, SM/POMP	Yes, 16%	16–79	91%	–	36% (5-year)	39% (5-year)
				<30	98%			54%
				30–49	89%			42%
				50–59	93%			29%
				>59	79%			17%
Rituximab-Hyper-CVAD*	73	C, Dox, V, Dex, R/HD-MTX, HD-Ara-C, R/POMP/MTX, A	No	15–79	92%	–	–	57% (3-year)

(*continued*)

Table 3-15 Conventional adult and pediatric/pediatric-inspired ALL regimens (*continued*)

STUDY	N	AGENTS	PH+, %	AGE	CR	EFS	DFS	OS
				Pediatric/Pediatric-Inspired				
GRAALL-2003	225	P/D, V, P, A, C/HD-AraC, Dex, A/HD-MTX, V, A, 6MP/C, E, M/POMP	No	15–60	93.5%	55% (3.5-year)	–	60% (3.5 year)
				<46	95%	58%	61%	64%
				46–60	87%	46%	53%	47%
DFCI ALL	92	Dox, V, P, HD-MTX, A/V, 6MP, Dox/V, Dex, Dox, 6MP, A, M	Yes, 20%	18–50	85%	–	69% (4 yr)	67% (4 yr)
USC ALL	51	D, V, P, pA/C, AraC, V, pA, P, 6MP/HD-MTX, pA, P/AraC, T/D, V, Dex, pA, C, AraC, TG/POMP	Yes, 22%	18–57	96%	–	58% (7-year)	51% (7-year)
PETHEMA ALL-96	81	D, V, P, A, C/HD-MTX, 6MP, E, ID-AraC/D, V, Dex, A, C/M, 6MP/V, P, A	No	15–30	98%	61% (6-year)	–	69% (6-year)
CALGB 10403**	318	D, V, P, pA/C, AraC, 6MP, V, pA/V, M, pA/Dox, V, Dex, pA, 6TG/DexOMP	No	17–39	–	66% (2-year)		78% (2-year)

*CD20+ B-cell ALL only defined as 20% or more CD20 expressing lymphoblasts in the bone marrow by flow cytometry.

**Study in progress, patients in follow-up.

6MP, 6-mercaptopurine; A, asparaginase; ACR, aclarubicin; AraC, cytarabine; C, cyclophosphamide; CR, complete remission; D, daunorubicin; Dex, dexamethasone; DexOMP, dexamethasone, vincristine, methotrexate, 6-mercaptopurine; DFS, disease-free survival; Dox, doxorubicin; E, etoposide; EFS, event-free survival; HD-AraC, high-dose cytarabine; HD-MTX, high-dose methotrexate; ID-AraC, intermediate-dose cytarabine; M, methotrexate; Mit, mitoxantrone; OS, overall survival; P, prednisone; pA, pegylated asparaginase; POMP, prednisone, vincristine, methotrexate, 6-mercaptopurine; Psl, prednisolone; R, rituximab; SM, solu-medrol; T, teniposide; TG, thioguanine; V, vincristine.

Elderly ALL

- Elderly patients with ALL, generally defined as patients older than 60 or 65 years of age, represent approximately one-third of all adult ALL. ALL in elderly patients are more likely to be precursor B-cell in origin and have high-risk cytogenetics including Ph+ ALL in 30% to 50% of cases, MLL rearranged disease in 5% to 10%, and complex cytogenetics. In addition, elderly patients have high rates of comorbidities placing them at high risk for treatment-related toxicity and death. Complete response rates to conventional adult chemotherapy regimens range from 40% to 81% with early death rates of 6% to 42% and 2-year overall survival ranging from 3% to 29%. For elderly patients treated on prospective studies specifically for older ALL, CR rates range from 43% to 90% with early death rates of 0% to 36% and 2-year overall survival ranging from 16% to 71%. The role of nonmyeloablative (NMA) and reduced-intensity conditioning (RIC) allogeneic HCT for elderly patients is an area of ongoing research and is discussed in detail in Chapter 4.
- For very elderly patients, frail elderly patients, and those with substantial comorbidities, the risks of even moderately intensive chemotherapy generally outweigh any expected benefit. When possible, these patients should be enrolled on clinical trials evaluating novel approaches and targeted therapies in the front-line setting. Otherwise, the use of palliative chemotherapy and potentially targeted therapies such as tyrosine kinase inhibitors or antibody-based therapies would be appropriate to minimize risk of early death.

Therapeutic Approaches to Philadelphia Chromosome Positive (Ph+) Acute Lymphoblastic

- Prior to the advent of tyrosine kinase inhibitors (TKIs) targeting BCR-ABL1, intensive chemotherapy alone was the only option to induce remission for Ph+ ALL with complete remission rates of approximately 80% and relapse rates exceeding 80%. The addition of TKIs (imatinib, dasatinib, nilotinib) has improved CR rates and improved outcomes for Ph+ ALL, principally by facilitating hematopoietic cell transplantation. Emerging data, however, suggest that some Ph+ ALL patients with deep responses to second-generation TKIs in combination with intensive chemotherapy may not derive additional benefit from allogeneic HCT, although longer follow-up and additional studies are needed to confirm this early finding.
- In elderly patients with Ph+ ALL, targeted therapies like TKIs have offered an opportunity to improve outcomes through improved response rates with the use of low-intensity or no chemotherapy. Second-generation TKIs appear as effective and tolerable as imatinib in elderly Ph+ ALL. Dasatinib in combination with prednisone or low-dose chemotherapy and nilotinib in combination with imatinib have reported CR rates of 94% to 100% and 2-year overall survival of approximately 65%.
- Given the success of both intensive chemotherapy + TKI, less-intensive chemotherapy + TKI, and corticosteroids + TKI, the ideal induction and postremission strategy for Ph+ ALL is unknown and future studies should aim to answer these questions in a randomized fashion. Allogeneic HCT in first remission is still considered a standard of care for eligible patients, although emerging evidence suggests that a response-based approach based on molecular response may help select patients who may not gain additional benefit from allogeneic HCT.

Allogeneic Hematopoietic Cell Transplantation in First Remission (See Also Chapter 4)

- Allogeneic hematopoietic cell transplantation is a recognized curative approach for adult patients with Ph-negative ALL in CR1 and leads to 5-year survival rates of about 50%. Whether allogeneic HCT is superior to chemotherapy alone for patients in first CR, especially the more intensive regimens currently being used for AYA Ph-negative ALL patients, is a subject of ongoing debate.

Table 3-16 Front-line studies of tyrosine kinase inhibitors in Ph+ ALL

REGIMEN	N	CR	EFS	RFS	OS	HCT RATE
			Imatinib			
UKALLXII/E2993						
Imatinib	175	92%	33% (4-year)	50% (4-year)	38% (4-year)	46%
Pre-imatinib	266	82%	18%	33%	22%	31%
NILG 09/00						
Imatinib	59	92%	–	39% (5-year)	38% (5-year)	72%
No imatinib	35	81%		25%	23%	54%
ALL202						
Imatinib	80	96%	60% (1-year)	–	76% (1-year)	49%
No imatinib (ALL93)	51	51%	≈18%		≈60%	–
GRAAPH-2005						
RI induction	135	98%	42% (5-year)		48% (5-year)	74%
Hyper-CVAD induction	133	91%	32%		43%	80%
MD Anderson: Imatinib+Hyper-CVAD	54	93%	–	43% (5-year)	43% (5-year)	30%
			Dasatinib/Nilotinib			
MD Anderson: Dasatinib + Hyper-CVAD	35	96%	42% (5-year)	44% (5-year)	46% (5-year)	17%
LAL1205 Dasatinib + Prednisone	53	100%	–	51% (20 months)	69% (20 months)	34%
Korea: Nilotinib + Chemotherapy	90	91%	–	72% (2-year)	72% (2-year)	70%

ALL, acute lymphoblastic leukemia; CR, complete remission; EFS, event-free survival; HCT, hematopoietic cell transplantation; Hyper-CVAD, hyperfractionated cyclophosphamide, vincristine, doxorubicin, dexamethasone; OS, overall survival; RFS, relapse-free survival; RI, reduced-intensity.

Management of MRD Positivity in First Remission: Allogeneic HCT and Blinatumomab

- Among available predictors of relapse, the presence of MRD by multiparameter flow cytometry or by quantitative PCR of a clonal T-cell receptor (TCR) or immunoglobulin gene rearrangement is highly predictive of subsequent relapse (see also Chapter 5). Conversely, MRD negativity predicted excellent disease-free and overall survival regardless of disease risk status at the time of diagnosis. For ALL patients with persistent MRD positivity, relapse rates are 80% to 90% with chemotherapy alone. For these patients, myeloablative chemotherapy and immunotherapies including allogeneic HCT are potential approaches to overcome mechanisms of chemotherapy resistance and potentially cure more patients with positive MRD. For MRD-positive ALL patients in first CR unable or unwilling to proceed to allogeneic HCT, therapy with the bifunctional T-cell engaging antibody blinatumomab appears to improve remission duration (see following text).

RELAPSED/REFRACTORY ALL

- Despite excellent response rates, approximately 10% of patients will be refractory to induction chemotherapy and relapse will occur in 30% to 40% of AYA ALL patients, with the majority of older ALL patients achieving a complete remission if consolidated with traditional moderate-intensity chemotherapy alone. Survival after relapse is very poor, with over 95% of adult patients succumbing to their disease or treatment-related death if unable to proceed to a potentially curative allogeneic HCT. For those able to proceed to allogeneic HCT, 5-year survival is approximately 20%. Even if CR is achieved with salvage chemotherapy, median relapse-free survival with salvage chemotherapy is only 4 to 9 months, with most CR patients dying within 1 year of relapse, so moving rapidly to allogeneic transplant after successful salvage is essential. Treatment choice is guided by a number of factors including time to relapse, type of prior therapy, ALL lineage, ALL immunophenotype, Ph/BCR-ABL1 status, ABL1 mutational status in Ph+ patients, age, availability of clinical trials, and eligibility for allogeneic HCT. The advent of more effective salvage therapies for ALL will hopefully translate into improved long-term survival.

- **Chemotherapy**
  - The use of conventional chemotherapy approaches for relapsed ALL yields response rates of about 30% to 50%. Choice of salvage therapy is determined at least in part by timing of relapse. For patients with late relapse, often defined as relapse occurring after completion of maintenance chemotherapy, treatment with the initial induction regimen is often recommended. For those with earlier relapse, alternative salvage is generally recommended with most providers selecting regimens containing agents to which the patient has not been previously exposed. The structures and mechanisms of action of the diverse chemotherapeutic agents are detailed in Chapter 7.
- **Targeted immune-based therapies (see also Immunology** in **Chapter 8)**
  - Many B-cell lymphoblastic leukemia antigens are restricted exclusively to B-lymphocytes in humans. This specificity for B-cell antigens permits targeting of B-lymphoblasts, as destruction of the only other target cell, B-lymphocytes, is generally manageable with low rates of serious infection. CD19 is expressed on the surface of nearly all B-cell ALL. Blinatumomab is a bifunctional T-cell engaging (BITE) antibody joining anti-CD3 and anti-CD19 variable regions from monoclonal antibodies with a short peptide linker. The resultant engineered molecule engages T-cells (through CD3) directly with CD19-expressing target cells including B-lymphoblasts. T-cell engagement leads to cytotoxic cell killing and T-cell proliferation. The major toxicity of blinatumomab is CNS toxicity including confusion, aphasia, ataxia, and seizure. A potentially life-threatening cytokine release syndrome can rarely occur.
  - Autologous T-cells engineered to express chimeric antigen receptors (CARs) targeting CD19 are proving to be an effective therapy for relapsed B-cell ALL. T-cells are typically infected with a lentiviral or retroviral vector expressing a chimeric T-cell receptor containing an extracellular single-chain variable fragment (scFv) targeting CD19, a transmembrane domain, an intracellular costimulatory domain(s), and a signaling domain (eg, CD3). The CD19-targeted CAR-expressing T-cells are then reinfused into the patient where the cells expand in response to stimulation by CD19 and kill cells expressing CD19, both normal B-lymphocytes and B-lymphoblasts. The rapid T-cell expansion is associated with a potentially fatal cytokine release syndrome (see Tumor Lysis and Cytokine Release Syndromes in Chapter 3) occurring within the first 3 weeks of therapy due to the release of cytokines such as IL-6, IFN-gamma, IL-10, and others seen with robust activation and proliferation of T-cells. Cytokine release syndrome may be rapidly reversed with the anti-IL-6 monoclonal antibody tocilizumab and may also respond to corticosteroids but with concern for decreased efficacy of the CAR T-cells. In addition, prolonged B-cell aplasia may occur after CAR19 T-cell therapy and patients may require supplementation with IV immunoglobulin to prevent infection. Relapse after CAR19 T-cell therapy is often associated with loss of CD19 expression.
- **Ph+/BCR-ABL1-positive disease**
  - Relapse of Ph+ ALL is frequently associated with mutations in the ATP-binding domain of ABL1 within the BCR-ABL1 fusion protein leading to resistance to TKIs. Depending on the specific mutation, a choice of an alternative TKI known to be active against that mutation is an option. In the setting of frank relapse, a TKI is usually combined with chemotherapy to try to recapture remission. The T315I BCR-ABL1 mutation is a common mechanism of resistance, and in patients treated with the second-generation TKI dasatinib the T315I

mutation was associated with relapse in 71% (12/17) of Ph+ ALL patients treated with dasatinib and prednisone. Ponatinib is a third-generation TKI active against the T315I-mutated BCR-ABL1, and has activity against dasatinib- or nilotinib-resistant ALL. As such, ponatinib may be useful as a bridge to allogeneic HCT if response can be achieved. Ponatinib is associated with arterial thrombosis, principally myocardial infarction, in patients with known cardiovascular disease or at least one cardiac risk factor. Chemotherapy, typically with the addition of a TKI, can get relapsed Ph+ ALL patients into remission. Targeted therapies such as blinatumomab and inotuzumab-ozagamycin may also have a role in treating relapsed Ph+ ALL. As with Ph-negative ALL, the best chance at long-term survival is allogeneic HCT for those who have not been previously transplanted.

Table 3-17 Therapeutics for relapsed or refractory adult acute lymphoblastic leukemia

REGIMEN	CR/CRI RATE	FDA APPROVED	BENEFITS	DRAWBACKS
Standard induction regimen		N/A	1. Familiarity 2. Ease of administration 3. Inexpensive	1. Cumulative toxicity of anthracyclines 2. Myelosuppressive
			Cytarabine-based	
FLAM FLAG-Ida HD-Ida, HiDAC	50% 39% 35%	N/A	1. Ease of administration 2. Inexpensive	1. Cumulative toxicity of anthracyclines 2. Myelosuppressive
Clofarabine containing	17%–50%	Yes	1. Good CR rates in some combinations	1. Prolonged myelosuppression 2. Expensive
Augmented Hyper-CVAD	47%	Yes	1. Familiarity with hyper-CVAD	1. Cumulative toxicity of anthracyclines 2. Myelosuppressive 3. Pegylated asparaginase toxicities
MOpAD	28%	Yes	1. Ease of administration 2. Outpatient 3. Minimally myelosuppressive 4. Inexpensive	1. Low CR rates 2. Pegylated asparaginase toxicities
Liposomal vincristine	20%	Yes	1. Single agent 2. Outpatient 3. Not myelosuppressive	1. Low CR rates 2. Expensive 3. Time-consuming to prepare
Nelarabine	≈30%–40%	Yes	1. Active single agent in T-cell ALL	1. Neurotoxicity 2. Expensive
Blinatumomab	43%	Yes	1. High CR rate in relapse with <50% marrow blasts 2. Durable remissions in MRD persistence/relapse	1. Neurotoxicity 2. Low CR rate with >50% marrow blasts 3. Continuous IV for 28 days each cycle 4. Requires hospitalization for initiation 5. Very expensive

(*continued*)

Table 3-17 Therapeutics for relapsed or refractory adult acute lymphoblastic leukemia (*continued*)

REGIMEN	CR/CRI RATE	FDA APPROVED	BENEFITS	DRAWBACKS
Inotuzumab-ozagamicin	58%–81%	No	1. High CR rates 2. Ease of administration 3. Outpatient	1. Hepatotoxicity including VOD/SOS 2. Short duration of response
CAR19 T-cells	80%–90%	No	1. High CR rates	1. Cytokine release syndrome 2. Complexity of preparation 3. Cost
Allogeneic HCT (refractory/relapse)	NR	N/A	1. 3-year OS 16%, 46% with 0 or 1 risk factor	1. High-relapse mortality (37%) 2. High nonrelapse mortality (51%) 3. Morbidity

ALL, acute lymphoblastic leukemia; CAR19, chimeric antigen receptor targeting CD19; CR, complete remission; CRi, complete remission with incomplete count recovery; FDA, Food and Drug Administration; FLAG-Ida, fludarabine, high-dose cytarabine, G-CSF, idarubicin; FLAM, fludarabine, cytarabine, mitoxantrone; HCT, hematopoietic cell transplantation; HD-Ida, high-dose idarubicin; HiDAC, high-dose cytarabine; Hyper-CVAD, hyperfractionated cyclophosphamide, vincristine, doxorubicin, dexamethasone; IV, intravenous; MOpAD, methotrexate, vincristine, pegylated asparaginase, dexamethasone; MRD, minimal residual disease; OS, overall survival; VOD/SOS, veno-occlusive disease and sinusoidal obstruction syndrome.

CNS Relapse

- The central nervous system is a site of relapse in about 10% of relapsed adult ALL. Of 609 adult Ph- and Ph+ ALL patients relapsed on the MRC UKALLXII/E2993, 523 (85.9%) had isolated bone marrow relapse, 33 (5.4%) bone marrow and CNS relapse, 22 (3.6%) isolated CNS relapse, 23 (3.8%) isolated extramedullary relapse, and 8 (1.3%) unknown site of relapse. Outcomes were very poor in patients with CNS involvement at relapse, with 84% dying at 1 year and no patient surviving beyond 3.5 years.
- Workup for CNS relapse should include an assessment for other sites of relapse and necessitates a bone marrow biopsy given the high rates of coincident CNS and bone marrow relapse. Assessment of extramedullary sites should be performed as indicated by ALL lineage, physical examination, and disease behavior at diagnosis. For Ph+ ALL, an assessment of BCR-ABL1 mutational status should be performed to guide TKI selection.
- In general, patients with CNS relapse receive both CNS- and systemic-directed therapy. For the CNS, intensified conventional intrathecal chemotherapy 2 to 3 times a week until clearance of blasts followed by a maintenance schedule is typical. Alternatively, liposomal cytarabine intrathecal given at 50 mg every 2 weeks is effective for eliminating CSF lymphoblasts. Cranial irradiation should be strongly considered as consolidation after response to intrathecal chemotherapy. Systemic chemotherapy should be administered with consideration given to the use of CNS-penetrating agents such as high-dose methotrexate and high-dose cytarabine as part of systemic therapy.
- Treatment for CNS relapse is inadequate with almost all patients succumbing to their disease. When possible, patients should be enrolled on clinical trials aimed at either reducing CNS relapse rates or treating active CNS relapse. As with any adult patient with relapsed ALL not having received an allogeneic HCT, attempts should be made to move the patient to allogeneic HCT with curative intent.

CONCLUSION

With the application of pediatric, pediatric-inspired, and intensive adult regimens to nearly all fit adult ALL patients, the intensity of conventional chemotherapy is reaching a boundary of tolerability for both adolescent, young adult, and older adult patients. Improved sequencing of active chemotherapy agents is one avenue to improving outcomes in adult ALL, although the application of novel targeted therapies holds the greatest promise for progress. Monoclonal antibodies, targeted chemotherapy in the form of antibody-drug conjugates, immunotherapies such as blinatumomab and CAR19 T-cells, liposomal drug formulations, and small molecule inhibitors for patients with targetable gene mutations, kinase fusions, or pathologically activated intracellular signaling pathways can likely be added safely to existing AYA and conventional adult chemotherapy regimens to overcome some mechanisms of resistance to front-line chemotherapy. How best to safely integrate these agents into front-line therapy without compromising efficacy of the targeted therapy or the backbone chemotherapy regimen is unclear, and ongoing studies aim to address these questions in the next decade. For elderly ALL, novel approaches to induction and consolidation that avoid the high rates of toxic death seen with conventional chemotherapy are needed. Allogeneic HCT remains a curative treatment for adult ALL and the standard of care for Ph+ ALL, with low rates of relapse but at the expense of high non-relapse mortality.

Selected References

Alvarnas JC, Brown PA, Aoun P, et al. Acute lymphoblastic leukemia, Version 2. *J Natl Compr Canc Netw*. 2015;13:1240–1279.

Bassan R, Spinelli O, Oldani E, et al. Improved risk classification for risk-specific therapy based on the molecular study of minimal residual disease (MRD) in adult acute lymphoblastic leukemia (ALL). *Blood*. 2009;113:4153–4162.

DeAngelo DJ, Stevenson K, Dahlberg SE, et al. Long-term outcome of a pediatric-inspired regimen used for adults aged 18–50 years with newly diagnosed acute lymphoblastic leukemia. *Leukemia*. 2015;29(3):526–534.

Dores GM, Devesa SS, Curtis RE, et al. Acute leukemia incidence and patient survival among children and adults in the United States, 2001–2007. *Blood*. 2011;119:34–43.

Douer D, Aldoss I, Lunning MA, et al. Pharmacokinetics-based integration of multiple doses of intravenous pegaspargase in a pediatric regimen for adults with newly diagnosed acute lymphoblastic leukemia. *J Clin Oncol*. 2014;32:905–911.

Fielding AK, Rowe JM, Buck G, et al. UKALLXII/ECOG2993: addition of imatinib to a standard treatment regimen enhances long-term outcomes in Philadelphia positive acute lymphoblastic leukemia. *Blood*. 2014;123:843–850.

Foa R, Vitale A, Vignetti M, et al. Dasatinib as first-line treatment for adult patients with Philadelphia chromosome-positive acute lymphoblastic leukemia. *Blood*. 2011;118:6521–6528.

Gökbuget N. How I treat older patients with ALL. *Blood*. 2013;122:1366–1375.

Gökbuget N, Kneba M, Raff T, et al. Adult patients with acute lymphoblastic leukemia and molecular failure display a poor prognosis and are candidates for stem cell transplantation and targeted therapies. *Blood*. 2012;120(9):1868–1876.

Goldstone AH, Richards SM, Lazarus HM, et al. In adults with standard-risk acute lymphoblastic leukemia, the greatest benefit is achieved from a matched sibling allogeneic transplantation in first complete remission, and an autologous transplantation is less effective than conventional consolidation/maintenance chemotherapy in all patients: final results of the International ALL Trial (MRC UKALL XII/ECOG E2993). *Blood*. 2008;111:1827–1833.

Huguet F, Leguay T, Raffoux E, et al. Pediatric-inspired therapy in adults with Philadelphia chromosome-negative acute lymphoblastic leukemia: the GRAALL-2003 study. *J Clin Oncol.* 2009;27(6):911–918.

Kantarjian HM, O'Brien S, Smith TL, et al. Results of treatment with hyper-CVAD, a dose-intensive regimen, in adult acute lymphocytic leukemia. *J Clin Oncol.* 2000;18:547–561.

Larson RA, Dodge RK, Burns CP, et al. A five-drug remission induction regimen with intensive consolidation for adults with acute lymphoblastic leukemia: cancer and leukemia group B study 8811. *Blood.* 1995;85:2025–2037.

Linker, C, Damon L, Ries C, Navarro W. Intensified and shortened cyclical chemotherapy for adult acute lymphoblastic leukemia. *J Clin Oncol.* 2002;20, 2464–2471.

Maude SL, Frey N, Shaw PA, et al. Chimeric antigen receptor T cells for sustained remissions in leukemia. *N Engl J Med.* 2014;371:1507–1517.

Ribera JM, Oriol A, Sanz MA, et al. Comparison of the results of the treatment of adolescents and young adults with standard-risk acute lymphoblastic leukemia with the Program Espanol de Tratamiento en Hematologia pediatric-based protocol ALL-96. *J Clin Oncol.* 2008;26:1843–1849.

Roberts KG, Li Y, Payne-Turner D, et al. Targetable kinase-activating lesions in Ph-like acute lymphoblastic leukemia. *N Engl J Med.* 2014;371(11):1005–1015.

Stock W, La M, Sanford B, et al. What determines the outcomes for adolescents and young adults with acute lymphoblastic leukemia treated on cooperative group protocols? A comparison of Children's Cancer Group and Cancer and Leukemia Group B studies. *Blood.* 2008;112:1646–1654.

Thomas DA, O'Brien S, Faderl S, et al. Chemoimmunotherapy with a modified hyper-CVAD and rituximab regimen improves outcome in de novo Philadelphia chromosome-negative precursor B- lineage acute lymphoblastic leukemia. *J Clin Oncol.* 2010;28:3880–3889.

Topp MS, Gökbuget N, Stein AS, et al. Safety and activity of blinatumomab for adult patients with relapsed or refractory B-precursor acute lymphoblastic leukaemia: a multicentre, single-arm, phase 2 study. *Lancet Oncol.* 2015;16(1):57–66.

Treatment of AML in Children/Adolescents

Jessica Knight-Perry and Lia Gore

DE NOVO AML

- Important challenges in the treatment of pediatric AML include disease heterogeneity, therapy toxicity, and relapse risk.
- With increased chemotherapeutic intensity, advances in supportive care, and the addition of allogeneic bone marrow transplant, 5-year overall survival is currently estimated between 60% and 70%.
- Genetic subtypes of AML are associated with different overall outcome and, therefore, are used for risk stratification and to assign risk-directed therapy:
  - AML with favorable cytogenetic characteristics that are amendable to chemotherapy alone.
  - AML with unfavorable cytogenetic characteristics requires both chemotherapy and allogeneic bone marrow transplant.
- Further increase in chemotherapeutic intensity is unlikely to improve overall survival, shifting the focus to broad-spectrum antileukemic agents with improved toxicity profiles as well as more directed agents aimed at specific cytogenetic abnormalities.

APML

- APML is a distinct AML subtype with the majority of cases demonstrating the 15;17 translocation and subsequent PLM/RARα fusion protein (see Acute Promyelocytic Leukemia (APL) Chapter 3 for additional details).
- The treatment regimen for APML is unique given the activity of agents that promote promyelocyte differentiation such as all-trans-retinoic acid (ATRA) and arsenic trioxide (ATO).
- Therapeutic regimens including ATRA and high doses of anthracyclines have yielded event-free survival ranging from 70% to 80%.
- The most recent pediatric clinical trials have focused on anthracycline dose reduction given the concern for cardiac toxicity and the well-established response to ATRA and ATO.

AML WITH TRISOMY 21

- Individuals with Trisomy 21 have an increased risk for AML and acute megakaryocytic leukemia in particular, with the most common cytogenetic abnormality in the GATA1 gene.
- Individuals with Trisomy 21 and AML have superior event-free survival and relapse rates when compared to those with AML who do not have Trisomy 21.
- Age at the time of diagnosis of AML is a known prognostic indicator for patients with Trisomy 21. Patients 4 years and older have significantly worse outcomes when compared to Trisomy 21 patients who are aged less than 4 years.
- Given their superior outcomes and increased susceptibility to therapy-related morbidity and mortality, therapeutic regimens for Trisomy 21 patients who are younger than 4 years are less intensive in comparison to the regimen for de novo AML.

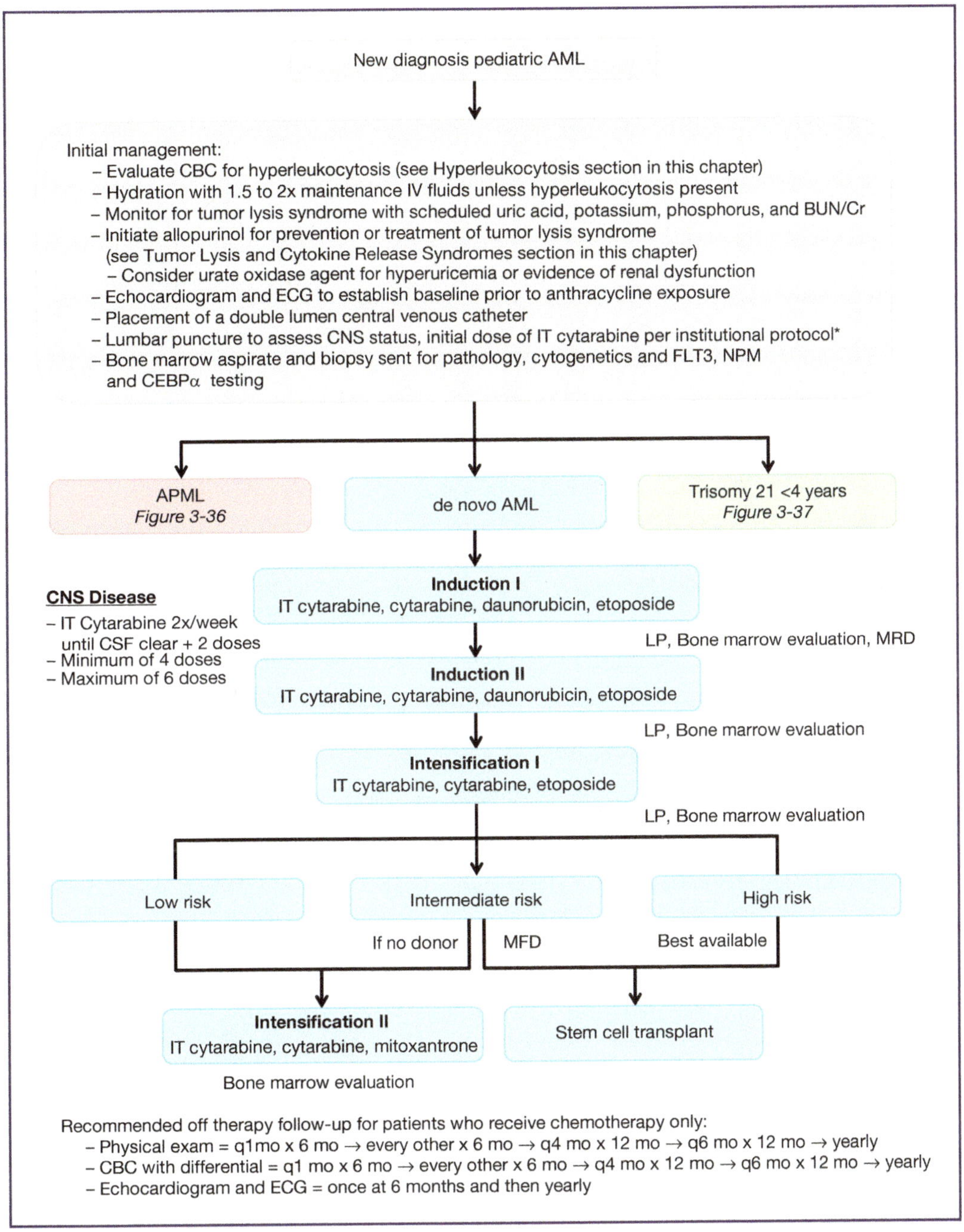

FIGURE 3-34: The current standard of care for the treatment of de novo AML includes three cycles of chemotherapy prior to risk stratification, Induction I (ADE 10 + 3 + 5), Induction II (ADE 8 + 3 + 5), and Intensification I. Pending risk stratification and donor availability, individuals either complete therapy with Intensification II or proceed on to allogeneic bone marrow transplant. In contrast, the active Children's Oncology Group (COG) trial has the previous regimen as the low-risk backbone with early risk stratification following Induction I. This risk stratification is based on cytogenetics as well as minimal residual disease (MRD) and defines individuals as high or low risk, with the removal of the intermediate-risk group. Low Risk: Trisomy 21 patients who are 4 years or older as well as individuals with inv(16), t(16;16) or t(8;21), regardless of the presence or absence of monosomy 7, monosomy 5 or 5q deletions. Intermediate Risk: Individuals who are neither low-risk nor high-risk features. High Risk: Individuals with monosomy 7, monosomy 5, 5q deletions, FLT3-ITD, and/or individuals with more than 15% blasts at the completion of Induction I.

*Defer LP if evidence of DIC, most common in APML.

ADE, ara-C(cytarabine), daunorubicin, etoposide; AML, acute myeloid leukemia; BUN/Cr, blood urea nitrogen/creatinine; CBC, complete blood count; CNS, central nervous system; ECG, electrocardiogram; FLT3-ITD, FMS-like tyrosine kinase 3 internal tandem duplication; IT, intrathecal; IV, intravenous; LP, lumbar puncture; MFD, matched, familial donor.

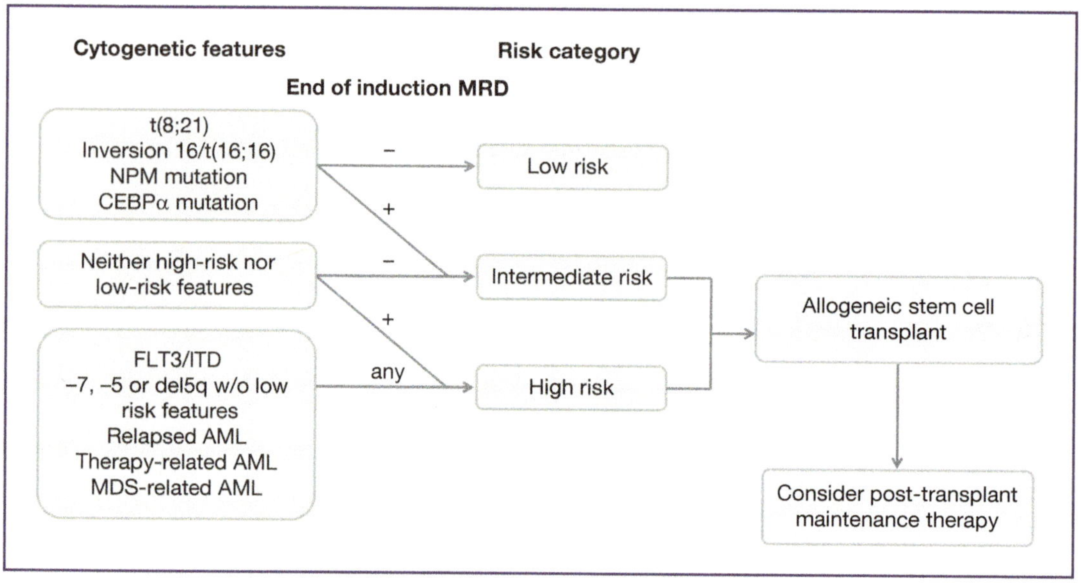

FIGURE 3-35: Risk stratification for de novo AML in pediatric population.

AML, acute myeloid leukemia; FLT3/ITD, FMS-like tyrosine kinase 3 internal tandem duplication; MDS, myelodysplastic syndrome; MRD, minimal residual disease; NPM, nucleophosmine.

- How best to manage AML in Trisomy 21 patients who are 4 years and older is not well defined; however, the majority of pediatric clinical trials enroll these individuals on the regimens designed for those without Trisomy 21. Enhanced supportive care and monitoring guidelines are often incorporated for Trisomy 21 patients, as they are shown to have increased incidence and severity of some toxicities (mucositis in particular).
- For patients with Trisomy 21 and congenital endocardial cushion defects, collaboration with a Pediatric Cardiology team for overall monitoring and management is recommended.

RELAPSED/REFRACTORY AML

- Outcome after relapse is dependent on a variety of factors, most prominent being cytogenetics and duration of first clinical remission.
- Therapeutic approach includes review of patient-specific disease characteristics, discussion of outcome with patient and family and, if deemed appropriate, reinduction chemotherapy followed by allogeneic bone marrow transplant with the best donor available (refer to Chapter 4 for additional information regarding stem cell transplantation).

COMMON COMPLICATIONS AND SUPPORTIVE CARE

- Supportive care is critical in pediatric AML therapy, given the significant treatment-related toxicities including prolonged neutropenia, leading to subsequent risk of Gram-negative and group A Streptococcal bacteremia as well as invasive fungal disease.
- Advances in supportive care in the past decades have contributed to improved pediatric AML outcomes.
- Areas of active research include use of prophylactic antimicrobials such as levofloxacin and identification of the most efficacious fungal prophylaxis.

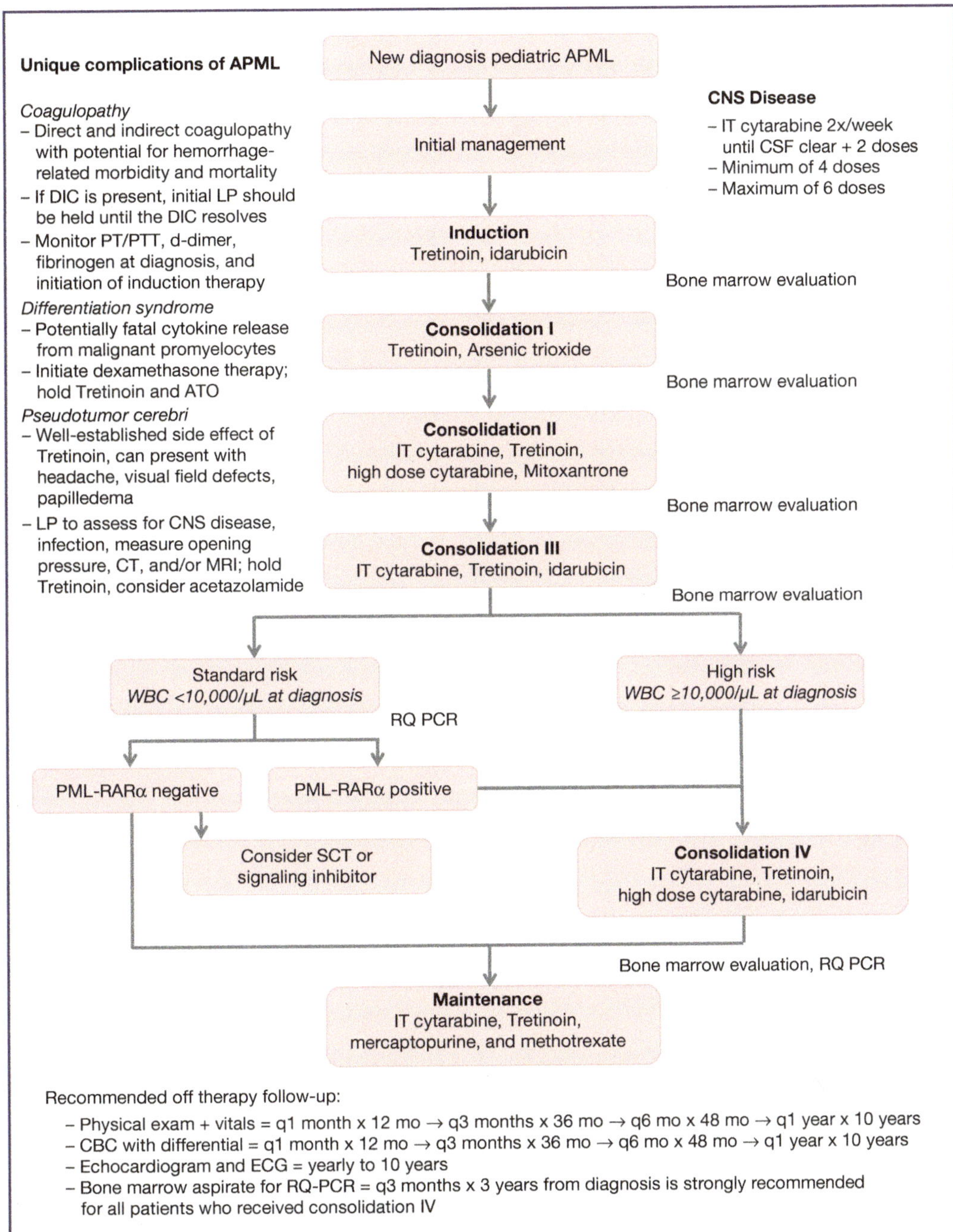

FIGURE 3-36: The current standard of care for pediatric APML consists of four to five cycles of chemotherapy of ATRA, ATO, and idarubicin followed by maintenance with ATRA and oral 6-MP (mercaptopurine) and methotrexate. Risk stratification is currently based on white blood cell count at diagnosis as well as the presence of the PML-RARα fusion protein at the end of Consolidation III. There are unique complications associated with APML, due in large part to the biology of the disease-specific promyelocytes. These complications include coagulopathy at the time of diagnosis and differentiation syndrome, which is most commonly seen at the beginning of induction therapy. Pseudotumor cerebri may occur at any time during therapy and is a well-established side effect of ATRA therapy.

APML (or APL), acute promyelocytic leukemia; ATO, arsenic trioxide; CBC, complete blood count; CNS, central nervous system; CSF, cerebral spinal fluid; DIC, disseminated intravascular coagulation; ECG, electrocardiogram; IT, intrathecal; IV, intravenous; LP, lumbar puncture; PT/PTT, prothrombin time/partial thromboplastin time; RQ-PCR, real-time quantitative polymerase chain reaction; SCT, stem cell transplantation; WBC, white blood cell.

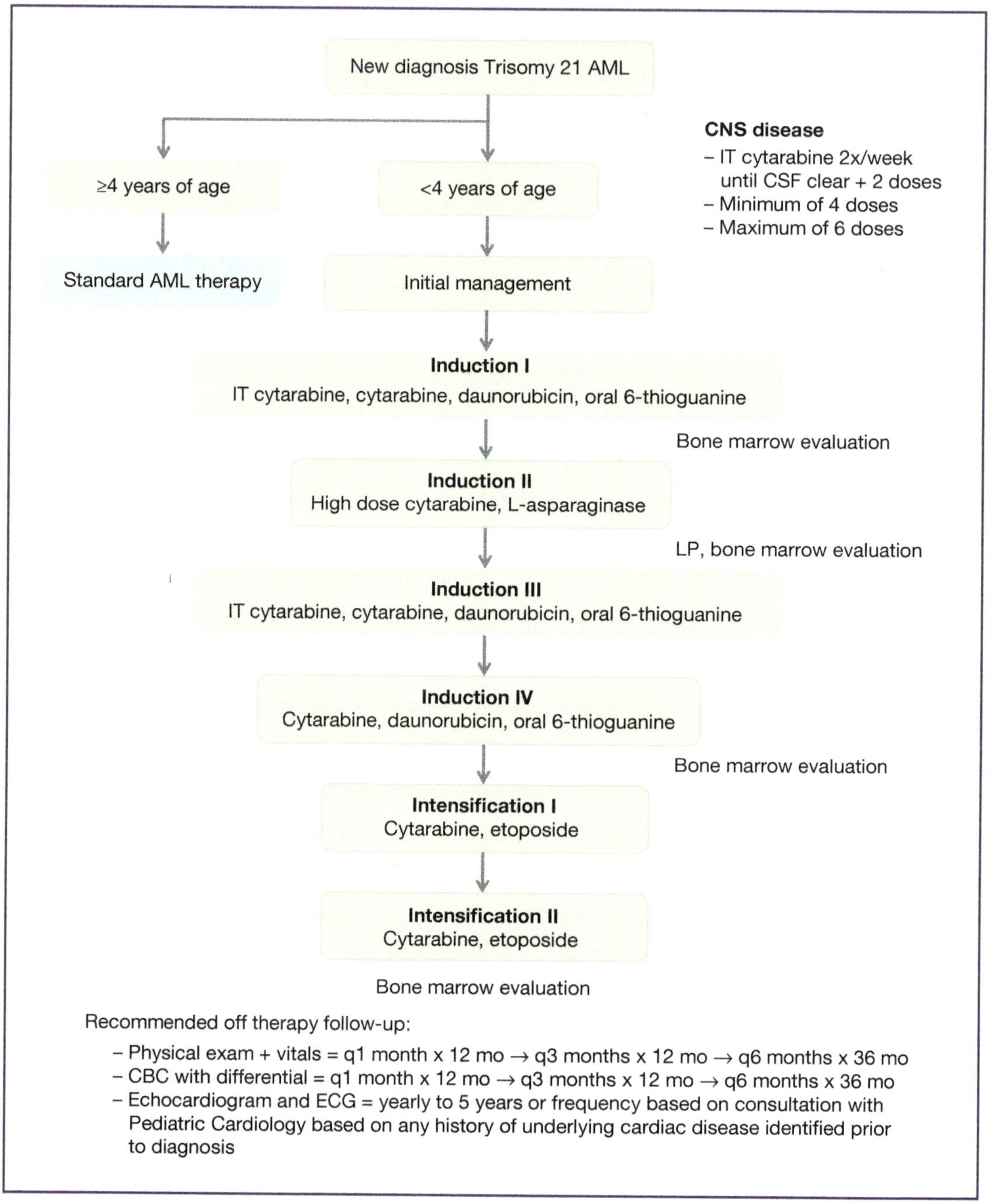

FIGURE 3-37: For individuals with Trisomy 21 and AML who are younger than 4 years of age, the current standard of care consists of six rounds of chemotherapy including high-dose cytarabine, daunorubicin, etoposide, and oral 6-thioguanine. This regimen does not include risk stratification. However, it is important to note that the current COG trial AAML1031 (ClinicalTrials.gov Identifier: NCT01371981) for this patient population uses MRD at the end of Induction I to stratify individuals into standard-risk and high-risk treatment arms with removal of high-dose cytarabine from the standard-risk arm and intensification of therapy for the high-risk population.

AML, acute myeloid leukemia; CBC, complete blood count; CNS, central nervous system; COG, Children's Oncology Group; CSF, cerebral spinal fluid; ECG, electrocardiogram; IT, intrathecal; MRD, minimal residual disease.

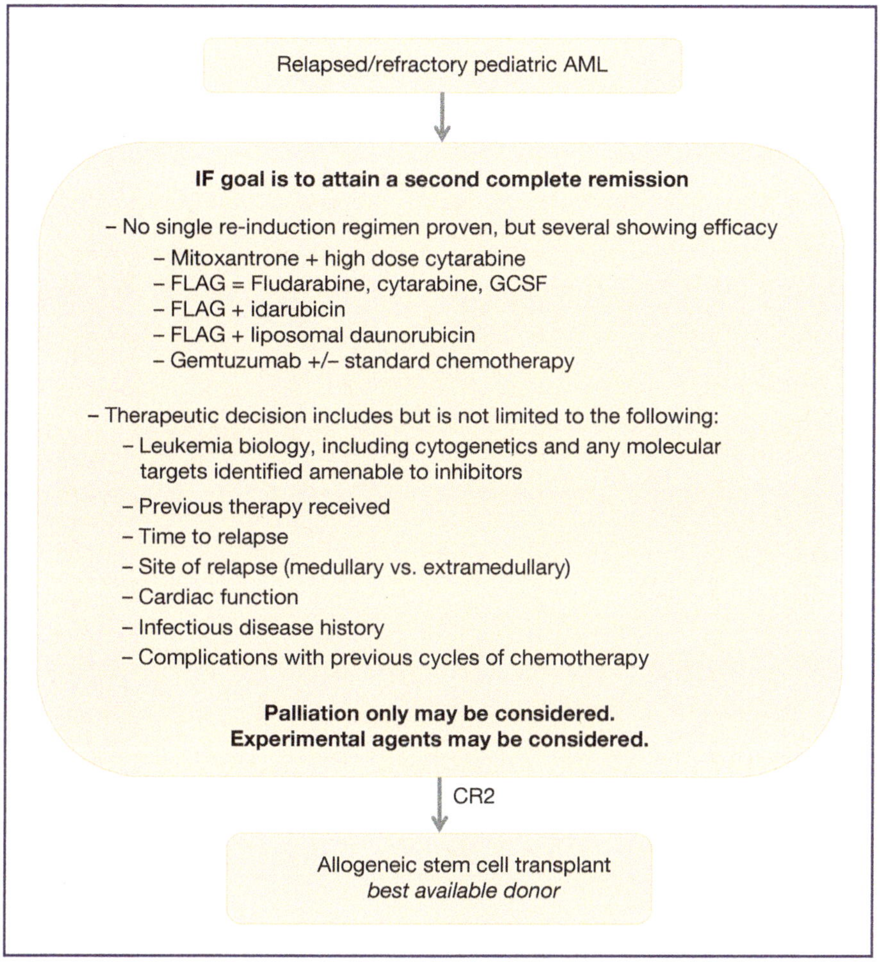

FIGURE 3-38: **Relapsed/refractory pediatric AML treatment algorithm.**
AML, acute myeloid leukemia; GCSF, granulocyte colony-stimulating factor.

Table 3-18 Common complications of AML therapy and relevant supportive care

COMPLICATIONS	SUPPORTIVE CARE
Bacterial Infection	
• Gram-negative organisms including *Pseudomonas* • Gram-positive organisms, most notably group A *Streptococcus* following high-dose cytarabine	• Broad-spectrum antibiotics for fever and neutropenia, including vancomycin following courses of high-dose cytarabine • Consider hospital admission until early signs of count recovery • Consider GCSF/cytokine support
Fungal Infection	
• Invasive fungal disease contributes to treatment-related morbidity and mortality, including *Candida* and *Aspergillus* species	• Antifungal prophylaxis • *Pneumocystis jiroveci* prophylaxis • Fungal disease workup of ≥5 days of fever
Viral Infection	
• Viral reactivation as well as primary infection with pathogens such as EBV, CMV, HSV	• Consider acyclovir for prevention of previously documented, mucocutaneous HSV

AML, acute myeloid leukemia; CMV, cytomegalovirus, EBV, Epstein-Barr virus, GCSF, granulocyte colony-stimulating factor; HSV, herpes simplex virus.

INDICATION FOR ALLOGENEIC STEM CELL TRANSPLANT

- Indications for allogeneic stem cell transplant after the first clinical remission have been a significant topic of debate (see Chapter 4).
- Risk stratification, chemotherapeutic efficacy and response, and acceptable donor availability are important considerations.
- In general, it is largely agreed that individuals with low-risk features, including APML and Trisomy 21 who are younger than 4 years of age, are best treated with chemotherapy alone, while individuals with high-risk features and/or positive residual disease at the end of induction are appropriate candidates for bone marrow transplant (refer to Chapter 4 for further details).

Table 3-19 Indications for allogeneic bone marrow transplant

INDICATIONS FOR ALLOGENEIC STEM CELL TRANSPLANT IN PEDIATRIC MYELOID LEUKEMIAS
In First Remission
MDS
Therapy-related or secondary MDS or AML
Refractory disease
MRD positivity at end of Induction I
FLT3/ITD with high allelic ratio
Monosomy 7, monosomy 5, or del5q MDS, without inv(16)/t(16;16), t(8;21), NPM or CEBPα
JMML
In Second Remission
Relapsed disease

AML, acute myeloid leukemia; JMML, juvenile myelomonocytic leukemia; MDS, myelodysplastic syndrome; MRD, minimal residual disease; NPM, nucleophosmine.

Emerging Therapies

- Further increase in chemotherapeutic intensity is unlikely to improve overall survival, shifting the focus to broad-spectrum antileukemic agents with improved toxicity profiles as well as agents directed at specific targetable cytogenetic or molecular abnormalities.
- Targeting of specific cytogenetic and molecular abnormalities provides a more directed approach to the marked heterogeneity observed in AML.
- Like conventional chemotherapy regimens, improved outcomes is likely to require combinations of agents with protean antileukemic effects for maximal benefit.

Table 3-20 Emerging therapies

Inhibitors of Signaling
CKD
FLT3
IDH1 and 2
JAK1 and 2
KIT
MEK1 and 2
PI-3 Kinase
TET2
Wee1
Wnt

(*continued*)

Table 3-20 Emerging therapies (*continued*)

Epigenetic Modifiers
DNA methyltransferase inhibitors
Histone deacetylase inhibitors
Histone methyltransferase inhibitors
Proteosome Inhibitors
Nuclear Export Inhibitors
Cell Signaling Inhibitors
JAK inhibitors
AKT inhibitors
Aurora kinase inhibitors
Cytotoxic Agents
Cell cycle inhibitors
Nucleoside analogues
Fusion nucleoside analog combinations
DNA intercalator + topoisomerase inhibitor
Liposomal encapsulated agents
Immunotherapy
Monoclonal antibodies
Antibody-drug conjugates
Natural killer cell therapy
Programmed death-1 inhibition
Stem cell transplantation including graft manipulation
Chimeric antigen receptor T-cells
Bi- and tri-specific antibodies

FLT3, FMS-like tyrosine kinase 3; IDH, isocitrate dehydrogenase; TET2, ten-eleven translocation 2.

Selected References

Abrahamsson J, Clausen N, Gustafsson G, et al. Improved outcome after relapse in children with acute myeloid leukeamia. *Br J Haematol*. 2007;136:229–236.

Avramis VI, Wiersma S, Krailo MD, et al. Pharmacokinetic and pharmacodynamics studies of fludarabine and cytosine arabinoside administered as loading boluses followed by continuous infusions after a phase I/II study in pediatric patients with relapsed leukemias. The children's cancer group. *Clin Cancer Res*. 1998;4(1):45–52.

Cooper TM, Franklin J, Gerbing RB, et al. AAML03P1, a pilot study of the safety of gemtuzumab ozogamicin in combination with chemotherapy for newly diagnosed childhood acute myeloid leukemia: a report from the Children's Oncology Group. *Cancer*. 2012;118:761–769.

Creutzig U, Reinhardt D, Diekamp S, et al. AML patients with Down syndrome have a high cure rate with AML-BFM therapy with reduced dose intensity. *Leukemia*. 2005;19:1355–1360.

Creutzig U, Zimmermann M, Bourquin JP, et al. Randomized trial comparing liposomal daunorubicin with idarubicin as induction for pediatric acute myeloid leukemia: results from study AML-BFM 2004. *Blood*. 2013;122:37–43.

Fenaux P, Chevret S, Guerci A, et al. Long-term follow-up confirms the benefit of all-trans retinoic acid in acute promyelocytic leukemia. European APL group. *Leukemia*. 2000;14(8):1371–1377.

Fleischhack G, Graf N, Hasan C, et al. IDA-FLAG (idarubicin, fludarabine, high dosage cytarabine and G-CSF)—an effective therapy regimen in treatment of recurrent acute myelocytic leukemia in children and treatment of relapsed and refractory pediatric AML 165 adolescents: initial results of a pilot study. *Klin Padiatr*. 1996;208(4):229–235.

Gamis AS, Howells WB, DeSwarte-Wallace J, et al. Alpha hemolytic streptococcal infection during intensive treatment for acute myeloid leukemia: a report from the children's cancer group study CCG-2891. *J Clin Oncol*. 2000;18:1845–1855.

Gamis AS, Woods WG, Alonzo TA, et al. Increased age at diagnosis has a significantly negative effect on outcome in children with Down syndrome and acute myeloid leukemia: a report from the Children's Cancer Group Study 2891. *J Clin Oncol*. 2003;21:3415–3422.

Gibson BE, Webb D, Wheatley K. Does transplant in first CR have a role in pediatric AML? A review of the MRC10 and 12 trials. *Blood*. 2000;96:522a.

Hiddemann W, Aul C, Maschmeyer G, et al. High-dose versus intermediate-dose cytarabine combined with mitoxantrone for the treatment of relapsed and refractory acute myeloid leukemia: results of an age-adjusted randomized comparison. *Semin Hematol*. 1991;28(3 Suppl 4):35–38.

Huhmann IM, Watzke HH, Geissler K, et al. FLAG (fludarabine, cytosine arabinoside, G-CSF) for refractory and relapsed acute myeloid leukemia. *Ann Hematol*. 1996;73(6):265–271.

Lehrnbecher T, Zimmermann M, Reinhardt D, et al. Prophylactic human granulocyte colony-stimulating factor in after induction therapy in pediatric acute myeloid leukemia. *Blood*. 2007;109:936–943.

Niewerth D, Creutzig U, Bierings MB, Kaspers GJ. A review on allogeneic stem cell transplantation for newly diagnosed pediatric acute myeloid leukemia. *Blood*. 2010;116:2205–2214.

Russo D, Piccaluga PP, Michieli M, et al. Liposomal daunorubicin (DaunoXome) for treatment of poor-risk acute leukemia. *Ann Hematol*. 2002;81(8):462–466.

Tavernier E, Le QH, Elhamri M, Thomas X. Salvage therapy in refractory acute myeloid leukemia: prediction of outcome based on analysis of prognostic factors. *Leuk Res*. 2003;27:205–214.

Wechsler J, Greene M, McDevitt MA, et al. Acquired mutations in GATA1 in the megakaryoblastic leukemia of Down syndrome. *Nat Genet*. 2002;32(1):148–152.

Zwaan CM, Reinhardt D, Zimmerman M, et al. Salvage treatment for children with refractory first or second relapse of acute myeloid leukaemia with gemtuzumab ozogamicin: results of a phase II study. *Br J Haematol*. 2010;148(5):768–776.

Adolescent and Young Adult (AYA) Patients With Acute Lymphoblastic Leukemia (ALL) and Lymphoblastic Lymphoma: Epidemiology, Survival Trends, and Optimal Therapy

Archie Bleyer

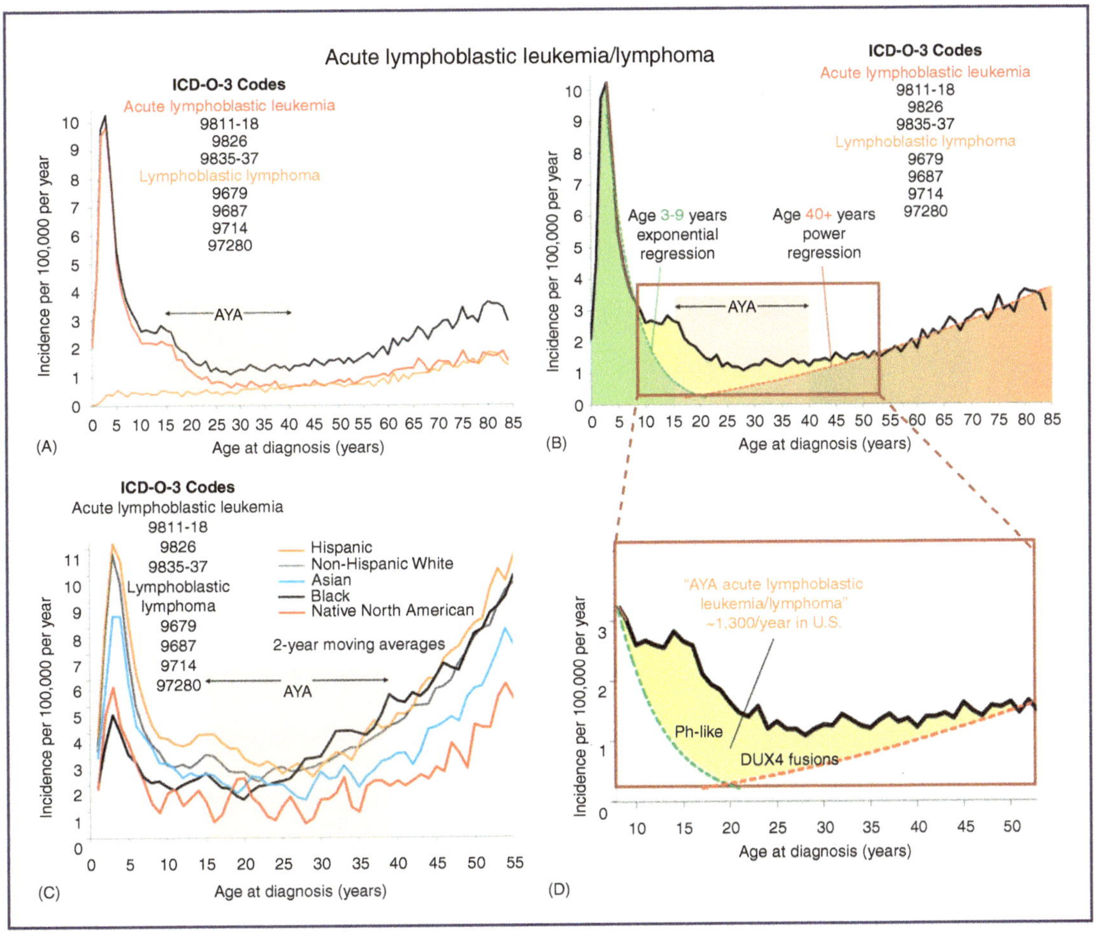

FIGURE 3-39: Incidence of ALL and lymphoblastic lymphoma in AYA Americans and their races/ethnicities. (A) Incidence of acute lymphoblastic leukemia/lymphoma by single years of age, 2000–2013, SEER18, regressions of incidence trends before and after AYA ages. (B, D) Area-under-the-curve (yellow) and above-the-regression curves that represents "AYA acute lymphoblastic leukemia/lymphoma" and estimated average annual number of newly diagnosed such patients in the United States for 2000 to 2013. (C) Incidence of AYA acute lymphoblastic leukemia/lymphoma by single years of age, 2000 to 2013, SEER18 by race/ethnicity. For all races/ethnicities, the incidence of ALL/LBL is lowest during the AYA years. At all ages up to 25, Hispanics have a higher incidence of ALL/LBL than any other race/ethnicity; in AYAs older than 25, Blacks have the highest incidence. Native North Americans have the lowest incidence of ALL/LBL in AYAs and older adults.

ALL, acute lymphoblastic leukemia; AYA, adolescent and young adult; LBL, lymphoblastic lymphoma.

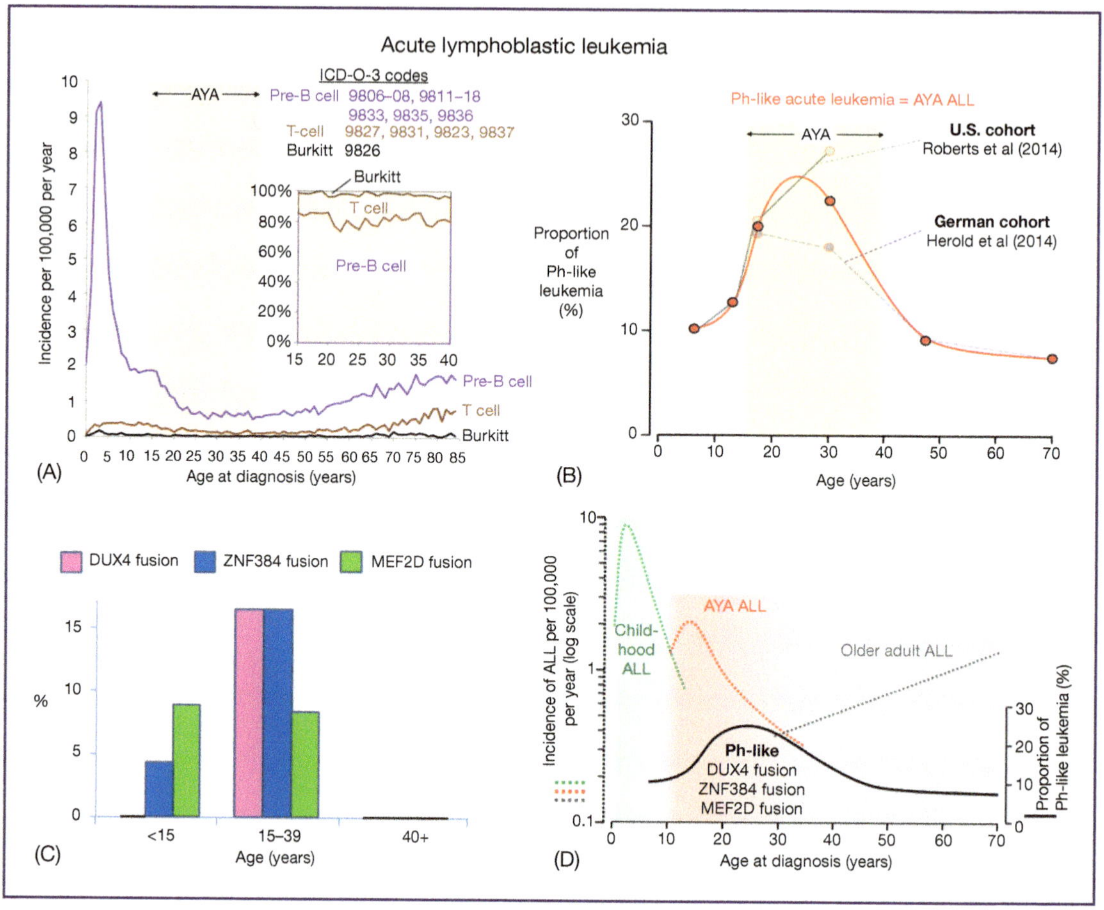

FIGURE 3-40: AYA ALL: Ph-like and DUX fusions. (A) The incidence of pre-B-cell, T-cell, and Burkitt ALL, SEER18, 2000–2013, by single year of age. The inset shows the distribution of the three basic immunophenotypes in AYAs. Pre-B-cell, T-cell, and Burkitt ALL account for 82%, 16% and 2% of all ALL in AYAs, and are relatively similar at all ages of AYAs. The adolescent peak is predominantly due to the pre-B-cell immunophenotype. (B) The proportion of all patients with ALL with Philadelphia chromosome like (Ph-like) type. The German cohort Herold et al was composed of patients who received treatment in the German Multicenter Study Group for Adult ALL trials, and the U.S. cohort was composed of the patients in the study reported by Roberts et al. The Ph-like incidence peak occurs between ages 20 and 30 years, and appears to account for ~1/4 of all cases of ALL in the age group. (C) A new "AYA ALL" based on DUX4 fusions has recently been described by Yasuda et al in Japan. DUX4 is an oncogenic driver of murine ALL and characterizes a "clinical entity distinct from ALL at other ages." (D) Comparison of the incidence of all ALL derived from 12,372 patients in SEER (dashed colored curves) and the proportion of all ALL that is Ph-like derived by Roberts et al (solid black curve). ALL, acute lymphoblastic leukemia; AYA, adolescent and young adult; SEER, surveillance, epidemiology, and end results.

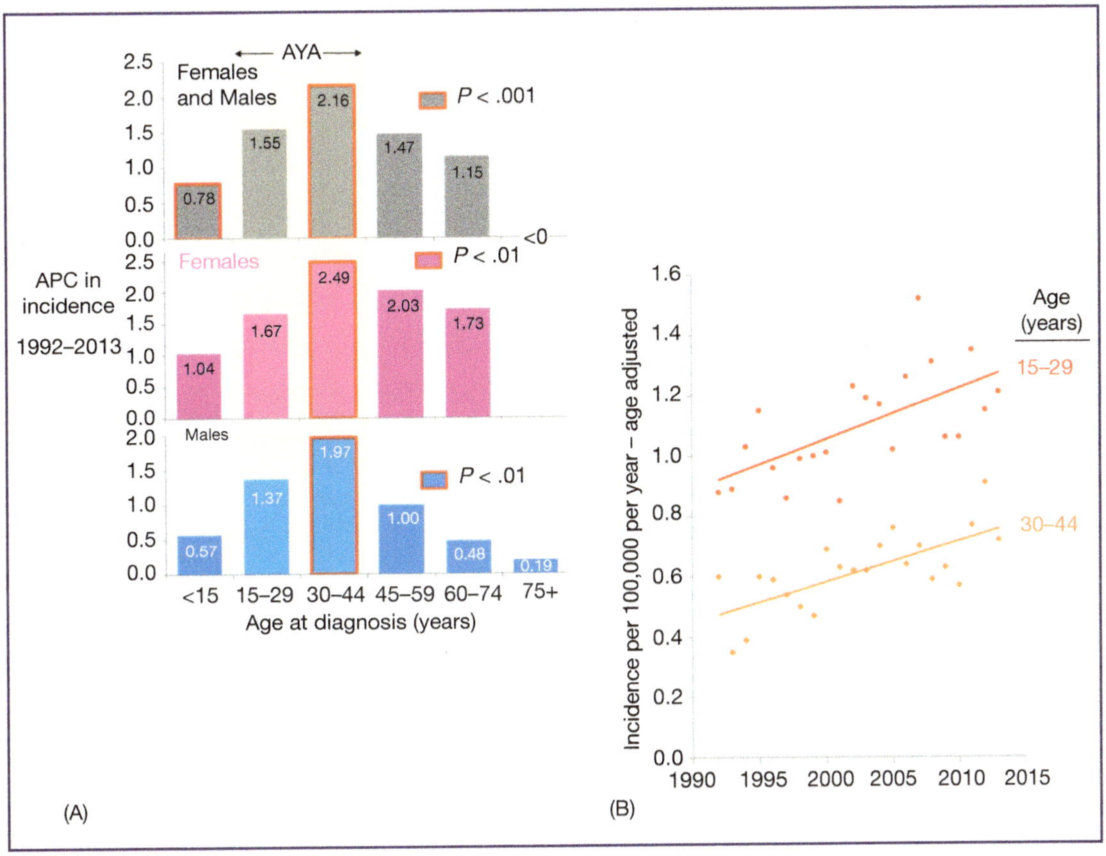

FIGURE 3-41: Increasing incidence of ALL in American AYAs. (A) Average annual percent change (APC) in incidence of ALL, 1992–2013, SEER13, by 15-year age intervals. AYAs have had, since at least 1992, a greater increase in the incidence of ALL than any other age group. AYA females have had a greater increase than AYA males, but in males AYAs have had a greater increase relative to other age groups. (B) Annual incidence of ALL in 15- to 29- and 30- to 44-year-olds, SEER13, 1992–2013. The annual incidence of ALL in AYAs has been steadily increasing since at least 1992 at a rate of 2.2% per year in 30- to 44-year-olds and 1.6% per year in 15- to 29-year-olds (Figure 3-41A).

ALL, acute lymphoblastic leukemia; APC, antigen-presenting cell; AYA, adolescent and young adult; SEER, surveillance, epidemiology, and end results.

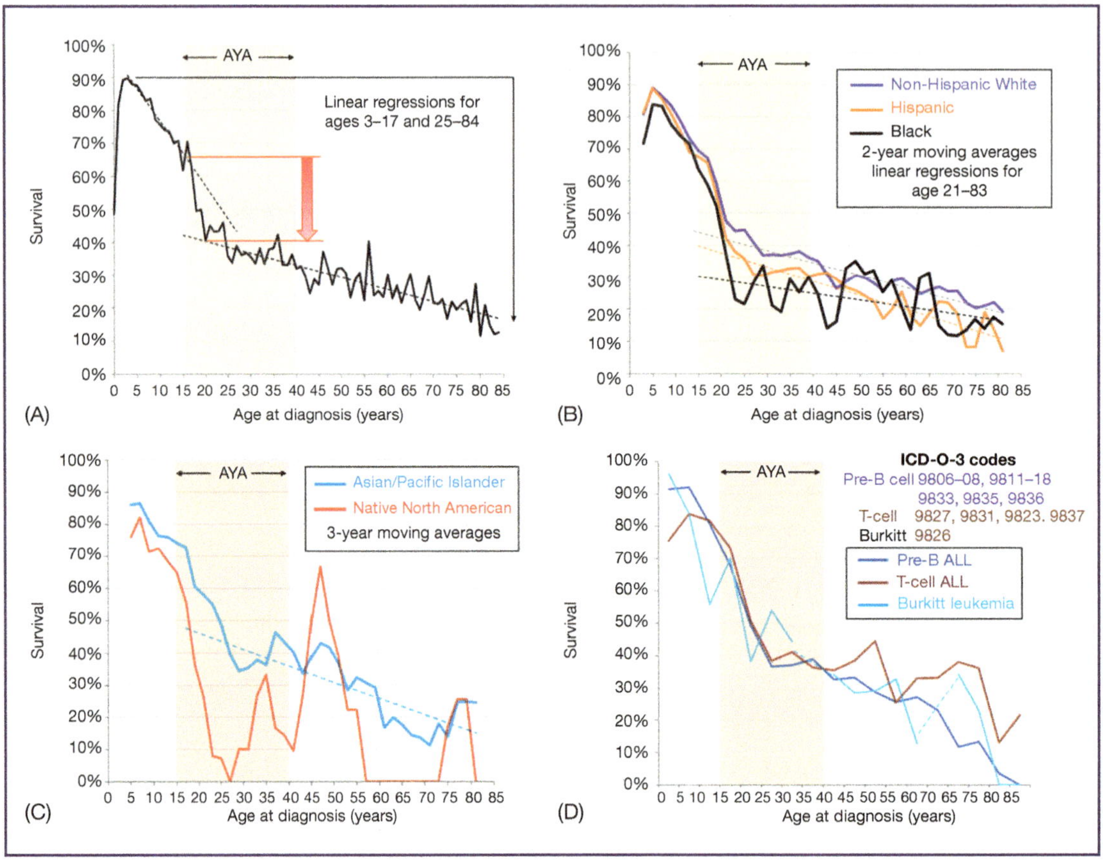

FIGURE 3-42: **Survival of Americans with ALL declines with age, especially in AYAs. (A) ALL: 5-year relative survival, 2000–2011, SEER18, at 1-year age intervals. The 5-year relative survival rate of ALL has its greatest decline between ages 16 and 21, during which the drop is an absolute 25%. By age 21, less than half the patients survive 5 years. The 25% absolute decrease that occurs from age 16 to 21 is one-third of the decrease over the entire age span, in just 5 years of age (arrow). (B) Since 2000, there has been little difference in the survival rate of non-Hispanic Whites, Hispanics, and Blacks younger than age 13. By age 16, however, survival diverges as a function of race/ethnicity, with African Americans having the worst survival, followed by Hispanics, non-Hispanic Whites, and Asians, in that order. The plummet in survival rate from age 16 to 21 is greatest in African Americans, with their 5-year survival being <30% by age 21. (C) In general, Asian/Pacific Islanders and native North Americans have a similar survival pattern to other race/ethnicities in the United States. The survival plummet from age 16 to 21 is less apparent in Asian/Pacific Islanders than it is in non-Hispanic Whites, Hispanics, and African Americans. (D) Since 2000, the three basic immunophenotypes of ALL have had a similar survival as a function of age. Each has evidence for the age 15 to 25 plummet.**

ALL, acute lymphoblastic leukemia; AYA, adolescent and young adult; SEER, surveillance, epidemiology, and end results.

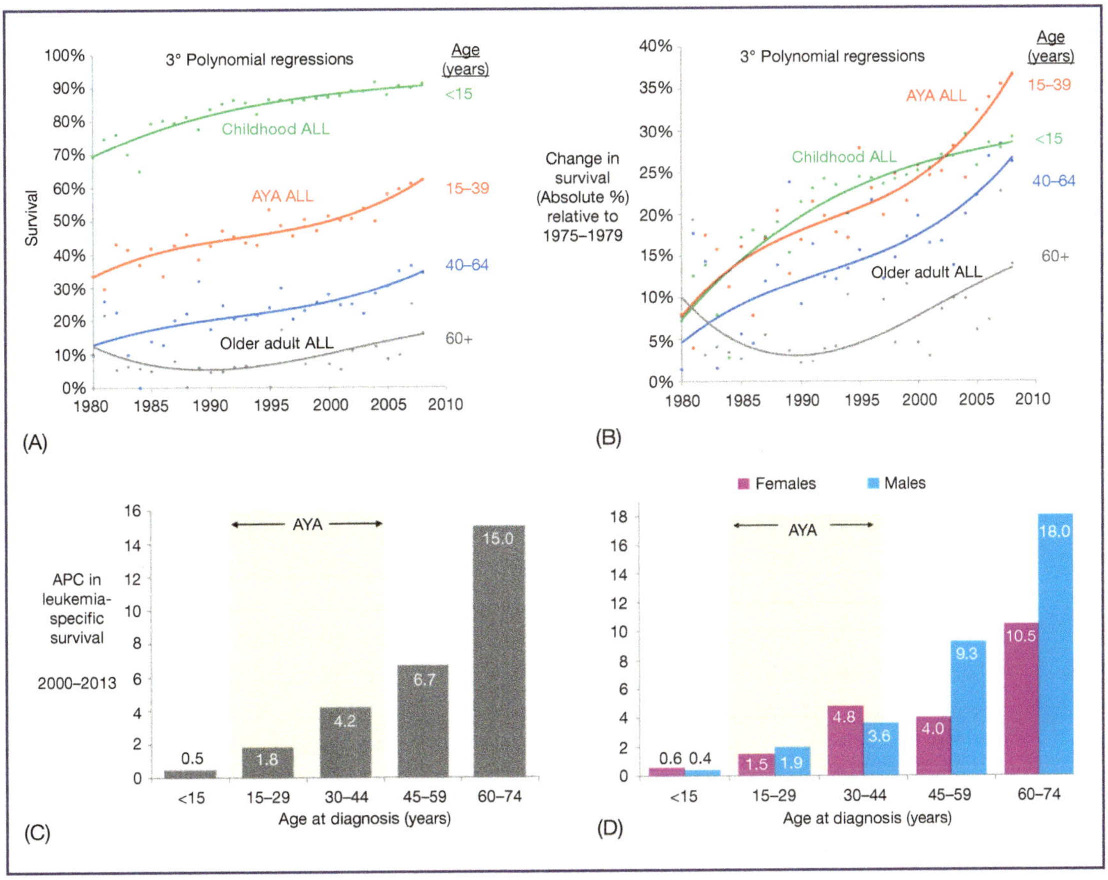

FIGURE 3-43: **Survival trends in American AYAs with ALL. (A) Since 1980, the 5-year leukemia-specific survival rate of ALL has steadily improved in children, AYAs, and adults <60 years of age. Until 2000, AYAs lagged behind the progress in children, and adults over 40 years of age had the least progress. In AYAs, the 5-year leukemia-specific survival nearly tripled during the three decades from 1980 to 2008, but more than 60% of the AYAs were still dying within 5 years after diagnosis, as of 2008. (B) In comparison with the survival rate during 1975–1979, children with ALL had the most progress until 2000 when AYAs surpassed children. (C) As indicated by the average percent change (APC) in 5-year leukemia-specific survival of ALL, 2000–2013, SEER, by 15-year age intervals, AYAs have had less improvement in their 5-year leukemia-specific survival since 2000 than any older patients. (D) Since 2000, older AYA females have had a greater increase than older females but AYA males of all ages have had distinctly less improvement than older males. The relatively greater improvement in older adults with ALL may be due to the incidence of Ph+ ALL being directly proportional to patient age (Figure 3-40A) and the tyrosine kinase inhibitors that are so effective in the treatment of Ph+ ALL being implemented since 2000. If so, the future bodes well for AYAs with Ph-like ALL.**

ALL, acute lymphoblastic leukemia; APC, antigen-presenting cell; AYA, adolescent and young adult; SEER, surveillance, epidemiology, and end results.

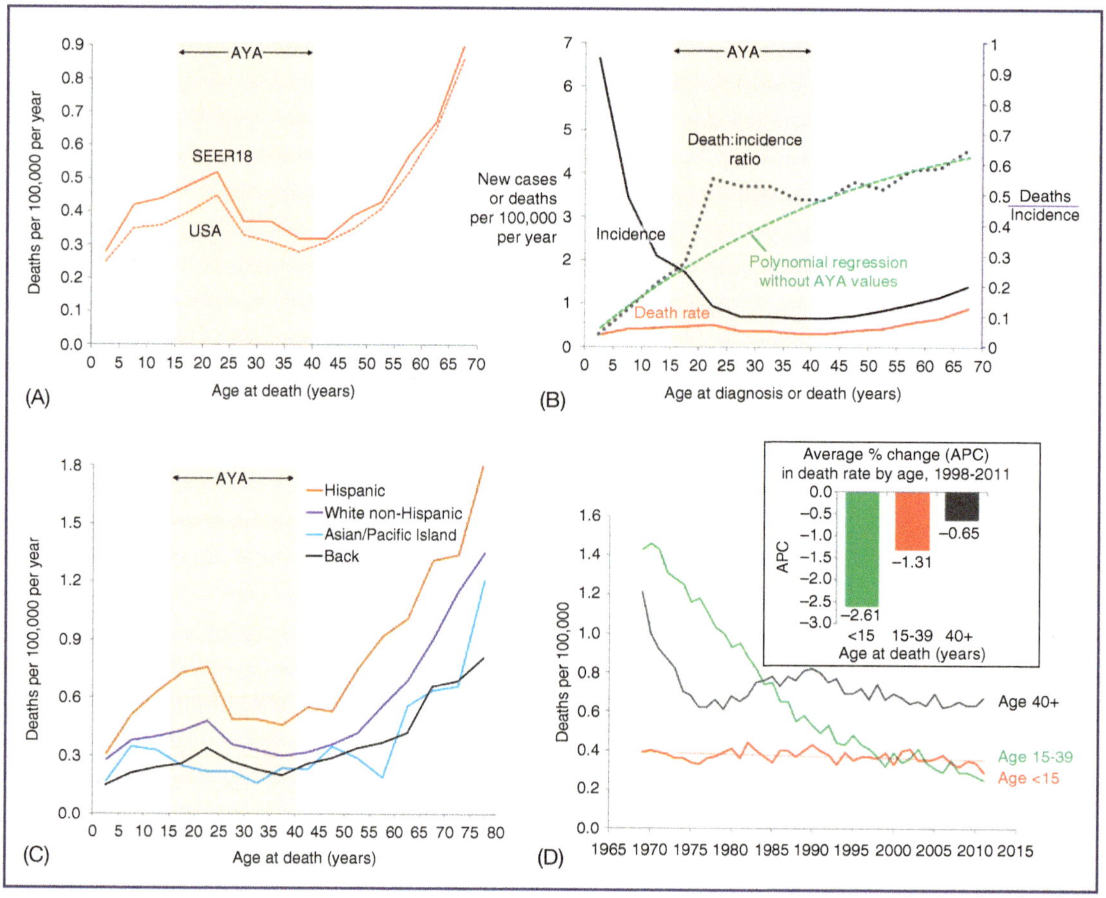

FIGURE 3-44: Age-dependent mortality of Americans with ALL. (A) The ALL death rate in SEER18, representing 28% to 29% of the United States, is indicative of the entire country. AYAs have a higher death rate from ALL than any other age group <55 years of age. The age group with the highest incidence (children) is also the age group with the lowest death rate. The younger the childhood age group, the lower the death rate. (B) The death to incidence ratio (dotted gray curve) for ALL increases with age, but nearly all of the increase occurs during childhood and adolescence. The excess of deaths relative to incidence in AYAs is apparent when the ratio is projected from younger and older ages (dashed green regression). In children <5 years of age, one ALL death occurs for every 25 cases diagnosed; by age 20, one death occurs for every two cases diagnosed. (C) For the entire United States, the ALL death rate peak in young AYAs is apparent in non-Hispanic Whites, Hispanics, Blacks, native North Americans (who have an insufficient number in SEER18 to be considered) but not in Asians. (D) For the entire United States, the ALL death rate in AYAs was >1/3 that of children <15 × in 1970 but has declined so much more slowly than in children that it became higher in the late 1990s and has been higher since.

ALL, acute lymphoblastic leukemia; AYA, adolescent and young adult; SEER, surveillance, epidemiology, and end results.

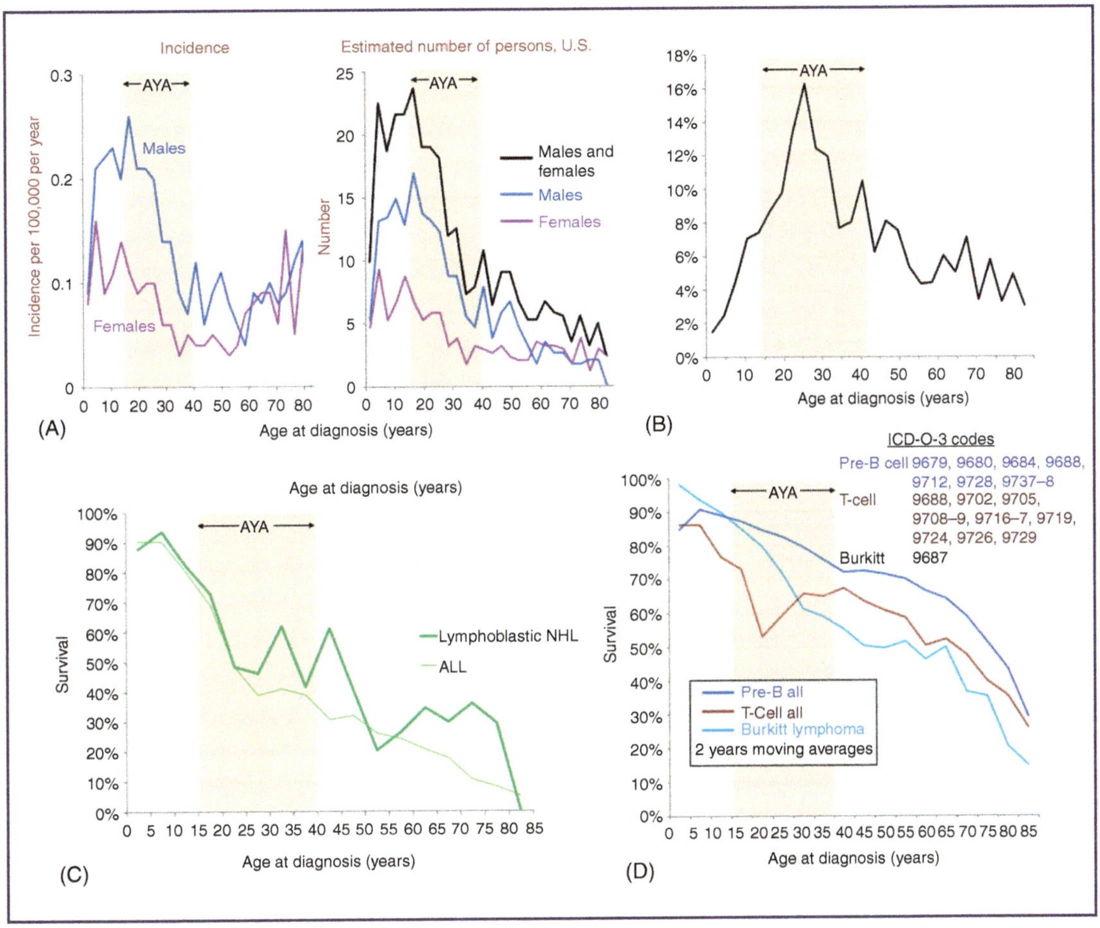

FIGURE 3-45: **Incidence and immunophenotype of lymphoblastic lymphoma in the United States. (A) The incidence of lymphoblastic lymphoma peaks and has the greatest number of Americans between 5 and 25 years of age. The incidence in children and AYAs is greater in males than in females, similar to ALL. (B) AYAs have the highest proportion, between 8% and 16%, of lymphoblastic malignancy (ALL + lymphoblastic lymphoma) that is lymphoblastic lymphoma. (C) The 5-year relative survival rate of lymphoblastic lymphoma has its greatest decline during adolescence. The survival rates of lymphoblastic lymphoma and ALL are identical during childhood and adolescence and similar in older patients, supporting the practice of treating both the same. (D) All three basic immunophenotypes of lymphoblastic lymphoma have a similar inverse survival function by age.**

ALL, acute lymphoblastic leukemia; AYA, adolescent and young adult; NHL, non-Hodgkin lymphoma.

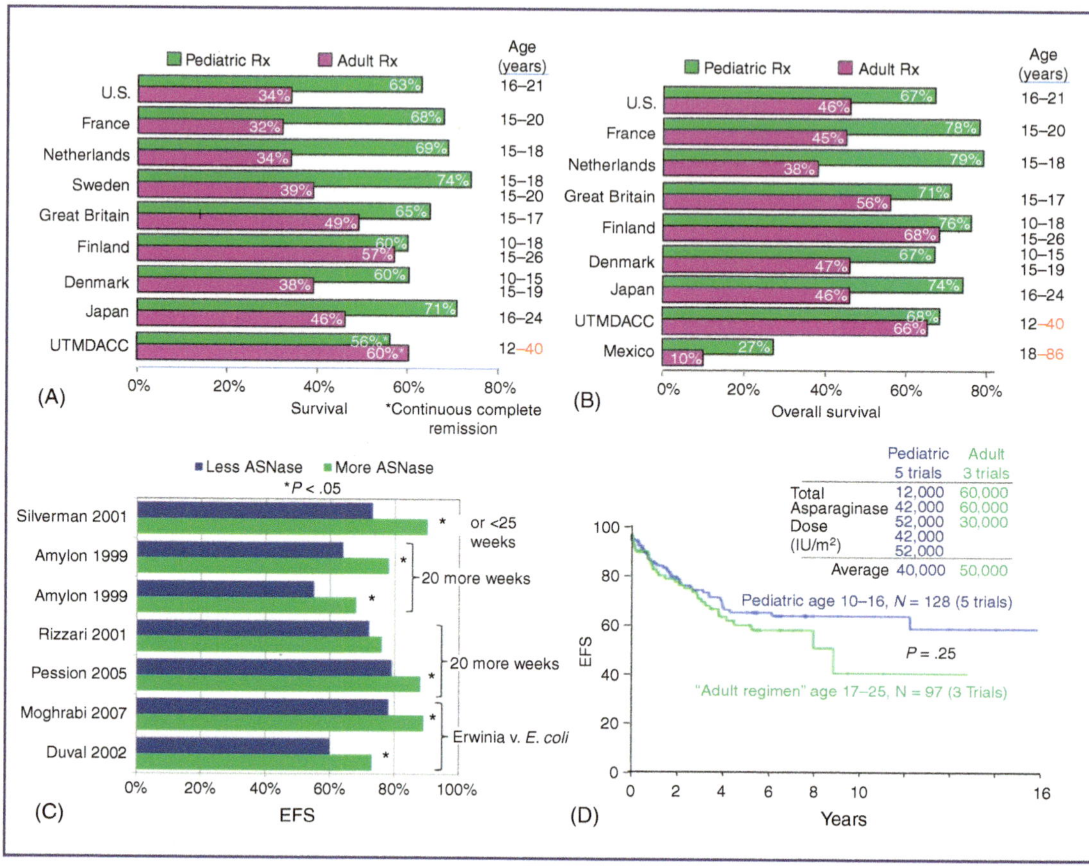

FIGURE 3-46: Treatment of AYAs with ALL: Pediatric-inspired versus adult treatment regimens. (A) Including reports from Norway and Italy not shown, there have been 11 comparisons of pediatric vs. adult regimens of the 4- to 7-year event-free or disease-free survival in AYAs with ALL treated by the same group with either an adult regimen or a pediatric-inspired regimen, all but one of which (UTMDACC) favors the pediatric regimen. (Data from Isakoff et al, with results from Denmark and the University of Texas MD Anderson Cancer Center [UTMDACC] added to the Isakoff report). (B) Including reports from Norway and Italy not shown, there have been 11 such comparisons of overall survival with the pediatric vs. adult regimens, all of which favor the pediatric regimen (Boissel et al, deBont et al, Hayakawa et al, Haïat et al, Nachman et al, Ramanujachar et al, Ribara et al, Ram et al, Ruiz-Delgado et al, Rytting et al, Schroeder et al, Stock et al, Testi et al, Usvasalo et al). (C) A major reason attributed for the better result with the pediatric type of regimen is the inclusion of asparaginase, which is rarely used in the adult regimens; when it is used, the interval of asparaginase therapy is shorter than in the typical pediatric regimen. All seven reported comparisons of relative total doses of asparaginase in the pediatric regimen indicate more asparaginase is better in providing higher rates of event-free survival (Amylon et al, Duval et al, Moghrabi et al, Pession et al, Rizzari et al, Silverman et al). (D) Of the two studies that had the least difference between the pediatric and adult regimens, from Finland and UTMDACC (Figures 3-46A & 3-46B), the adult regimens in the Finnish study included total doses of asparaginase that exceeded those used in their pediatric regimens.

ALL, acute lymphoblastic leukemia; AYA, adolescent and young adult; EFS, event-free survival.

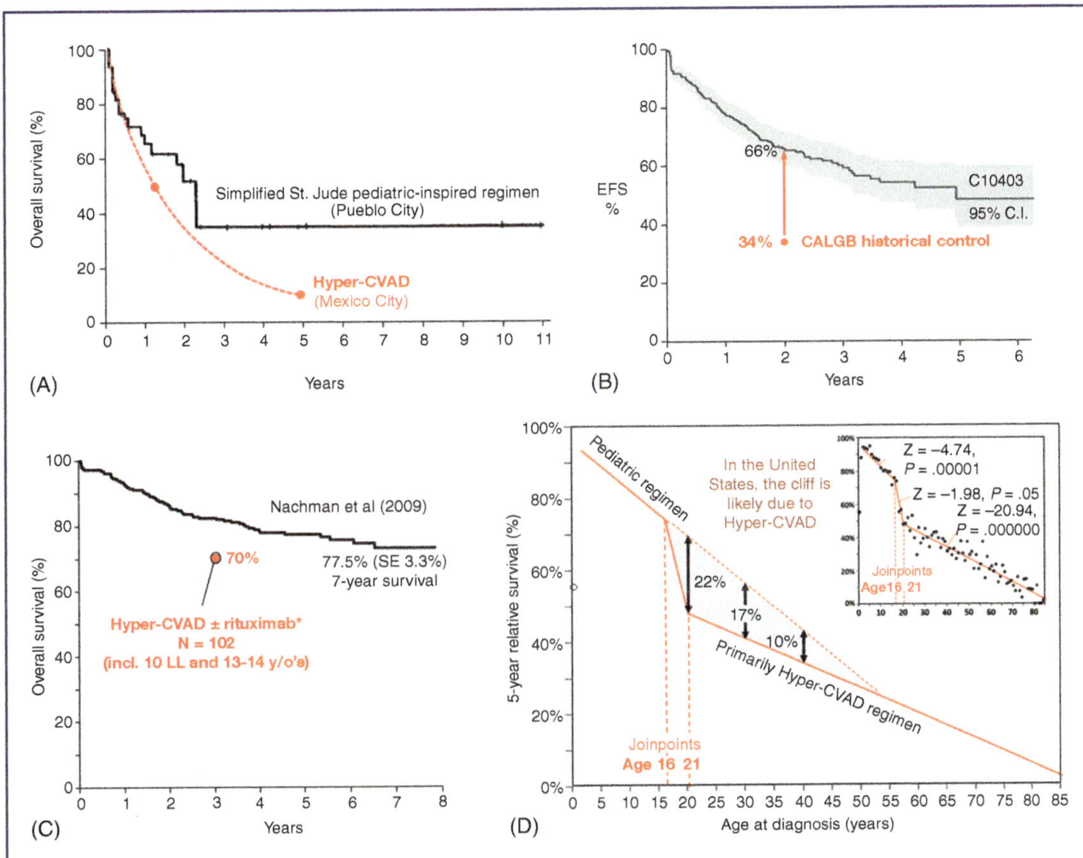

FIGURE 3-47: Treatment of AYAs with ALL: Pediatric-inspired regimens versus hyper-CVAD. (A) A report from Mexico (at the bottom of Figure 3-46B) in adults up to the age of 86 also reported a better overall survival with a simplified St. Jude pediatric regimen. (B) The NCI Intergroup Trial C10403 conducted by The Alliance (CALGB), SWOG, and ERG (ECOG) had better results in 18- to 30-year-olds than their historical control experience. (C) Comparison of overall survival of 16- to 21-year-olds treated by the Children's Cancer Group on CCG-1962 and by MD Anderson Cancer Center with hyper-CVAD, with or without rituximab. (D) The SEER 5-year relative survival cliff (Figure 3-47A) has joinpoints at 16 and 21 years of age. The linear regression from age 21 in American adults with ALL is primarily due to the use of hyper-CVAD since it is the most widely used regimen in the United States. Since the linear regression in pediatric patients under the age of 16 would predict for a higher survival rate in AYAs (the dashed extension of the linear regression), the 50-year overall survival of AYAs with ALL could be expected to improve by 10% to 22% if the pediatric regimen was the primary regime in these patients instead of hyper-CVAD.

*Thomas et al. also Rytting et al.

ALL, acute lymphoblastic leukemia; AYA, adolescent and young adult; CALGB, Cancer and Leukemia Group B; ECOG, Eastern Cooperative Oncology Group; hyper-CVAD, hyperfractionated cyclophosphamide, vincristine, doxorubicin, dexamethasone; NCI, National Cancer Institute; SEER, surveillance, epidemiology, and end results.

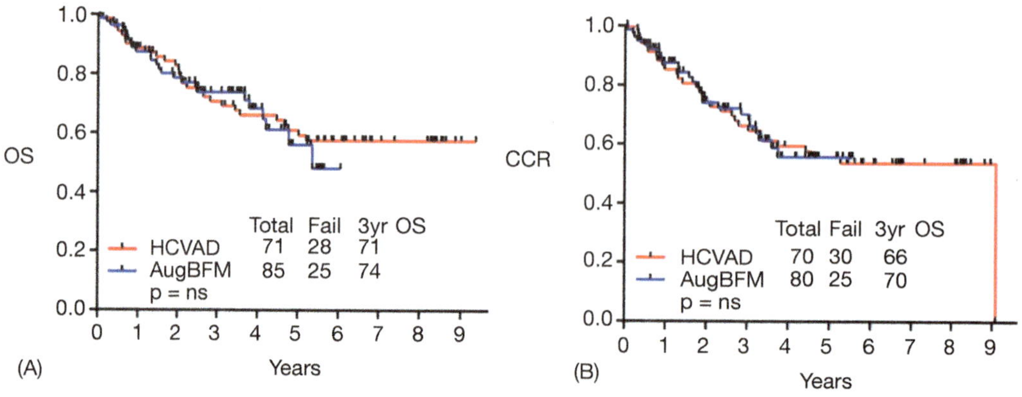

	ABFM	Hyper-CVAD
Rituximab	0	52%
T-cell	19%	?
Downs	4%	?

(C)

	BFM	Hyper-CVAD
Adults	20	30
Median age (years)	25	30
Age <25	45%	30%
M:F	15:5	17:3
B-Lineage	80%	70%
CR	95%	96%
5-Year survival	59%	34%

(D)

FIGURE 3-48: Treatment of AYAs with ALL: Pediatric-inspired regimen versus hyper-CVAD. (A, B) A report by Rytting of regimens used at UTMDACC suggests that in comparison with their historical control experience with hyper-CVAD, modified COG pediatric regimen (augmented Berlin-Frankfurt-Munster [BFM]) did not have better continuous remission (Figure 3-48A) and overall survival (Figure 3-48B) rates. (C) In the Rytting report, 71 patients were selected post-hoc to compare with the augmented BFM regimen. The comparison was thereby not randomized, not concurrent (≥4 calendar year difference), with all patients treated at a single institution, and 52% of whom received eight doses of rituximab since their ALL was CD20+. (D) A comparison of BFM and hyper-CVAD regimens at two centers in Turkey resulted in a superior result with the pediatric regimen (59% vs. 34% 5-year survival), leading the adult-treating oncologists to switch to the pediatric-inspired regimen(s).

ALL, acute lymphoblastic leukemia; AYA, adolescent and young adult; COG, Children's Oncology Group; hyper-CVAD, hyperfractionated cyclophosphamide, vincristine, doxorubicin, dexamethasone; UTMDACC, University of Texas MD Anderson Cancer Center.

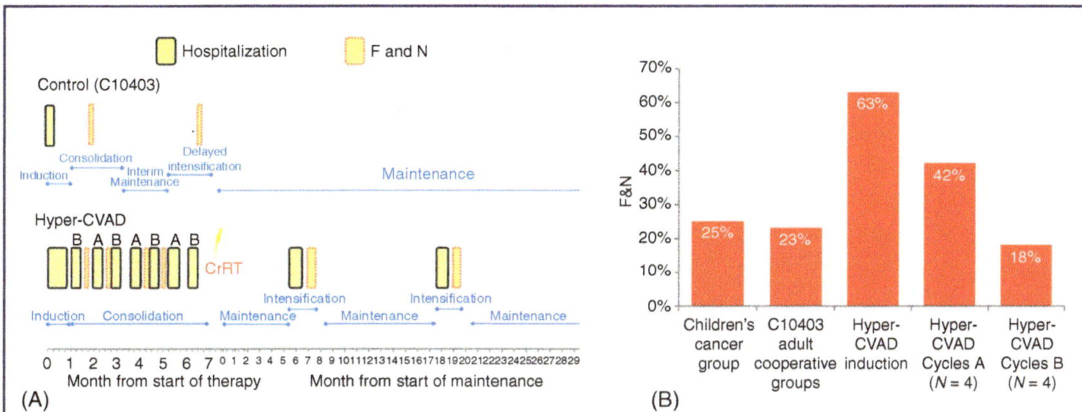

	Pediatric (C10403)	Hyper-CVAD
Hospitalization after initial diagnosis	Not required	Required for 8 cycles
Readmission for fever and neutropenia	Uncommon	Frequent
Prolonged cytopenia	Rare	Limiting
Infertility	Low risk	High risk (few successful pregnancies reported)
Neurotoxicity-Central	Cognition problematic	More problematic
Neurotoxicity-Peripheral	Acceptable	? More problematic
Cardiomyopathy potential	Moderate	? More problematic
Secondary malignancy potential	Rare	Myelodysplasia and AML
Financial cost	All outpatient Rx; all maintenance PO except vincristine	15+ hospitalizations, ↑↑ drug costs, only 2 drugs PO, . . .

(C)

PubMed search terms	ALL QOL Children	ALL QOL Adult Hyper-CVAD
Publications	268	0

PubMed search terms	ALL Infertility Children	ALL Infertility Adult Hyper-CVAD
Publications	47	1

(D)

FIGURE 3-49: Additional hyper-CVAD results and adverse effects and quality-of-life comparison with pediatric-inspired regimens. (A) Hyper-CVAD requires far more frequent hospital admission (all of the induction and cycles of hyper-CVAD are administered in the inpatient setting) and readmission to treat complications than does the pediatric-inspired regimens. (B) The hyper-CVAD regimen is more myelosuppressive than the pediatric regimens such that multiple hospital admission for treatment of fever and neutropenia occurs in most patients after induction and in 18% to 42% of patients after cycles A and B, respectively. (C) In addition, the total cumulative doses of most of the agents in hyper-CVAD are considerably greater than the comparable agents in pediatric regimens. Hyper-CVAD is thereby associated with greater rates of myelodysplasia, secondary acute myeloid leukemia, infertility, residual cognitive dysfunction, and a potential for greater cardiotoxicity and peripheral neurotoxicity (60). (D) Efforts to reduce long-term and delayed adverse effects of therapy have been a priority of the pediatric treatment investigators since 1955, more than 60 years ago. In the United States, more than 160 regimens were evaluated during the last half century in phase 3 trials by COG. Multiple regimens were also studied in Europe. Since 2000, the COG has conducted 10 randomized controlled trials in newly diagnosed patients. In contrast, less than 10 randomized controlled trials have been conducted in adult patients. The relative difference is manifest in the number of peer-reviewed publications on quality of life and infertility: 268 versus 0 and 47 versus 1, respectively.

ALL, acute lymphoblastic leukemia; COG, Children's Oncology Group; hyper-CVAD, hyperfractionated cyclophosphamide, vincristine, doxorubicin, dexamethasone.

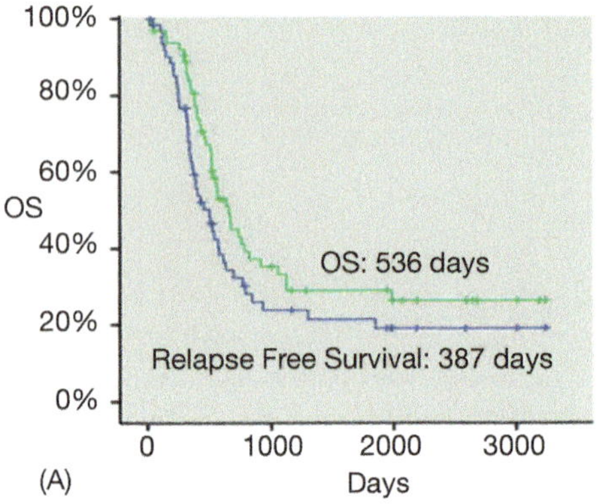

(A)

	Regimen Included ASNase	
	Yes	No
Patients	30	14
Median OS (Months)	48	18
	$P = .7$	

(B)

	Pediat BFM	Hyper-CVAD
Adults	20	30
Median Age (Years)	25	30
Age <25	45%	30%
M:F	15:5	17:3
B-Lineage	80%	70%
CR	95%	96%
5-Year Survival	59%	34%

(C)

In T-cell ALL, Swedish investigators treated 19 patients with a median age of 32 years (range 18–72 years)

- Hyper-CVAD "resulted in a high CR rate and appeared safe."
- But it "showed poor efficacy at preventing relapse."
- Hyper-CVAD is no longer recommended for adults with T-cell ALL in Sweden.

(D)

FIGURE 3-50: Additional hyper-CVAD results and adverse effects and quality-of-life comparison with pediatric-inspired regimens. (A) Investigators at the Winship Cancer Institute of Emory University, University of Alabama-Birmingham, and Moffitt Cancer Center & Research Institute reported (61) an unacceptable outcome of their T-cell ALL and lymphoblastic lymphoma patients treated with hyper-CVAD. (B) Investigators at the University of Texas Southwestern Medical Center and at Parkland Hospital Retrospective analyzed 197 consecutive adult patients treated during 2004–2014 for newly diagnosed ALL. Their mean age was 26 years and 77% were Hispanic. Hyper-CVAD was administered to 57% of the patients, CALGB 10403 to 11%, and 32% were treated with various other pediatric protocols or their therapy was unknown. The median survival was more than 3 times longer with asparaginase-containing regimens. (C) At two centers in Turkey, a retrospective analysis of the outcomes of BFM pediatric regimen and hyper-CVAD chemotherapy was reported to have a 59% 5-year overall survival rate with the pediatric type of regimen and a corresponding 34% rate for hyper-CVAD. (D) In Sweden, hyper-CVAD is no longer used to treat adult T-cell ALL because of the low disease-survival rate.

ALL, acute lymphoblastic leukemia; BFM, Berlin-Frankfurt-Munster Group; CALGB, Cancer and Leukemia Group B; hyper-CVAD, hyperfractionated cyclophosphamide, vincristine, doxorubicin, dexamethasone.

Selected References

Alacacioglu I, Medeni SS, Ozsan GH, et al. Is the BFM regimen feasible for the treatment of adult acute lymphoblastic leukemia? A retrospective analysis of the outcomes of BFM and hyper-CVAD chemotherapy in two centers. *Chemotherapy*. 2014;60(4):219–223.

Amylon MD, Shuster J, Pullen J, et al. Intensive high-dose asparaginase consolidation improves survival for pediatric patients with T-cell acute lymphoblastic leukemia and advanced stage lymphoblastic lymphoma: a Pediatric Oncology Group study. *Leukemia*. 1999;13(3):335–342.

Boissel N, Auclerc MF, Lheritier V, et al. Should adolescents with acute lymphoblastic leukemia be treated as old children or young adults? Comparison of the French FRALLE-93 and LALA-94 trials. *J Clin Oncol*. 2003;21(5):774–780.

DeAngelo DJ, Stevenson K, Dahlberg SE, et al. Long-term outcome of a pediatric-inspired regimen used for adults aged 18–50 years with newly diagnosed acute lymphoblastic leukemia. *Leukemia*. 2015;29(3):526–534.

DeAngelo DJ, Stevenson K, Neuberg DS, et al. A multicenter phase II study using a dose intensified pegylated-asparaginase pediatric regimen in adults with untreated acute lymphoblastic leukemia: a DFCI ALL consortium trial. *Blood*. 2015;126:80.

de Bont JM, van der Holt B, Dekker AW, et al. Adolescents with acute lymphatic leukaemia achieve significantly better results when treated following Dutch paediatric oncology protocols than with adult protocols. *Ned Tijdschr Geneeskd*. 2005;149(8):400–406.

Douer D, DeAngelo DJ, Advani A, et al. Applying pediatric therapeutic strategies to adults with acute lymphoblastic leukemia and lymphoma. II. Comparison with adult treatment regimens, including hyper-CVAD. *Amer Oncol & Hemat Rev*. 2014;47–53.

Duval M, Suciu S, Ferster A, et al. Comparison of Escherichia coli-asparaginase with Erwinia-asparaginase in the treatment of childhood lymphoid malignancies: results of a randomized European Organisation for Research and Treatment of Cancer-Children's Leukemia Group phase 3 trial. *Blood*. 2002;99(8):2734–2739.

Haïat S, Marjanovic Z, Lapusan S, et al. Outcome of 40 adults aged from 18 to 55 years with acute lymphoblastic leukemia treated with double-delayed intensification pediatric protocol. *Leuk Res*. 2011;35(1):66–72.

Hallböök H, Gustafsson G, Smedmyr B, et al. Treatment outcome in young adults and children >10 years of age with acute lymphoblastic leukemia in Sweden: a comparison between a pediatric protocol and an adult protocol. *Cancer*. 2006;107(7):1551–1561.

Hayakawa F, Sakura T, Yujiri T, et al. Markedly improved outcomes and acceptable toxicity in adolescents and young adults with acute lymphoblastic leukemia following treatment with a pediatric protocol: a phase II study by the Japan Adult Leukemia Study Group. *Blood Cancer J*. 2014;4(10):e252.

Herold T, Baldus CD, Gökbuget N. Ph-like acute lymphoblastic leukemia in older adults. *N Engl J Med*. 2014;371(23):2235.

Huguet F, Leguay T, Raffoux E, et al. Pediatric-inspired therapy in adults with Philadelphia chromosome-negative acute lymphoblastic leukemia: the GRAALL-2003 study. *J Clin Oncol*. 2009;27(6):911–918.

Isakoff MS, Freyer DF, Bleyer A. Young adults with acute lymphoblastic leukemia treated with a pediatric-inspired regimen do not need a bone marrow transplant in first remission. *Blood*. 2013;121:5253–5255.

Kantarjian HM, O'Brien S, Smith TL, et al. Results of treatment with hyper-CVAD, a dose-intensive regimen, in adult acute lymphocytic leukemia. *J Clin Oncol*. 2000;18:547–561.

Kota VS, Hathaway AR, Shah BD, et al. Poor outcomes with hyper CVAD for T-cell acute lymphoblastic leukemia and lymphoblastic lymphoma. *Blood*. 2015;126:(abstract 3762).

Moghrabi A, Levy DE, Asselin B, et al. Results of the Dana-Farber Cancer Institute ALL Consortium Protocol 95-01 for children with acute lymphoblastic leukemia. *Blood*. 2007;109(3):896–904.

Nachman JB, La MK, Hunger SP, et al. Young adults with acute lymphoblastic leukemia have an excellent outcome with chemotherapy alone and benefit from intensive postinduction treatment: a report from the children's oncology group. *J Clin Oncol*. 2009;27(31):5189–5194.

Pession A, Valsecchi MG, Masera G, et al. Long-term results of a randomized trial on extended use of high dose L-asparaginase for standard risk childhood acute lymphoblastic leukemia. *J Clin Oncol*. 2005;23(28):7161–7167.

Ram R, Wolach O, Vidal L, et al. Adolescents and young adults with acute lymphoblastic leukemia have a better outcome when treated with pediatric-inspired regimens: systematic review and meta-analysis. *Am J Hematol*. 2012;87(5):472–478.

Ramanujachar R, Richards S, Hann I, et al. Adolescents with acute lymphoblastic leukaemia: outcome on UK national paediatric (ALL97) and adult (UKALLXII/E2993) trials. *Pediatr Blood Cancer*. 2007;48(3):254–261.

Ribera JM, Oriol A, Sanz MA, et al. Comparison of the results of the treatment of adolescents and young adults with standard-risk acute lymphoblastic leukemia with the Program Espanol de Tratamiento en Hematologia pediatric-based protocol ALL-96. *J Clin Oncol*. 2008;26:1843–1849.

Rizzari C, Valsecchi MG, Aricò M, et al. Effect of protracted high-dose L-asparaginase given as a second exposure in a Berlin-Frankfurt-Münster-based treatment: results of the randomized 9102 intermediate-risk childhood acute lymphoblastic leukemia study—a report from the Associazione Italiana Ematologia Oncologia Pediatrica. *J Clin Oncol*. 2001;19(5):1297–1303.

Roberts KG, Li Y, Payne-Turner D, et al. Targetable kinase-activating lesions in Ph-like acute lymphoblastic leukemia. *N Engl J Med*. 2014;371(11):1005–1015.

Ruiz-Delgado GJ, Macías-Gallardo J, Lutz-Presno JA, et al. Outcome of adults with acute lymphoblastic leukemia treated with a pediatric-inspired therapy: a single institution experience. *Leuk Lymphoma*. 2011;52(2):314–316.

Rytting ME, Thomas DA, O'Brien S, et al. Augmented Berlin-Frankfurt-Muenster based therapy for young adults with acute lymphoblastic leukemia (ALL). *Blood*. 2013;122:1400.

Rytting ME, Thomas DA, O'Brien SM, et al. Augmented Berlin-Frankfurt-Münster therapy in adolescents and young adults (AYAs) with acute lymphoblastic leukemia (ALL). *Cancer*. 2014;120(23):3660–3668.

Schroeder H. *Pediat Blood Cancer*. 2005;45(Special Supplement 6):578. 37th Annual Conference of the International Society of Paediatric Oncology SIOP 2005, Vancouver, Canada (21–24 September, 2005).

Silverman LB, Gelber RD, Kimball Dalton V, et al. Improved outcome for children with acute lymphoblastic leukemia: results of Dana-Farber Consortium Protocol 91-01. *Blood*. 2001;97(5):1211–1218.

Stock W, Douer D, Deangelo DJ, et al. Prevention and management of asparaginase/pegasparaginase-associated toxicities in adults and older adolescents: recommendations of an expert panel. *Leuk Lymph*. 2011;52(12):2237–2253.

Stock W, La M, Sanford B, et al. What determines the outcomes for adolescents and young adults with acute lymphoblastic leukemia treated on cooperative group protocols? A comparison of Children's Cancer Group and Cancer and Leukemia Group B studies. *Blood*. 2008;112:1646–1654.

Stock W, Luger SM, Advani AS, et al. Favorable outcomes for older adolescents and young adults with acute lymphoblastic leukemia: early results of U.S. Intergroup Trial C10403. *Blood*. 2014;124:796.

Testi AM, Valsecchi MG, Conter V, et al. Difference in outcome of adolescents with acute lymphoblastic leukemia enrolled in pediatric (AIEOP) and adult (GIMEMA) protocols. *Blood*. 2004;104:1954.

Thomas DB, O'Brien S, Rytting M, et al. Acute lymphoblastic leukemia (ALL) or lymphoblastic lymphoma (LL) after frontline therapy with hyper-CVAD regimens. *Blood*. 2008;112:1930.

Usvasalo A, Raty R, Knuutila S, et al. Acute lymphoblastic leukemia in adolescents and young adults in Finland. *Haematologica*. 2008;93(8):1161–1168.

Yasuda T, Tsuzuki S, Kawazu M, et al. Recurrent DUX4 fusions in Pre-B Ph-negative acute lymphoblastic leukemia of adolescents and young adults. *Nat Genet*. 2016;48:569–574.

Treatment of ALL in Children and Adolescents

Susan R. Rheingold and Stephen P. Hunger

- Acute lymphoblastic leukemia (ALL) is the most common childhood malignancy, accounting for 25% of cancer in children younger than 15 years and 19% in those younger than 20 years.
- While lymphoblasts appear very similar under the microscope, pediatric ALL is an extremely heterogeneous disease.
- ALL therapy is tailored based upon age at diagnosis, leukemia phenotype (B- vs. T-cell), early response to therapy based primarily on minimal residual disease (MRD), and detailed genetic and molecular typing, which are integrated to determine "risk" and tailor treatment intensity (Figure 3-51).
- The 5-year event-free survival (EFS) and overall survival (OS) rates for children and adolescents with ALL are now 80%–85% and greater than 90%. Low-risk subgroups can be defined with a 5-year EFS rate of almost 95% and 5-year OS rate of 98% or better.

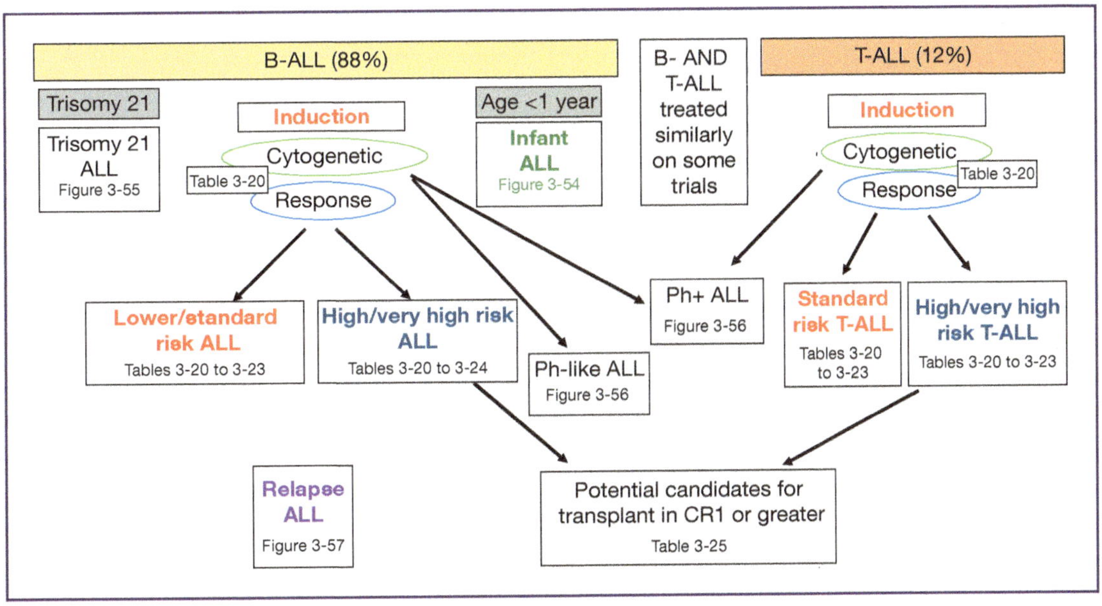

FIGURE 3-51: Newly diagnosed ALL treatment algorithm based on clinical factors, biologic features of the leukemia, and early response to therapy.

B-ALL, B acute lymphoblastic leukemia; T-ALL, T acute lymphoblastic leukemia.

PROGNOSTIC INDICATORS/RISK STRATIFICATION

- Although many factors go into determining a patient's ultimate risk stratification and resultant intensity of chemotherapy, MRD testing is the strongest single predictor of outcome. In every subgroup, patients who are MRD negative (defined by each cooperative group but generally less than 0.1% to 0.01% blasts) after an initial month of therapy have better outcomes than those who remain MRD positive. Among those who are MRD positive at end induction, patients that subsequently become MRD negative after an additional 1 to 2 months of therapy fare substantially better than those that remain MRD positive.

- The lowest-risk patients are between the ages of 1 and 10, present with a low initial WBC, have the best risk cytogenetics (*ETV6-RUNX1* fusion or hyperdiploidy with specific chromosome trisomies [4,10 +/− 17]), and have negative-MRD at end induction. These patients have expected EFS/OS rates of >95%.
- Standard-risk patients, sometimes labeled as average or intermediate risk, have expected EFS/OS ranging from 85% to 95% with current chemotherapy and include patients <13 without good risk cytogenetics who are MRD negative at the end of induction (EOI).
- Higher-risk patients include those who remain MRD positive after the first month of induction therapy, teenagers, and those with certain genetic findings [*MLL* rearrangements, intrachromosomal amplification of chromosome 21 (iAMP21)] and have expected EFS/OS ranging from 70% to 85%.
- Very high-risk subgroups exist, which still have very poor outcomes with conventional chemotherapy and attention is being focused on targeted therapy for these groups. The very high-risk patients may be candidates for bone marrow transplant (BMT) although no definitive randomized trials have directly compared chemotherapy alone to BMT.

Table 3-21 Prognostic factors for ALL in children and adolescents

	PREDICTED OUTCOME >95%	PREDICTED OUTCOME 85%–95%	PREDICTED OUTCOME 70%–85%	PREDICTED OUTCOME <70%
Risk	Low	Standard/Intermediate	High	Very high
Demographics				
Age at Diagnosis	>1 and <10	≥10 and <13	>13 years	<1 year, ≥18 years
Clinical Factors				
Initial WBC	<50,000/microliter	>50,000/microliter	B-ALL <200,000/microliter	B-ALL ≥200,000/microliter
Immunophenotype	pre-B-ALL	T-ALL	T-ALL ≥200,000/microliter Early thymic precursor T-ALL	
Extramedullary Disease		CNS 2	CNS 3/testicular ALL	
Genetic/Molecular	*ETV6-RUNX1*	*TCF3-PBX1 (E2A-PBX1)*	Down syndrome	Philadelphia chromosome-like
	Hyperdiploidy with favorable trisomies 4,10,17		*BCR-ABL1* *MLL* *iAMP21*	Hypodiploidy (<44 chromosomes)
Early Response	MRD negative at EOI	MRD negative at EOI	MRD positive EOI and MRD negative at EOC	MRD persistently positive at 2–3+ months
	Good prednisone response (<1,000 blasts/microliter)	Good prednisone response (<1,000 blasts/microliter)	Poor prednisone response (≥1,000 blasts/microliter)	Induction failure (>25% blasts morphologically at EOI)

ALL, acute lymphoblastic leukemia; CNS, central nervous system; EOC, end of consolidation; EOI, end of induction; MLL; mixed lineage leukemia; MRD; minimal residual disease; WBC, white blood cell.

ALL THERAPY

- Over the past 5 decades, pediatric ALL therapy has evolved considerably. Most, but not all, treatment regimens are based on the Berlin-Frankfurt-Munster (BFM) regimen, which has been adapted and modified by the COG. Most pediatric oncology cooperative groups include four intensive phases of therapy (Induction, Consolidation, Interim Maintenance, and Delayed Intensification or Protocol I, II, etc.) lasting 6 to 8 months, followed by 18 to 30 months of low-intensity Maintenance or Continuation therapy (Table 3-22).

- The COG has separate clinical trials for B- and T-ALL, but many cooperative groups combine these populations for study.
- Therapy is primarily given in the outpatient setting, including oral chemotherapy taken at home.
- Most pediatric trials include at least one randomized question attempting to improve outcome by (a) adding a new agent, (b) changing dosing of conventional chemotherapy, or (c) attempting to decrease therapy-related toxicity.

Table 3-22 Sample chemotherapy combinations used in different blocks of ALL therapy by two major cooperative groups, Children's Oncology Group (COG) and Berlin-Frankfurt-Munster (BFM)

		COG	BFM	COG	BFM
BLOCK (COG/BFM)	**GOAL**	**LOW/STANDARD RISK**	**STANDARD/ INTER RISK**	**HIGH/VERY HIGH RISK**	**HIGH RISK**
Induction/protocol 1A	Induce a morphologic remission and possible MRD-negative remission	Dex x 28 days VCR d 1,8,15,22 PEG d4 IT d1,8,29	P prophase d1-7 P or Dex d8-28 VCR & D d8,15,22,29 PEG d12, 26 IT d1,12,33	P d1-28 or Dex d1-15 VCR & D d 1,8,15,22 PEG d4 IT d1,8,29 (CNS 3 also d15,22)	P prophase d1-7 P or Dex d8-28 VCR & D d8,15,22,29 PEG d12,26 IT d1,12,33
Consolidation/ protocol IB	Consolidate the remission and intensive CNS-directed therapy	VCR d1 6-MP d1-28 IT d1,8,15	CPM d36,64 AraC d38-41,45-48,52-55,59-62 6MP d36-63 IT d45,59	CPM d1,29 AraC d1-4,8-11, 29-32,36-39 6-MP d1-14,29-42 VCR d15,22,43,50 PEG d15,43 IT d1,8,15,22	CPM d36,64 AraC d38-41,45-48,52-55,59-62 6MP d36-63 IT d45,59
Interim maintenance/ protocol M	Methotrexate intense cycle, often without myelo-suppression	VCR d1,11,21,31, 41 Escalating MTX d1,11,21,31,41 IT d31	HD-MTX d8,22,36,50 6-MP d1-56 IT d8,22,36,50	HD-MTX d1,15,29,43 VCR d1,15,29, 43 6-MP d1-56 IT d1,29	**HR Block 1:** Dex d1-5, VCR d1&6, HD-MTX d1, CPM d2-4, HD AraC d5, PEG d6, IT d1 **HR Block 2:** Dex d1-5,Vind d1&6, HD-MTX d1,Ifos d2-4, D d5, PEG d6, IT d1 **HR Block 3:** Dex d1-5, HD AraC d1&2, ETOP d3-5, PEG d6, IT d1
Delayed intensification/ protocol IIA and IIB	Re-intensificiation and reconsolidation period; repeats first 2 months with some drug substitutions	Dex d1-8 & 15-22 VCR & DOX d 1,8,15 PEG d4 CPM d29 AraC d29-32 & 36-39 6-TG d29-42 IT d1,29	Dex d1-21 VCR & DOX d8,15,22,29 PEG d8 CPM d36 AraC d38-41, 45-47 6-TG d36-49 IT d38,45	Dex d1-7, 15-21 VCR d1,8,15,43,50 DOX d1,8,15 PEG d4,43 CPM d29 AraC d29-32 & 36-39 6-TG d29-42 IT d1,29,36	**Protocol III x 3 (alt with IM)** Dex d1-15 VCR & DOX d1,8 PEG d1 CPM d15 AraC d17-20,24-27 6-TG d15-28 IT d17,24

(*continued*)

Table 3-22 Sample chemotherapy combinations used in different blocks of ALL therapy by two major cooperative groups, Children's Oncology Group (COG) and Berlin-Frankfurt-Munster (BFM) (*continued*)

		COG	BFM	COG	BFM
BLOCK (COG/BFM)	GOAL	LOW/STANDARD RISK	STANDARD/ INTER RISK	HIGH/VERY HIGH RISK	HIGH RISK
2nd Interim maintenance	Depending upon phenotype and risk	VCR d1,11,21,31, 41 Escalating MTX d1,11,21,31,41 IT d1,31	N/A	VCR d1,11,21,31, 41 Escalating MTX d1,11,21,31,41 PEG d2,22 IT d1,31	6-MP daily MTX weekly PEG every other week
Maintenance/ continuation	Long-term less intense outpatient therapy to prevent relapse	VCR d1,29,57 Dex d1-5,29-33,57-61 6-MP daily MTX weekly IT d1	6-MP daily MTX weekly	VCR d1,29,57 P d1-5,29-33,57-61 6-MP daily MTX weekly IT d1	6-MP daily MTX weekly
		~18/~30 months for girls/boys	2 years from diagnosis	~18/~30 months for girls/boys	2 years from diagnosis

6-MP, mercaptopurine; 6-TG, thioguanine; AraC, cytarabine; ASP, l-asparginase; CPM, cyclophosphamide; D, daunorubicin; Dex, dexamethasone; DOX, doxorubicin; ETOP, etoposide; HD-MTX, high-dose methotrexate with leucovorin rescue; IT, intrathecal; MTX, methotrexate; PEG, PEG-asparaginase; P, prednisone; VCR, vincristine; Vind, vindesine.

RADIATION THERAPY

Radiation is another modality used in treating extramedullary disease in a small fraction of children and adolescents with ALL.

Table 3-23 Use of radiation in pediatric ALL

CENTRAL NERVOUS SYSTEM

- In the early 1970s, craniospinal radiation was used for the first time in childhood ALL with a significant improvement in survival (60%) through the reduction of CNS relapse.
- In the ensuing 50 years, cranial radiation has been replaced by intensive intrathecal therapy to reduce long-term neurologic toxicity and decrease the risk of secondary CNS malignancies. In conjunction, spinal irradiation has largely been eliminated.
- A recent meta-analysis showed that with modern chemotherapy cranial radiation reduced the risk of relapse only in patients who were CNS 3 at diagnosis (63). Patients who are CNS 3 at diagnosis currently receive 18 cGy cranial radiation in most cooperative groups.
- Prophylactic cranial radiation 12 to 18 cGy is still used in certain high-risk B- and T-ALL subgroups by many cooperative groups.
- Due to its significant neurologic toxicity, cranial radiation is often omitted in children younger than 3 to 5 years of age and is rarely used in infant ALL.
- St. Jude Children's Research Hospital has replaced all cranial radiation in protocols for newly diagnosed ALL with 25 to 30 intrathecal triples (cytarabine, methotrexate, and hydrocortisone).
- Several European cooperative groups (UKALL MRC, DCOG, EORTC) have also eliminated cranial irradiation in all or almost all patients.

TESTICULAR

- Males with testicular involvement at diagnosis traditionally received 24 cGy testicular radiation during consolidation therapy. Many cooperative groups have successfully omitted testicular radiation in males who have complete resolution of testicular leukemia by the end of induction.

CNS, central nervous system; T-ALL, T acute lymphoblastic leukemia.

OUTCOME

Successive generations of North American pediatric cooperative group trials have improved 5-year overall survival from less than 20% in the early 1970s to the current expected survival rates of more than 90%.

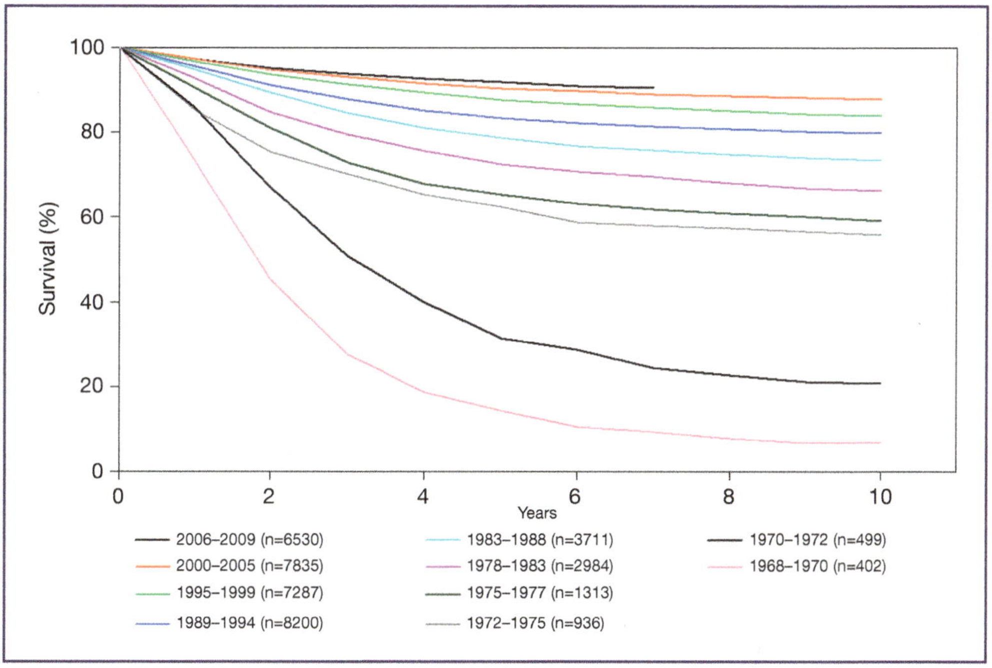

FIGURE 3-52: Overall survival of children with ALL enrolled in COG clinical trials 1968 to 2009.
***Source:* Adapted from Hunger SP, Mullighan CG. Acute lymphoblastic leukemia in children. *N Engl J Med.* 2015;373:1541–1552.**
ALL, acute lymphoblastic leukemia; COG, Children's Oncology Group.

With the exclusion of infants less than 1 year of age, age correlates with overall survival, with pediatric and adolescent patients having a significantly better chance of survival than adults over 40. The use of pediatric-based regimens for patients 20 to less than 40 years of age is improving outcomes. International Cooperative group outcomes are similar (Table 3-23).

INFANT ALL

- ALL in children less than 1 year of age is extremely rare (<5%) and is almost always precursor B-cell ALL. Babies are more likely to have elevated WBC at diagnosis, hepatosplenomegaly, skin chloromas, and 20% will have CNS involvement.
- In 80% of cases, infant ALL is associated with rearrangement of the 11q23 *mixed lineage leukemia (MLL* or *KMT2A)* gene. Almost all babies aged less than 3 months are *MLL*r.
- On flow cytometry, the *MLL*r blasts are often CD10 negative and express myeloid antigens such as CD13 and CD33; therapy is more of an ALL/AML hybrid (Figure 3-54).
- Outcome for infants has not improved at the rate of children older than 1 year, with an overall survival of 50% to 60% and <50% for those with *MLL* rearrangements.
- Therapy targeting the *MLL* leukemogenic pathway is being actively investigated, including targeting FLT3-ITD, aberrant methylation, and histone modification, as well as *MLL* fusion proteins.

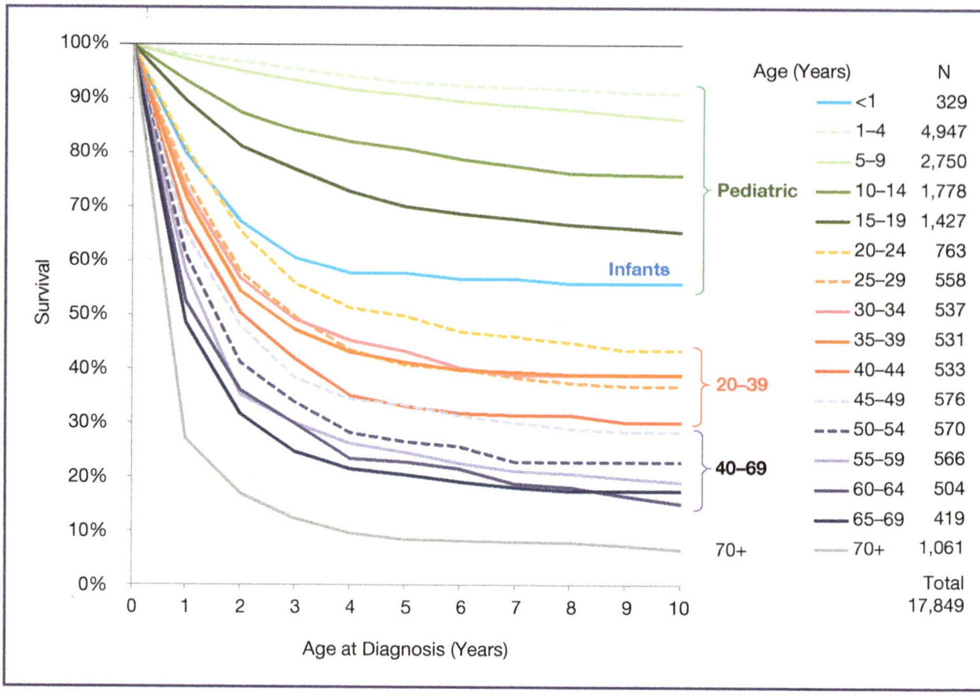

FIGURE 3-53: Relative Survival by age at diagnosis of ALL in 18 SEER Regions during 2000–2013 [SEER].

***Source*: Used with the approval of Archie Bleyer, MD and Eric Tai, MD.**

ALL, acute lymphoblastic leukemia; SEER, surveillance, epidemiology, and end results.

Table 3-24 International pediatric ALL cooperative group outcomes

GROUP	TRIAL	YEARS	IMMUNO-PHENOTYPE	EVENT-FREE SURVIVAL*	OVERALL SURVIVAL*
COG–U.S., Canada, Australia, New Zealand	AALL0232/0331	2002–2014	B-ALL (5,845)	0331–89% 0232–78%	92.30%
	AALL0434		T-ALL (1,995)	85.1%^	91.5%^
SJCRH–U.S.	Total XV	2000–2007	B-ALL (422)	86.90%	94.60%
			T-ALL (76)	78.40%	87.60%
DFCI–U.S., Canada	00-01	2000–2004	B-ALL (443)	82.00%	91%
			T-ALL (49)	69.00%	
AIEOP-BFM–Western Europe	AIEOP-BFM 2000	2000–2006	B-ALL (4,016)	80.4%#	91.8%#
			T-ALL (464)	75.9%#	80.7%#
NOPHO–Denmark, Finland, Iceland, Norway, and Sweden	ALL-2000	2000–2007	B-ALL (906)	81%	91%
			T-ALL (115)	64%	72%
DCOG–the Netherlands	ALL-9	1997–2004	B-ALL (701)	82%	86%
			T-ALL (90)	72%	
MRC/NCRI–UK	UKALL 2003	2003–2011	All patients (3,126)	87.20%	91.50%
EORTC–Belgium, France	CLG 58591	1998–2008	All patients (1,940)	82.70%	89.70%

*Survival values at 5-years except ^= 4 years and #= 7 years.

AIEOP, Associazione Italiana Ematologia Oncologia Pediatric Group; B-ALL, B acute lymphoblastic leukemia; BFM, Berlin-Frankfurt-Munster Group; CLG, Children's Leukemia Group; COG, Children's Oncology Group; DCOG, Dutch Childhood Oncology Group; DFCI, Dana Farber Cancer Institute Consortium; EORTC, European Organisation for Research and Treatment of Cancer; MRC, Medical Research Council; NCRI, National Cancer Research Institute; NOPHO, Nordic Society of Pediatric Hematology and Oncology; SJCRH, St. Jude Children's Research Hospital; T-ALL, T acute lymphoblastic leukemia.

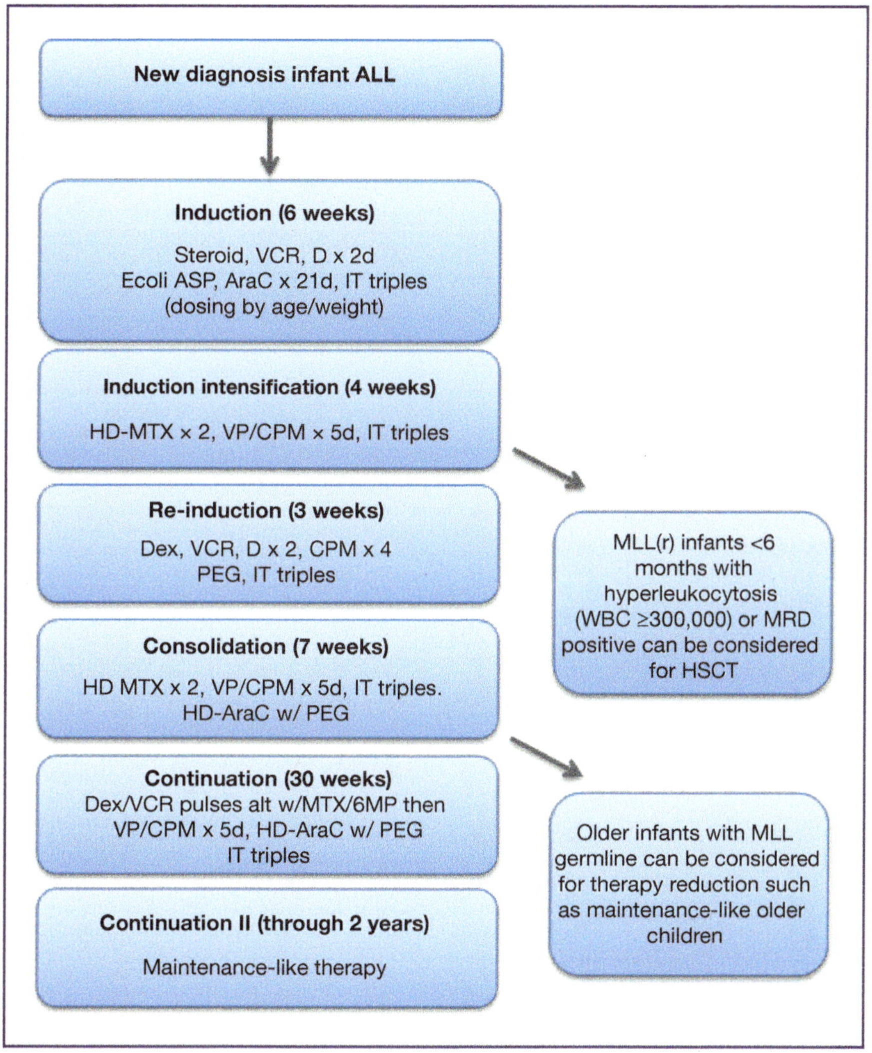

FIGURE 3-54: **Tailored ALL therapy for infants <1 year with ALL.**

ALL, acute lymphoblastic leukemia; AraC, Cytarabine; ASP, l-asparginase; CPM, cyclophosphamide; D, daunorubicin; Dex, dexamethasone; HD-AraC, high-dose cytarabine; HD-MTX, high-dose methotrexate; HSCT, hematopoietic stem cell transplant; IT, intrathecal; MLL, mixed lineage leukemia; MRD, minimal residual disease; PEG, PEG-asparaginase; VCR, vincristine; VP, etoposide; WBC, white blood cell.

DOWN SYNDROME-ASSOCIATED ALL

- Children with Down syndrome (DS) have a fivefold increased risk of developing ALL and account for about 3% of all children with ALL. DS-ALL children rarely develop T-ALL and have much lower rates of favorable leukemia cytogenetics.
- Therapeutic regimens for Down syndrome patients are less intensive in comparison to the regimen for their age-matched peers given their increased susceptibility to therapy-related morbidity and mortality (Figure 3-55).
- The outcome for patients with DS-ALL is inferior to that of children without Down syndrome, with an overall survival rate of about 65%.
- At least half of DS-ALL patients have *CRLF2* gene rearrangements and half of those will have concomitant activation of the JAK/STAT pathway. Targeting of this pathway may increase cure rates and permit a reduction in toxicity from chemotherapy.

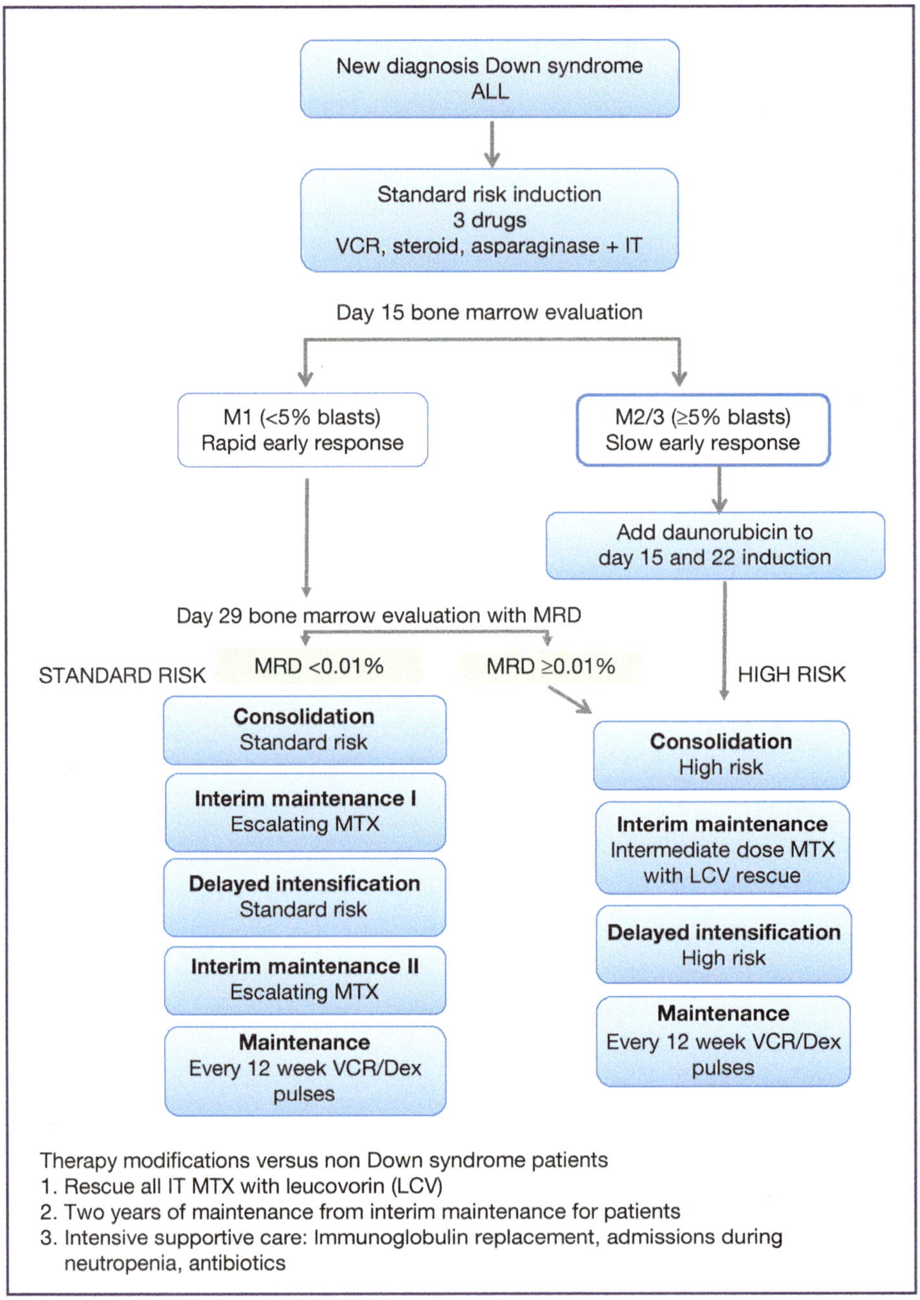

FIGURE 3-55: **Children's Oncology Group modified therapy for newly diagnosed Down syndrome-associated ALL (DS-ALL).** ALL, acute lymphoblastic leukemia; Dex, dexamethasone; IT, intrathecal; MRD, minimal residual disease; MTX, methotrexate; VCR, vincristine.

PHILADELPHIA CHROMOSOME POSITIVE (PH+) AND PHILADELPHIA CHROMOSOME-LIKE ALL

- The Philadelphia chromosome, which creates a *BCR-ABL1* fusion gene and protein, was the first cytogenetic abnormality identified that was involved in the pathogenesis of cancer. Imatinib, a targeted BCR-ABL1 TKI, was FDA-approved for use in chronic myeloid leukemia in 2000. Addition of imatinib and related TKIs has revolutionized therapy for children with Ph+ ALL (Figure 3-56).

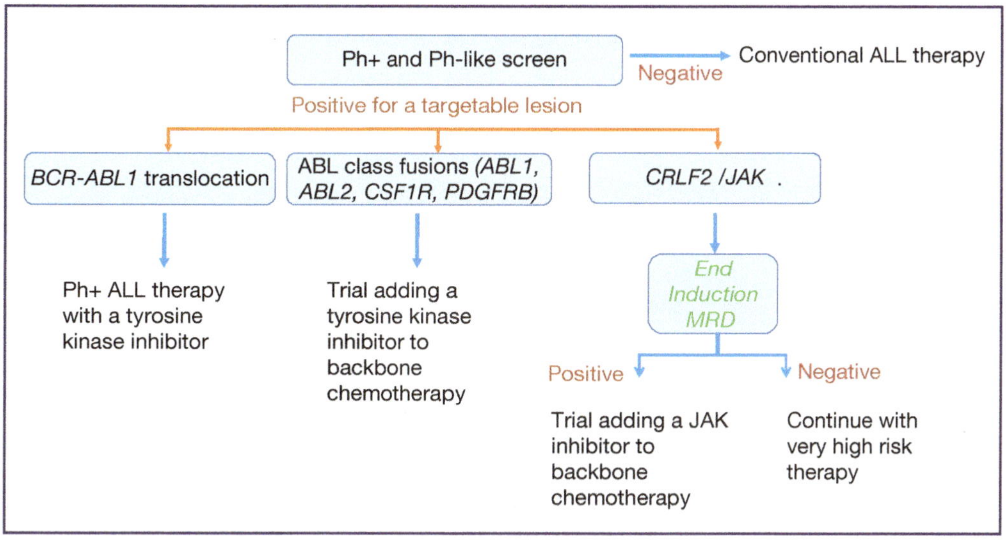

FIGURE 3-56: Addition of targeted therapy to backbone chemotherapy for Ph+ or Ph-like ALL in Children's Oncology Group high-risk ALL trials.

ALL, acute lymphoblastic leukemia.

Table 3-25 Therapies under investigation in current trials, both for de novo and relapsed ALL

AGENT	MECHANISM OF ACTION	TARGET
Immune therapy		
CAR-T 19	T-cells engineered to target CD19	B-ALL
CAR-T 22	T-cells engineered to target CD22	B-ALL
Blinatumomab	Bispecific antibody to CD19 and CD3 targets cytotoxic T-cells to blasts	B-ALL
Rituximab	Unconjugated antibody to CD20	B-ALL
Inotuzumab	Antibody to CD22 linked to calicheamycin	B-ALL
Small molecule inhibitors		
Imatinib	Inhibition of BCR-ABL and related ABL class kinases (ABL1, CSF1R, C-KIT, PDGFBR)	Ph+ and Ph-like ALL
Dasatinib	Inhibition of Bcr-Abl, SRC, and related ABL class kinases (ABL1, CSF1R, C-KIT, PDGFBR)	Ph and Ph-like ALL
Nilotinib	Inhibition of Bcr-Abl and related ABL class kinases (ABL1, CSF1R, C-KIT, PDGFBR)	Ph+ ALL
Ruxolitinib	Inhibition of JAK/CRLF2	Ph-like ALL
Bortezomib	28S protease & NF-κB inhibition	B- and T-ALL
FLT3 inhibitors	Inhibition of FLT3	Infant MLL
Gamma secretase inhibitors	Inhibition of NOTCH1	T-ALL
mTOR inhibitors	Inhibition of mTOR	B- and T-ALL
Epigenetic modifiers		
Vorinostat	Histone deacetylase inhibition	B- and T-ALL
Panobinostat	Histone deacetylase inhibition	Infant MLL
Azacitidine	Methytransferase inhibition	Infant MLL
Decitabine	Methytransferase inhibition	Infant MLL

(*continued*)

Table 3-25 Therapies under investigation in current trials, both for de novo and relapsed ALL (*continued*)

AGENT	MECHANISM OF ACTION	TARGET
Nucleoside analogues		
Nelarabine	Deoxyguanosine analog	T-ALL
Clofarabine	Deoxyadenosine analog	B- and T-ALL, Infant MLL

ALL, acute lymphoblastic leukemia; B-ALL, B acute lymphoblastic leukemia; FLT3, FMS-like tyrosine kinase 3; MLL, mixed lineage leukemia; mTOR, mechanistic target of rapamycin; T-ALL, T acute lymphoblastic leukemia.

- Ph+ ALL accounts for about 3% of childhood ALL, but Ph-like ALL affects 15% of patients <21 years and 1 in 5 teenagers and young adults. Ph-like patients are more likely to be of Hispanic or Native American ancestry. Current outcomes are less than 50% for these patients.
- Detailed genetic studies have shown a high frequency (about 50%) of *CRLF2*-rearrangements in Ph-like ALL (about half with concomitant JAK1 or JAK2 mutations), potentially targetable by JAK2 inhibitors such as ruxolitinib. Another 10% to 20% of Ph-like ALL cases have rearrangements of the erythropoietin receptor gene (*EPOR*) or *JAK2* fusion genes, also potentially targetable by JAK2 inhibitors. About 20% of Ph-like ALL cases have gene fusions involving *ABL1, ABL2, CSF1R,* or *PDGFRB,* which phenocopy BCR-ABL1 and are highly sensitive to TKIs such as imatinib or dasatinib *in vitro.*
- Targeting of specific genetically defined subsets of Ph-like ALL with a TKI will hopefully improve outcome in these groups similarly to TKI therapy of Ph^+ ALL.

TARGETED THERAPIES

- Alternative means of targeting leukemic blasts have been under investigation for years. Signal transduction inhibitors target cell signaling pathways activated in ALL and epigenetic modifiers can alter gene expression in leukemia cells.
- Immune-based therapies include monoclonal antibodies that deliver toxins, chemotherapy or cytotoxic T-cells directly to the leukemia blasts.
- Most recently, immune therapy using a patient's own T-cells genetically modified to express chimeric antigen receptors (CAR T-cells) that recognize proteins present on the surface of normal and malignant B-cells (CD19 and CD22) has revolutionized therapy for relapsed and refractory B-ALL and there is significant enthusiasm for testing CAR T-cells in earlier phases of leukemia therapy.

RELAPSED/REFRACTORY ALL

- Despite a significant improvement in ALL outcomes, 10% to 15% of children with ALL will relapse.
- Outcome following relapse correlates with leukemia immunophenotype, time from diagnosis to relapse, location of relapse, and response to therapy. Overall survival varies from 75% in patients with isolated extramedullary relapses >18 months from diagnosis to <20% in patients with bone marrow relapses <18 months from diagnosis.
- Each cooperative group has their own classification for risk post relapse and stratification to allogeneic bone marrow transplant versus continued chemotherapy +/– radiation therapy. A general algorithm is presented in Figure 3-57.

- Chemotherapy is intensified and includes increased dose of conventional agents, chemotherapy not typically used in front-line therapy (etoposide, ifosfamide, mitoxantrone, idarubicin) and experimental agents.
- Outcome for second or subsequent relapse was traditionally less than 10% but newer therapies such as CAR T targeted against CD19 may drastically alter that.

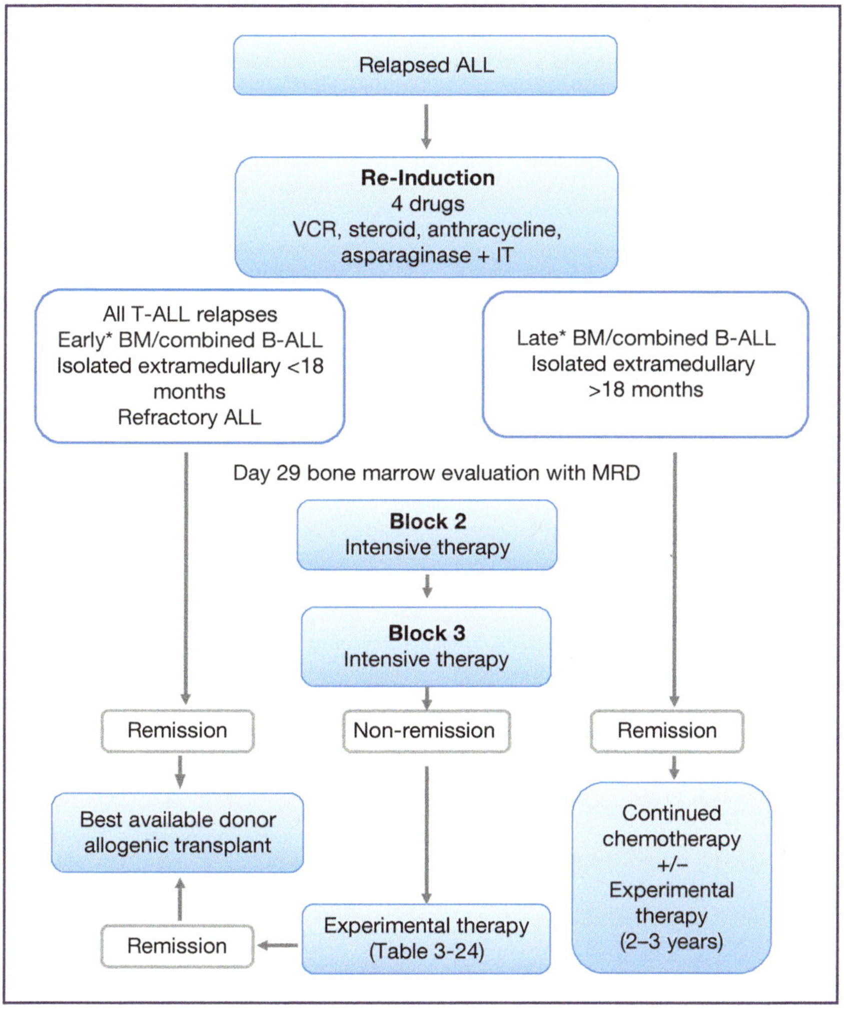

FIGURE 3-57: Treatment algorithm for relapsed ALL.

*Definitions of early and late relapse will differ by cooperative group.

ALL, acute lymphoblastic leukemia; B-ALL, B acute lymphoblastic leukemia; BM, bone marrow; IT, intrathecal; MRD, minimal residual disease; T-ALL, T acute lymphoblastic leukemia; VCR, vincristine.

INDICATIONS FOR ALLOGENEIC STEM CELL TRANSPLANT

Table 3-26	Potential candidates for allogenic stem cell transplant
FIRST COMPLETE REMISSION	
	Hypodiploid ALL (<44 chromosomes)
	t(4;11) with high WBC or slow early response
	Induction failures
	High-risk B- or T-ALL who remain MRD >0.01% after 3 to 6 months of treatment
	Very high-risk infant ALL
SECOND OR GREATER COMPLETE REMISSION	
	Any relapse of T-ALL
	Bone marrow relapse <36 months from diagnosis for B-cell ALL
	Bone marrow relapse ≥36 months from diagnosis for B-cell ALL with MRD positive after reinduction therapy
	Hypodiploid, Ph+, Ph-like ALL
	Any subsequent relapse (>CR2)

B-ALL, B acute lymphoblastic leukemia; MRD, minimal residual disease; T-ALL, T acute lymphoblastic leukemia; WBC, white blood cell.

Selected References

Buitenkamp TD, Izraeli S, Zimmermann M, et al. Acute lymphoblastic leukemia in children with Down syndrome: a retrospective analysis from the Ponte di Legno study group. *Blood.* 2014;123:70–77.

Conter V, Bartram CR, Valsecchi MG, et al. Molecular response to treatment redefines all prognostic factors in children and adolescents with B-cell precursor acute lymphoblastic leukemia: results in 3184 patients of the AIEOP-BFM ALL 2000 study. *Blood.* 2010;115:3206–3214.

Grupp SA, Kalos M, Barrett D, et al. Chimeric antigen receptor-modified T cells for acute lymphoid leukemia. *N Engl J Med.* 2013;368:1509–1518.

Hunger SP, Loh ML, Whitlock JA, et al. Children's oncology group's 2013 blueprint for research: acute lymphoblastic leukemia. *Pediatr Blood Cancer.* 2013;60:957–963.

Hunger SP, Mullighan CG. Acute lymphoblastic leukemia in children. *N Engl J Med.* 2015;373:1541–1552.

Larsen EC, Devidas M, Chen S, et al. Dexamethasone and high-dose methotrexate improve outcome for children and young adults with high-risk B-acute lymphoblastic leukemia: a report from children's oncology group study AALL0232. *J Clin Oncol.* 2016;34:2380–2388.

Maloney KW, Carroll WL, Carroll AJ, et al. Down syndrome childhood acute lymphoblastic leukemia has a unique spectrum of sentinel cytogenetic lesions that influences treatment outcome: a report from the children's oncology group. *Blood.* 2010;116:1045–1050.

Maude SL, Frey N, Shaw PA, et al. Chimeric antigen receptor T cells for sustained remissions in leukemia. *N Engl J Med.* 2014;371:1507–1517.

Pui CH, Campana D, Pei D, et al. Treating childhood acute lymphoblastic leukemia without cranial irradiation. *N Engl J Med.* 2009;360:2730–2741.

Pui CH, Yang JJ, Hunger SP, et al. Childhood acute lymphoblastic leukemia: progress through collaboration. *J Clin Oncol.* 2015;33:2938–2948.

Roberts KG, Li Y, Payne-Turner D, et al. Targetable kinase-activating lesions in Ph-like acute lymphoblastic leukemia. *N Engl J Med.* 2014;371(11):1005–1015.

Roberts KG, Morin RD, Zhang J, et al. Genetic alterations activating kinase and cytokine receptor signaling in high-risk acute lymphoblastic leukemia. *Cancer Cell.* 2012;22:153–166.

Schrappe M, Valsecchi MG, Bartram CR, et al. Late MRD response determines relapse risk overall and in subsets of childhood T-cell ALL: results of the AIEOP-BFM-ALL 2000 study. *Blood*. 2011;118:2077–2084.

Schultz KR, Carroll A, Heerema NA, et al. Long-term follow-up of imatinib in pediatric Philadelphia chromosome-positive acute lymphoblastic leukemia: children's oncology group study AALL0031. *Leukemia*. 2014;28:1467–1471.

Smith MA, Reaman GH. Remaining challenges in childhood cancer and newer targeted therapeutics. *Pediatr Clin North Am*. 2015;62:301–312.

Surveillance, Epidemiology, and End Results (SEER) Program. National Cancer Institute. Software version 8.1.2. www.seer.cancer.gov/seerstat

Tasian SK, Loh ML, Hunger SP. Childhood acute lymphoblastic leukemia: integrating genomics into therapy. *Cancer*. 2015;121:3577–3590.

Tomizawa D. Recent progress in the treatment of infant acute lymphoblastic leukemia. *Pediatr Int*. 2015;57:811–819.

Vora A, Goulden N, Wade R, et al. Treatment reduction for children and young adults with low-risk acute lymphoblastic leukaemia defined by minimal residual disease (UKALL 2003): a randomised controlled trial. *Lancet Oncol*. 2013;14:199–209.

Vrooman LM, Stevenson KE, Supko JG, et al. Postinduction dexamethasone and individualized dosing of *Escherichia Coli* L-asparaginase each improve outcome of children and adolescents with newly diagnosed acute lymphoblastic leukemia: results from a randomized study–Dana-Farber Cancer Institute ALL Consortium Protocol 00-01. *J Clin Oncol*. 2013;31:1202–1210.

Winter SS, Devidas M, Chen S, et al. Capizzi-style methotrexate with pegasparagase (C-MTX) is superior to high-dose methotrexate (HDMTX) in T-lineage acute lymphoblastic leukemia (T-ALL): results from Children's Oncology Group (COG) AALL0434. *Blood*. 2015;126:794.

4

Allogeneic Transplant in Adults and Children for AML and ALL

Allen R. Chen, Gordon Cohen, Sawa Ito, Heather Symons, and Nancy M. Hardy

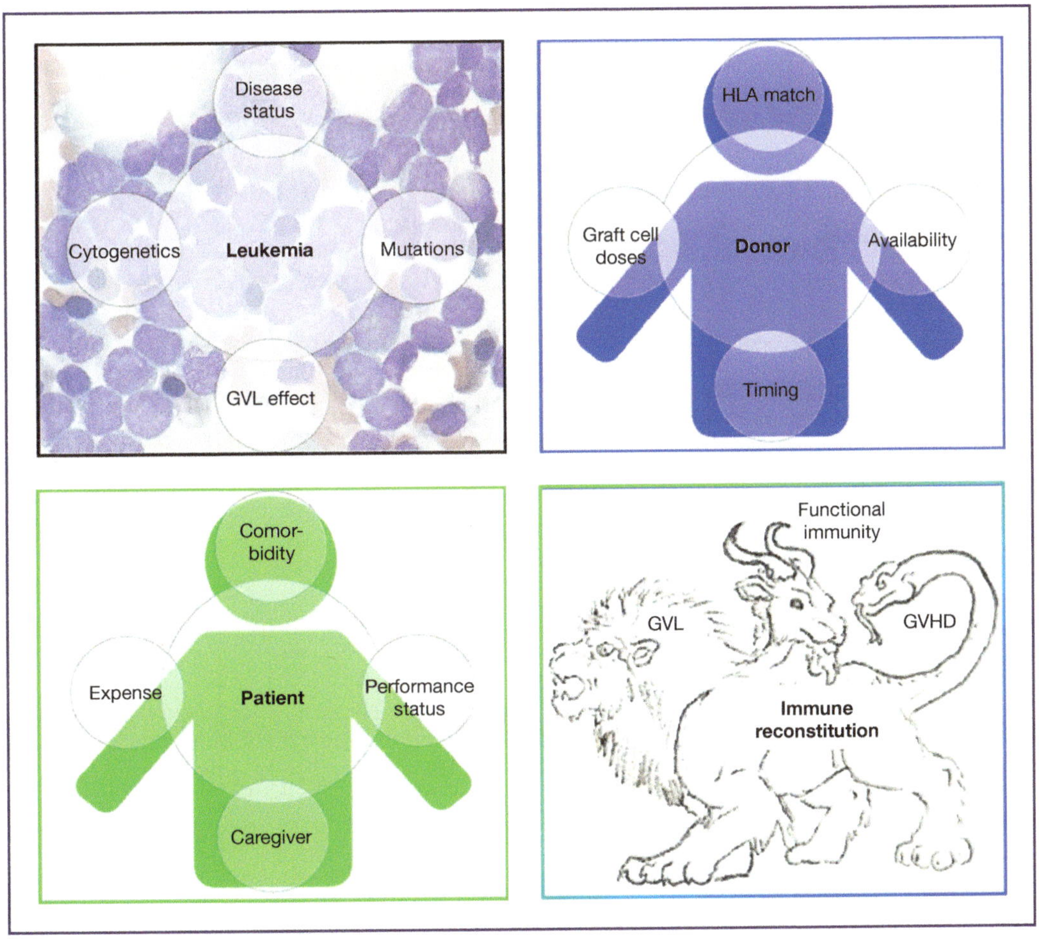

FIGURE 4-1: Essentials for successful transplant outcomes.
GVL, graft-versus-leukemia; HLA, human leukocyte antigen.

Allogeneic hematopoietic stem cell transplantation improves a patient's chance of survival after leukemia. The leukemia is susceptible to myeloablative chemotherapy/radiation doses and/or the immunologic graft-versus-leukemia (GVL) effect; a suitable and timely allograft donor is available; and the patient's performance status and organ function can withstand the anticipated transplant-related toxicities after an effective conditioning regimen and can be sustained through reestablishment of hematopoiesis and immunity.

Leukemia. There are distinct differences in transplant outcomes between leukemia subtypes and adult and pediatric patients; nonetheless, there are some broadly applicable benefits of transplantation. First, transplant allows for the use of myeloablative chemotherapy. While transplant employing reduced-intensity conditioning can improve survival over conventional chemotherapy and extends the benefit of transplant to individuals who cannot tolerate a myeloablative preparative regimen, an advantage of high-dose conditioning is killing leukemia cells that might be resistant to standard doses of chemotherapy. Second, the transplanted donor immune system can recognize the host's leukemia cells as being foreign and generate an antitumor immune response through the GVL effect. In general, outcomes after transplant are best for patients who undergo transplant in remission, so that a robust GVL effect can be established and effectively prevent recurrence. While transplant outcomes for patients with active leukemia are inferior, with fewer than 20% of patients with acute leukemia surviving at 3 years, a retrospective analysis of registry data suggests that myeloablative transplantation may offer benefit to a subset of these individuals. Novel diagnostic tools, eg, molecular methods of rapidly assessing leukemia gene mutations and detecting minute residual disease, are increasingly accessible and affordable. Ongoing investigation is defining how these diagnostic tools will permit individualized assessment of relapse risk and potential benefit of transplantation. Disease risk algorithms are being refined and increasingly employed to inform decisions about whether and when to transplant and to help optimize conditioning intensity, graft selection, and immune suppression.

Patient. Even with significant improvements in supportive care, transplantation remains an extremely challenging therapy with significant risk. The risk/benefit assessment of whether to pursue transplantation must include evaluation of the patient's overall condition, eg, whether an individual can tolerate the transplant process, whether active infections can be effectively controlled through the anticipated period of immunosuppression, and whether an individual's anticipated transfusion needs can be supported through marrow recovery. Progress in understanding the GVL effect on cure has permitted refinement of conditioning therapy and employment of less toxic, reduced-intensity, or nonmyeloablative regimens. Less-intensive conditioning often results in less tissue and organ damage and a shorter duration of marrow aplasia, but the risk of leukemia relapse is increased and risks of graft-versus-host disease (GVHD) and its therapies remain problematic. In adults, there is renewed interest in increased-intensity conditioning to enhance leukemic control; prognostic algorithms are increasingly employed in an attempt to individualize optimal conditioning.

Donor. Selecting the best donor takes into consideration the donor–recipient HLA match, with better matching reducing GVHD, immune suppression, and infection and greater disparity increasing the potency of GVL. Historically, the degree of HLA matching has been a key determinant of transplant outcome, with better matching yielding improved survival. However, donor selection must take into account the risk of relapse while searching for the optimal donor. If the risk of relapse is high and the chance of finding a perfect match is low, then proceeding quickly with a known mismatch may be preferable to a lengthy search for a full match. Recent strides permit transplantation across HLA barriers, with reliable engraftment and lower rates of GVHD; the impact of novel alloprophylaxis approaches on GVL and relapse is the subject of active investigation.

Immune Reconstitution. Allogeneic transplantation ideally results in stable, complete engraftment of donor-derived blood and immune cells. Optimally, the donor graft maintains active antitumor immune surveillance–the GVL effect–while providing functional immunity against pathogens and tolerating often-beneficial commensal organisms. Poor graft function can result in immune deficiency and infections. Establishment of a dysfunctional immune response can result in GVHD, in which the donor immune system attacks noncancerous patient tissues, as will be described in other figures.

It is important to refer individuals who may benefit from bone marrow/stem cell transplant (BMT) for evaluation as early as feasible, to permit enough time for careful donor selection and planning, ideally providing 3 to 4 months' lead time. Realistically, this is rarely an achievable timeframe for ALL. Timing of referral is quite different between pediatric and adult patients with ALL, reflecting markedly better treatment outcomes with conventional chemotherapy and radiation approaches in childhood ALL. All adults with ALL who have a good performance status should be considered for BMT evaluation as soon as feasible following diagnosis, given the high incidence of relapse with chemotherapy and improved outcomes after remission consolidation with allogeneic BMT.

In contrast, the prognosis in childhood ALL is generally much better and referral for BMT evaluation can often be deferred. In fact, late relapses in pediatric B-lineage ALL do not necessarily require BMT

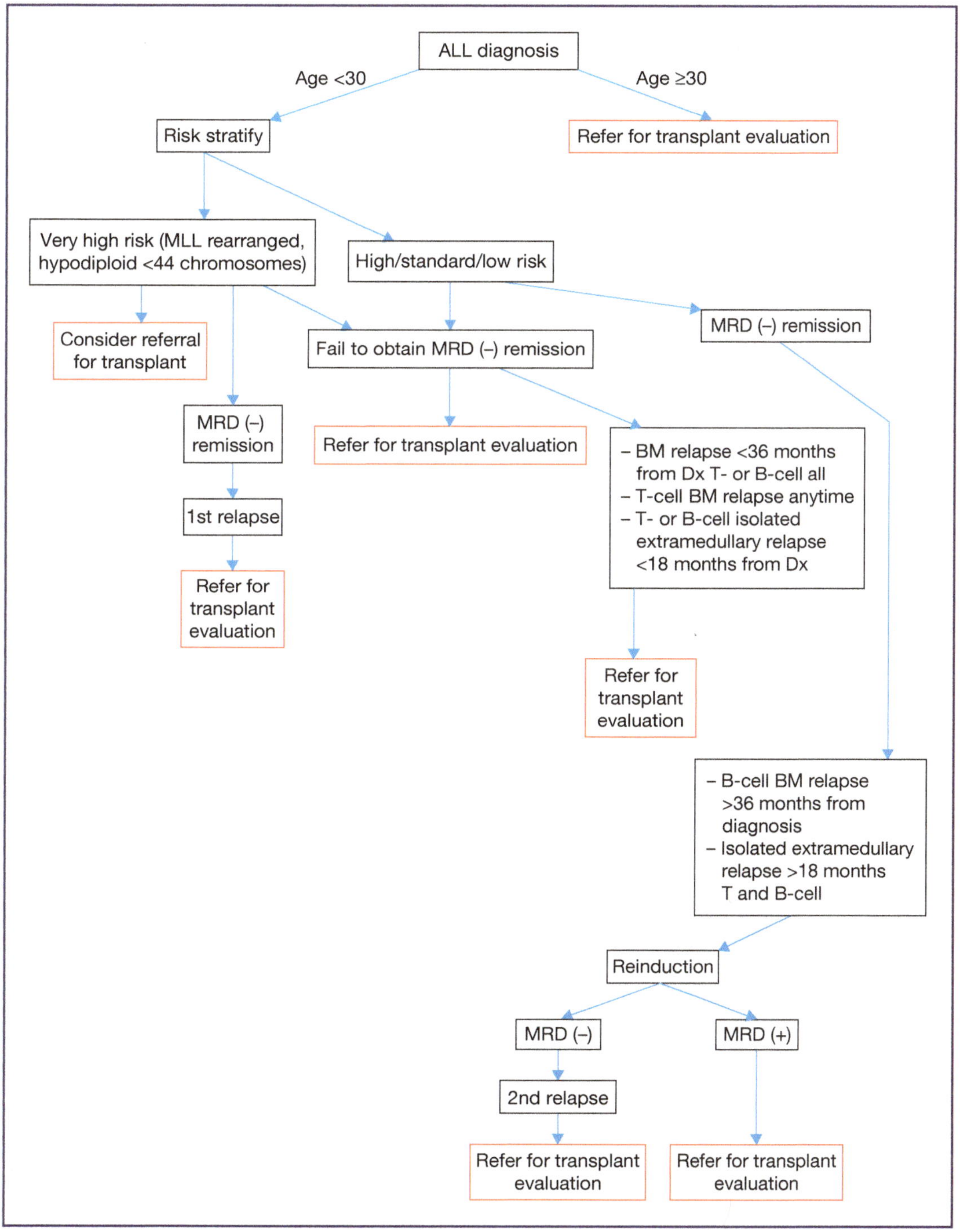

FIGURE 4-2: When to refer a patient with acute lymphoblastic leukemia for transplant consultation. ALL, acute lymphoblastic leukemia; BM, bone marrow; MLL, mixed lineage leukemia; MRD, minimal residual disease.

evaluations, as the prognosis may still be acceptable with conventional therapy. Only children with very high-risk ALL at diagnosis need be considered for a BMT evaluation at initiation of therapy (eg, infant leukemia with MLL gene rearrangements and hypodiploid ALL), given the high incidence of relapse and poor treatment outcomes in these ALL subtypes following chemotherapy alone. Children with intermediate-risk ALL at diagnosis, but who have minimal residual disease (MRD) after induction therapy, are also at very high risk of relapse and should be expeditiously referred for BMT consultation.

Arguably, the most important prognostic indicator of successful allogeneic transplant for ALL is the depth of remission at the time of transplant. Highly sensitive measurements of MRD, typically measured by flow cytometry or polymerase chain reaction (PCR), are useful to assess the depth of remission. Patients with ALL in an MRD-negative remission have significantly superior long-term outcomes compared with those with detectable MRD at the time of allogeneic BMT.

Table 4-1 Outcomes of patients with ALL with and without transplant

ALL SUBGROUP	WITHOUT TRANSPLANT		WITH TRANSPLANT	
Pediatric		Outcome		Outcome
Infant MLL rearranged	45%–50%	EFS (5Y)	45%–50%	EFS (5Y)
Philadelphia chromosome+	~70%	DFS (5Y)	60%–65%	DFS (5Y)
Hypodiploid	37%–69%	OS (8Y)	38%–71%	OS (5Y)
Induction failure	26.50%	DFS (5Y)	56%	DFS (5Y)
Early relapse	20%	EFS (10Y)	36%	EFS (10Y)
Late relapse	49%	EFS (10Y)	52%	EFS (10Y)
Adult				
Low-risk, CR1	52%	OS (5Y)	62%	OS (5Y)
High-risk, CR1	35%	OS (5Y)	41%	OS (5Y)
Relapsed ALL	0%	OS (1Y)	38%	OS (3Y)
Philadelphia chromosome+	19%	OS (4Y)	50%	OS (4Y)

ALL, acute lymphoblastic leukemia; DFS, disease-free survival; EFS, event-free survival; MLL, mixed lineage leukemia; OS, overall survival.

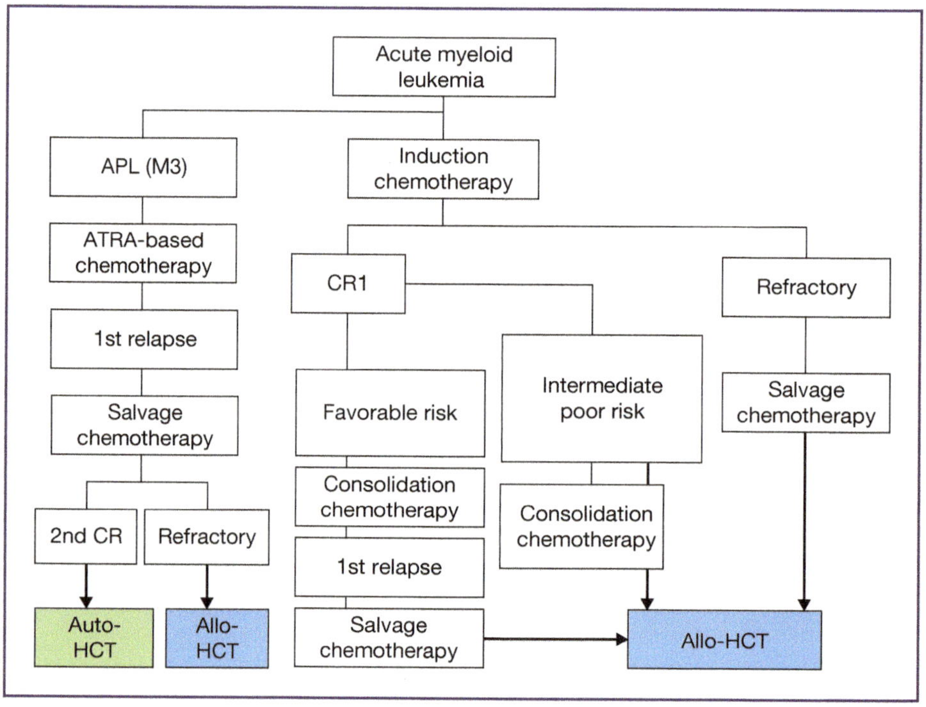

FIGURE 4-3: When to refer a patient with acute myeloid leukemia for transplant consultation.
APL, acute promyelocytic leukemia; ATRA, all-trans retinoic acid; CR, complete remission; HCT, hematopoietic cell transplantation.

While new insights hold promise for new targeted therapies, allogeneic BMT remains the best curative therapy for most patients with AML. In the past decade, the safety and accessibility of BMT has dramatically improved by (a) refined management of infectious complications and GVHD and (b) expanded donor availability with the increasing application of haploidentical and cord blood transplants. Early BMT referral of suitable candidates is key to maximizing its curative potential for AML. BMT should be considered for postremission therapy in all AML patients except those with favorable-risk AML who are likely to achieve long-term remission with conventional chemotherapy. For intermediate- to high-risk AML, the BMT referral is best initiated as soon after diagnosis as feasible. Close communication between the leukemia and transplant teams is essential to optimize timing for successful transplant. For patients in whom complete remission (CR) cannot be achieved, BMT may still be an option, with up to 20% long-term survival. In refractory AML, novel approaches employing sequential cytoreduction and BMT appear promising.

Table 4-2 Outcomes of patients with AML with and without transplant

		AML SUBGROUP	ESTIMATED OS WITHOUT TRANSPLANT	ESTIMATED OS WITH TRANSPLANT
Pediatric AML	**Favorable risk**	inv(16)/t(16;16) t(8;21) NPM mutation CEBPA mutation Negative MRD (<0.1%) at end of Induction I (no high-risk features)	70%–80%	73%
	High risk	FLT3/ITD + with high allelic ratio (>0.4) Monosomal karyotype* del5q* Clinical or radiographic evidence of progressive extramedullary AML end induction* MRD ≥0.1% end induction*	27%–35%	33%–50%
Adult AML	**Favorable risk**	t(8;21) inv (16)/t(16;16) Mutated CEPBA(biallelic) Mutated NPM1 (no FLT3-ITD mutation)	64%–67%	54%–81%
	Intermediate risk	Normal cytogenetics +8 alone t(9;11) t(8;21), inv(16), t(16;16) with c-kit mutation Other nondefined	CR1: 28%–45%	CR1: 52%–56%
	High risk	Complex cytogenetics Monosomal karyotype 11q23 (non-t(9;11)) inv(3), t(3;3) t(6;9) t(9;22) FLT3-ITD+	CR1: 0%–20%	CR1: 31%–54%

*without inv(16)/t(16;16), t(8;21), NPM or CEPBA mutations.

AML, acute myeloid leukemia; CR, Complete remission; FLT3, FMS-like tyrosine kinase 3; ITD, internal tandem duplication; MRD, minimal residual disease; OS, overall survival.

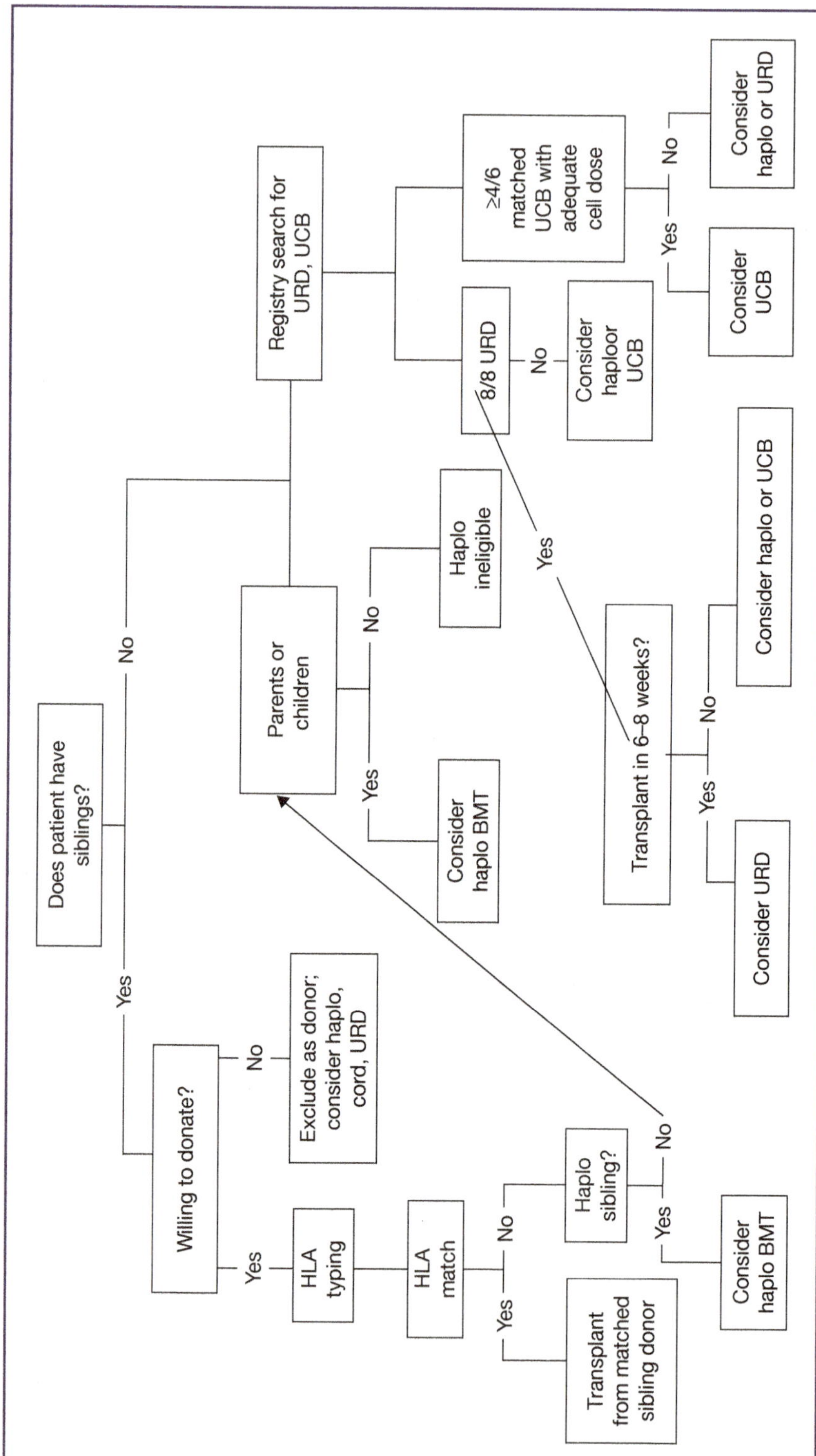

FIGURE 4-4: Donor selection.

BMT, bone marrow transplantation; HLA, human leukocyte antigen; UCB, unrelated cord blood; URD, unrelated donor.

An HLA-identical sibling donor (6/6 matching of HLA-A, B, DR haplotypes) is considered the gold standard BMT donor. Alternative donors include matched unrelated donors (8/8, HLA-A, B, C, DRB1), mismatched unrelated donors, umbilical cord blood units (HLA-A, B, C, DRB1), and HLA-haploidentical (at least one matching HLA-haplotype) donors. There are relative risks and benefits for each of these alternative donor sources as compared to HLA-matched sibling donors. Almost every patient will have a haploidentical donor and there is increased availability of umbilical cord blood products given the permissibility for HLA mismatches (ie, 4/6) as well as double-cord blood protocols, although it is more difficult to find 5/6 or 6/6 HLA-matched single-cord blood products of adequate cell dose for patients over 20 years of age. For unrelated donors, the probability of identifying an 8/8 HLA match varies with ethnicity. In the United States, Caucasians of European descent have about a 75% chance of having a matched donor in the registry, whereas minorities have a much lower probability, eg, about 37% for Mexican Americans and 19% for African Americans. The National Marrow Donor Program (NMDP) search algorithm HapLogic uses data on the frequencies of alleles and haplotypes in human populations to predict the probability of high-resolution matches at individual HLA loci and at all key loci simultaneously for the patient and each potential donor. This is especially helpful when there are many potential unrelated adult donors or cord blood units but only sufficient resources and/or time to type a few of the potential donors/units at higher resolution.

Once an allogeneic BMT is recommended for a patient, the first step is to identify a suitable donor. The search typically starts within the patient's family by typing available siblings for shared identity at several HLA loci of the major histocompatibility complex. Mendelian genetics dictate that each sibling has a one-in-four chance of being HLA identical to the patient and a two-in-four chance of being haploidentical. If an HLA-identical sibling is not available, one must consider searching for a matched unrelated, mismatched unrelated, umbilical cord blood, or haploidentical donor. Often, simultaneous searches for an alternative donor are performed with time being a major factor in which alternative donor to ultimately select, with the goal of waiting no longer than 6 to 8 weeks to transplant. If there is more than one donor option, additional factors include ABO blood type (preference of ABO compatible over minor incompatibility over major incompatibility), CMV status (preference of a CMV seronegative donor for a CMV seronegative patient), and gender (preference of a male donor for male patient). In the haploidentical setting with multiple related donor options, emerging data support consideration of donor age, killer immunoglobulin-like receptor (KIR) haplotype, HLA-DQB1 and DPB1 matching, and cost.

Although transplant is potentially curative and improves overall outcomes for patients with many acute leukemias, most deaths after transplant are the result of leukemia recurrence. Relapse after transplant is extremely difficult to treat, with fewer than 25% of patients surviving 1 year. Relapse is particularly challenging when disease recurs within the first 6 months after transplant.

The discovery that the GVL effect is a key contributor to the curative benefit of allogeneic transplantation allows us to fine-tune the major components of transplant therapy, eg, conditioning, immune suppression, and allograft. The intensity of each may be dialed up or down in anticipation of (or response to) relapse.

A risk-adapted transplant approach takes into account factors from the time of initial diagnosis, with risk of leukemic relapse estimated from the clinical presentation, cytogenetic abnormalities, and genetic mutations. Response to induction therapy further affects relapse risk, with increasingly sensitive methods of detecting residual disease contributing to decision making with regard to whether, when, and how to proceed with transplantation. Indeed, the disease status at transplantation is a potent predictor of relapse risk, lowest in first remission without detectable MRD, higher in second (and subsequent) remissions and/or detectable MRD, and very high in patients transplanted with active leukemia. A disease risk index (DRI) has been developed as a research tool to study survival of adult patients treated with allogeneic SCT across cancer diagnoses. The DRI can predict survival after transplant based on disease characteristics independent of age (adults only), conditioning intensity, or graft/donor source. In AML, risk is assigned based on cytogenetic risk and disease status at the time of transplant; in ALL, risk is assigned based on disease status alone. The DRI may provide a useful prognostic assessment for patients, but treatment decisions remain based on individualized estimated risk of relapse. Optimal leukemic control may be defined by individual disease sensitivity to chemotherapeutic, radiation, and immune effects, and thus to conditioning intensity, combined-modality utilization, donor HLA disparity, and immune suppression. For example, patients with higher risk may benefit from incorporating one or more

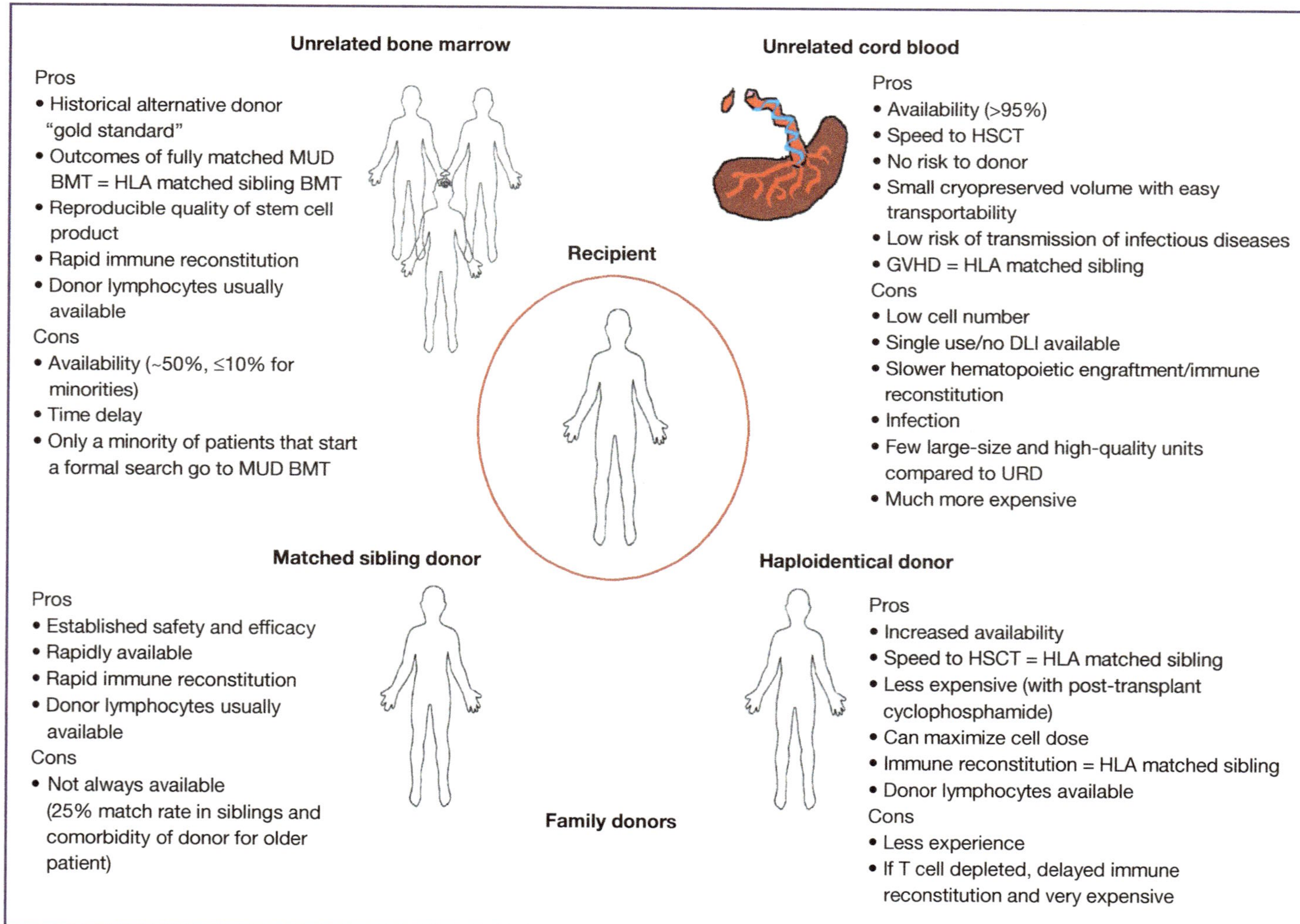

FIGURE 4-5: **Pros and cons about donors.**

BMT, bone marrow transplantation; DLI, donor lymphocyte infusion; GVHD, graft-versus-host disease; HLA, human leukocyte antigen; HSCT, hematopoietic stem cell transplant; MUD, matched unrelated donor; URD, unrelated donor.

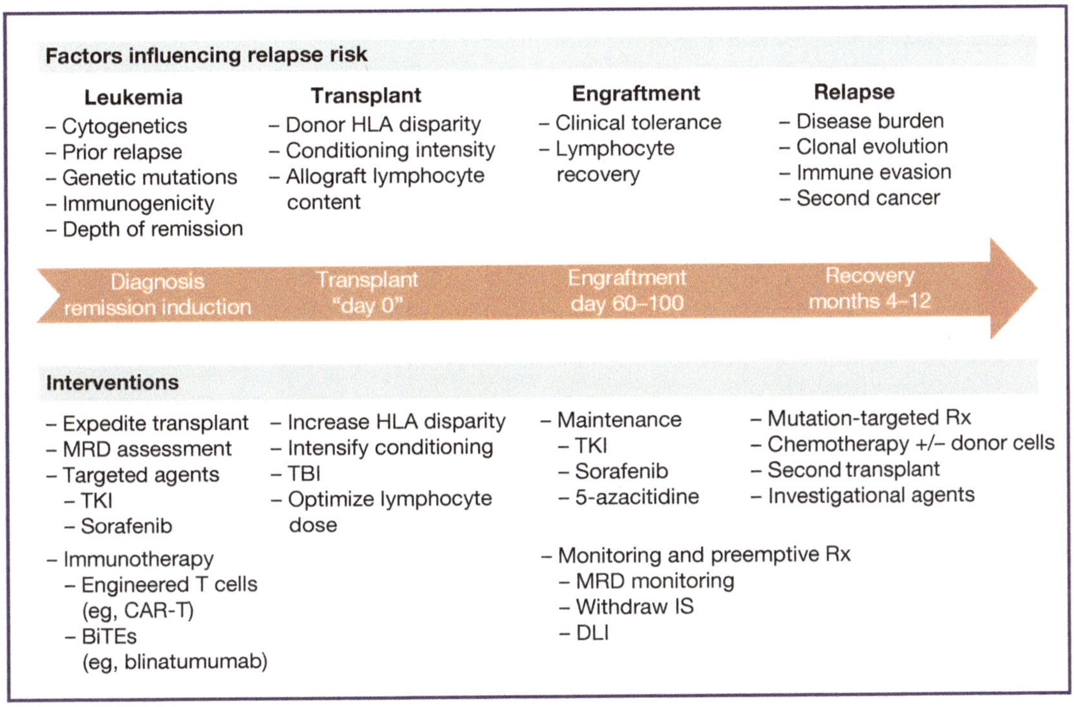

FIGURE 4-6: Strategies to prevent and treat relapse after transplant.

DLI, donor lymphocyte infusion; HLA, human leukocyte antigen; MRD, minimal residual disease; TBI, total body irradiation; TKI, tyrosine kinase inhibitors.

of the following strategies: intensification of conditioning, incorporating radiation into conditioning, HLA-disparate allografts, limited in vivo T-cell depletion, or early withdrawal of immune suppression.

Efforts to promote leukemic control must be balanced against higher treatment toxicities; large studies demonstrate that while transplant intensification strategies may reduce the incidence of relapse, treatment-related deaths often mitigate the overall survival benefit. The age-comorbidity index has been validated in adults as a predictor of nonrelapse mortality after allogeneic transplant with nonmyeloablative, reduced-intensity, or high-dose conditioning; this assessment can be used to optimize transplant conditioning for individual patients.

Posttransplant intervention to prevent relapse may be particularly important for patients with high-risk leukemia and/or after lower-intensity transplant approaches. However, potential benefits must be carefully weighed against risks of graft failure and GVHD. Prevention strategies are an area of emerging interest, including administration of prophylactic donor cell infusions, maintenance with immunomodulatory drugs (eg, azacytadine), and targeted therapy (eg, sorafenib for FLT3-ITD). Premature closure of a lenalidomide maintenance trial due to a high incidence of acute GVHD highlights the importance of clinical-trial evaluation of posttransplant maintenance therapies. Ongoing studies show promise in patients with leukemia relapse after transplant including chimeric antigen receptor (CAR) T cells engineered to express anti-CD19 antibodies and bispecific antibodies (or bispecific T-cell engagers, BiTEs), eg, blinatumumab, which engages both CD3 on T cells and CD19 on B-ALL cells to initiate an antileukemic T-cell immune response. Alternatively, close monitoring for MRD or very early relapse after transplant may permit preemptive therapy in patients at risk of imminent relapse while sparing others potential treatment-related toxicity.

Treatment of overt relapse after transplant remains very challenging, especially within the first 6 months; patients relapsing later fare somewhat better, especially if relapse occurs a year or more after transplant. Long-term disease control appears to be possible with combined cytotoxic and donor cell therapies, including donor lymphocyte infusion with or without a stem cell boost or second transplant with the same or a different donor. Establishment of remission prior to cell therapy appears to be essential to successful outcomes.

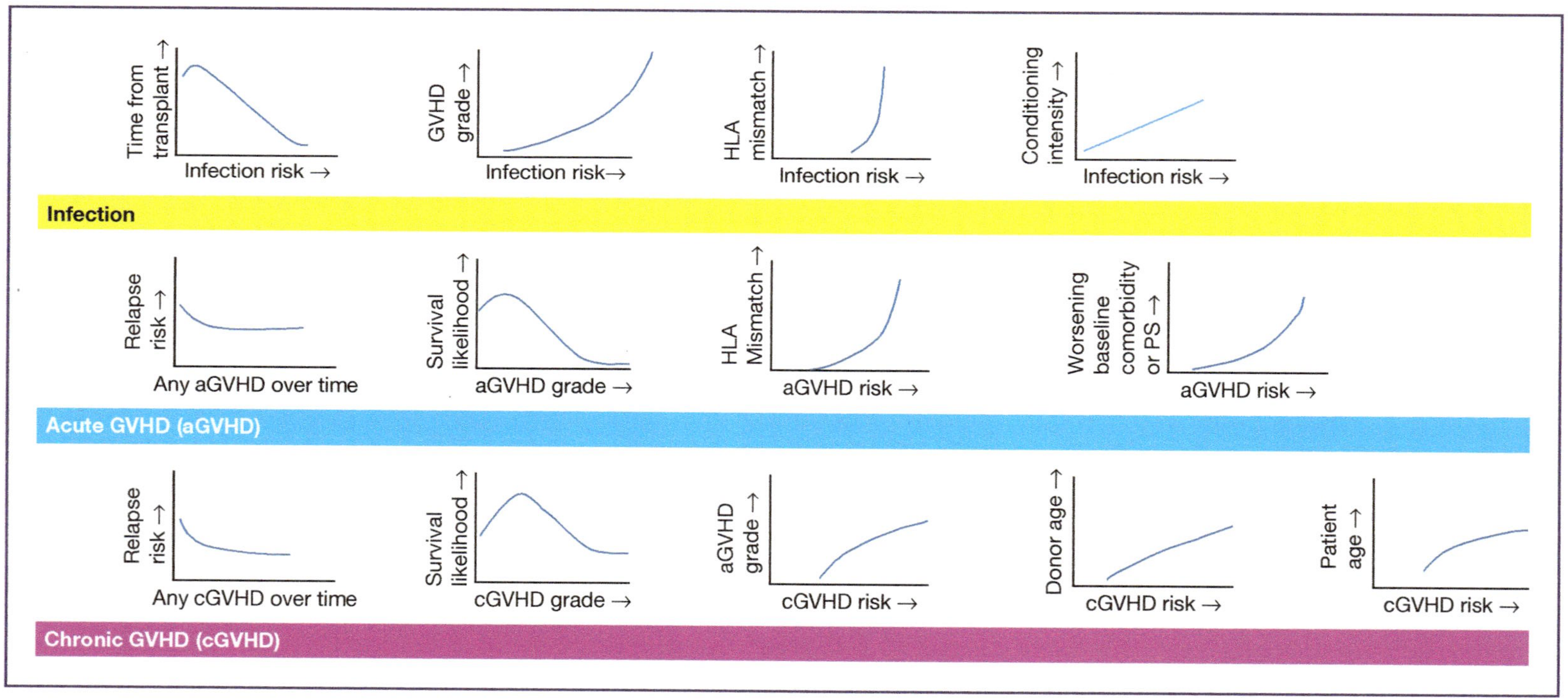

FIGURE 4-7: Immune dysregulation in allogeneic transplant. The graphs illustrate general relationships between important clinical outcomes and the immunologic compromise and dysregulation, which follows allogeneic BMT.

BMT, bone marrow transplantation; GVHD, graft-versus-host disease; HLA, human leukocyte antigen.

Infection: Following an allogeneic BMT, patients are at increased risk for all types of infections (viral, bacterial, and fungal). There are many factors contributing to the timing and degree of susceptibility to infection, including the patient's underlying disease, prior therapies, and pretransplant comorbidities, especially in the peritransplant period; the effects of transplant conditioning (chemotherapy, radiation) on host defense, eg, neutropenia, damage to the skin and gastrointestinal mucosa, with higher-intensity regimens causing greater tissue damage, more profound immune suppression, and increased risk for infections; the degree of donor and recipient HLA match and intensity of immunosuppressive prophylaxis, with the risk of infection increasing with increasing HLA disparity due to greater immune suppression and delayed B- and T-cell reconstitution as well as due to increased risk of GVHD.

GVHD: GVHD occurs when the transplanted donor immune system identifies the patient's ("host") organs or tissues as foreign, resulting in a damaging immune response. GVHD can be distinguished both clinically and histologically by characteristic patterns of tissue damage. Historically, acute GVHD was defined as GVHD occurring within the first 100 days after transplant, based on typical patterns of injury to the skin, gastrointestinal tract, and liver observed during this early period. Chronic GVHD, with pleomorphic manifestations, was historically defined as GVHD after Day 100. With evolution of conditioning regimens and immune suppression strategies, these temporal definitions no longer adequately describe the manifestations of GVHD, which can present classically, as "late-acute," with typical clinical acute GVHD arising or persisting beyond Day 100, or as part of an "overlap syndrome" in which typical acute GVHD features present along with chronic-type features.

Acute GVHD requiring intervention, ie, Grades II–IV acute GVHD, occurs in up to 60% of allogeneic hematopoietic stem cell transplants. There have been many studies on the impact of acute GVHD on transplant outcomes; apparent inconsistencies reflect heterogeneity in patient populations, disease indications, conditioning regimens, and prevention and treatment approaches. In general, it appears that the development of acute GVHD may reduce relapse risk, due to the GVL effect; this has been better established in pediatric ALL and in adults receiving reduced-intensity conditioning. Low-grade acute GVHD has been associated with improved survival in some studies (also better established in the pediatric population). Because of increased immune suppression and therapy as well as resulting tissue damage, higher-grade acute GVHD increases the risk of nonrelapse mortality (NRM), diminishing the GVL effect on overall survival.

Chronic GVHD: Chronic GVHD usually presents between 4 and 6 months after BMT. It can involve almost any organ system, although it most frequently involves the skin and mouth. The incidence varies depending on patient, disease, and transplant characteristics, occurring in 30% to 70% of allogeneic transplant recipients. There are more data supporting an association between chronic GVHD (than acute GVHD) and decreased relapse risk–due to presumed GVL effect–and net benefit in relapse-free and overall survival, especially in younger patients transplanted for chronic myelogenous leukemia. More recent studies encompassing broader patient, disease, and transplant characteristics challenge the association between chronic GVHD and beneficial outcomes. Factors that increase chronic GVHD risk are increasing age of recipient or donor, increasing HLA mismatch, and history of acute GVHD.

The pretransplant period begins with evaluations and ends with delivery of the conditioning regimen that cytoreduces or ablates the leukemia and eliminates the immunologic barrier to engraftment, counting down to Day 0, defined as the day of graft infusion. Concerns during this period include immediate toxicities such as nausea and vomiting, fluid shifts, and seizures. Preparative regimen toxicities, such as mucositis, veno-occlusive disease of the liver, and pancytopenia, tend to peak in the first week or two after BMT.

The combination of injury to mucocutaneous barriers and pancytopenia and intense immune suppression lead to invasive infections by organisms that colonize the GI tract and skin and recrudescence of preexisting infections. These problems become life-threatening if neutrophil engraftment does not ensue promptly, typically around 10 days after PBSC infusion, 18 days after marrow infusion, and 35 days after cord blood infusion.

As donor T-cells proliferate and encounter recipient antigen-presenting cells in the inflammatory milieu of tissue injured by the conditioning regimen, they can proliferate in response to alloantigen and produce acute GVHD. Although Day 100 was classically regarded as the watershed between acute and chronic GVHD, we now recognize distinct syndromes and may diagnose late acute GVHD or early

	Organ Systems	Common Clinical Manifestations	Representative Pictures
Acute GVHD	Skin	Erythema Maculopapular rash	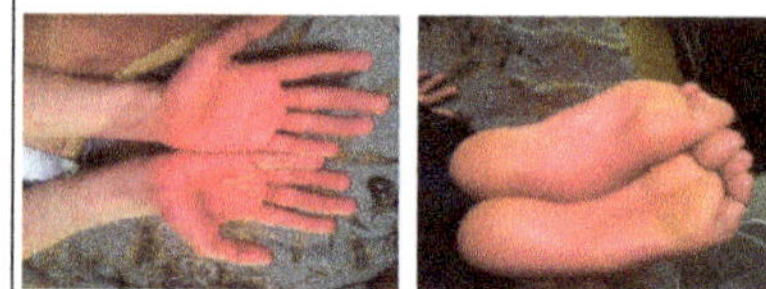 Erythema of palms and feet
	GI tract	Profuse diarrhea Vomiting Anorexia Nausea Ileus	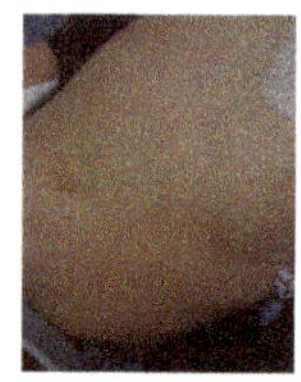 Diffuse maculopapular rash 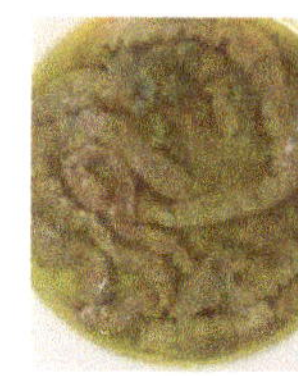 Diarrhea w/sloughing of intestinal lining
	Liver	Cholestatic liver disease with hyperbilirubinemia	
Chronic GVHD	Skin	Poikiloderma Lichen planus–like eruption Deep sclerotic features Morphea-like superficial sclerotic features Lichen sclerosus–like lesions	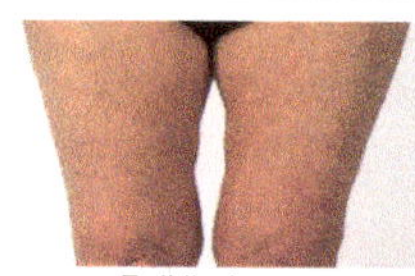 Poikiloderma
	Nails	Dystrophy Brittleness or ridging Onycholysis Pterygium unguis Nail loss	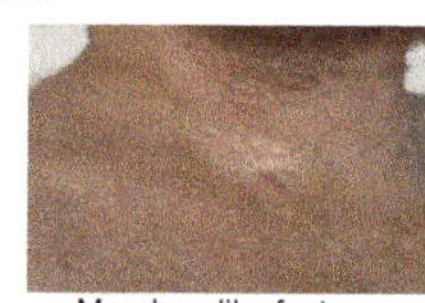 Morphea-like features
	Hair	New scarring or nonscarring scalp alopecia body hair loss	
	Mouth	Lichun planus-like changes Xerostomia Ulcers Pseudomembranes	
	Eyes	Dry, gritty, pain Cicatricial conjunctivitis Keratoconjunctivitis sicca Confluent areas of punctate keratopathy Blepharitis Photophobia	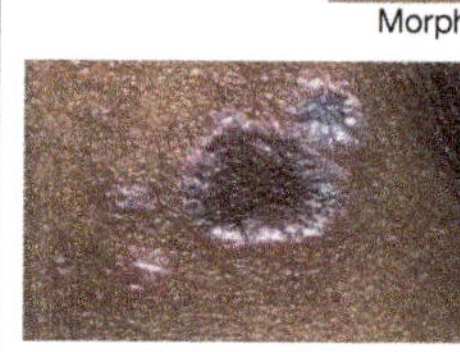 Lichen sclerosis
	Genitalia-male	Phimosis Urethral or meatus scarring or stenosis	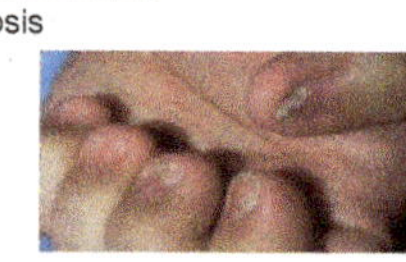 Nail dystrophy
	Genitalia-female	Vaginal scarring Clitoral/labial agglutination	
	GI tract	Esophageal web, strictures or stenosis	
	Liver	Hepatitis-like disorder Slowly progressive cholestatic disorder	
	Lungs	Bronchiolitis obliterans syndrome Cryptogenic organizing pneumonia	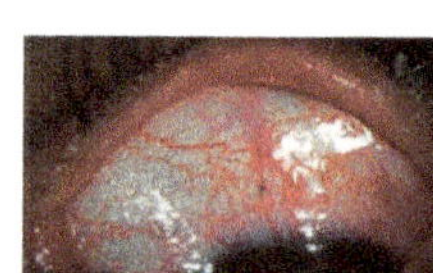
	Musculoskeletal system	Fasciitis Joint stiffness or contractures Myositis	
	Hematopoietic and immune systems	Cytopenias Hypereosinophilia Autoantibodies	Blepharitis

FIGURE 4-8: Clinical manifestations of acute and chronic GVHD.

Source: Adapted from Chronic GVHD Photographs courtesy of NMDP website: Chronic GVHD. (n.d.). https://bethematchclinical.org/Post-Transplant-Care/Chronic-GVHD

GVHD, graft-versus-host disease.

chronic GVHD. On engraftment, the risk of bacterial infections rapidly decreases in patients without active GVHD, but resistance to fungus develops more gradually, and resistance to viral infections still slower, with immunity approaching normal in 1 to 2 years.

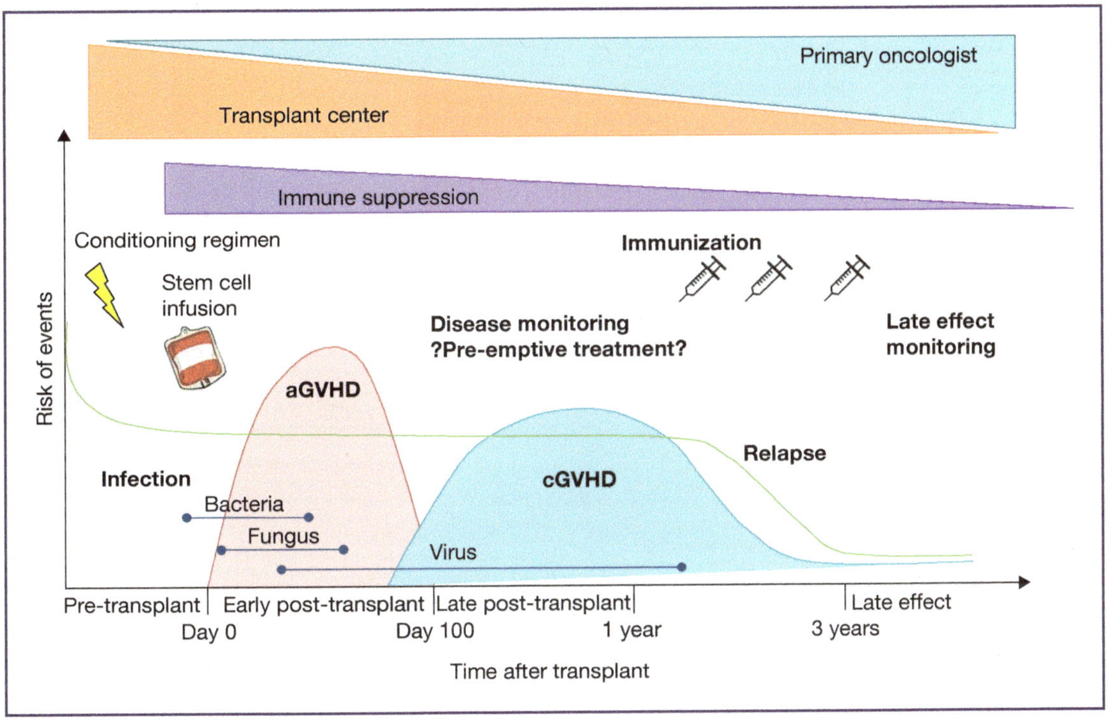

FIGURE 4-9: Transplant timeline indicating the evolution of major risks after allogeneic BMT, with the risk of GVHD shown as prevalence and the risk of relapse indicated as a hazard rate.

BMT, bone marrow transplantation; GVHD, graft-versus-host disease.

Immune recovery tends to be more rapid in younger patients with younger donors. Patients with untreated active GVHD are severely immunocompromised, and often have more severe infectious complications than those whose GVHD is controlled—even with potent immunosuppressive agents. It is important to provide patients with active GVHD and those on intensive immunosuppressive therapy with prophylaxis against opportunistic pathogens, such as pneumocystis and other fungi. Viral infections can be devastating in the first months after BMT; during this period, antiviral prophylaxis and, in the case of CMV, viral monitoring and preemptive therapy have clear benefit. The risk of relapse is transiently reduced in the first few weeks after transplant by the preparative regimen, but then rapidly increases until about 6 months after transplant, when it begins a gradual decline over a 2-year period. Expert panels have assembled recommended practices for the long-term follow-up after BMT is performed in adults.

Table 4-3 Late effects and long-term care after transplant

	MINIMAL ASSESSMENT	MANAGEMENT IF INDICATED
Eye	Screening cataract and sicca symptoms	Referral to ophthalmologist Artificial tear Topical immunosuppressant Cataract surgery
Dental	Screening dry mouth, oral GVHD, secondary malignancy	Referral to dentist Artificial saliva Oral dexamethasone rinse

(continued)

Table 4-3 Late effects and long-term care after transplant (*continued*)

	MINIMAL ASSESSMENT	MANAGEMENT IF INDICATED
Cardiology	Blood pressure Coronary artery disease risk	Echocardiogram/EKG Coronary artery assessment Antihypertensive medications Adjustment of calcineurin inhibitors
Pulmonary	Pulmonary function test 6-minute walk test if applicable	Chest CT scan Bronchoscopy Inhaled steroid or systemic immunosuppressant Treatment underlying infections
Nephrology	Serum creatinine Urine protein or albumin	ACE inhibitors or ARB Screen for nephrotic syndrome or TMA
Nutritional	Screening for malnutrition or obesity	Counseling with dietitian
Bone and Joint	Bone density scanning with DEXA Screening symptoms of avascular necrosis and joint cGVHD	Calcium and vitamin D Bisphosphonate Adjust steroid dose Referral to orthopedic surgeon
Diabetes	Fasting blood sugar Hemoglobin A_1C if applicable	Control blood sugars
Dyslipidemia	Fasting lipid panel Coronary artery disease risk	Antilipid medication
Thyroid Function	TSH	Thyroid replacement
Infections	Neutrophil and lymphocyte count Quantitative immunoglobulin	Prophylaxis (virus, fungus, PCP) IVIG for selected population Posttransplant immunization
Iron Overload	Ferritin and iron saturation	Phlebotomy if tolerated Iron chelation
Psychiatry	Screening adjustment disorder, anxiety, and depression	Referral to psychiatrist Adjust steroid dose
Physiatry	Screening physical capacity and flexibility	Exercise program Treatment of cGVHD Referral to rehabilitation medicine
Fertility	History and previous conditioning regimen	Referral to reproductive specialist
Female Hypogonadism	Screening symptoms and amenorrhea FSH, LH	Estrogen replacement
Male Hypogonadism	Screening symptoms Total and free testosterone	
Second Malignancies	Skin, oropharyngeal examination Thyroid examination Liver US for HBV+ recipient Annual Pap and HPV DNA test Follow general guidelines for breast, lung, colon cancer screening	Refer to dermatologist for suspicious lesions Fine-needle aspiration if suspicious for thyroid mass
Quality of Life	Screening socioeconomic challenges Emotional needs assessment	Refer to social worker

ACE, angiotensin-converting enzyme; ARB, angiotensin II receptor blockers; DEXA, bone density scanning with dual-energy x-ray absorptiometry; FSH, follicle-stimulating hormone; GVHD, graft-versus-host disease; LH; luteinizing hormone; PCP, pneumocystis pneumonia; TMA, thrombotic microangiopathy; TSH, thyroid-stimulating hormone; US, ultrasound.

The number of transplant survivors is increasing at an unprecedented rate due to improved patient survival and extension of transplant options to older patients, identification of transplant benefit in intermediate-risk acute leukemias, and better outcomes with alternative donor sources. The long-term health care needs of this population are unique, and so establishment of a cadre of providers with expertise in late effects of transplantation is urgently needed.

Late effects can involve multiple organs, depending on pretransplant therapies, preexisting conditions, the conditioning chemotherapy and radiation regimen, acute and chronic GVHD, the side effects of immunosuppressive agents, and infectious complications. A comprehensive and systematic approach is required to identify complications early and apply effective prevention and treatment measures, as summarized in Table 4-3. Despite the challenges in developing specialized survivor clinics, some workable strategies have been proposed. Good communication between the transplant physician, the multidisciplinary team, the primary care provider, and, perhaps most importantly, the survivors themselves is critical to meeting the long-term health care needs for this growing population.

Selected References

Apperley J, Niederwieser D, Huang XJ, et al. Haploidentical hematopoietic stem cell transplantation: a global overview comparing Asia, the European Union, and the United States. *Biol Blood Marrow Transplant*. 2016;22(1):23–26.

Armand P, Gibson CJ, Cutler C, et al. A disease risk index for patients undergoing allogeneic stem cell transplantation. *Blood*. 2012;120(4):905–913.

Armand P, Kim HT, Logan BR, et al. Validation and refinement of the disease risk index for allogeneic stem cell transplantation. *Blood*. 2014;123(23):3664–3671.

Bader P, Kreyenberg H, Henze GH, et al. Prognostic value of minimal residual disease quantification before allogeneic stem-cell transplantation in relapsed childhood acute lymphoblastic leukemia: the ALL-REZ BFM Study Group. *J Clin Oncol*. 2009;27(3):377–384.

Bader P, Kreyenberg H, von Stackelberg A, et al. Monitoring of minimal residual disease after allogeneic stem-cell transplantation in relapsed childhood acute lymphoblastic leukemia allows for the identification of impending relapse: results of the ALL-BFM-SCT 2003 trial. *J Clin Oncol*. 2015;33(11):1275–1284.

Baker KS, Chow E, Steinberger J. Metabolic syndrome and cardiovascular risk in survivors after hematopoietic cell transplantation. *Bone Marrow Transplant*. 2012;47(5):619–625.

Balduzzi A, Valsecchi MG, Uderzo C, et al. Chemotherapy versus allogeneic transplantation for very-high-risk childhood acute lymphoblastic leukaemia in first complete remission: comparison by genetic randomisation in an international prospective study. *Lancet*. 2005;366(9486):635–642.

Barrett J, Gluckman E, Handgretinger R, et al. Point-counterpoint: haploidentical family donors versus cord blood transplantation. *Biol Blood Marrow Transplant*. 2011;17(1 Suppl):S89–S93.

Bejanyan N, Weisdorf DJ, Logan BR, et al. Survival of patients with acute myeloid leukemia relapsing after allogeneic hematopoietic cell transplantation: a Center for International Blood and Marrow Transplant research study. *Biol Blood Marrow Transplant*. 2015;21(3):454–459.

Besse K, Maiers M, Confer D, et al. On modeling human leukocyte antigen-identical sibling match probability for allogeneic hematopoietic cell transplantation: estimating the need for an unrelated donor source. *Biol Blood Marrow Transplant*. 2016;22(3):410–417.

Boyiadzis M, Arora M, Klein JP, et al. Impact of chronic graft-versus-host disease on late relapse and survival on 7,489 patients after myeloablative allogeneic hematopoietic cell transplantation for leukemia. *Clin Cancer Res*. 2015;21(9):2020–2028.

Buckley SA, Appelbaum FR, Walter RB. Prognostic and therapeutic implications of minimal residual disease at the time of transplantation in acute leukemia. *Bone Marrow Transplant*. 2013;48(5):630–641.

Cancer Genome Atlas Research Network. Genomic and epigenomic landscapes of adult de novo acute myeloid leukemia. *N Engl J Med*. 2013;368(22):2059–2074.

Chronic GVHD photographs for Figure 4-8 courtesy of NMDP website: Chronic GVHD. (n.d.). Retrieved from https://bethematchclinical.org/Post-Transplant-Care/Chronic-GVHD

Copelan EA, Avalos BR, Ahn KW, et al. Comparison of outcomes of allogeneic transplantation for chronic myeloid leukemia with cyclophosphamide in combination with intravenous busulfan, oral busulfan, or total body irradiation. *Biol Blood Marrow Transplant*. 2015;21(3):552–558.

Copelan EA, Hamilton BK, Avalos B, et al. Better leukemia-free and overall survival in AML in first remission following cyclophosphamide in combination with busulfan compared with TBI. *Blood*. 2013;122(24):3863–3870.

Cornelissen JJ, Gratwohl A, Schlenk RF, et al. The European leukemia net AML working party consensus statement on allogeneic HSCT for patients with AML in remission: an integrated-risk adapted approach. *Nat Rev Clin Oncol*. 2012;9(10):579–590.

Cornelissen JJ, Versluis J, Passweg JR, et al. Comparative therapeutic value of post-remission approaches in patients with acute myeloid leukemia aged 40–60 years. *Leukemia*. 2015;29(5):1041–1050.

de Lima M, Giralt S, Thall PF, et al. Maintenance therapy with low-dose azacitidine after allogeneic hematopoietic stem cell transplantation for recurrent acute myelogenous leukemia or myelodysplastic syndrome: a dose and schedule finding study. *Cancer*. 2010;116(23):5420–5431.

Dohner H, Weisdorf DJ, Bloomfield CD. Acute myeloid leukemia. *N Engl J Med*. 2015;373(12):1136–1152.

Dreyer ZE, Dinndorf PA, Camitta B, et al. Analysis of the role of hematopoietic stem-cell transplantation in infants with acute lymphoblastic leukemia in first remission and MLL gene rearrangements: a report from the Children's Oncology Group. *J Clin Oncol*. 2011;29(2):214–222.

Duncan CN, Majhail NS, Brazauskas R, et al. Long-term survival and late effects among one-year survivors of second allogeneic hematopoietic cell transplantation for relapsed acute leukemia and myelodysplastic syndromes. *Biol Blood Marrow Transplant*. 2015;21(1):151–158.

Duval M, Klein JP, He W, et al. Hematopoietic stem-cell transplantation for acute leukemia in relapse or primary induction failure. *J Clin Oncol*. 2010;28(23):3730–3738.

Eckert C, von Stackelberg A, Seeger K, et al. Minimal residual disease after induction is the strongest predictor of prognosis in intermediate risk relapsed acute lymphoblastic leukaemia–long-term results of trial ALL-REZ BFM P95/96. *Eur J Cancer*. 2013;49(6):1346–1355.

Fielding AK, Rowe JM, Buck G, et al. UKALLXII/ECOG2993: addition of imatinib to a standard treatment regimen enhances long-term outcomes in Philadelphia positive acute lymphoblastic leukemia. *Blood*. 2014;123(6):843–850.

Filipovich AH, Weisdorf D, Pavletic S, et al. National Institutes of Health consensus development project on criteria for clinical trials in chronic graft-versus-host disease: I. Diagnosis and staging working group report. *Biol Blood Marrow Transplant*. 2005;11(12):945–956.

Flowers ME, Inamoto Y, Carpenter PA, et al. Comparative analysis of risk factors for acute graft-versus-host disease and for chronic graft-versus-host disease according to National Institutes of Health consensus criteria. *Blood*. 2011;117(11):3214–3219.

Gokbuget N, Kneba M, Raff T, et al. Adult patients with acute lymphoblastic leukemia and molecular failure display a poor prognosis and are candidates for stem cell transplantation and targeted therapies. *Blood*. 2012;120(9):1868–1876.

Gokbuget N, Stanze D, Beck J, et al. Outcome of relapsed adult lymphoblastic leukemia depends on response to salvage chemotherapy, prognostic factors, and performance of stem cell transplantation. *Blood*. 2012;120(10):2032–2041.

Goldstone AH, Richards SM, Lazarus HM, et al. In adults with standard-risk acute lymphoblastic leukemia, the greatest benefit is achieved from a matched sibling allogeneic transplantation in first complete remission, and an autologous transplantation is less effective than conventional consolidation/maintenance chemotherapy in all patients: final results of the International ALL Trial (MRC UKALL XII/ECOG E2993). *Blood*. 2008;111(4):1827–1833.

Gooley TA, Chien JW, Pergam SA, et al. Reduced mortality after allogeneic hematopoietic-cell transplantation. *N Engl J Med*. 2010;363(22):2091–2101.

Gragert L, Eapen M, Williams E, et al. HLA match likelihoods for hematopoietic stem-cell grafts in the U.S. registry. *N Engl J Med*. 2014;371(4):339–348.

Griffith ML, Savani BN, Boord JB. Dyslipidemia after allogeneic hematopoietic stem cell transplantation: evaluation and management. *Blood*. 2010;116(8):1197–1204.

Grochow LB, Jones RJ, Brundrett RB, et al. Pharmacokinetics of busulfan: correlation with veno-occlusive disease in patients undergoing bone marrow transplantation. *Cancer Chemother Pharmacol*. 1989;25(1):55–61.

Gustafsson JA, Remberger M, Ringden O, et al. Graft-versus-leukaemia effect in children: chronic GVHD has a significant impact on relapse and survival. *Bone Marrow Transplant*. 2003;31(3):175–181.

Gyurkocza B, Sandmaier BM. Conditioning regimens for hematopoietic cell transplantation: one size does not fit all. *Blood*. 2014;124(3):344–353.

Hahn T, McCarthy PL, Jr, Zhang MJ, et al. Risk factors for acute graft-versus-host disease after human leukocyte antigen-identical sibling transplants for adults with leukemia. *J Clin Oncol*. 2008;26(35):5728–5734.

Handgretinger R. Haploidentical transplantation: the search for the best donor. *Blood*. 2014;124(6):827–828.

Harrison CJ, Hills RK, Moorman AV, et al. Cytogenetics of childhood acute myeloid leukemia: United Kingdom Medical Research Council Treatment trials AML 10 and 12. *J Clin Oncol*. 2010;28(16):2674–2681.

Hashmi S, Carpenter P, Khera N, et al. Lost in transition: the essential need for long-term follow-up clinic for blood and marrow transplantation survivors. *Biol Blood Marrow Transplant*. 2015;21(2):225–232.

Heidegger S, van den Brink MR, Haas T, et al. The role of pattern-recognition receptors in graft-versus-host disease and graft-versus-leukemia after allogeneic stem cell transplantation. *Front Immunol*. 2014;5:337.

Holtick U. Albrecht M, Chemnitz JM, et al. Bone marrow versus peripheral blood allogeneic haematopoietic stem cell transplantation for haematological malignancies in adults. *Cochrane Database Syst Rev*. 2014;4:CD010189.

Horan JT, Alonzo TA, Lyman GH, et al. Impact of disease risk on efficacy of matched related bone marrow transplantation for pediatric acute myeloid leukemia: the Children's Oncology Group. *J Clin Oncol*. 2008;26(35):5797–5801.

Horowitz MM, Gale RP, Sondel PM, et al. Graft-versus-leukemia reactions after bone marrow transplantation. *Blood*. 1990;75(3):555–562.

Ichinohe T. Long-term feto-maternal microchimerism revisited: microchimerism and tolerance in hematopoietic stem cell transplantation. *Chimerism*. 2010;1(1):39–43.

Inamoto Y, Shah NN, Savani BN, et al. Secondary solid cancer screening following hematopoietic cell transplantation. *Bone Marrow Transplant*. 2015;50(8):1013–1023.

Jagasia M, Arora M, Flowers ME, et al. Risk factors for acute GVHD and survival after hematopoietic cell transplantation. *Blood*. 2012;119(1):296–307.

Jagasia MH, Greinix HT, Arora M, et al. National Institutes of Health consensus development project on criteria for clinical trials in chronic graft-versus-host disease: I. The 2014 diagnosis and staging working group report. *Biol Blood Marrow Transplant*. 2015;21(3):389–401 e1.

Jan M, Snyder TM, Corces-Zimmerman MR, et al. Clonal evolution of preleukemic hematopoietic stem cells precedes human acute myeloid leukemia. *Sci Transl Med*. 2012;4(149):149ra118.

Joshi S, Savani BN, Chow EJ, et al. Clinical guide to fertility preservation in hematopoietic cell transplant recipients. *Bone Marrow Transplant*. 2014;49(4):477–484.

Kasamon YL, Luznik L, Leffell MS, et al. Nonmyeloablative HLA-haploidentical bone marrow transplantation with high-dose posttransplantation cyclophosphamide: effect of HLA disparity on outcome. *Biol Blood Marrow Transplant*. 2010;16(4):482–489.

Kekre N, Koreth J. Novel strategies to prevent relapse after allogeneic haematopoietic stem cell transplantation for acute myeloid leukaemia and myelodysplastic syndromes. *Curr Opin Hematol*. 2015;22(2):116–122.

Kochenderfer JN, Dudley ME, Carpenter RO, et al. Donor-derived CD19-targeted T cells cause regression of malignancy persisting after allogeneic hematopoietic stem cell transplantation. *Blood*. 2013;122(25):4129–4139.

Koreth J, Schlenk R, Kopecky KJ, et al. Allogeneic stem cell transplantation for acute myeloid leukemia in first complete remission: systematic review and meta-analysis of prospective clinical trials. *JAMA*. 2009;301(22):2349–2361.

Laport GG, Alvarnas JC, Palmer JM, et al. Long-term remission of Philadelphia chromosome–positive acute lymphoblastic leukemia after allogeneic hematopoietic cell transplantation from matched sibling donors: a 20-year experience with the fractionated total body irradiation–etoposide regimen. *Blood*. 2008;112(3):903–909.

Lee SJ, Flowers ME. Recognizing and managing chronic graft-versus-host disease. *Hematology Am Soc Hematol Educ Program*. 2008:134–141.

Locatelli F, Masetti R, Rondelli R, et al. Outcome of children with high-risk acute myeloid leukemia given autologous or allogeneic hematopoietic cell transplantation in the aieop AML-2002/01 study. *Bone Marrow Transplant*. 2015;50(2):181–188.

Locke F, Agarwal R, Kunnavakkam R, et al. A novel clofarabine bridge strategy facilitates allogeneic transplantation in patients with relapsed/refractory leukemia and high-risk myelodysplastic syndromes. *Bone Marrow Transplant*. 2013;48(11):1437–1443.

Lowenberg B, Pabst T, Vellenga E, et al. Cytarabine dose for acute myeloid leukemia. *N Engl J Med*. 2011;364(11):1027–1036.

Luger SM, Ringden O, Zhang MJ, et al. Similar outcomes using myeloablative vs reduced-intensity allogeneic transplant preparative regimens for AML or MDS. *Bone Marrow Transplant*. 2012;47(2):203–211.

Majhail NS, Rizzo JD, Lee SJ, et al. Recommended screening and preventive practices for long-term survivors after hematopoietic cell transplantation. *Biol Blood Marrow Transplant*. 2012;18(3):348–371.

Malard F, Labopin M, Stuhler G, et al. Sequential intensified conditioning regimen allogeneic hematopoietic stem cell transplantation in adult patients with high-risk AML in complete remission: a survey from the ALWP of the EBMT. *Blood*. 2015;126(23):3105.

Mardis ER, Ding L, Dooling DJ, et al. Recurring mutations found by sequencing an acute myeloid leukemia genome. *N Engl J Med*. 2009;361(11):1058–1066.

Marr KA, Bow E, Chiller T, et al. Fungal infection prevention after hematopoietic cell transplantation. *Bone Marrow Transplant*. 2009;44(8):483–487.

Mehta PA, Zhang MJ, Eapen M, et al. Transplantation outcomes for children with hypodiploid acute lymphoblastic leukemia. *Biol Blood Marrow Transplant*. 2015;21(7):1273–1277.

Migliaccio AR, Adamson JW, Stevens CE, et al. Cell dose and speed of engraftment in placental/umbilical cord blood transplantation: graft progenitor cell content is a better predictor than nucleated cell quantity. *Blood*. 2000;96(8):2717–2722.

Mikulska M, Del Bono V, Viscoli C. Bacterial infections in hematopoietic stem cell transplantation recipients. *Curr Opin Hematol*. 2014;21(6):451–458.

Nachman JB, Heerema NA, Sather H, et al. Outcome of treatment in children with hypodiploid acute lymphoblastic leukemia. *Blood*. 2007;110(4):1112–1115.

Oran B, Jimenez AM, De Lima M, et al. Age and modified European leukemianet classification to predict transplant outcomes: an integrated approach for acute myelogenous leukemia patients undergoing allogeneic stem cell transplantation. *Biol Blood Marrow Transplant*. 2015;21(8):1405–1412.

Oyekunle AA, Kroger N, Zabelina T, et al. Allogeneic stem-cell transplantation in patients with refractory acute leukemia: a long-term follow-up. *Bone Marrow Transplant*. 2006;37(1):45–50.

Patriarca F, Luznik L, Medeot M, et al. Experts' considerations on HLA-haploidentical stem cell transplantation. *Eur J Haematol*. 2014;93(3):187–197.

Pratz KW, Gojo I, Karp JE, et al. Prospective study of peri-transplant use of sorafenib as remission maintenance for FLT3-ITD patients undergoing allogeneic transplantation. *Blood*. 2015;126(23):3164.

Pulsipher MA, Langholz B, Wall DA, et al. The addition of sirolimus to tacrolimus/methotrexate GVHD prophylaxis in children with ALL: a phase 3 Children's Oncology Group/pediatric blood and marrow transplant consortium trial. *Blood*. 2014;123(13):2017–2025.

Pulsipher MA, Skinner R, McDonald GB, et al. National Cancer Institute, National Heart, Lung and Blood Institute/Pediatric Blood and Marrow Transplantation Consortium First International Consensus Conference on late effects after pediatric hematopoietic cell transplantation: the need for pediatric-specific long-term follow-up guidelines. *Biol Blood Marrow Transplant*. 2012;18(3):334–347.

Rollig C, Bornhauser M, Kramer M, et al. Allogeneic stem-cell transplantation in patients with NPM1-mutated acute myeloid leukemia: results from a prospective donor versus no-donor analysis of patients after upfront HLA typing within the SAL-AML 2003 trial. *J Clin Oncol*. 2015;33(5):403–410.

Rubnitz JE. How I treat pediatric acute myeloid leukemia. *Blood*. 2012;119(25):5980–5988.

Saber W, Opie S, Rizzo JD, et al. Outcomes after matched unrelated donor versus identical sibling hematopoietic cell transplantation in adults with acute myelogenous leukemia. *Blood*. 2012;119(17):3908–3916.

Sanchez-Garcia J, Serrano J, Serrano-Lopez J, et al. Quantification of minimal residual disease levels by flow cytometry at time of transplant predicts outcome after myeloablative allogeneic transplantation in ALL. *Bone Marrow Transplant*. 2013;48(3):396–402.

Savani BN, Griffith ML, Jagasia S, et al. How I treat late effects in adults after allogeneic stem cell transplantation. *Blood*. 2011;117(11):3002–3009.

Schechter T, Gassas A, Chen H, et al. The outcome of allogeneic hematopoietic cell transplantation for children with FMS-like tyrosine kinase 3 internal tandem duplication-positive acute myelogenous leukemia. *Biol Blood Marrow Transplant*. 2015;21(1):172–175.

Schmid C, Labopin M, Nagler A, et al. Treatment, risk factors, and outcome of adults with relapsed AML after reduced intensity conditioning for allogeneic stem cell transplantation. *Blood*. 2012;119(6):1599–1606.

Schmid C, Labopin M, Socie G, et al. Outcome of patients with distinct molecular genotypes and cytogenetically normal AML after allogeneic transplantation. *Blood*. 2015;126(17):2062–2069.

Schmid C, Labopin M, Veelken H, et al. Efficacy, safety and long term results of prophylactic and preemptive donor lymphocyte infusion after allogeneic stem cell transplantation for acute leukemia: a registry-based evaluation on 343 patients by the acute leukemia working party of EBMT. *Blood*. 2015;126(23):863.

Schultz KR, Carroll A, Heerema NA, et al. Long-term follow-up of imatinib in pediatric Philadelphia chromosome-positive acute lymphoblastic leukemia: Children's Oncology Group study AALL0031. *Leukemia*. 2014;28(7):1467–1471.

Shlush LI, Zandi S, Mitchell A, et al. Identification of pre-leukaemic haematopoietic stem cells in acute leukaemia. *Nature*. 2014;506(7488):328–333.

Sockel K, Bornhaeuser M, Mischak-Weissinger E, et al. Lenalidomide maintenance after allogeneic HSCT seems to trigger acute graft-versus-host disease in patients with high-risk myelodysplastic syndromes or acute myeloid leukemia and del(5q): results of the LENAMAINT trial. *Haematologica*. 2012;97(9):e34–e35.

Sorror ML, Martin PJ, Storb RF, et al. Pretransplant comorbidities predict severity of acute graft-versus-host disease and subsequent mortality. *Blood*. 2014;124(2):287–295.

Sorror ML, Storb RF, Sandmaier BM, et al. Comorbidity-age index: a clinical measure of biologic age before allogeneic hematopoietic cell transplantation. *J Clin Oncol*. 2014;32(29):3249–3256.

Tallen G, Ratei R, Mann G, et al. Long-term outcome in children with relapsed acute lymphoblastic leukemia after time-point and site-of-relapse stratification and intensified short-course multidrug chemotherapy: results of trial ALL-REZ BFM 90. *J Clin Oncol*. 2010;28(14):2339–2347.

Tarlock K, Chang B, Cooper T, et al. Sorafenib treatment following hematopoietic stem cell transplant in pediatric FLT3/ITD acute myeloid leukemia. *Pediatr Blood Cancer*. 2015;62(6):1048–1054.

Tichelli A, Rovo A, Gratwohl A. Late pulmonary, cardiovascular, and renal complications after hematopoietic stem cell transplantation and recommended screening practices. *Hematology Am Soc Hematol Educ Program*. 2008;125–133.

Tomblyn M, Chiller T, Einsele H, et al. Guidelines for preventing infectious complications among hematopoietic cell transplantation recipients: a global perspective. *Biol Blood Marrow Transplant*. 2009;15(10):1143–1238.

Topp MS, Gökbuget N, Stein AS, et al. Safety and activity of blinatumomab for adult patients with relapsed or refractory B-precursor acute lymphoblastic leukaemia: a multicentre, single-arm, phase 2 study. *Lancet Oncol*. 2015;16(1):57–66.

Topp MS, Gökbuget N, Zugmaier G, et al. Phase II trial of the anti-CD19 bispecific T cell–engager blinatumomab shows hematologic and molecular remissions in patients with relapsed or refractory B-precursor acute lymphoblastic leukemia. *J Clin Oncol*. 2014;32(36):4134–4140.

Vigorito AC, Campregher PV, Storer BE, et al. Evaluation of NIH consensus criteria for classification of late acute and chronic GVHD. *Blood*. 2009;114(3):702–708.

Vyas P, Appelbaum FR, Craddock C. Allogeneic hematopoietic cell transplantation for acute myeloid leukemia. *Biol Blood Marrow Transplant*. 2015;21(1):8–15.

Weisdorf D, Zhang M-J, Arora M, et al. Graft-versus-host disease induced graft-versus-leukemia effect: greater impact on relapse and disease-free survival after reduced intensity conditioning. *Bio Blood Marrow Transplant*. 2012;18(11):1727–1733.

Wingard JR, Majhail NS, Brazauskas R, et al. Long-term survival and late deaths after allogeneic hematopoietic cell transplantation. *J Clin Oncol*. 2011;29(16):2230–2239.

5

Measurable (Minimal) Residual Disease

The Mechanics of Quantized Hematopoiesis

Michael R. Loken

- Normal hematopoiesis is an ideal model system for the study of gene product regulation. Intact, single cells are available in peripheral blood or bone marrow without the need for tissue disaggregation required for other cellular systems. All stages of maturation from the hematopoietic stem cells to mature peripheral blood cells are readily obtained for study. The antigen expression patterns for different lineages have been well characterized with the monoclonal antibodies.
- Flow cytometry can be used to precisely quantify the expression of several antigens (cell surface gene products) simultaneously, allowing for the analysis of multiple cell types of different maturational stages.
- By comparing neoplastic cells to the normal well-regulated patterns of hematopoiesis, leukemic cell populations can be characterized based on how they differ from their normal counterparts. This approach of "difference from normal" can be used to identify residual disease following therapy, even without a diagnostic specimen or if the phenotype changes.
- Most of the available monoclonal antibodies that are used to study hematopoiesis recognize cell surface antigens that are glycoproteins. These antigens are the functional end products of genes and therefore are ideal for understanding the regulation of gene product expression under both normal and neoplastic control. Antibodies that recognize carbohydrates or phospholipids do not necessarily identify a single specific gene product and are therefore not utilized for flow cytometric studies of gene product regulation.
- In this chapter, the normal development of hematopoietic cells is modeled as a steady state. A constant turnover of cells occurs with immature cells from the bone marrow replacing the dying mature blood cells. By patterning this developmental process as a steady state, the appearance and disappearance of cellular antigens and the precise relationships between cellular events can be related to specific times in the maturational process. Gene products assayed in a quantitative manner can elucidate the underlying principles of regulation of the maturational process from uncommitted progenitor cell to mature, functional blood cell.

FUNDAMENTALS OF QUANTITATIVE ANTIGEN EXPRESSION

Most antigens expressed on populations of mature cells are represented by a normal, Gaussian distribution when plotted on a log scale (Figure 5-1). This distribution is characterized by the mean and standard deviation (SD) of the events. The distribution of the amounts of gene products around the mean can be broad (Figure 5-1A) or narrow (Figure 5-1B). A narrower distribution, reflecting a tighter regulation around the mean, suggests that the amount of that specific gene product is more important from an evolutionary standpoint than a gene product with a broad distribution.

The standard deviation of gene product expression may also be the result of multiple cell lineages or cell lines all expressing the same antigen, but at different levels, such as CD45. Even a relatively tight

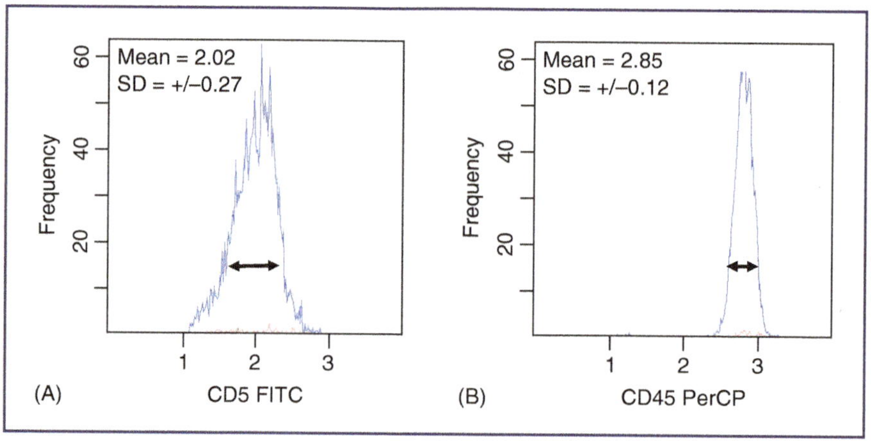

FIGURE 5-1: Gene product (antigen) expression on mature normal cells is a log normal distribution (defined by a mean and standard deviation) for the majority of antigens/gene products. The expression of CD5 on mature T cells (A) is broad as compared to the expression of CD45 on mature lymphocytes (B). The units for the x axes are log10; where 1 = 10, 2 = 100, 3 = 1000.

FITC, fluorescein; PerCP, peridinin chlorophyll protein; SD, standard deviation.

distribution such as CD45, which is expressed on mature lymphocytes, may be the result of population heterogeneity (Figure 5-2). This composite nature of antigen expression on a population of cells is demonstrated by comparing the CD45 expression of mature B cells, NK cells, CD4+, and CD8+ T cells (Figure 5-2). Although the width of CD45 intensity distribution is narrow, the distribution of CD45 on the individual lymphoid lineages is even tighter (Figure 5-2). The shape and mean of CD45 intensity for all lymphocytes is then a reflection of the relative proportions of each of these mature lymphoid lineages. Interestingly, the tight regulation of CD45 on mature lymphocytes is independent of the multiple isoforms of this gene found on these different lymphoid cells, a result from the differences of gene splicing.

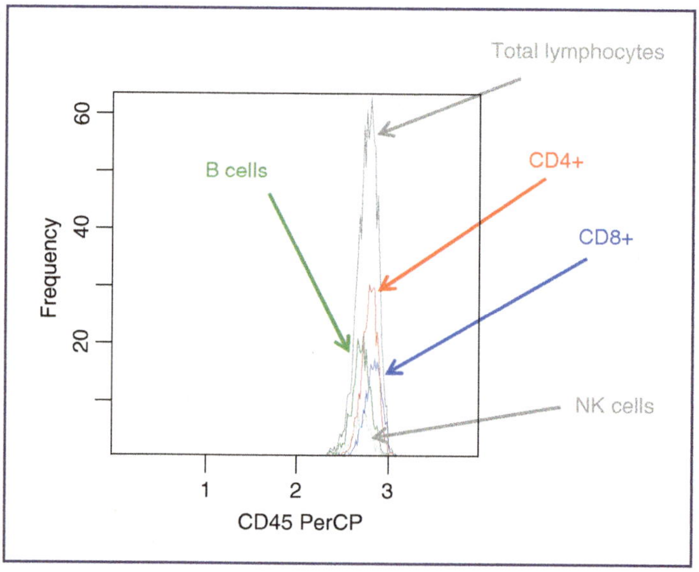

FIGURE 5-2: CD45 intensity distribution is a composite of the distributions observed for different mature lymphoid subsets. The mean intensity of CD45 is lowest for the CD19+ B cells, followed by the NK cells, CD4+ lymphocytes, and the CD8+ lymphocytes. The regulation of CD45 for each of these lymphoid subsets is tighter than that observed for the entire lymphoid population, indicating a high degree of regulation of amount of CD45 around the mean.

Differences in amounts of antigen expression between cells are not simply a function of cell size. Forward light scatter (FWD Scatter) is measured on a flow cytometer at low angles, looking back into the laser beam. This characteristic is dominated by diffraction, which is related to the cross-sectional area of the cell, ie, cell size. Lymphocytes are small and have low FWD Scatter but have the highest level of CD45 (Figure 5-3). The larger eosinophils, monocytes, and neutrophils express lower amounts of CD45, indicating that the difference in gene product expression is independent of cell size. Even within a lineage, there is minimal variability in antigen intensities between the smallest and largest cells. Similarly, the expression of CD33 is not related to size. Lymphocytes do not express CD33, while different intensities of CD33 expression are observed on eosinophils, neutrophils, and the high-expressing monocytes (Figure 5-3B). No relationship or correlation between FWD and the amount of these two antigens is obvious on mature cells in normal peripheral blood.

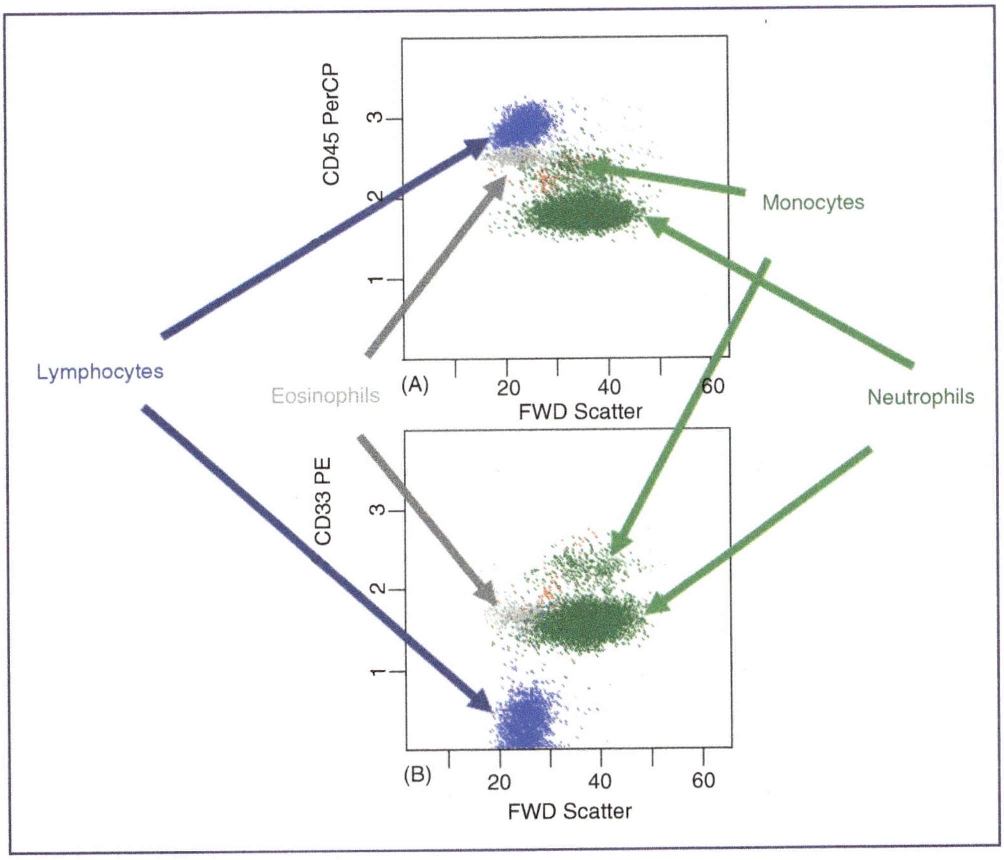

FIGURE 5-3: **Intensity differences in gene product expression are not simply a consequence of size. FWD Scatter provides a measure of cell size in the flow cytometer. (A) CD45 expression is highest on the lymphocytes (Blue) although they are the smallest cells, as compared to neutrophils (green), monocytes (green), and eosinophils (gray). (B) CD33 is not expressed on lymphocytes but is found on myeloid cells at different intensities depending upon the lineage. The intensities of CD33 are not related to cell size as identified by light scatter.**

FWD Scatter, forward light scatter.

The relationship of intensities between CD45 and CD33 illustrates that each gene product is independently regulated (Figure 5-4). The independence of these two antigens on each of the cell populations is identified by the lack of a correlation in intensities between one antigen and the other. This lack of correlation between multiple cell surface antigens is observed for all gene products, with an exception of those antigens that are expressed as large, multigene complexes, such as CD3 and T-cell receptor.

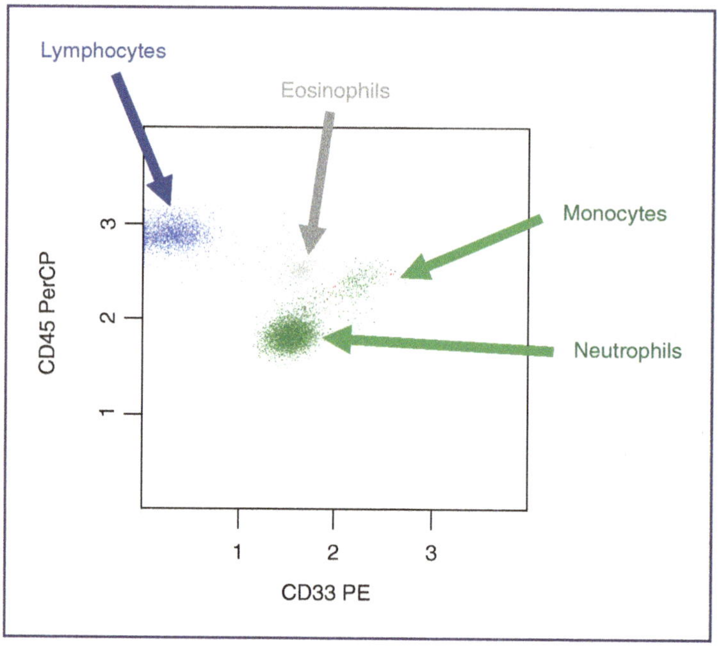

FIGURE 5-4: The lack of correlation between the expression of CD45 and CD33 on different mature cell lineages illustrates that each gene product is independently regulated with respect to amount.
PE, phycoerythrin; PerCP, peridinin chlorophyll protein.

The amounts of many cell surface antigens are surprisingly constant from individual to individual. The consistency of antigen expression can be demonstrated by the expression of CD4 on T lymphocytes. As part of the comprehensive quality control system for flow cytometry, lymphocytes were stained with the same monoclonal antibody CD4, conjugated to various fluorochromes [fluorescein (FITC), phycoerythrin (PE), peridinin chlorophyll protein (PerCP), allophycocyanin (APC)]. These cells were used to establish proper spectral compensation *prior to* data acquisition on the flow cytometer. Although fluorescence intensities of these cells were not the primary goal of this assessment, a comparison of the fluorescence histograms of 12 normal individuals collected over a period of 18 months showed minimal variability (Figure 5-5). The CD4+ cells (Blue, Figure 5-5) demonstrated a tight distribution that was located in an almost identical position for each individual. These data show that the amount of CD4 expressed on lymphocytes is the same from individual to individual.

The mean position of CD4 from randomly selected individuals from a period of October 2003 until June 2015 obtained on two separate flow cytometers shows minimal variability (Figure 5-6, average SD = 0.06 log units). Similar data have been obtained in laboratories in Argentina and Taiwan demonstrating constancy of CD4 intensity for individuals with diverse genetic backgrounds. These data demonstrate that the analytic system is stable over long periods of time, allowing quantitative immunofluorescence to be compared in a properly controlled data set, even if the specimens were collected at different times. In addition, it shows that the amount of some gene products is tightly regulated and invariant from person to person, indicating that CD4 intensity is highly conserved in evolution. The amounts of certain gene products expressed on cell surfaces are a **biologic constant.**

MATURATION IN HEMATOPOIESIS IS CHARACTERIZED BY QUANTIZED STEPS

It has been a daunting problem to unravel the antigen expression patterns in bone marrow composed of such a complex heterogeneous mixture of cells (11 different lineages or distinct cell types and their maturational stages: T, B, and NK lymphoid cells; plasma cells; erythrocyte; monocyte; neutrophil; eosinophil; basophil; mast cells; and plasmacytic dendritic cells). The identification of all of these cell

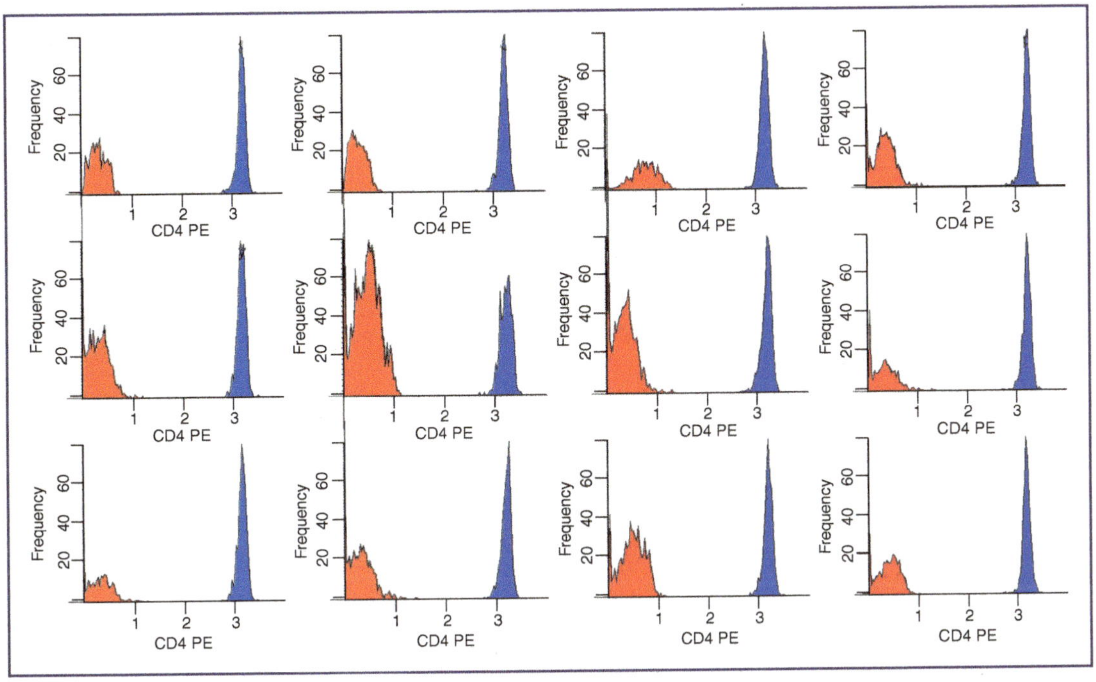

FIGURE 5-5: CD4 intensity histograms for 12 individuals collected over a period of 18 months. The CD4 positive cells (Blue) exhibit a tight peak of fluorescence, well separated from the other lymphocytes (Red). The mean position of the peaks is almost identical from individual to individual.

PE, phycoerythrin.

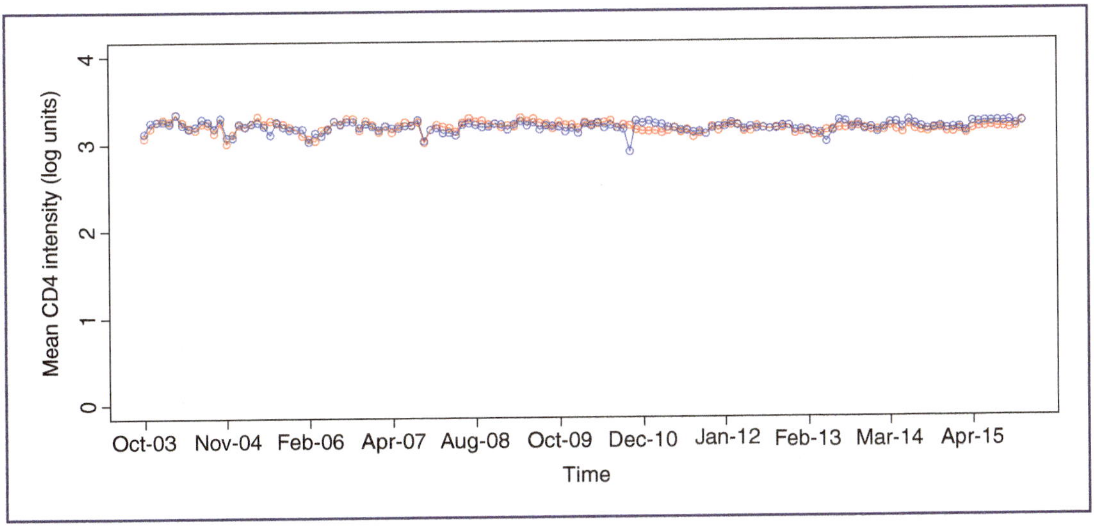

FIGURE 5-6: The CD4 intensity for normal individuals is the same even when assayed over a long period of time and on two different flow cytometers (Red vs. Blue). As part of the QC of the analytic system, CD4-stained normal blood specimens were used to establish proper spectral compensation. The mean positions of CD4 were not used to establish instrument settings, but only to measure overall performance. These data illustrate that the amount of CD4 expressed on normal, mature T cells is invariant from person to person [Mean SD = 0.062 (Blue); 0.059 (Red)] and demonstrate that the analytic system is stable over long periods of time.

types and their maturational stages was made feasible by focusing on a single lineage of cells at a time, using a lineage-specific marker, such as glycophorin A on the erythroid cells or CD19 on the B cells. The complexity of the mixture could be simplified only by studying cells expressing this lineage-specific marker, providing a more intuitive approach to follow the maturation of individual cell lineages. The maturational sequence of antigen expression can be defined by quantitative flow cytometry, focusing on a single lineage of cells from the least mature cells in the bone marrow to the mature cells in the blood and modeling normal maturation as a steady state.

An analogy of this procedure could be made for morphology. On a microscope slide of a bone marrow smear, hematopoetic cells from multiple lineages and multiple maturational stages are admixed together. Imagine instead of analyzing the cells in their intermingled state, one could place each lineage separately in different regions of the microscope slide and align the cells of a single lineage according to maturational sequence. The morphologist could then review the cells starting with the least mature cells of the lineage and move down the line with progressively more and more mature cells. Abnormal cells or dyspoiesis could then be more readily detected by a comparison to their corresponding normal counterparts.

Single lineage maturational analysis by quantitative flow cytometry accomplishes the same process by studying the sequential change in antigen expression following cells from hematopoietic stem cell to the mature functional blood cell. These studies originally began with the erythroid lineage, followed by the B lymphoid lineage and then the monocyte and neutrophil lineages.

B lymphoid development was particularly useful in defining maturation based on quantitative gene product expression. The lineage-specific antigen, CD19, is expressed on the most immature, terminal deoxynucleotidyl transferase (TdT) positive, CD34 positive B lineage cells. The expression of CD19 is maintained throughout maturation to the mature B lymphocytes and is even identified on normal plasma cells. The lymphoid cells and progenitor cells were first identified on the basis of CD45 and Side Scatter (light scattered at right angles to the laser, which measures cellular granules), thereby eliminating monocytes, neutrophils, and erythroid cells from the analysis (Figure 5-7A). Within these cells the entire maturing B-cell lineage could be identified using CD19 (Figure 5-7B). The remainder of the displays of the cell populations illustrated in Figure 5-7 are limited to the CD19+ lymphocytes and progenitor cells identified in Figure 5-7B. Four clearly distinct populations of cells could be identified using combinations of CD45, CD19, CD10, CD20, CD34, and CD38. The least mature cells, Stage I (colored gold), express the lowest amount of CD45, reduced CD19, high CD10, and CD34. These cells have low Side Scatter and are slightly larger than the remainder of B lymphoid precursors as identified by FWD Scatter (Figure 5-7C). These cells have been shown to express TdT. The next stage of B-cell development, Stage II (colored red), exhibits higher levels of CD45 and CD19, slightly reduced CD10, and heterogeneous CD20. CD34 is lost on these cells at Stage II (Figure 5-7G). The cells in Stage II have been shown to express cytoplasmic but not surface immunoglobulin (corresponding to the classic pre-B-cell). The next stage of B-cell development, Stage III (colored light blue), demonstrates a further increase in CD45, continued expression of CD19, maximal expression of CD20, and heterogeneous expression of CD10. This population now has surface immunoglobulin appearing on the cells. The final stage of B-cell development, Stage IV (colored dark blue), corresponds to mature B lymphocytes expressing high levels of CD45, CD19, CD22, CD20, and reduced CD38.

These data contain a wealth of information about the underlying regulation of gene products during maturation. As the B cells mature, changes in multiple antigens occur at the same time of development. Comparing the gold and red population, CD10 is reduced, while CD45 increases in intensity. CD34 is lost, while CD20 begins to be expressed. The CD45 expressed on the B lineage cells has an additional exon as compared to the myeloid and T-cell CD45. In addition, the gold, red, and light blue populations are undergoing rapid cell division as measured in an increase in DNA content with 25% of the cells in S, G2, and M phase of the cell cycle. The dark blue cells are not proliferating and have reduced CD38 expression. The cellular proliferation is also observed in cell size differences, especially within the red population (Figure 5-7C). In summary, the maturation of the B cells is marked by several mechanisms of coordinated regulation: gene product down-regulation (CD10), gene product up-regulation (CD45), gene products being shut off (CD34), gene products being turned on (CD20), differential splicing (CD45), and a change in DNA synthesis. Some antigens, such as CD20, may require a significant amount of time to reach their predetermined intensities, resulting in a broad fluorescence distribution within a

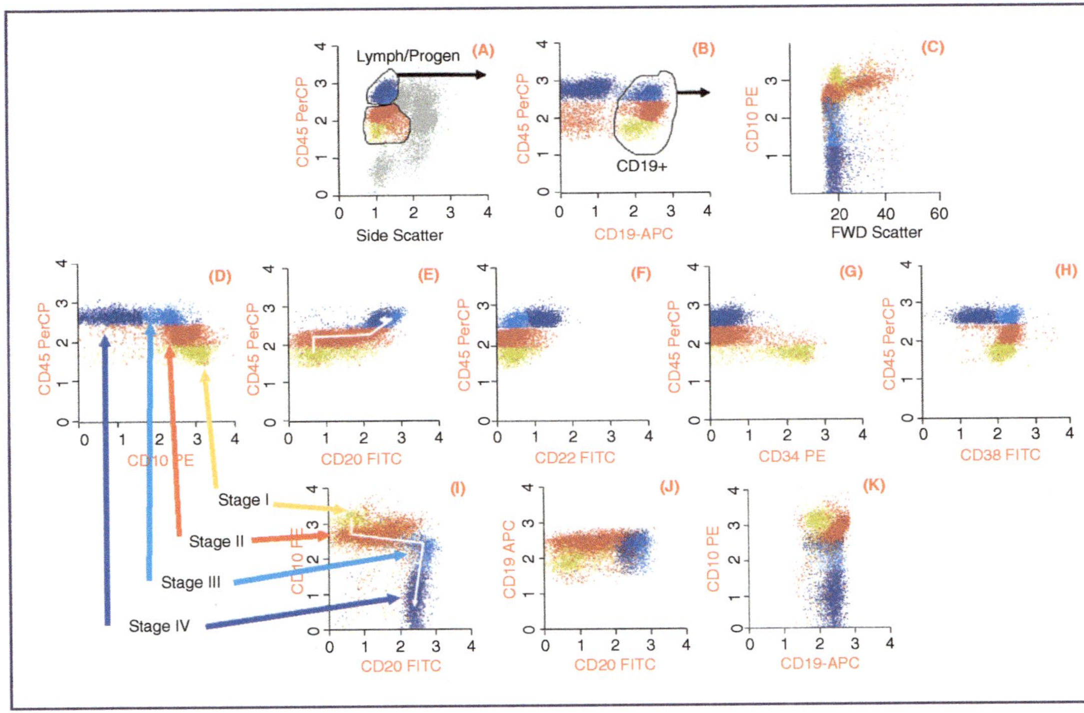

FIGURE 5-7: Maturation of B lineage cells in normal bone marrow is observed as a series of steps identified by the expression of multiple cell surface antigens. The composite figure illustrates the data from three separate 4-color tubes (CD20-FITC/CD10-PE/CD45-PerCP/CD19-APC; CD22-FITC/CD34-PE/CD45-PerCP/CD19-APC; CD38-FITC/CD34-PE/CD45-PerCP/CD19-APC). The lymphocytes and progenitor cells are identified by CD45 vs. log Side Scatter (A). The entire B-cell lineage was identified using CD19 (B). The remainders of the plots (C–K) are gated to display only the B lineage cells. The same populations are identified by multiple physical characteristics and expression of gene products. The least mature cells, Stage I, gold, express low levels of CD19, low CD45, high CD10, high CD38, and high CD34 without expression of CD20 or CD22. These cells also express nuclear terminal deoxynucleotidyl transferase (data not shown). A second population (Stage II, red) exhibits higher levels of CD19 and CD45, lower levels of CD10, and heterogeneous CD20 without expression of CD34 or CD22. A third population of B lymphoid cells (Stage III, light blue) show increased CD45, CD19, high levels of CD20 and CD38, as well as CD10. The last group of cells corresponds to mature B lymphocytes (Stage IV, dark blue) detectable by high levels of CD45, CD19, CD20, and expression of CD22 with reduced CD38. The relatively discrete nature of these populations shows that multiple gene products are regulated together in a coordinated fashion. Therefore, the progression from least mature B lymphoid precursors (gold) to the mature B lymphocytes (blue) occurs in a stepwise fashion identifiable by changes in multiple gene products at each step.

APC, allophycocyanin; FITC, fluorescein; FWD Scatter, forward light scatter; PE, phycoerythrin; PerCP, peridinin chlorophyll protein.

maturational stage. In a reciprocal manner, the loss of an antigen from the cell surface requires either active degradation or simply dilution with each cell division. Boundaries between stages, therefore, are defined based on the initial change of intensities of expression.

The transitions between Stages I and IV are rapid, relative to the total time required for B-cell maturation. Very few events separate one developmental stage from the next, indicating the transitions in cellular characteristics occur not only at the same time but are also very fast. These attributes are not only found among B lineage cells but are also identified within the myeloid cells and the erythroid cells as they mature. These data indicate that the maturational process for cells of a single lineage is stepwise or **quantized**, not continuous, as a precisely coordinated series of changes in gene product expression are required for cells to transition from one stage to the next.

Identifying the quantized nature of development of neutrophils was further complicated as no lineage-specific antibody is available to distinguish between monocytes, neutrophils, eosinophils, basophils, and dendritic cells. The analytic process requires working backward from peripheral blood cells maintaining all relationships between each monoclonal antibody, in a process called multidimensional analysis. Key aspects of neutrophil development can be visualized by combining CD16/CD13/CD45/CD34 (Figure 5-8). The cells in the entire neutrophil lineage are confined to the progenitor and neutrophil regions identified by CD45 and Side Scatter (Figure 5-8A). The heterogeneity of the cells within these regions can be reduced by examining other cell surface antigens (Figures 5-8B and 5-8C). Identification of these populations by linking all combinations of assayed parameters simultaneously is the basis of multidimensional data analysis. In this example, four colors of immunofluorescence and two light scattering parameters result in a six-dimensional data space. Identification of the maturational sequence requires relating all of the data to observe the small populations of interest.

The uncommitted progenitor cell population, shown in gold (Figure 5-8), is characterized by high expression of CD34 and intermediate expression of CD13. These cells include not only the quiescent hematopoietic stem cells but also the multipotent progenitor cells. These cells are undergoing the decision to differentiate into individual lineages but have not yet acquired the cell surface antigens indicating commitment down any maturational pathway.

Once these immature cells become committed to a specific lineage, CD34 intensity begins to decrease (Figure 5-8B). Cells destined to become neutrophils increase in the amount of CD13, while cells developing to monocytes slightly decrease their CD13 expression. Commitment to basophils and plasmacytic dendritic cells as well as B lymphocytes causes a rapid decrease in CD13 expression. Characterization of the first steps of neutrophil maturation can be achieved by selecting the uncommitted progenitor cells and the progenitor cells with increased CD13 (Figure 5-8D). The cells expressing CD34 are observed as red, while the cells with increased Side Scatter and included in the blue neutrophil region (Figure 5-8A) are colored light blue (Figure 5-8H and 5-8I). The change in Side Scatter is a result of the acquisition of the primary granules. The relationship of these three cell populations with respect to other characteristics are shown in Figures 5-8E to 5-8I.

The cells residing between red and blue dashed lines (Figure 5-8D) are designated "neutrophilic myeloid progenitor cells," while the light blue population is termed "granular neutrophilic blasts" and corresponds to the type III granular blasts identified by morphology. The remainder of the neutrophil development can be visualized by combining CD13 and CD16 (Figure 5-8G). After CD13 reaches a maximum intensity, this antigen rapidly drops in amount only to reappear later in development and in concert with CD16. Therefore, during neutrophil development, CD13 first increases to a maximum; then granules begin to appear. Subsequently, this gene product is turned off only to be reactivated at a later stage of development when CD16 begins to appear (metamyelocytes). The transition from the uncommitted myeloid progenitor cell to high expression of CD13 is very rapid, as demonstrated by the relative infrequency of the population (red) as compared to the relatively slow increase in expression observed later in maturation (Figure 5-8G).

The transition from the uncommitted progenitor cells to the neutrophilic myeloid progenitor cells can also be observed by multiple other gene products, including an increase in CD33 as well as a decrease in expression of HLA-DR (data not shown). Both the neutrophilic myeloid progenitor and the neutrophilic granular progenitor cells have detectible low levels of HLA-DR. The transitional boundary between

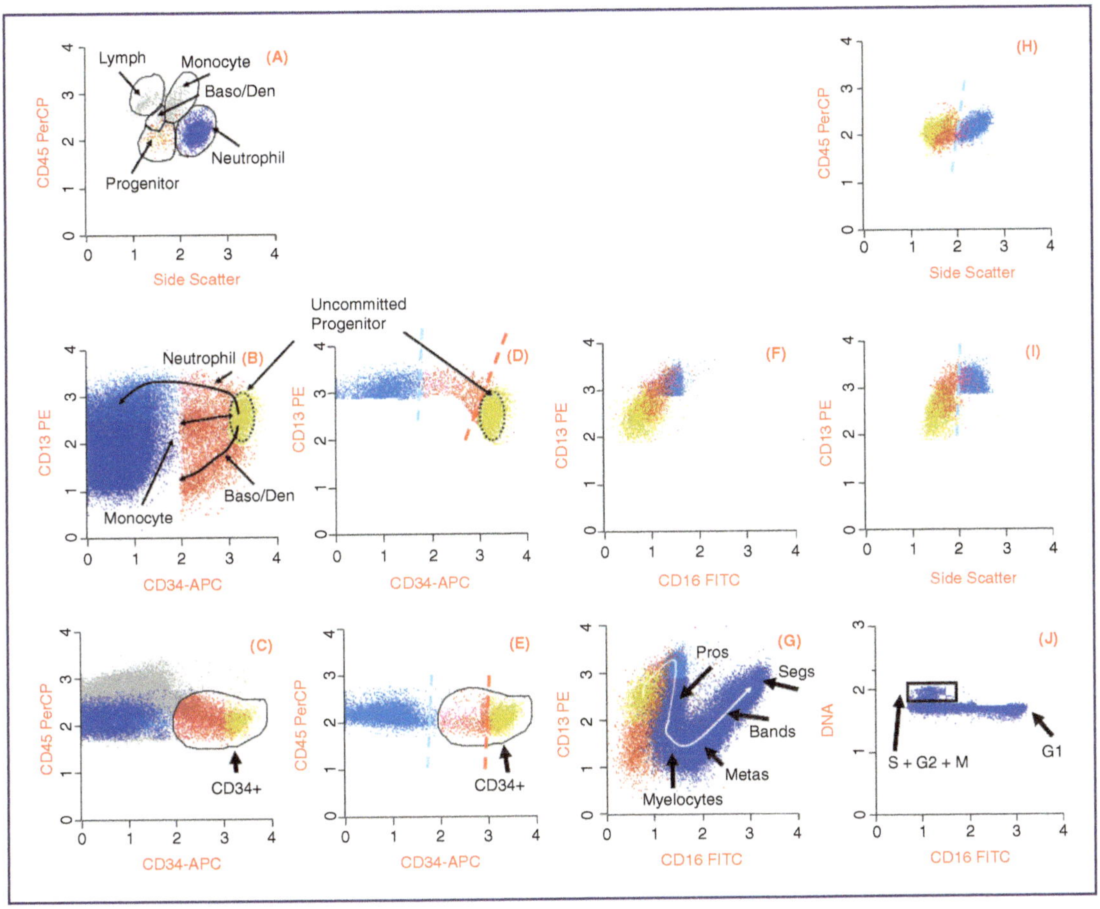

FIGURE 5-8: The earliest stages of neutrophil maturation in normal bone marrow can also be divided into discrete steps based on the expression of multiple gene products and physical characteristics. A normal bone marrow specimen was stained with CD16-FITC/CD13-PE/CD45-PerCP/CD34-APC (A–I). The progenitor and neutrophil populations were identified using CD45 and log Side Scatter (A). Cells expressing CD34 were colored red or gold, while cells with increased Side Scatter were colored light or dark blue. The relationships between CD13, CD34, and CD45 for the progenitor cells and neutrophils are shown in B, C. The uncommitted progenitor cells (gold) express high levels of CD34 and intermediate CD13 and CD45. When these cells become committed to specific lineages, the CD34 expression decreases. Cells committed to the neutrophil lineage increase the amount of CD13 (B), while cells maturing to monocytes retain the same amount of CD13 in contrast to the cells differentiating to basophils and dendritic cells, which decrease the amount of CD13 (B). The earliest identifiable neutrophilic myeloid progenitor cells (red) and granular blasts (light blue) were identified by the regions in D. The corresponding populations are shown in other projections of the multidimensional data (E–I). The progression of maturation from the uncommitted progenitor cells (gold) to the neutrophilic myeloid progenitor cells (red) to the granular blasts (light blue) are noted by the dashed lines in D, E, H, and I. All of these early populations are negative for CD16 (G), which appears later during neutrophil maturation. The location of morphologically distinct maturational steps is noted on the CD13 vs. CD16 plot, G (Pros: Promyelocytes, Myelocytes, Metas: metamyelocytes, Bands, Segs: segmented neutrophils). A different bone marrow specimen was stained with CD16-FITC, CD13-PE, and DRAQ-5, a quantitative DNA stain, here exhibited as a log scale (J). Cells that exhibit high levels of DNA corresponding to S, G-2, and M phases of the cell cycle are confined to the CD16-negative population of the maturing neutrophils, indicating that DNA synthesis stops at the same time as CD16 appears on the cell surface.

APC, allophycocyanin; FITC, fluorescein; PE, phycoerythrin; PerCP, peridinin chlorophyll protein.

the neutrophilic myeloid progenitor cells and the neutrophilic granular progenitor cells can also be observed in the decrease of expression of CD117 (data not shown).

The next stage of maturation, promyelocyte, is best defined phenotypically by a different set of reagents, HLA-DR and CD11b, in combination with high Side Scatter. The use of different combinations of reagents to assess distinct steps of development is analogous to changing the magnification on a microscope in order to better see a specific cellular morphology or the neighboring cells around a unique cell. Different reagent combinations can focus on different steps in the maturation of each lineage. Promyelocytes lack HLA-DR and CD11b, but exhibit high levels of Side Scatter and correspond to the next stage of development illustrated in Figure 5-8G. Promyelocytes, however, are not clearly identifiable by their expression of CD13 and CD16.

At the later stage of maturation when CD16 and CD13 are expressed together, the maturing neutrophils stop dividing. This can be observed in Figure 5-8J where a normal bone marrow specimen was stained for CD16-FITC, CD13PE, and DRAQ-5, a quantitative DNA stain (here displayed on a logarithmic scale). The only cells with the combined properties of high Side Scatter and DNA content greater than G1 lack expression of CD16, demonstrating that the coordinated expression of CD13 and CD16 in the second half of neutrophil maturation is also accompanied by the cessation of DNA synthesis.

The stages of neutrophil development defined by immunophenotype have direct correspondence to the developmental stages identified by morphology. Experiments using cell sorting demonstrated that the different steps of development each have homogeneous morphology and these corresponded to traditional maturational stages of neutrophil development identified by that morphology.

The complexity of gene product regulation underlying stepwise or quantized nature of hematopoietic development is illustrated in the schematic diagram shown in Figure 5-9. This diagram symbolizes

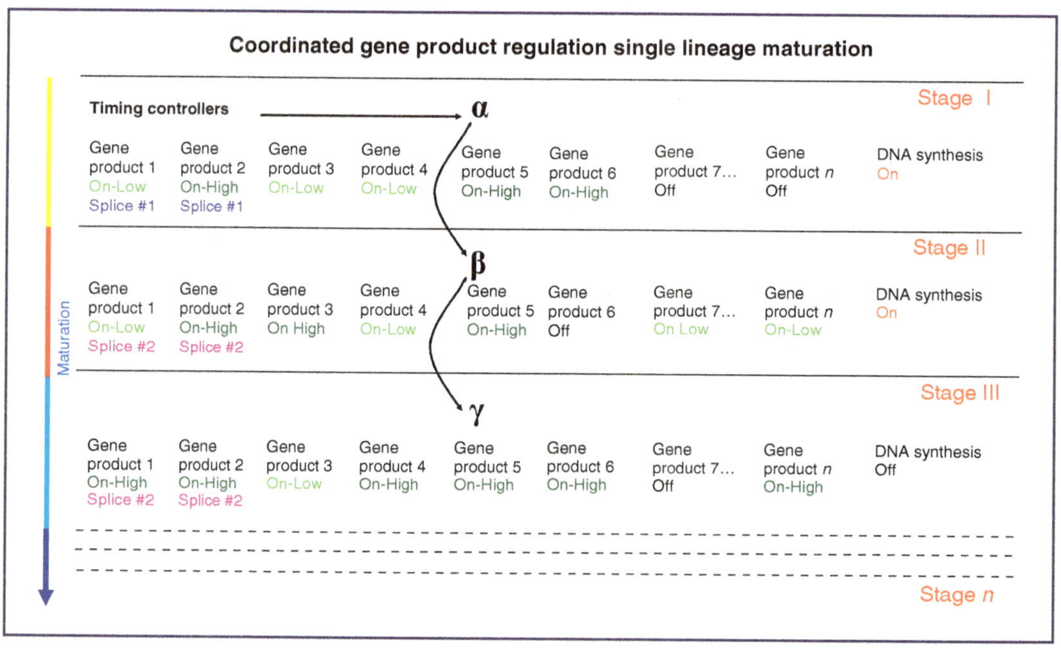

FIGURE 5-9: **Hypothetical processes required to result in stepwise maturation in a single lineage of cells. Once a cell becomes committed to a specific lineage, a "timing controller" (α, β, γ) regulates a group of genes to produce gene products at different amounts at a specific time during cellular maturation. Stepwise maturation requires changing the regulation of multiple gene products simultaneously by a new "timing controller," resulting in the coordination of diverse cellular processes, turning genes on or off, up- or down-regulating the amounts of gene products, changing splicing, and initiating or terminating DNA synthesis. At each step during the developmental process, a different "timing controller" links the multiple processes to occur at the same time.**

the maturation of a single lineage of cells after the commitment step. The first stage of maturation is characterized by a group of gene products (1–*n*) and DNA synthesis, all of which are all synchronously activated by a hypothetical "timing controller" α. Each gene product illustrated is expressed at a specific amount, with a specific isoform, for the sufficient allotted time required for the cells to mature sufficiently to move to the next state. After some predetermined period of time (or accumulation of some crucial component), the next stage is activated (Figure 5-9, Stage II). These groups of gene products change in concert to different amounts or different isoforms that are turned on or off, regulated by a new hypothetical timing controller, β. Again, the cells mature until a crucial component accumulates to trigger the next stage of development (Figure 5-9, Stage III). This group of gene products changes again in their expression as controlled by a third hypothetical timing controller, γ.

Although most of the genes studied by flow cytometry are cell surface antigens, cytoplasmic antigens such as TdT, myeloperoxidase, and CD79a also follow similar steps in quantitative regulation. It is not difficult to extrapolate these data to all cellular processes both external and internal, especially when the control of DNA synthesis is considered to also be regulated in coordination with the cell surface gene products.

The number of identifiable steps varies between cell lineages; the erythroid lineage appears to have only two stages, the B lymphoid cells have four stages, while the neutrophils exhibit seven stages. The cells at each of these stages are almost separate entities, with some similarities to the preceding and subsequent steps, but are unique in their repertoire of gene product expression.

The process of cellular maturation can be graphically illustrated by comparing the conceptual difference between a continuous model and a stepwise (quantized) model for cellular maturation (Figure 5-10). During normal development, hematopoiesis is a steady state with constant turnover of cells. The number of cells at any given maturational stage is the same in a steady state [$d(n)/d(t) = 0$]. In the continuous model, gene products a–f appear sequentially in the ever-broadening river depicting cellular division and expansion (Figure 5-10A). The observed kinetic data of hematopoiesis suggest a different model of maturation, akin to a series of pools connected by waterfalls (Figure 5-10B). In this graphical representation of B-cell development, multiple gene products are co-regulated at exactly the same time during development. The transitions between maturational stages are rapid and multivariable. The size of each pool is related to the time required for the cell to mature sufficiently to proceed to the next stage. The number of stages and the size of each pool differ from lineage to lineage. Cell division occurs within each pool or stops at the boundary between stages; for example, Stage III B cells are dividing, while Stage IV B cells are quiescent.

NEOPLASTIC TRANSFORMATION RESULTS IN DISRUPTION OF MATURATION

Once the normal pathways of cellular development were delineated based on quantitative gene product expression, comparisons between normal and neoplastic phenotypes were made. It was found that for both acute lymphoblastic leukemia (ALL) and acute myeloid leukemia (AML), the leukemia phenotypes did not fit into any part of the normal developmental sequence and therefore were not a frozen state of maturation (the dominant concept of cancer at the time of these studies). Instead, the phenotype of each leukemia exhibited aberrant relationships between cellular antigens, making them clearly different from their normal counterparts. *Leukemia is different from normal.* In addition, a comparison between different leukemia phenotypes showed that quantitative antigen expression was unique with regard to the absolute amounts of each antigen and their relationships to other lineage-associated gene products. Although similarities of phenotypes were identified, a detailed, quantitative comparison of multiple gene products showed that each leukemia was unique. **Each leukemia phenotype is different from every other leukemia.** These data show that the neoplastic transformation disrupts the precise regulation of gene products found in normal development and that the pathways to create these differences are highly variable even between similar types of leukemia.

Neoplastic transformation is not the result of a single mutational event, but requires multiple sequential genetic mutations to generate a cancerous cell. These genetic abnormalities can occur to any of the genes, promoters, splicing variants, or regulators that control the appropriate amounts of each of the

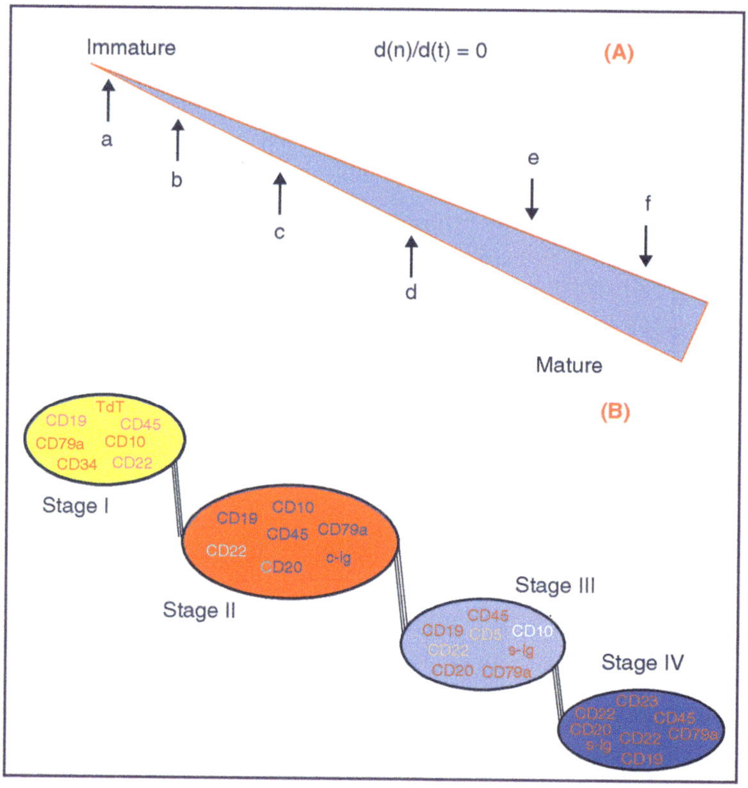

FIGURE 5-10: Schematic diagrams of maturation of cells assuming steady-state production. (A) Sequential appearance of different gene products (a–f) during development was the initial model analogous to a flowing river. However, the recognition that the multiple gene products are coordinated during the developmental process leads to a different schematic where multiple stages of development are recognizable and the transition between the stages is rapid. (B) The flow of B lymphoid cells from immature to mature is better represented by a series of pools and waterfalls than a flowing river. The colors of the stages illustrated here match those depicted in Figure 5-7.
TdT, terminal deoxynucleotidyl transferase.

specific gene products at the exact time of development, illustrated in Figure 5-9. The types of antigenic abnormalities observed in leukemia include lineage infidelity (lymphoid antigens on myeloid cells or vice versa), quantitative expression differences (over- or underexpression of antigens), antigenic absence (loss of an antigen that should be there), and antigenic asynchrony (immature antigens expressed on mature cells).

The underlying mechanisms for each of these phenotypic abnormalities can be deduced based on the maturational model illustrated in Figure 5-9. Lineage infidelity can arise on immature B cells (characteristic of precursor B ALL) if the regulators controlling the shutdown of either CD13 or CD33 are inhibited since these antigens are both present on the uncommitted progenitor cells, which is the maturational step just prior to the commitment to the B lineage. Detection of CD7 or CD19 on myeloid leukemia may result from the inappropriate activation of these antigens that should normally be quiescent during myeloid development. Quantitative antigen abnormalities can occur within each gene product or could be the result of a mutation that affects the hypothetical timing controllers. Antigenic absence, for example, absence of CD45 often observed on precursor B ALL, may be the result of that gene not being properly activated, or could result from improper splicing that occurs in the transition from the uncommitted progenitor cell to the earliest B-cell lineage precursor. Asynchronous antigen expression results from the loss of the regulator(s) that turns a specific early gene off. The large variability between phenotypes of leukemia reflects the accumulation of different genetic mutational events that can occur in any of the regulators, promoter regions, or structural genes affected in the generation of the leukemia. If any one of the numerous genes regulated during maturation receives a mutation or deletion that results in that gene product being improperly expressed, proper maturation may not proceed. The target of the mutational events may be more detrimental if they affect regulatory genes as compared to structural genes.

The progressive, sequential accumulation of genetic abnormalities observed during the evolution of myelodysplastic syndrome to acute myeloid leukemia provides a working hypothesis for the effect of additional mutations, illustrated schematically in Figure 5-11. The difference in gene product regulation between normal hematopoiesis and early MDS in this figure is depicted as a diminution of gene product D between Stages II and III and a loss of expression of gene product E. These abnormalities result in a decrease in production of the final, mature cells. The more mature cells are phenotypically abnormal as well as demonstrate dyspoiesis morphologically. These cells may coexist with normal hematopoietic cells in the early stages of MDS. A further accumulation of genetic abnormalities occurs over time in this scheme, resulting in hypothetical overexpression of gene product B and a loss of gene product C. These changes result in the accumulation of immature cells, observed as a shift to the left, with an increase in progenitor cells/blasts that may exceed the 20% threshold for the definition of AML. Maturation is not blocked, per se, but the cells are unable to properly mature. *De novo* AML may be the result of a more catastrophic genetic abnormality affecting multiple gene products such as might be expected if abnormalities occur in the hypothetical "timing controllers" (Figure 5-9).

Phenotypic heterogeneity, often observed in leukemia, can be ascribed to disruption of maturation rather than the presence of multiple clones. The intensity of CD34 provides a measure of maturation within the progenitor cell compartment, with the loss of this antigen marking commitment and maturation to one of several lineages. Three examples of maturational heterogeneity in AML are shown in Figure 5-12. Specimens A, B, and D were seen in sequence in the laboratory on the same day. Patient A was submitted on day 28 post-induction chemotherapy and exhibited normal maturation with no evidence of AML (comparable to Figure 5-8B). The diagnostic specimen for

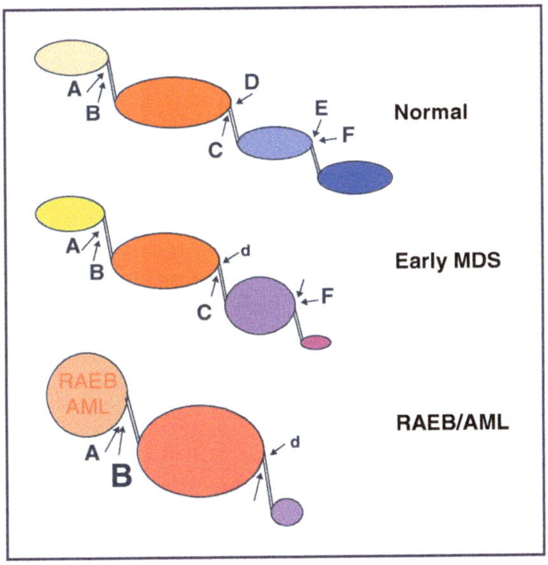

FIGURE 5-11: Schematic diagram illustrating the effect of mutations on the development of hematopoietic cells. In early myelodysplastic syndromes, the dysregulation of gene products is illustrated by a reduction in the amount of gene product D and loss of gene product E as compared to the schematic normal development shown in the top figure. Continued acquisition of mutations results in further changes in the regulation of gene products, resulting in the increase in immature, abnormal cells and the lack of normal development. Mutations that affect gene product expression can hypothetically occur in any of the genes or regulators illustrated in Figure 5-9.

MDS, myelodysplastic syndrome; RAEB/AML, refractory anemia with excess myeloblasts/acute myeloid leukemia.

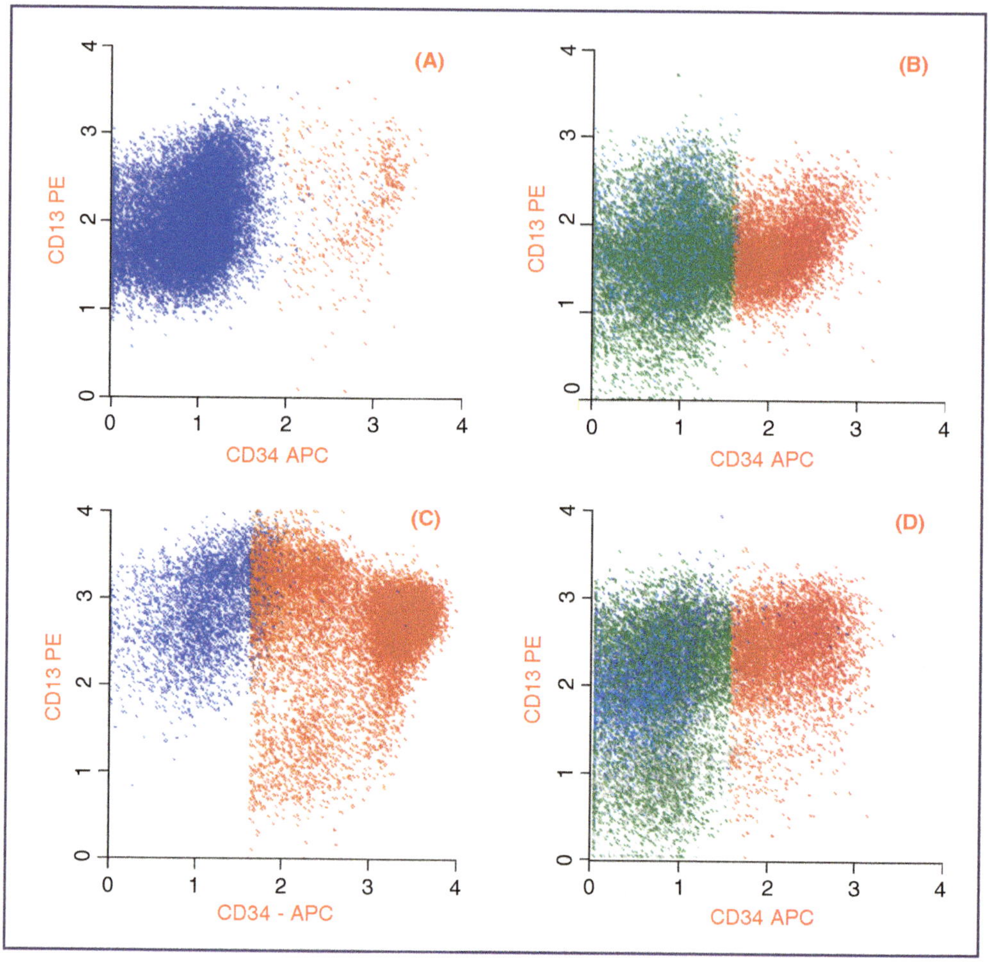

FIGURE 5-12: Comparison of antigen expression from three different acute myeloid leukemia patients (obtained in sequence on the same day). A patient at the end of induction #1 showed no evidence of residual disease (A) with 3.2% CD34-positive cells (Gating is identical to Figure 5-8B). The diagnostic specimen for this patient (C) demonstrated 37% abnormal myeloblasts with maturation to the neutrophil lineage (increasing CD13 and increased granularity, blue). In comparison, the diagnostic leukemia shown in (B) (62% abnormal myeloid progenitor cells) is maturing to monocytes with decreased CD13 and maturation to the monocyte region by CD45/log SSC (green dots). The diagnostic leukemia illustrated in (D) (50% abnormal myeloid progenitor cells) demonstrates maturation to both the monocytes and neutrophils, green and blue dots.

APC, allophycocyanin; PE, phycoerythrin.

this patient is shown in Figure 5-12C, where 37% of the bone marrow cells were leukemia, with abnormal maturation toward neutrophils as denoted by an increase in CD13 and some cells exhibiting granules identified by the blue dots. In contrast, the patient with a presumed diagnosis of AML is illustrated in Figure 5-12B, with 62% AML where the cells were maturing toward monocytes with a decrease in CD13 expression and an increase in CD45 consistent with abnormal monocyte development (green dots). The third patient, also a diagnostic specimen with 50% AML, exhibited abnormal development to both monocytes and neutrophils as indicated by both green and blue dots (Figure 5-12D).

The phenotypic heterogeneity observed among AML cases most often reflects abnormal maturation of AML when a comparison is made to the corresponding normal antigen expression. This can only be observed when quantitative antigen expression is used to define phenotypic differences. Using traditional flow cytometric techniques in which % positive cells are reported, leukemias B, C, and D are all the same with partial expression of CD34 with coexpression of CD13. By understanding the maturational sequence of these antigens, the differences and relationships in the diagnostic phenotypes can become readily apparent.

The importance of quantitative immunophenotyping can also be demonstrated in precursor B ALL (Figure 5-13). The normal maturational pattern of the B lymphoid cells is illustrated in Figure 5-13A. This specimen is different from the individual that is shown in Figure 5-7; however, the populations appear identical in both location and frequency. Three separate diagnostic specimens from patients with ALL are shown in Figure 5-13B, 5-13C, and 5-13D. Each leukemia specimen (leukemic cells shown in green) has a small proportion of normal developing B lymphoid cells that serve as an internal reference. In patient B, CD10 is highly overexpressed with some maturation observed by the expression of dim

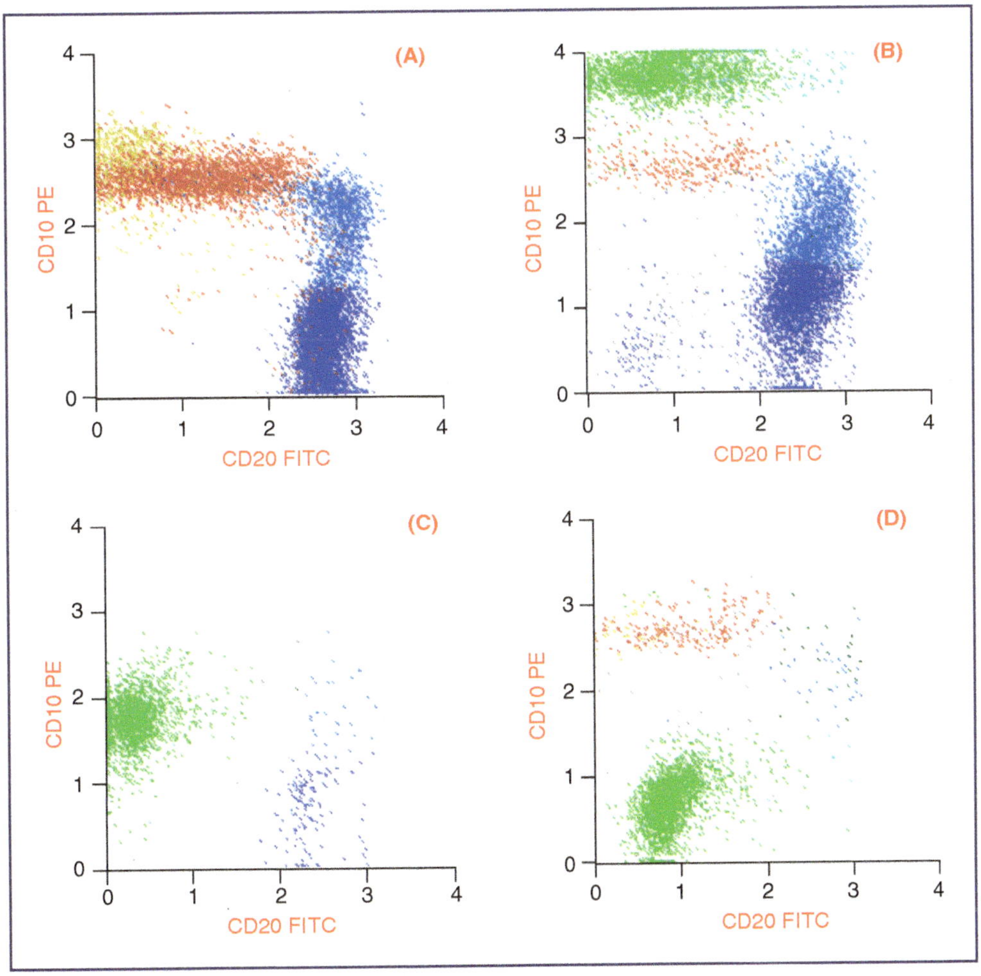

FIGURE 5-13: **Comparison of antigen expression of normal bone marrow (A) with three different acute lymphoblastic leukemia diagnostic specimens (B–D) stained with CD20-FITC/CD10-PE/CD45-PerCP/CD19-APC. Although the normal bone marrow looks like the specimen in Figure 5-7, it is from a different patient demonstrating the consistency of antigen intensities. The leukemia populations (green) are distinct from the normal cells that are also within the submitted bone marrow specimens, and which provide important quality control for the entire analytic process. The leukemia in B overexpresses CD10, while the leukemia in C underexpresses CD10, which is absent from leukemia D. CD20 is dimly expressed in B and D, while absent from C.**

FITC, fluorescein isothiocyanate; PE, phycoerythrin.

CD20. In patient C, CD10 is underexpressed without expression of CD20. In contrast, the leukemia in patient D does not express CD10 but does exhibit a low level of CD20. The scenarios for the mutational events that cause these different patterns can be hypothesized from the model illustrated in Figure 5-9. In patient B, the regulator of amount of CD10 is abnormally high, while CD20 is barely expressed. In patient C, the regulator of CD10 intensity is abnormally low with no triggering of maturation to Stage II. In contrast, in patient D, no CD10 is expressed but the cells are attempting to mature because of the dim expression of CD20. A more complete understanding of the process of neoplastic transformation can be made when the diagnostic phenotype is compared to the precise regulation observed for normal maturing cells within that same lineage.

SUMMARY

Quantitative antigen changes observed in maturing hematopoietic cells in normal bone marrow are reproducible, consistent from individual to individual, and independent of age or marrow stress. Pediatric and adult bone marrows exhibit identical phenotypic patterns as do patients who have undergone chemotherapy or even stem cell transplantation. Although the intensity relationships are the same, the proportions of cells in each maturational step may vary depending on the established steady state, age of the individual, or state of marrow stress with an attempt to return to steady state. The combined relationships of antigen expression suggest that the process of maturation is quantized: best identified as a series of steps, requiring coordination of multiple cellular processes. The maturational process for each lineage is denoted by coordinated gene product expression in which multiple antigens change in appearance or intensities at exactly the same times of development. The coordination of cellular events also involves a control of such diverse processes as DNA synthesis and m-RNA splicing. Neoplastic transformation variably affects this coordination of gene product regulation, resulting in acute leukemia with aberrant phenotypes that are unique for that leukemia. By linking detailed phenotypes with genotype it may be possible to unravel the precise effect that each mutational event contributes to the dysregulation of gene product expression, which may then lead to better treatment regimens for each individual patient.

Selected References

Foster JH, Hawkins DS, Loken MR, et al. Minimal residual disease detected prior to hematopoietic cell transplantation. *Pediatr Blood Cancer*. 2011;57:163–165.

Goasguin JE, Bennett JM, Cox C, et al. Prognostic implication and characterization of the blast cell population in the myelodysplastic syndrome. *Leuk Res*. 1991;15(12):1159–1165.

Hollander Z, Shah VO, Civin CI. Loken MR. Assessment of proliferation during maturation of the B lymphoid lineage in normal human bone marrow. *Blood*. 1988;71:528–531.

Horan PK, Loken MR. A practical guide for the use of flow systems in flow cytometry. In Van Dilla MA, ed. *Instrumentation and Data Analysis*. San Diego, CA. Academic Press. 1985;260–280.

Hurwitz CA, Loken MR, Graham ML, et al. Asynchronous antigen expression in B lineage acute lymphoblastic leukemia. *Blood*. 1988;72(1):299–307.

Loken MR. Residual disease in AML, a target that can move in more than one direction. *Cytometry B Clin Cytom*. 2014;86(1):15–17.

Loken MR, Alonzo TA, Pardo ML, et al. Residual disease detected by multidimensional flow cytometry signifies high relapse risk in patients with de novo acute myeloid leukemia: a report from the Children's Oncology Group. *Blood*. 2012;120(8):1581–1588.

Loken MR, Shah VO, Dattilio KL, Civin CI. Flow cytometric analysis of human bone marrow: II. Normal B lymphoid development. *Blood*. 1987;70:1316.

Loken MR, Shah VO, Dattilio KL, Civin CI. Flow cytometric characterization of human bone marrow: I. Normal Erythroid Development. *Blood*. 1987;69:255–263.

Loken MR, Terstappen LWMM, Civin CI, et al. Flow cytometric characterization of erythroid, lymphoid and monomyeloid lineages in normal human bone marrow. In: Laerum OD, Bjerksnes R, eds. *Flow Cytometry in Hematology*. New York, NY: Academic Press; 1992:31–42.

Loken MR, Wells DA. Normal antigen expression in hematopoiesis: Basis for interpreting leukemia phenotypes. In: Stewart C, Nicholson J, eds. *Immunophenotyping*. New York, NY: Wiley Liss, Inc; 2000:133–160.

Olweus J, Lund-Johanson F, Terstappen LWMM. CD64/FcgRi Is a granulo-monocytic lineage marker on CD34+ hematopoietic progenitor cells. *Blood*. 1995;85(9):2402–2413.

Salzman GC, Crowell JM, Martin JC, et al. Cell classification by laser light scattering: identification and separation of unstained leukocytes. *Acta Cytol*. 1975;19(4):374–377.

Shah VO, Civin CI, Loken MR. Flow cytometric analysis of human bone marrow: IV. Differential quantitative expression of T200 common leukocyte antigen during normal hematopoiesis. *J. Immunol.* 1988;140:1861–1867.

Shulman HM, Wells D, Gooley T, et al. The biologic significance of rare peripheral blasts after hematopoietic cell transplantation is predicted by multidimensional flow cytometry. *Am J Clin Pathol.* 1999;112(4):513–523.

Stelzer GT, Shults KE, Loken MR. CD45 Gating for routine flow cytometric analysis of human bone marrow specimens. *Ann NY Acad Sci*. 1993;677:265–280.

Streuli M, Hall LR, Saga Y, et al. Differential usage of three exons generates at least five different mRNAs encoding human leukocyte common antigens. *J Exp Med*. 1987;166(5):1548–1566.

Terstappen LWMM, Hollander Z, Meiners H, Loken M. Quantitative comparison of myeloid antigens on five lineages of mature peripheral blood cells. *J Leuk Biology*. 1990;48:138–148.

Terstappen LWMM, Huang S, Safford M, Lansdorp PM, Loken MR. Sequential generations of hematopoietic colonies derived from single nonlineage-committed CD34+CD38- progenitor cells. *Blood*. 1991;77:1218–1227.

Terstappen LWMM, Loken MR. Myeloid cell differentiation in normal bone marrow and acute myeloid leukemia assessed by multi-dimensional flow cytometry. *Anal Cell Path*. 1990;2(1):229–240.

Terstappen LWMM, Safford M, Konemann S, et al. Flow cytometric characterization of acute myeloid leukemia. Part II. Phenotypic heterogeneity at diagnosis. *Leukemia*. 1992;6(1):70–80.

Terstappen LWMM, Safford M, Loken MR. Flow cytometric analysis of human bone marrow: III. Neutrophil maturation. *Leukemia*. 1990;4:657–663.

Thomas ML, Lefrançois L. Differential expression of the leucocyte-common antigen family. *Immunol Today*. 1988;9(10):320–326.

Wells DA, Sale GE, Shulman HE, et al. Multidimensional flow cytometry of marrow can differentiate leukemic lymphoblasts from normal lymphoblasts and myeloblasts following chemotherapy and/or bone marrow transplant. *Am J Clin Path*. 1998;110(1):84–94.

Minimal Residual Disease (MRD) in Acute Lymphoblastic Leukemia (ALL): An Important Prognostic Indicator and Efficacy/Response Biomarker in Children and Adults

Gregory H. Reaman and Franklin O. Smith III

Multiple reports during the past decade demonstrate that detection of minimal residual disease (MRD) at an early time point (ie, during/following induction or consolidation therapy) is a powerful and independent prognostic indicator of prolonged event-free survival (EFS) in children and adults with acute lymphoblastic leukemia (ALL). In most cases of children with ALL treated with current, state-of-the-science, multiagent chemotherapy regimens, early detection of MRD has surpassed in importance other widely used and accepted prognostic indicators. As a prognostic biomarker, assessment of MRD has had a profound impact worldwide on the design and conduct of risk-adjusted clinical trials in ALL for all risk groups of patients, currently defined by long-standing, accepted clinical and biological prognostic factors.

As standardized methodologies for MRD detection have improved, the evaluation of MRD as an in vivo marker of early therapeutic efficacy has allowed for the allocation of patients to different risk-based treatments in an attempt to both improve outcome and mitigate the risk of short- and long-term toxicity of therapy (Table 5-1).

Early response to treatment is increasingly being measured by assessing the number of residual ALL cells by their clonal rearrangement of immunoglobulin (Ig) and T-cell receptor (TcR) genes, fusion gene expression, and/or leukemia-associated immunophenotype (LAIP). Sensitive methods (ie, 1 leukemia cell in 10,000 to 100,000 normal cells in a clinical sample) for detection of MRD using assays based on the real-time, quantitative polymerase chain reaction (RQ-PCR) and/or flow cytometry (FCM) are being used to risk stratify patients on therapeutic trials designed to adapt treatment for individual patients relative to their risk for treatment failure. More recently, next-generation sequencing (NGS) techniques

Table 5-1 Characteristics of the three classical MRD methods

MRD TECHNIQUE	ESTIMATED SENSITIVITY	APPLICABILITY	ADVANTAGES	DISADVANTAGES
RQ-PCR of IG/TR genes or breakpoint regions of fusion transcripts	10^{-4}–10^{-5}	BCP-ALL: 95% T-ALL: 90%–95%	Applicable in virtually all BCP-ALL and T-ALL. Sensitive. Well standardized + regular international QA rounds.	Time-consuming. Expensive. Requires extensive experience and knowledge.
RQ-PCR of fusion transcripts and other aberrances	10^{-4}–10^{-6}	BCP-ALL: 25%–40% (age dependent) T-ALL: 10%–15%	Relatively easy. Sensitive. Applicable for specific leukemia subgroups, such as BCR-ABL or MLL-AF4.	Limited standardization (only harmonization). Limited QA rounds (with conversion factors). Limited applicability in ALL (absence of targets in >50% of cases). Risk of contamination
Conventional flow cytometry	3–4 colors: 10^{-3}–10^{-4} 6–8 colors: 10^{-4}	BCP-ALL: >90% T-ALL: >90%	Fast analysis at cell population level or single cell level. Easy storage of data. Information about the whole sample cellularity.	Variable sensitivity, because of similarities between normal (regenerating) cells and malignant cells. Limited standardization, no QA results.

Source: Adapted from van Dongen JJ, van der Velden VH, Brüggemann M, Orfao A. Minimal residual disease diagnostics in acute lymphoblastic leukemia: need for sensitive, fast, and standardized technologies. *Blood.* 2015;125:3996–4009.

ALL, acute lymphoblastic leukemia; BCP, B-cell precursor; IG/TR, immunoglobulin/T-receptor; MLL, mixed lineage leukemia; MRD, minimal residual disease; QA, quality assurance; RQ-PCR, real-time quantitative polymerase chain reaction.

measuring immunoglobulin heavy chain (IgH)-variable diversity, joining (V[D]J), or T-cell receptor clonal rearrangements have been introduced. This methodology expands the sensitivity of MRD measurement from 1 in 10^4 to 10^5 to 1 in 10^7 cells and is predictive of relapse in children with ALL. However, it is not yet clear whether this increased sensitivity has immediate implications for prognosis and risk classification. Finally, in the setting of minimal disease burden following allogeneic hematopoietic stem cell transplantation (HSCT), early MRD assessed using NGS appears highly predictive of relapse and poor survival. The decisions for selection of one methodology over another are complex and dependent on a number of factors. Detailed descriptions of these methodologies are provided in Chapter 2.

CLINICAL SIGNIFICANCE OF MRD DETECTION

Early response to therapy has traditionally been one of the most important prognostic factors in children with ALL. As a predictor of outcome, early response encompasses host factors, biology of the leukemia, and the specifics of treatment. Early response can be assessed by the reduction/absence of leukemic cells in the bone marrow (measured morphologically) at early time points during multiagent induction therapy, by the clearance of leukemic blasts in the peripheral blood with a 1-week prednisone prophase, and more recently using sensitive techniques to detect MRD. More sensitive measure of early response by assessment of MRD using FCM and PCR techniques to identify Ig/TcR rearrangements or fusion transcripts have provided unequivocal evidence of the prognostic importance of MRD levels determined at an early time point in therapy.

The importance of MRD as a prognostic indicator has also been evaluated in T-cell ALL. In the AEIOP-BFM 2000 study, patients with T-cell ALL were observed to have delayed kinetics of MRD clearance

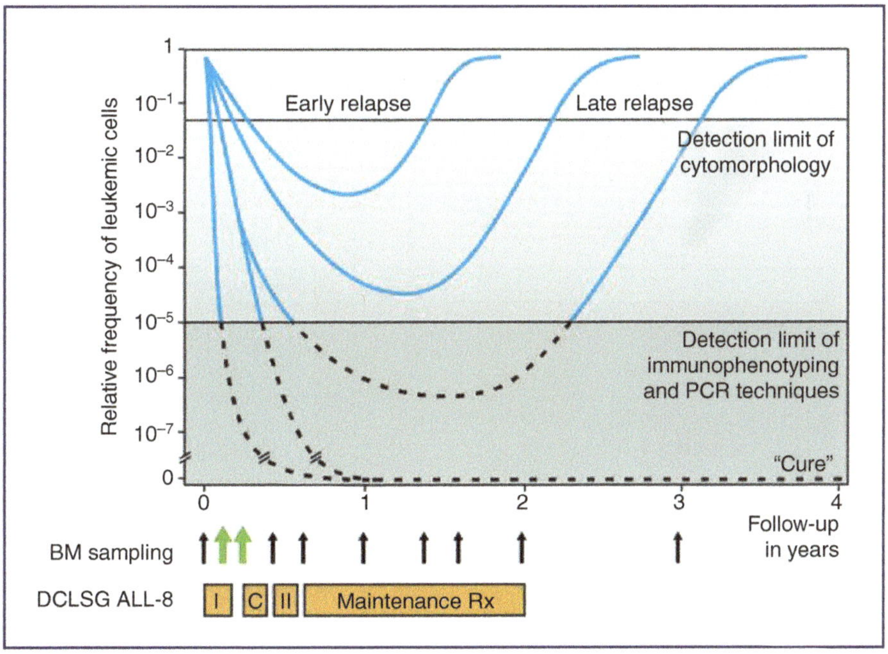

FIGURE 5-14: Detection of MRD during follow-up of ALL patients. Schematic diagram of relative frequencies of ALL cells in bone marrow during and after treatment. Detection limits of cytomorphology and immunophenotyping and PCR techniques are presented.

Source: **Republished with permission of American Society Of Hematology from van Dongen JJ, van der Velden VH, Brüggemann M, Orfao A. Minimal residual disease diagnostics in acute lymphoblastic leukemia: need for sensitive, fast, and standardized technologies. *Blood.* 2015;125:3996–4009.**

ALL, acute lymphoblastic leukemia; BM, bone marrow; C, consolidation treatment; I, induction treatment; II, reinduction treatment; MRD, minimal (or measurable) residual disease; PCR, polymerase chain reaction.

when compared to B precursor ALL patients. Nonetheless, negative MRD levels at either/both days 33 and 78 were highly predictive of a favorable outcome. Only 16% of T-cell ALL patients were MRD negative at day 33 and experienced a relapse rate of 7%; 32% of patients who were MRD positive at day 33 achieved negative MRD levels by day 78. This group had a relapse rate of 9%.

In the largest prospective evaluation of more than 3,000 patients enrolled in the AIEOP-BFM 2000 study, MRD detected by standardized and centralized RQ-PCR analysis at two specific early time points, day 33 and day 78, was highly predictive of relapse, replacing nearly all of the conventional clinical and biological factors currently used. Only the known adverse cytogenetic features, hypodiploidy, t(4;11), and t(9;22), remained independently poor prognostic factors. Absence of MRD by RQ-PCR at the end of induction was the strongest predictor for an excellent outcome (5-year EFS >90%). The investigation of early (day 15) MRD by FCM in a series of more than 800 patients by the AEIOP group suggests that early MRD clearance identifies a group of patients with an excellent outcome (5-year EFS >95%). The kinetics

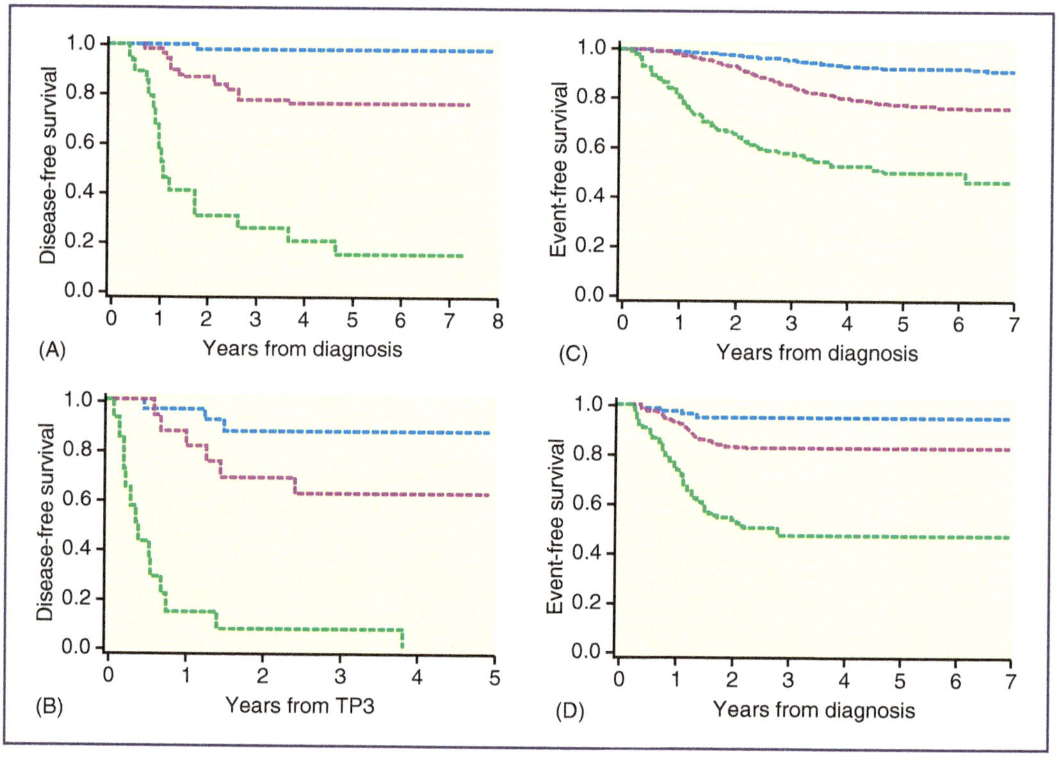

FIGURE 5-15: **Long-term follow-up in childhood ALL patients, based on MRD measurements. (A) Disease-free survival (DFS) of 129 patients classified according to three MRD-based risk groups in the International BFM study; low risk, no MRD detected at day 33 and day 78 (blue dashed line); high risk MRD >10^{-3} at day 78 (green dashed line); intermediate risk, MRD <10^{-3} at day 78 (purple dashed line). (B) DFS of 54 infants with ALL treated according to the INTERFANT-99 protocol; low risk, MRD <10^{-4} at all time points (blue dashed line); high risk, MRD >10^{-4} at week 22 (green dashed line). (C) EFS of 3,184 B-cell precursor (BCP) patients in the AIEOP-BFM 2000 study. Standard risk (SR), if no MRD detected at days 33 and 78 (blue dashed line); intermediate risk (MR), MRD positive at day 33 and/or day 78 but <10^{-3} at day 78 (purple dashed line); high risk (HR), MRD >10^{-3} at day 78 (green dashed line). (D) EFS of 464 T-ALL patients of the AIEOP-BFM 2000 study. SR, MR, HR as for BCP patients in (C).**

Source: Adapted from van Dongen JM, van der Velden VHJ, Bruggemann M, et al. Minimal residual disease diagnostics in acute lymphoblastic leukemia; need for sensitive, fast, and standardized technologies. *Blood.* 2015;125:3996–4009.

AIEOP, Associazione Italiana Ematologia Oncologia Pediatric Group; ALL, acute lymphoblastic leukemia; BFM, Berlin-Frankfurt-Munster Group; EFS, event-free survival; MRD, minimal residual disease.

of MRD clearance, assessed by changes in MRD level between days 33 and 78, also demonstrated predictive ability; persistent low levels of MRD beyond consolidation also portend a poor outcome.

In the COG study P9900, MRD assessed by FCM in peripheral blood at day 8 and bone marrow at day 29 (end of induction) in nearly 2,000 patients predicted long-term EFS. Informative end-induction MRD results with a sensitivity of 0.01% performed in a central reference laboratory were available for 92% of patients within 48 hours of specimen receipt. End-induction MRD level was highly prognostic, with 5-year EFS of 88% ± 1%, 59% ± 5%, and 30% ± 8% for MRD levels of 0.01%–0.1%, 0.1%–1%, and greater than 1%, respectively. These results confirmed a threshold of 0.01% as the optimal cutoff level for risk stratification in risk-adjusted treatment studies. End-induction MRD was again found to be the most important prognostic variable in multivariate analysis. Current risk stratification in COG ALL studies of low-risk B-cell precursor ALL includes both day 8 peripheral blood and day 29 bone marrow MRD. This approach now defines a group of patients with a predicted 5-year EFS exceeding 95%.

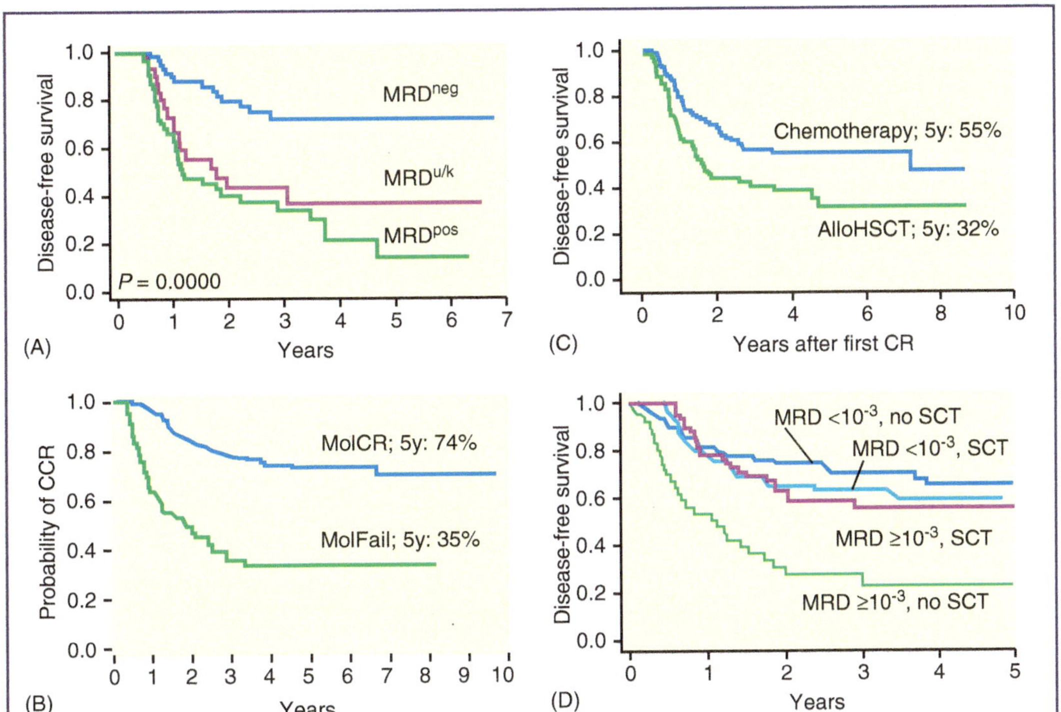

FIGURE 5-16: Results of prospective clinical trials for Philadelphia chromosome negative ALL classified by MRD detection. (A) DFS stratified by MRD levels at weeks 16 and 22. MRD^{neg}, <10^{-4} at week 16 and no detectable MRD at week 22, MRD^{pos}, all others with evaluable results, MRD$^{u/k}$, MRD risk class unknown. (B) Probability of continuous complete remission (CR) stratified by MRD at week 16; MolCR, MRD negativity with an assay sensitivity of greater than 10^{-4}; MolFail, quantifiable MRD positivity >10^{-4}. (C) DFS for high risk patients stratified by intention to treat (ITT) with chemotherapy compared with allogeneic hematopoietic stem cell transplantation (AlloHSCT) patients for early morphologic response but with post-consolidation flow cytometric MRD (weeks 16–18). Patients were assigned to chemotherapy if <10% marrow blasts on day 14 and flow MRD < 5 × 10^{-4} (weeks 16–18) and to AlloHSCT if >10% marrow blasts on day 14 and/or flow MRD > 5 × 10^{-4} weeks (16–18). (D) Relapse-free survival (RFS) according to MRD at week 6 and type of post-CR treatment (AlloHSCT vs. no AlloHSCT) in high risk patients with Philadelphia chromosome negative ALL.

Source: Adapted from van Dongen JM, van der Velden VHJ, Bruggemann M, et al. Minimal residual disease diagnostics in acute lymphoblastic leukemia; need for sensitive, fast, and standardized technologies. *Blood*. 2015;125:3996–4009.

ALL, acute lymphoblastic leukemia; CCR, conventional care regimen; CR, complete remission; DFS, disease-free survival; MRD, minimal residual disease; SCT, stem cell transplantation.

There is increasing evidence for the prognostic significance of early MRD detection in adults with ALL treated with intensive, multiagent regimens similar to those utilized in the pediatric population. This has been clearly demonstrated especially, by the German Multicenter ALL (GMALL) Group. The finding of MRD levels less than 0.01% within the first 3 weeks of therapy was associated with a 3-year relapse rate of 0%, in contrast to a 94% relapse rate in patients with persistent MRD levels of 0.01% up to week 16 of therapy. The use of early MRD assessment in risk stratification of adult patients with ALL treated with modern multiagent chemotherapy on clinical trials of the GMALL study group and the Northern Italy Leukaemia Group (NILG) have resulted in marked improvement in long-term outcomes for adult patients. In addition, results of the ALL 4-2002 study of the Polish Adult Leukemia Group demonstrated the independent prognostic value of end-induction MRD assessed by multiparametric FCM.

Negative early MRD levels appear to have prognostic significance in the setting of first hematological relapse and in isolated extramedullary relapse. Negative MRD levels prior to HSCT in both patients with relapsed disease and in those transplanted in first remission are associated with superior relapse-free survival when compared to the outcomes of patients with persistent MRD positivity at the time of transplant. Extending the predictive utility of post-induction MRD to treatment planning and decision making, incorporating specific transplantation strategies, provides a rationale for future clinical investigations and confirms the role of MRD as a useful biomarker for in vivo response to therapy.

ROLE OF MRD AS A DRUG DEVELOPMENT TOOL IN ALL (SEE ALSO CHAPTER 9)

The evidence base to indicate that early MRD status is the strongest predictor of long-term EFS in ALL is unequivocal. The magnitude of the importance of its current, critical role in risk stratification for treatment decisions has raised the consideration of its potential as a surrogate end point for clinical trials of investigational therapeutic interventions. The significant increase in sensitivity afforded by accepted techniques to assess MRD compared to standard techniques to define objective response and complete remission in this disease could influence future considerations and standards for response assessment and hasten the development timeline for new drugs and biologics for ALL. The use of an early response biomarker in evaluating early interventions based on increased risk could afford a new strategy for leukemia drug development. Adopting an important prognostic biomarker and a reliable response biomarker as a surrogate for new agent efficacy requires a large retrospective meta-analysis or careful prospective evaluation in future controlled trials to confirm the predictive ability of MRD for later traditional end points of EFS and OS and standardization of sensitive techniques for which exacting performance standards have been established.

Selected References

Attarbaschi A, Mann G, Panzer-Grumayer R, et al. Minimal residual disease values discriminate between low and high relapse risk in children with B-cell acute lymphoblastic leukemia and intrachromosomal amplification of chromosome 21: the Austrian and German acute lymphoblastic leukemia Berlin-Frankfurt-Muenster (ALL-BFM) trials. *J Clin Oncol*. 2008;26:3046–3050.

Bader P, Kreyenberg H, Henze G, et al. Prognostic value of minimal residual disease quantification before allogeneic stem cell transplantation in relapsed childhood acute lymphoblastic leukemia: the ALL-REZ BFM Study Group. *J Clin Oncol*. 2009;27:377–384.

Bassan R, Hoeltzer D. Modern therapy of acute lymphoblastic leukemia. *J Clin Oncol*. 2011;29:532–543.

Bassan R, Spinelli O, Oldani E, et al. Improved risk classification for risk-specific therapy based on the molecular study of minimal residual disease in adult acute lymphoblastic leukemia. *Blood*. 2009;113:4153–4162.

Basso G, Veltroni M, Valsecchi MG, et al. Risk of relapse of childhood acute lymphoblastic leukemia is predicted by flow cytometric determination of residual disease on day 15 bone marrow. *J Clin Oncol*. 2009;27:5168–5174.

Borowitz MJ, Wood BL, Devidas M, et al. Prognostic significance of minimal residual disease in high risk B-ALL: a report from the Children's Oncology Group study AALL0232. *Blood*. 2015;126:964–971.

Campana D. Minimal residual disease in acute lymphoblastic leukemia. *Hematology*. 2010;2010:7–12.

Cave H, van der Werff ten Bosch J, Suciu S, et al. Clinical significance of minimal residual disease in childhood acute lymphoblastic leukemia. European Organization for Research and the Treatment of Cancer–Childhood Leukemia Cooperative Group. *N Engl J Med*. 1998;339:591–598.

Cazzaniga G, Valsecchi MG, Gaipa G, et al. Defining the correct role of minimal residual disease tests in the management of acute lymphoblastic leukemia. *Br J Haematol*. 2011;155:45–52.

Conter V, Bartram CR, Valsecchi MG, et al. Molecular response to treatment redefines all prognostic factors in children and adolescents with B-cell precursor aciute lymphoblastic leukemia: results in 3184 children in the AEIOP-BFM ALL 2000 study. *Blood*. 2010;115:3206–3214.

Coustan-Smith E, Campana D. Immunological minimal residual disease detection in acute lymphoblastic leukemia: a comparative approach to molecular testing. *Best Pract Res Clin Haematol*. 2010;23:347–358.

Flohr T, Schrauder A, Cazzaniga G, et al. Minimal residual disease-directed risk stratification using real time quantitative PCR analysis of immunoglobulin and T-cell receptor gene rearrangements in the international multicenter trial AEIOP-BFM 2000 for childhood acute lymphoblastic leukemia. *Leukemia*. 2008;22:771–782.

Foster JH, Hawkins DS, Loken MR, et al. Minimal residual disease detected prior to hematopoietic cell transplantation. *Pediatr Blood Cancer*. 2011;57:163–165.

Gaynon PS, Bleyer WA, Steinherz PG, et al. Day 7 marrow response and outcome for children with acute lymphoblastic leukemia and unfavorable presenting features. *Med Pediatr Oncol*. 1990;11:2234–2242.

Paganin M, Zecca M, Fabbri G, et al. Minimal residual disease is an important predictive factor of outcome in children with relapsed "high risk" acute lymphoblastic leukemia. *Leukemia*. 2008;22:2193–2200.

Pui CH, Campana D, Pei D, et al. Treating childhood acute lymphoblastic leukemia without cranial irradiation. *N Engl J Med*. 2009;360:2730–2741.

Pulsipher MA, Carlson C, Langholz B, et al. IgH-V(D)J NGS MRD measurement pre- and early post-allotransplant defines very low- and very high-risk ALL patients. *Blood*. 2015;125:3501–3508.

Riehm H, Gadner H, Henze G, et al. Results and significance of six randomized trials in four consecutive ALL-BFM studies. *Haematol Blood Transf*. 1990;33:439–450.

Schmiegelow K, Forestier E, Hellebostad M, et al. Long-term results of NOPHO ALL-92 and ALL-2000 studies of childhood acute lymphoblastic leukemia. *Leukemia*, 2010;24:345–354.

Stow P, Key L, Chen X, et al. Clinical significance of low levels of minimal residual disease at the end of remission induction therapy in childhood acute lymphoblastic leukemia. *Blood*. 2010;115:4657–4663.

van der Velden VH, Corral L, Valsecchi MG, et al. Prognostic significance of minimal residual disease in infants with acute lymphoblastic leukemia treated within the Interfant-99 protocol. *Leukemia*. 2009;23:1073–1079.

van Dongen JM, van der Velden VHJ, Bruggemann M, et al. Minimal residual disease diagnostics in acute lymphoblastic leukemia; need for sensitive, fast, and standardized technologies. *Blood*. 2015;125:3996–4009.

Wilemse MY, Seriu T, Hettinger K, et al. Detection of minimal residual disease identifies differences in treatment response between T-ALL and precursor B-ALL. *Blood*, 2002;99:4386–4393.

Sequence-Specific MRD for ALL

Aaron C. Logan

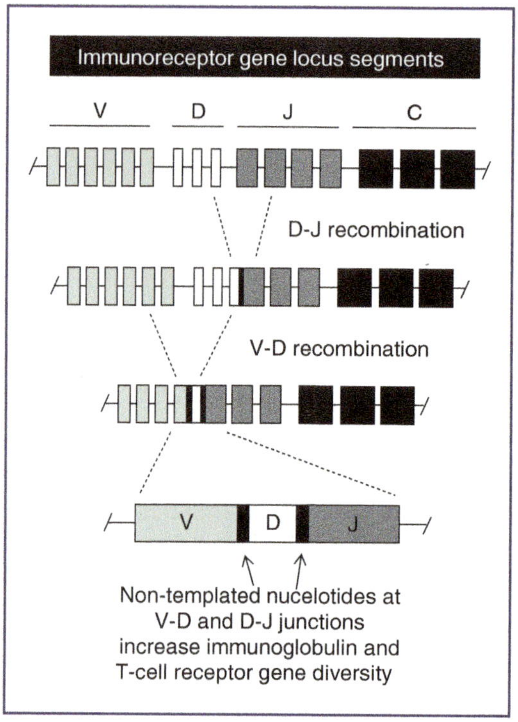

FIGURE 5-17: The immunoreceptor loci are composed of gene segments which undergo rearrangement to create a unique contiguous coding sequence. In this example, the immunoglobulin heavy chain locus is demonstrated, with Variable, Diversity, Joining, and Constant segments that are sequentially brought together in the process of VDJ recombination. Additional diversity in VDJ sequences arise from non-templated nucleotide insertions and deletions at the V-D and D-J junctions.

VDJ, variable, diversity, and joining.

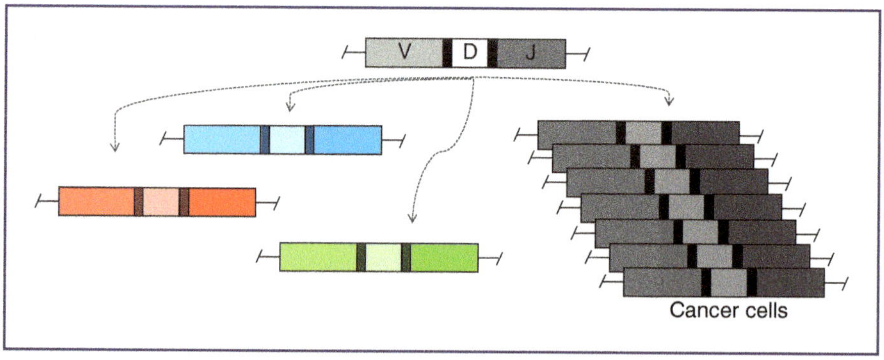

FIGURE 5-18: Each lymphocyte bears a unique VDJ sequence, or clonotype, in one or more of its immunoreceptor genes. When a lymphocyte population expands clonally, such as in a lymphoid malignancy, the overrepresentation of that population's unique VDJ clonotype within the immunoreceptor repertoire can be quantified. The malignancy-specific VDJ clonotype(s) can be used for subsequent quantification of malignant cells during the course of treatment.

VDJ, variable, diversity, and joining.

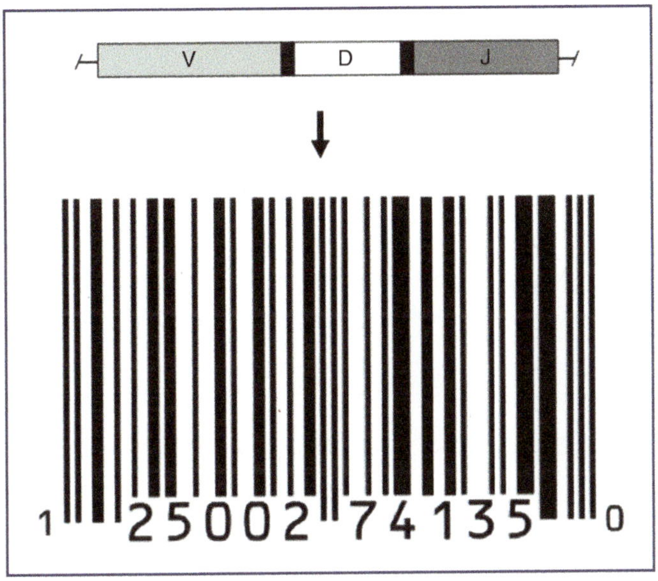

FIGURE 5-19: The unique VDJ clonotype(s) within a lymphoid malignancy can be thought of as naturally occurring genetic barcodes which can be used to quantify disease burden.

VDJ, variable, diversity, and joining.

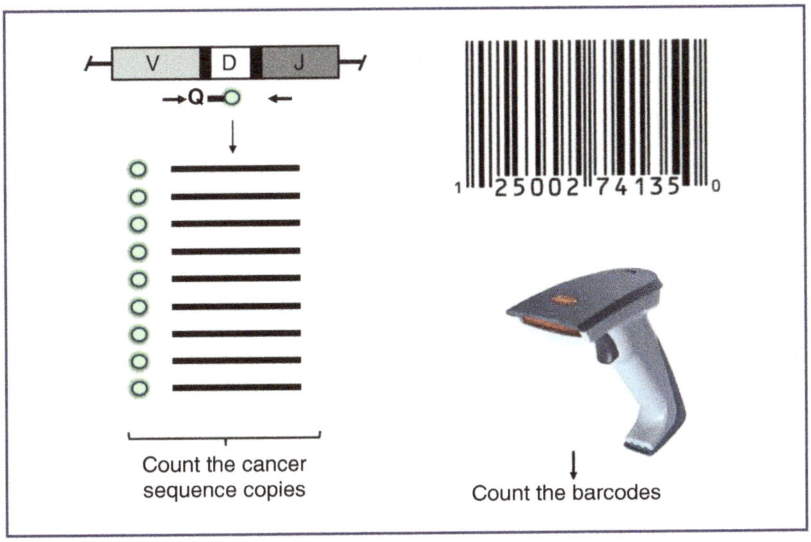

FIGURE 5-20: Allele-specific oligonucleotide (ASO)-PCR is a ***patient-specific*** barcode reader. ASO-PCR utilizes quantitative PCR methods to enumerate the number of specific VDJ clonotype templates present in a clinical DNA sample. This process relies on specific primers (arrows) and a quencher (Q)-bound probe that anneal to a patient's malignancy-specific VDJ sequence. Each time a copy of the VDJ clonotype is made, the quencher is released from the fluorophore, allowing the thermocycler to detect each copy as it is produced. In this way, ASO-PCR is analogous to a VDJ barcode counter. This method is highly sensitive and specific, but the need for patient-specific assays is costly and laborious.

PCR, polymerase chain reaction; VDJ, variable, diversity, and joining.

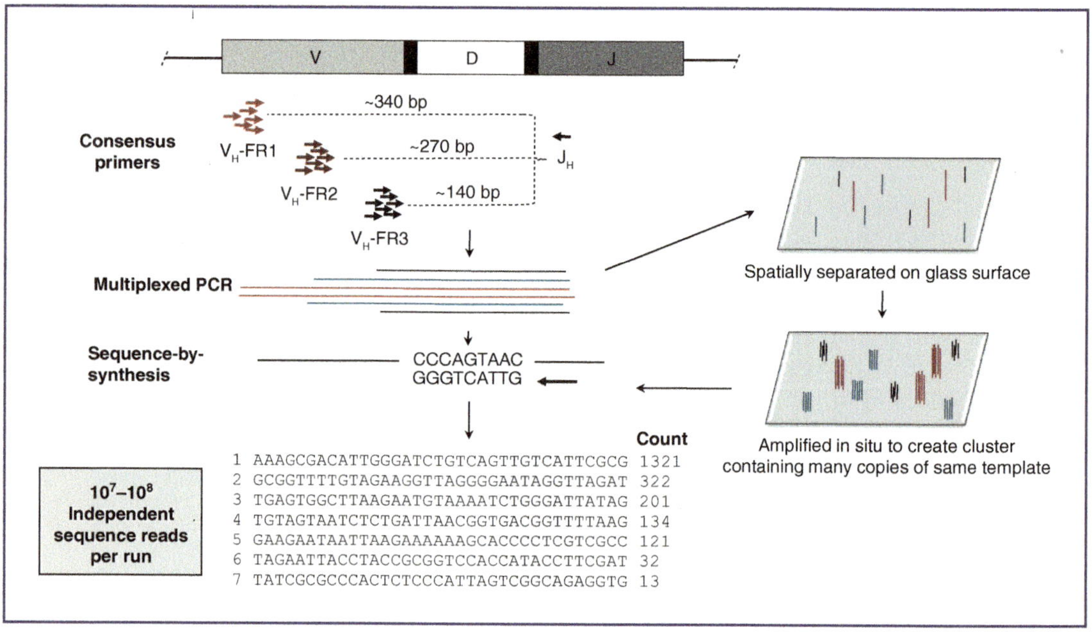

FIGURE 5-21: **NGS quantification of MRD utilizes mixtures of consensus primers (arrows) that facilitate amplification of the entire repertoire of a specific immunoreceptor's VDJ region. No patient-specific reagents are required. The amplimers resulting from multiplexed PCR are then spatially separated by fixation on a glass plate (eg, in an Illumina sequencer) and amplified in situ to create clusters. Each cluster is then sequenced by synthesis during a process in which solutions of individual nucleotides bound to fluorophores are sequentially flowed across the glass plate (flow cell). Each time a nucleotide is added in a template-directed manner, a fluorophore is released and quantified by the sequencer, yielding a sequence for each cluster. Tens or hundreds of thousands of sequences can be simultaneously determined and quantified using this NGS method, yielding a quantitative assessment of the immunoreceptor repertoire.**

MRD, minimal residual disease; NGS, next-generation sequencing; PCR, polymerase chain reaction; VDJ, variable, diversity, and joining.

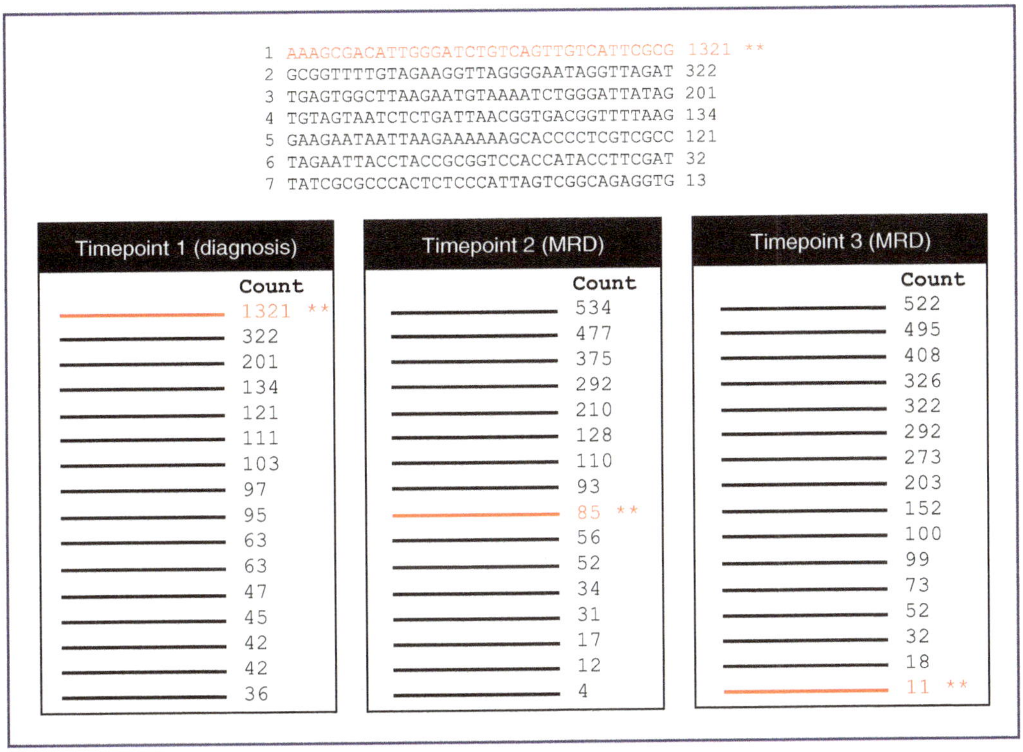

FIGURE 5-22: **Once a dominant VDJ clonotype (**) is identified at the time of diagnosis of a lymphoid malignancy (Timepoint 1), using the NGS platform, the presence of that same clonotype can be enumerated within the VDJ repertoire at subsequent timepoints through the course of therapy, thus serving as a means for quantifying MRD.**

MRD, minimal residual disease; NGS, next-generation sequencing; VDJ, variable, diversity, and joining.

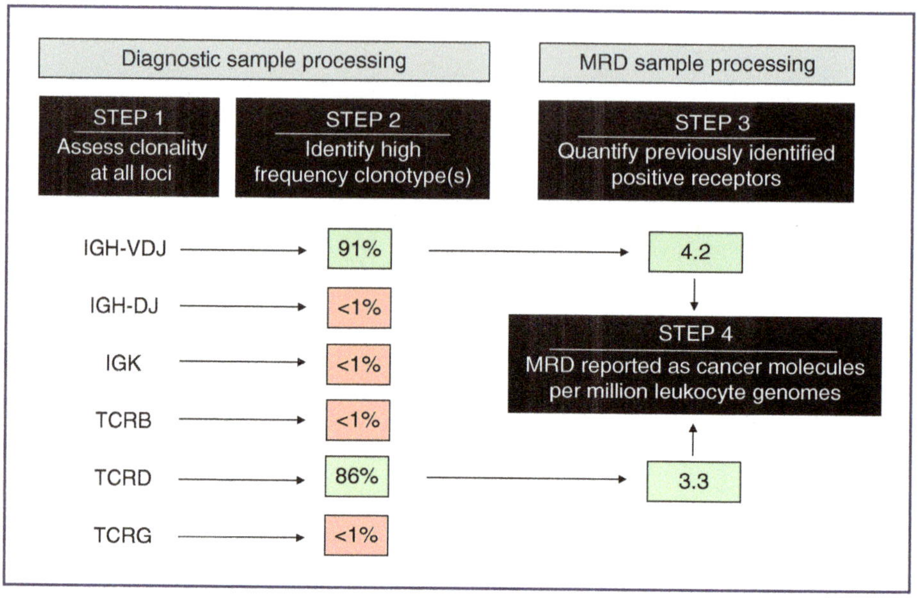

FIGURE 5-23: The NGS approach for MRD quantification relies on assessment of clonality at one or more immunoreceptor gene loci in a diagnostic specimen. Consensus primers for multiple loci can be used to assess clonality, including the IGH, with complete VDJ or partial DJ rearrangements; the immunoglobulin light chain kappa (IGK); and TCRB, delta (TCRD), and gamma (TCRG) loci. The high frequency clonotype(s) marking the malignant cell population identified in a diagnostic specimen are recorded for subsequent MRD quantification in which the repertoire of the malignancy-specific immunoreceptor loci are again sequenced, and the number of malignancy specific molecules are determined.

IGH, immunoglobulin heavy chain; MRD, minimal residual disease; NGS, next-generation sequencing; TCRB, T-cell receptors beta; VDJ, variable, diversity, and joining.

Measurable Residual Disease for AML

Christopher S. Hourigan and Aaron C. Logan

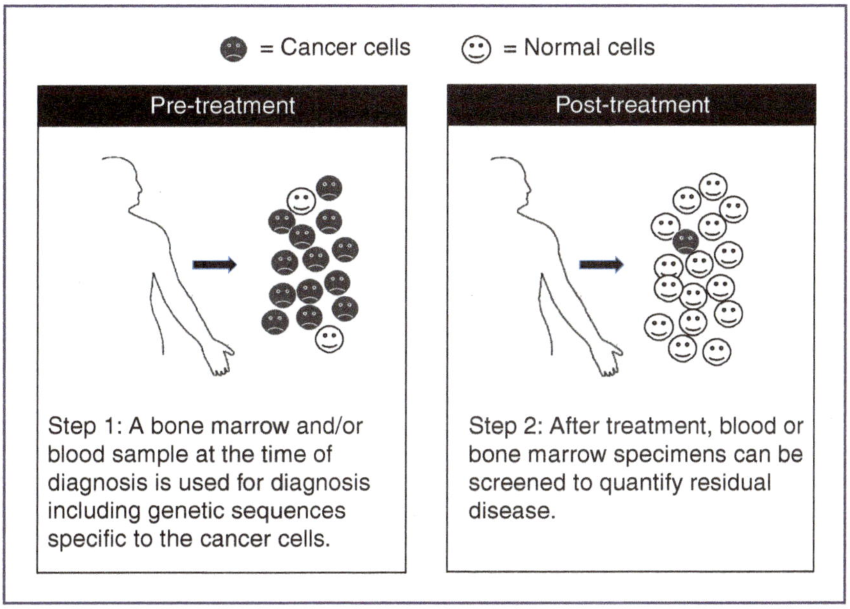

FIGURE 5-24

STANDARD CRITERIA FOR COMPLETE REMISSION HAS CHANGED LITTLE OVER TIME DESPITE DEVELOPMENT OF BETTER TECHNOLOGY FOR DETECTING AML

Table 5-2 Evolution of criteria for complete remission in adult patients with AML

RESPONSE CRITERIA	1956	2012
Bone marrow	Less than 5% blasts and absence of cells that can be individually identified as leukaemic	Less than 5% blasts including no blasts with Auer rods
Extramedullary disease	Subsidence of all evidence of leukaemic infiltration	No residual evidence of extramedullary disease
Platelets	>100,000	>100,000
Neutrophil count	>200/mm^3	>1,000/mcL
Haemoglobin	>12 gm/d1 for 1 month	Transfusion-free
Clinical	No symptoms attributable to leukaemia	

An additional category of cytogenetics normal in those with previously abnormal cytogenetics is listed, but not required, for a morphological complete response in the complete remission category of 2012 National Comprehensive Cancer Network guidelines and is "commended primarily for use in clinical research studies" in the current International Working Group criteria that those guidelines are based on. There is evidence, however, that persistence of cytogenetic abnormalities in patients with AML in complete remission is associated with a worse prognosis.
Source: From Hourigan CS, Karp JE. Minimal residual disease in acute myeloid leukaemia. *Nat Rev Clin Onc.* 2013;10(8):460–471.
AML, acute myeloid leukemia.

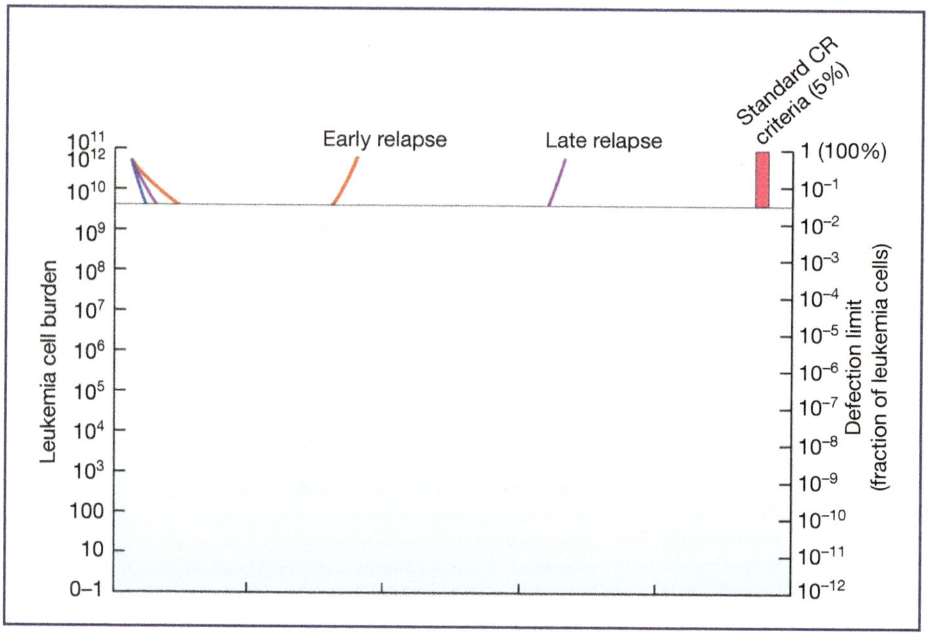

FIGURE 5-25: **Clinical detection of leukemia based on morphologic criteria provides only a partial understanding of leukemia cell disease burden and risk and timing for relapse.**

Source: From Hourigan CS, Karp JE. Minimal residual disease in acute myeloid leukaemia. *Nat Rev Clin Onc*. 2013;10(8):460–471.

CR, complete remission.

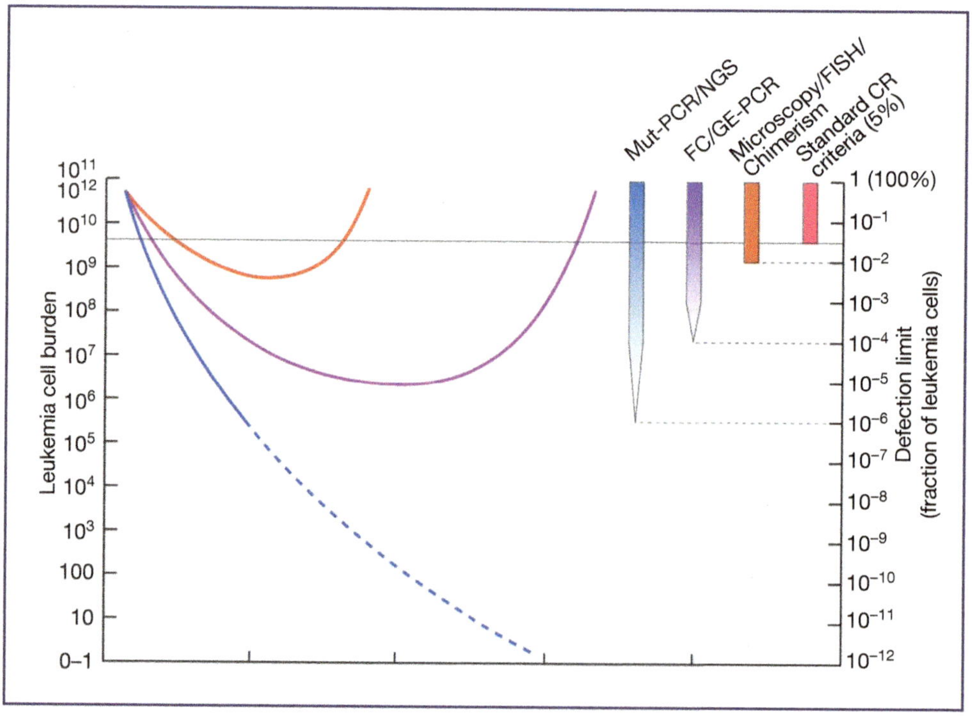

FIGURE 5-26: **Higher sensitivity tools may allow a more complete clinical picture.**

Source: From Hourigan CS, Karp JE. Minimal residual disease in acute myeloid leukaemia. *Nat Rev Clin Onc*. 2013;10(8):460–471.

CR, complete remission; FISH, fluorescence in situ hybridization; NGS, next generation sequencing; PCR, polymerase chain reaction.

"Oh Honey, there is nothing complete about a complete remission."
—Heard on ward round in 2008, Professor Judy Karp, Johns Hopkins

- Complete remission, as defined by conventional morphological criteria, is a highly heterogeneous state with a wide range of residual leukemia burden.
- Due to the low sensitivity of morphological assessment, many patients in "complete" remission have residual disease that will lead to clinically evident relapse without additional treatment.

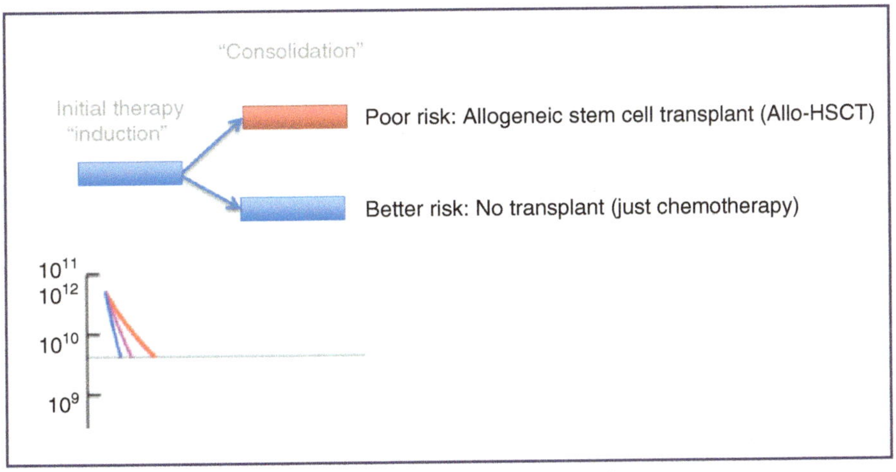

FIGURE 5-27: Current risk stratification for AML.
"Consolidation"—additional therapy given to patients in "complete remission" to prevent relapse. Triaged based on pretreatment surrogates of disease biology and NOT on how effective initial induction therapy was.

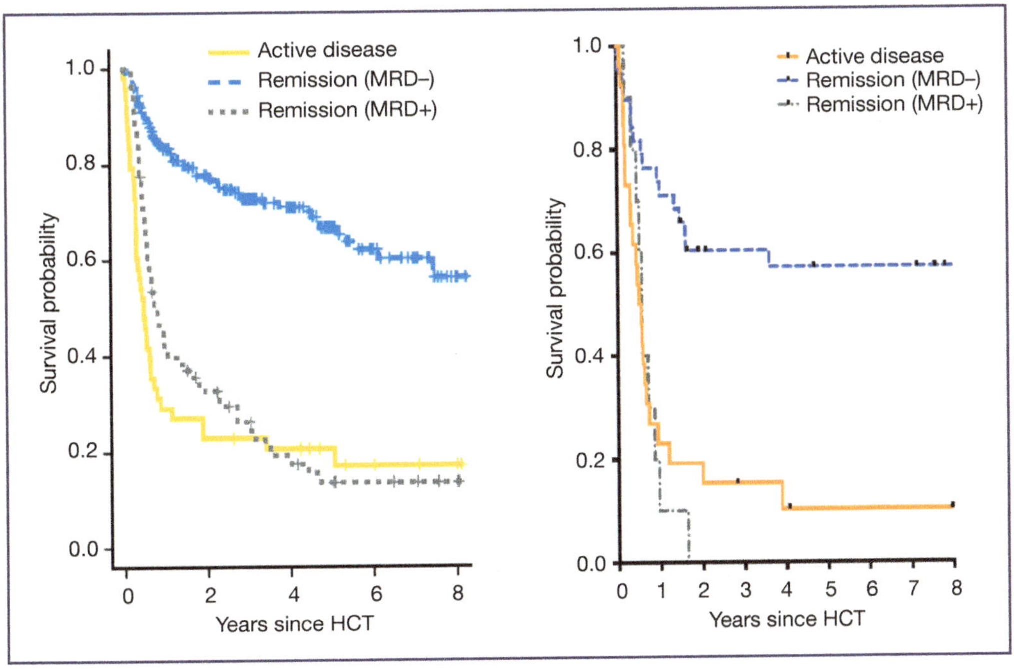

FIGURE 5-28: Presence of AML MRD before allo-HSCT is associated with poor outcomes.
Source: Araki et al, JCO (2016) and Hourigan et al, JCO (2016).
AML, acute myeloid leukemia; HCT, hematopoietic cell transplantation; MRD, minimal residual disease.

Table 5-3 Many ways to measure residual disease in AML

	PRO	CON
Morphology	Commonly used standard. Easy to perform.	Low sensitivity (~5%), many false negatives.
Flow Cytometry	High sensitivity technique for determining residual AML in the right hands. Applicable to most patients.	Requires specialist expertise and equipment. Variation between centers and operators. Often requires diagnostic sample.
Cytogenetics/FISH	Clinically available.	Low sensitivity. Chromosomal abnormalities may persist from founder clone long after leukemia has been eradicated.
Chimerism	Clinically available.	Post Allo-SCT patients only.
RQ-PCR (Gene Expression)	Does not require diagnostic information. Simple to perform.	Not applicable to all AML patients.
RQ-PCR (Mutated Sequence)	Extremely high sensitivity for detecting residual transcript that may be found in AML.	Limited to inv(16), t(8,21), t(15:17) and NPM1 mutation currently.
Next-Gen Sequencing	Most AMLs have a genetic abnormality that could be tracked.	Technique not validated yet for MRD. Intrinsic error rate of NGS.

AML, acute myeloid leukemia; FISH, fluorescence in situ hybridization; MRD, minimal residual disease; NGS, next generation sequencing; RQ-PCR, real-time quantitative polymerase chain reaction.

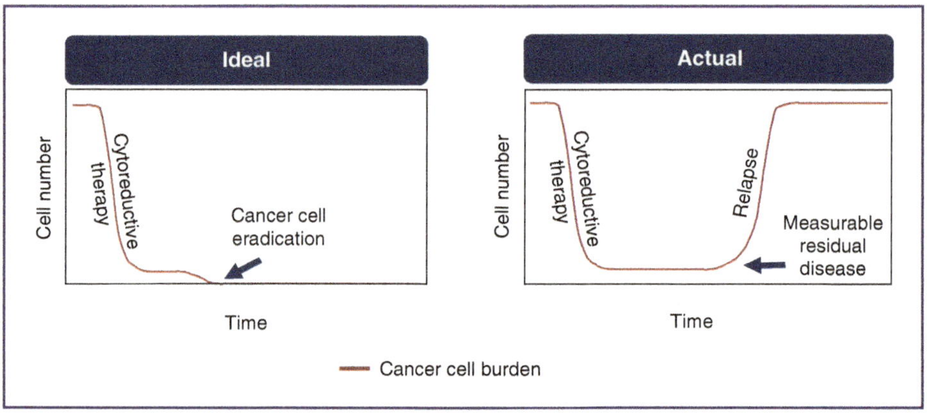

FIGURE 5-29: Ideally, cytoreductive therapy leads to complete cancer cell eradication and cure. However, in actuality, cytoreductive therapy leaves a variable amount of MRD that eventually leads to relapse.
MRD, minimal residual disease.

SOME POTENTIAL USES FOR MRD IN AML

1. **Serial monitoring**: For early prediction of hematological relapse after completion of treatment.
2. **Risk stratification:** At key treatment landmarks—eg, postinduction and pretransplant.
3. **Adjunct therapy:** To determine eligibility for, and efficacy of, eg, maintenance therapy for patients in a morphological complete remission but at continued risk of relapse.
4. **As a surrogate end point?** Role of AML MRD in drug development and approvals is controversial. Not currently accepted as a surrogate end point.

MRD IN AML

1. "CR" and "relapse" are artificial constructs—disease burden is at first approximation a continuous variable and our measurement of it is limited by the sensitivity of the tools we use.

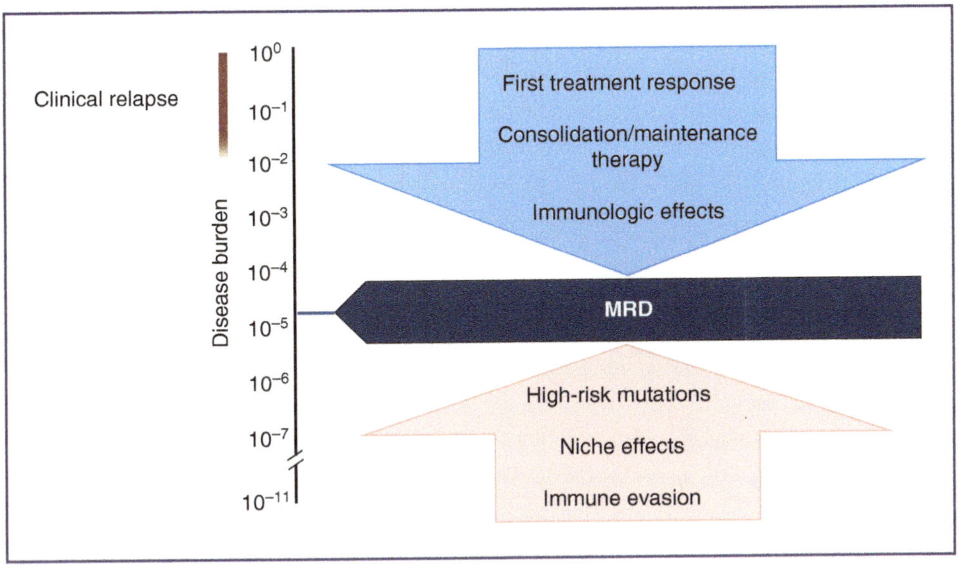

FIGURE 5-30: **Leukemia cell burden and MRD are determined by 2 opposing influences. Initial and consolidation/maintenance therapies and immunologic effects decrease MRD, while high risk mutations, niche effects and immune evasion lead to persistence of MRD.**

MRD, minimal residual disease.

2. MRD tests aren't always perfect—but they provide additional information about those in CR, allowing better estimates of those with high and low risks of "relapse."
3. Repeated MRD measurements longitudinal add power to assessment. Serial monitoring may be the most powerful application of these tools.
4. MRD tracks help triage to, and help evaluate efficacy of, treatment given to patients in a morphological remission.
5. While "dose response" is seen in some blood cancers, in AML *any* detectable leukemia prior to allo-HSCT appears to be associated with poor prognosis.

Selected References

Araki D, Wood BL, Othus M, et al. Allogeneic hematopoietic cell transplantation for acute myeloid leukemia: time to move toward a minimal residual disease-based definition of complete remission? *J Clin Oncol*. 2016;34(4):329–336.

Hourigan CS, Goswami M, Battiwalla M, et al. When the minimal becomes measurable. *J Clin Oncol*. 2016;34(21):2557–2558.

Hourigan CS, Karp JE. Minimal residual disease in acute myeloid leukaemia. *Nat Rev Clin Onc*. 2013;10(8):460–471.

6

Psychosexual Aspects of Management of Acute Leukemia

Nancy Corbitt and Trisha Kendall

Management of acute leukemias is not all about bone marrow biopsies, cytogenetics, and molecular mutations inquiries. This chapter provides the health care professional with insight into caring for the whole person with a diagnosis of acute leukemia, with a focus on overall health-related quality of life (HRQoL) issues, including sexuality and fertility. Each patient and his/her family represents a unique opportunity to make a difference by developing a holistic treatment plan, with artful listening, and taking time to consider the profound changes that the diagnosis and treatment of leukemia exert on quality of life. These HRQoL issues are distinctive at different life stages, with special considerations for the young adult patients.

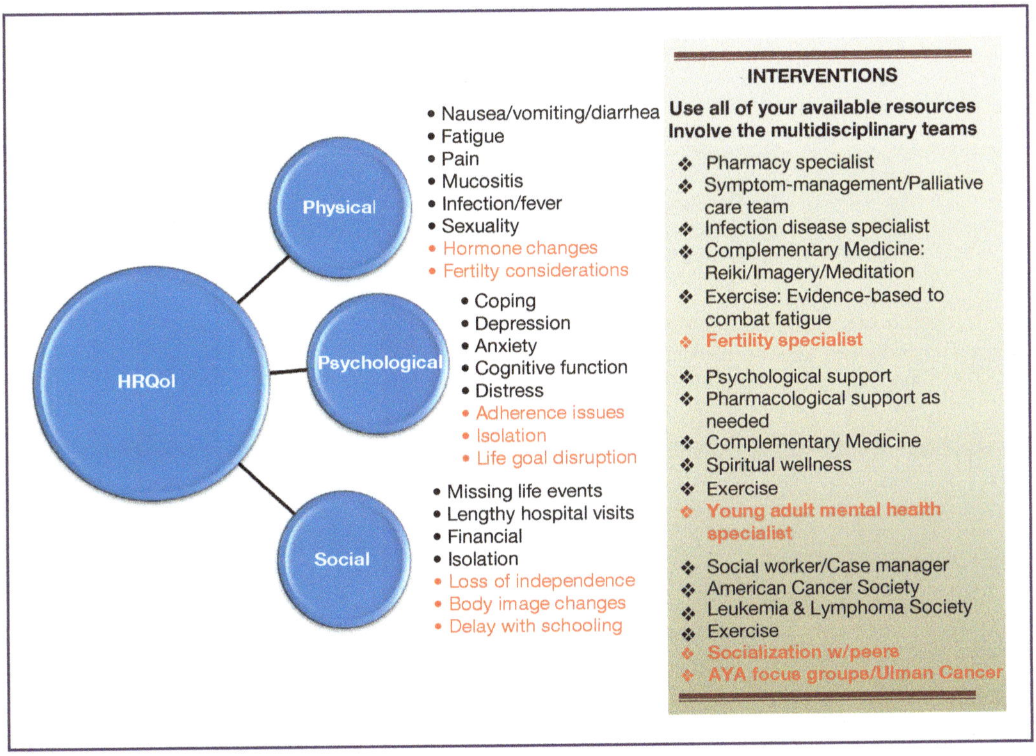

FIGURE 6-1: Health-related quality of life issues for patients with acute leukemia. Special issues for adolescents and young adults (AYA) are highlighted in red. It is important to consider the developmental stage of each patient in order to anticipate his/her needs.

Gender identity, sexual preference, and types of sexual acts will influence the education needed to provide to the patient. Discussions about platelet and neutrophil counts will be influenced by whether the patient participates in anal, oral, and/or vaginal sex. Infection concerns arise even with oral sex, so patients should be advised to use condoms or dental dams. These are just a few of the types of open, frank, and informative conversations that are needed between patient and health care provider in order to provide holistic care.

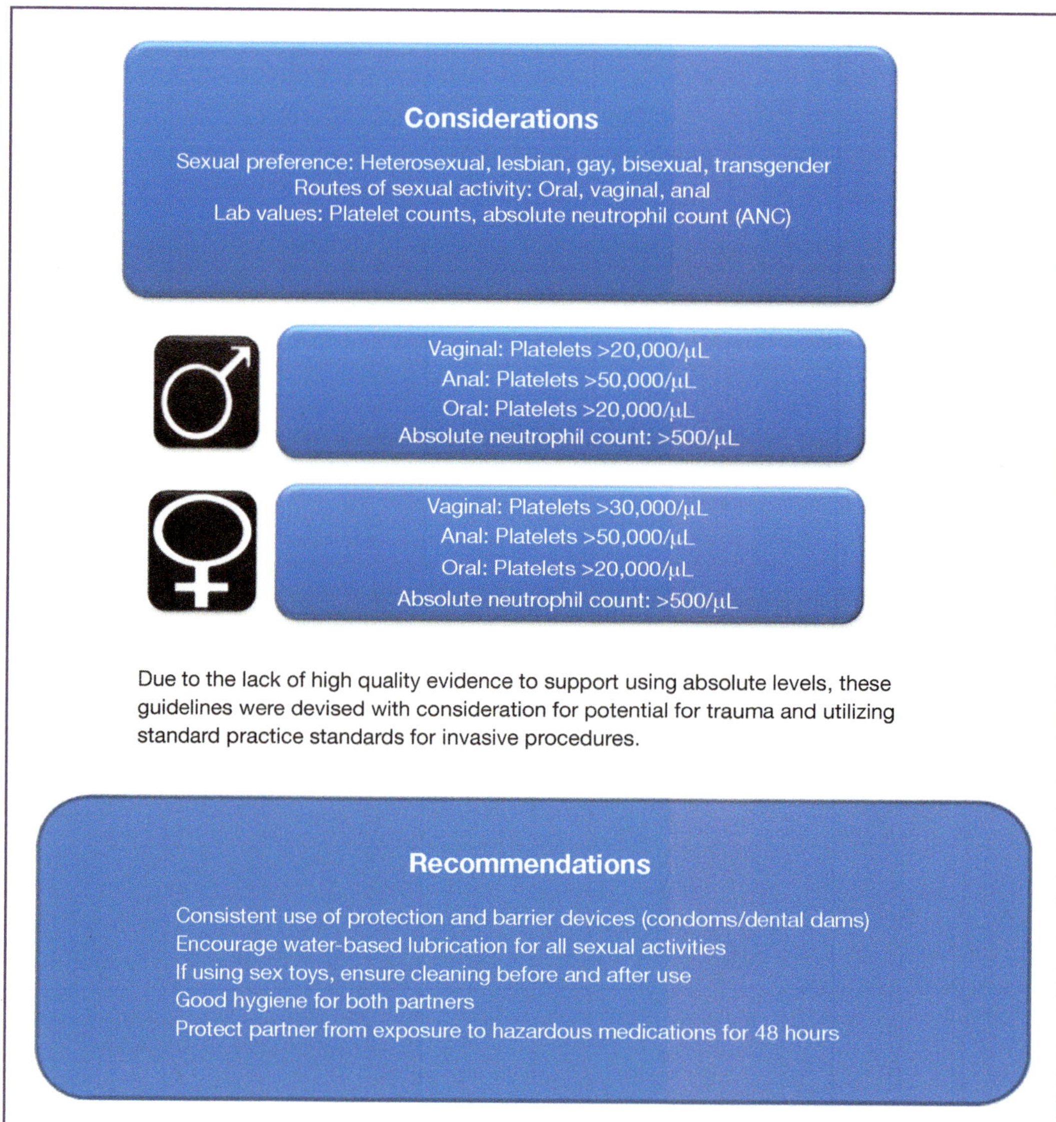

FIGURE 6-2: Guidelines for sexual activity for patients with acute leukemia.

Leukemia is one of the top diagnosed cancers for young adults. Seventy-five percent of female patients with ALL are in their child-bearing years, with a 64% survival rate. Fertile females diagnosed with AML and chronic myeloid leukemia (CML) comprise roughly 20% of the total affected female patients. Therefore, a discussion about fertility options is required at diagnosis.

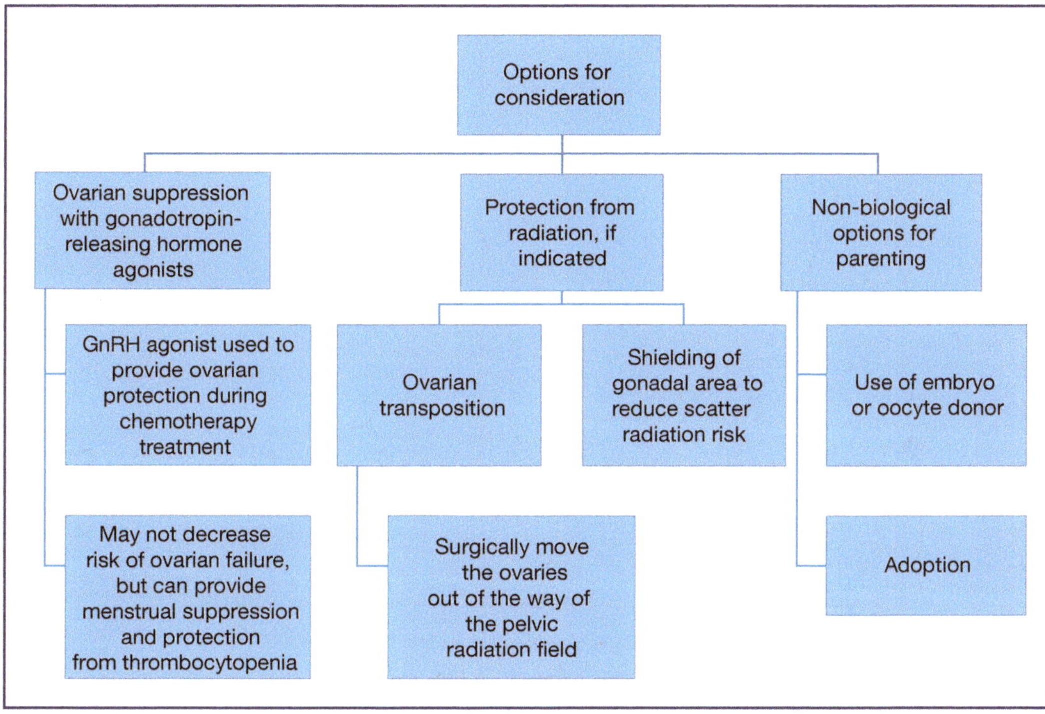

FIGURE 6-3: Recommended fertility options for women. Please note that, at this time, the following strategies are not recommended: embryo cryopreservation, oocyte cryopreservation, and ovarian tissue cryopreservation.

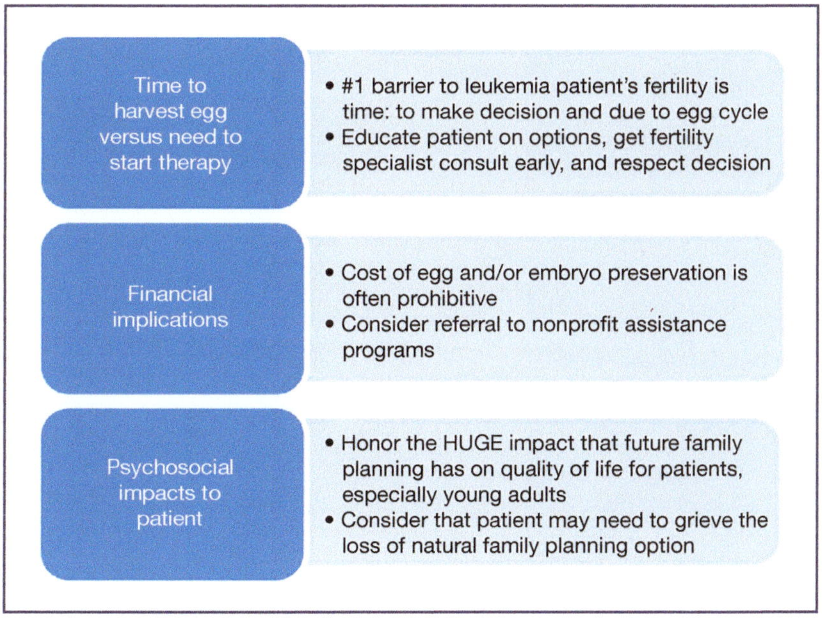

FIGURE 6-4: Special considerations for female patients.

Postpubescent males have a distinctive set of concerns, even though fertility options are often easier to accomplish for this group of patients.

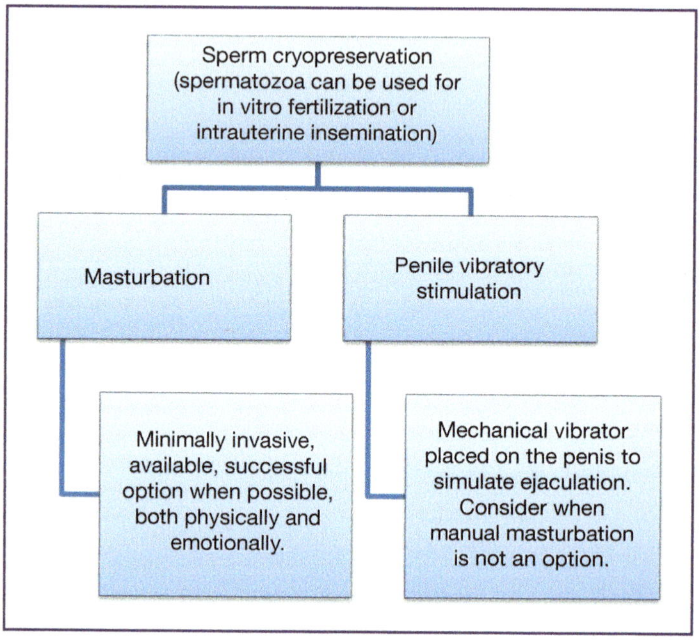

FIGURE 6-5: Recommended fertility options for postpubescent males. Please note that, at this time, the following strategies are not recommended: rectal electrostimuation, testicular or epididymal aspiration under anesthesia, or experimental manipulation of spermatogonial stem cells.

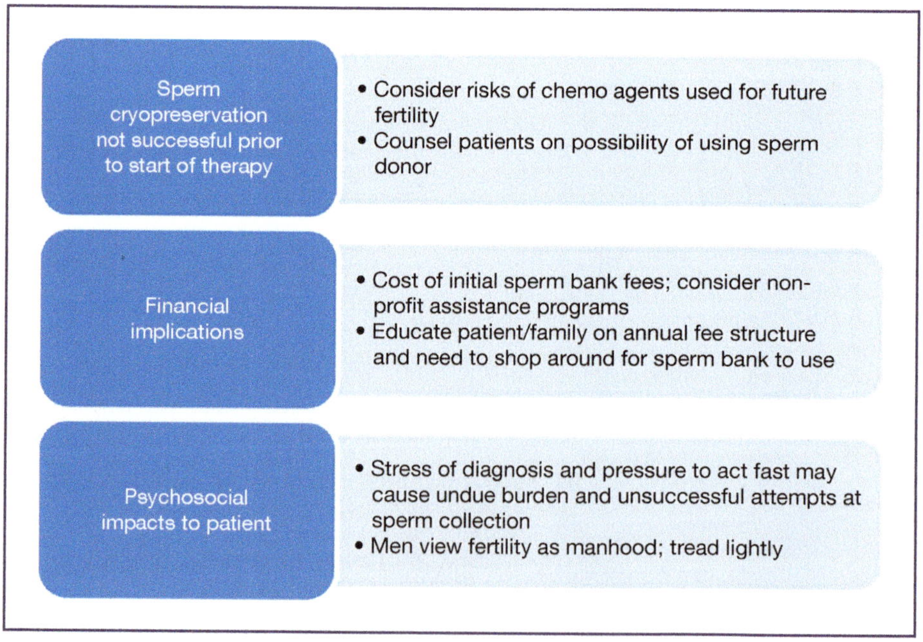

FIGURE 6-6: Special considerations for male patients.

For young adults newly diagnosed and survivors, the hope of having a family is often at the top of the list of things that concerns them. Addressing the psychological quality-of-life issues that arise when initially diagnosed, such as coping, depression, anxiety, and isolation, by consulting with the interdisciplinary team may assist the patient and family members throughout treatments and physical recovery periods.

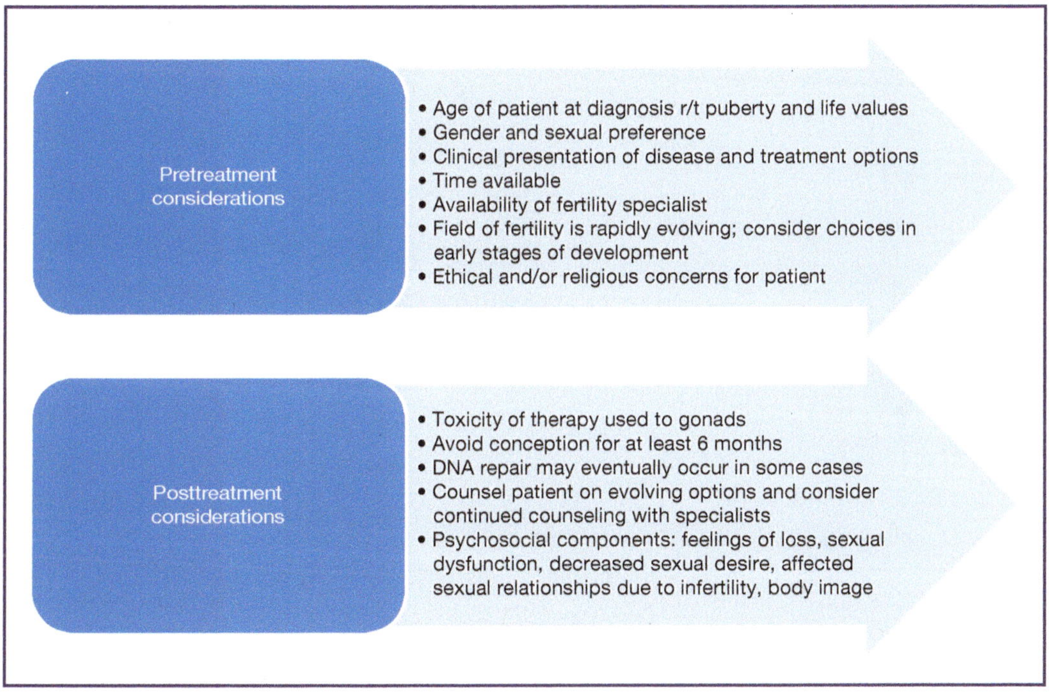

FIGURE 6-7: Guidelines for fertility for patients with acute leukemia: Developing a holistic plan.

In the end, the patient, in consultation with the oncologist, will guide the decision about which fertility options and sexual behaviors are best for them. It is the responsibility of all health care providers to present the options available. An acute leukemia diagnosis changes lives, but our role is to treat the whole patient and consider his or her unique quality-of-life needs.

Selected References

Albrecht T. Physiologic and psychological symptoms experienced by adults with acute leukemia; an integrative literature review. *Oncol Nurs Forum*. 2014;41(3):286–295.

Albrecht T, Rosenzweig M. Distress in patients with acute leukemia. *Cancer Nurs*. 2014;37(3):218–226.

Cheng J, Hourigan C, Smith T. Adult acute myeloid leukemia long-term survivors. *J Leuk*. 2014;2(2):1–7.

Lange S, Tait D, Matthews M. Oncofertility: an emerging discipline in obstetrics & gynecology. *ObstetGynecol Surv*. 2013;68(8):582–593.

Park E, Norris R, Bober S. Sexual health communication during cancer care: barriers and recommendations. *Cancer J*. 2009;15(1):74–77.

Rodriquez-Wallberg K, Oktay K. Fertility preservation during cancer treatment: clinical guidelines. *Cancer Manag Res*. 2014;6:105–117.

Smith A, Bellizzi K, Keegan T, et al. Health-related quality of life on adolescent and young adult patients with cancer in the United States: the adolescent and young adult health outcomes and patient experience study. *J Clin Oncol*. 2013;31(17):2136–2145.

7

Chemotherapeutic Agents for Treatment of AML and ALL

Ashkan Emadi, Noa G. Holtzman, Matthew J. Wieduwilt, and Judith E. Karp

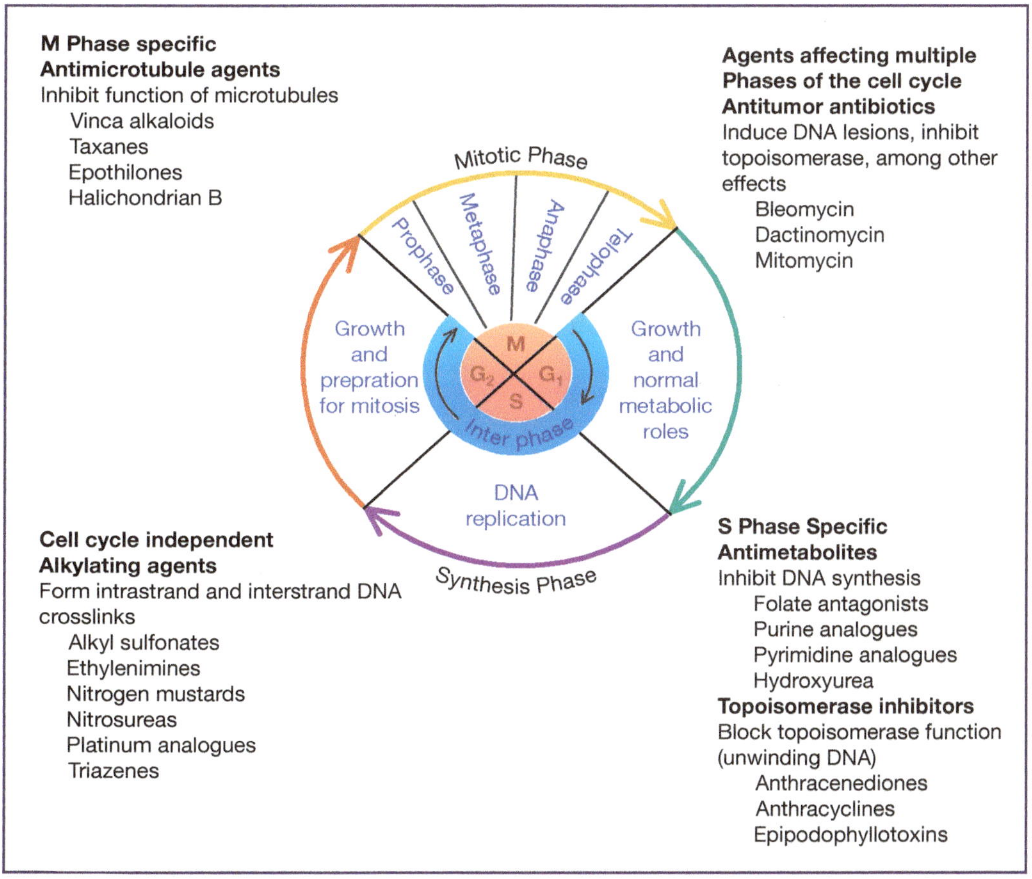

FIGURE 7-1: Cell cycle-specific (ie, schedule-dependent) vs. nonspecific (ie, dose-dependent) chemotherapeutic agents.

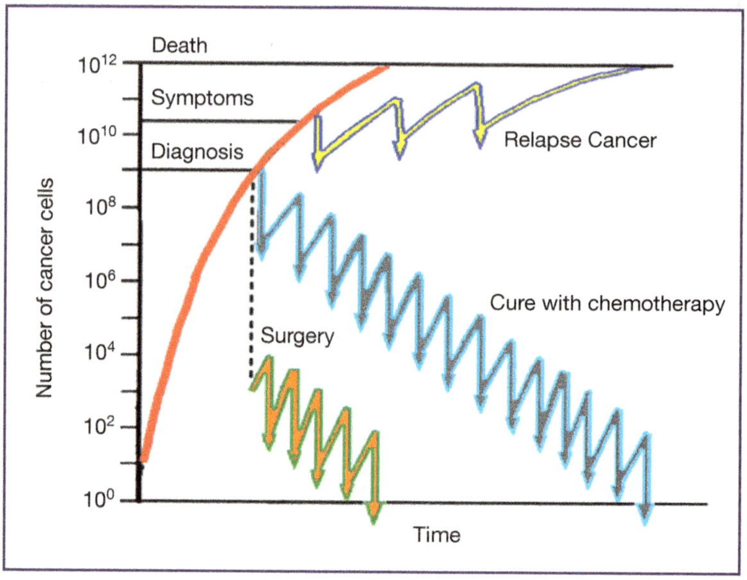

FIGURE 7-2: **Log kill hypothesis. The CELL KILL HYPOTHESIS proposes that the actions of cancer chemotherapy drugs follow first-order kinetics, ie, a given dose kills a constant PROPORTION of a tumor cell population (rather than a constant NUMBER of cells).**

Classification of Cytotoxic Chemotherapy Drugs

ALKYLATING AGENTS

- These agents directly damage DNA to prevent the cancer cell from reproducing.
- They are not cell cycle specific.
- They are used to treat leukemia, lymphoma, Hodgkin's disease, multiple myeloma, sarcoma, and cancers of the lung, breast, and ovary.
- In rare cases, they can cause long-term damage to the bone marrow, ie, treatment-related AML (t-AML).
- The risk of t-AML from alkylating agents is "dose-dependent," meaning that the risk is small with lower doses, but goes up as the total amount of the drug used gets higher.
- The risk of leukemia after receiving alkylating agents is highest about 5 to 7 years after treatment and usually involves abnormality of chromosomes 5 and 7.

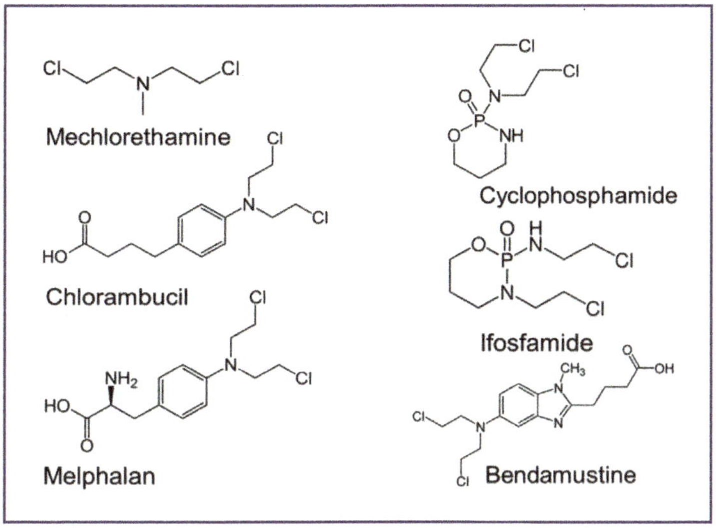

FIGURE 7-3: Nitrogen mustards.

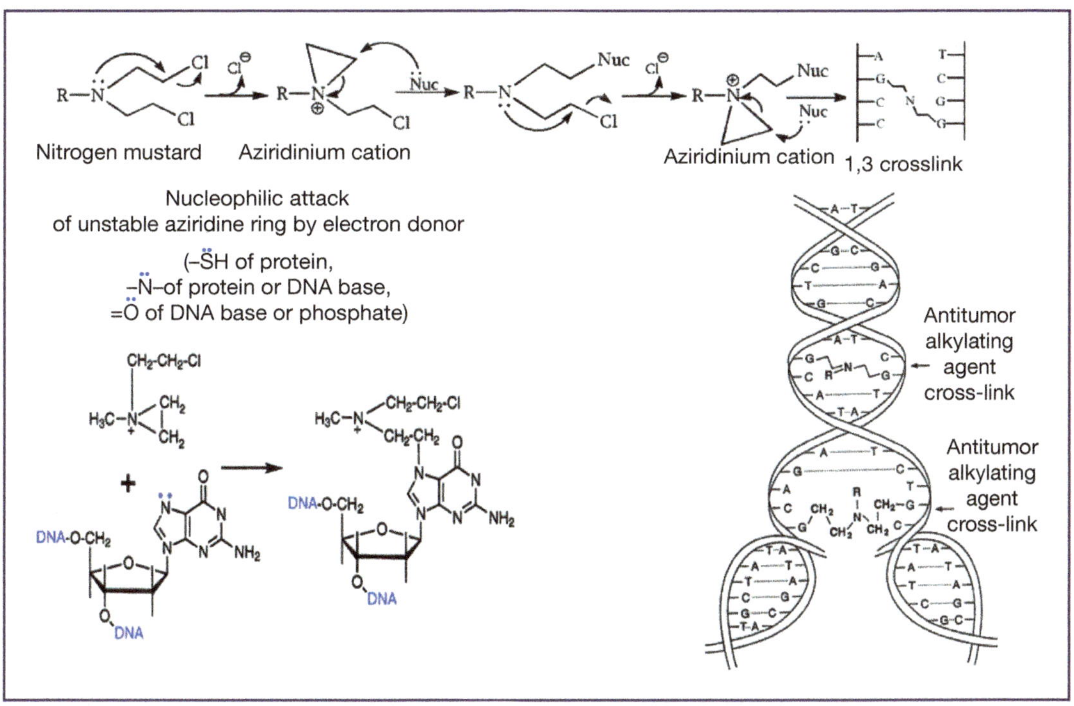

FIGURE 7-4: Mechanism of action of nitrogen mustards. In nitrogen mustard, the nitrogen atom displaces the chloride to result in a strained, three-membered intermediate cation, called aziridinium. This ion reacts easily with nucleophiles. The N-7 position of guanine in DNA is strongly nucleophilic and can be readily alkylated by the aziridium cation. The second chemical transformation of nitrogen mustard provides another aziridinium ion, which, upon reaction with another DNA nucleophile, forms a DNA crosslink.

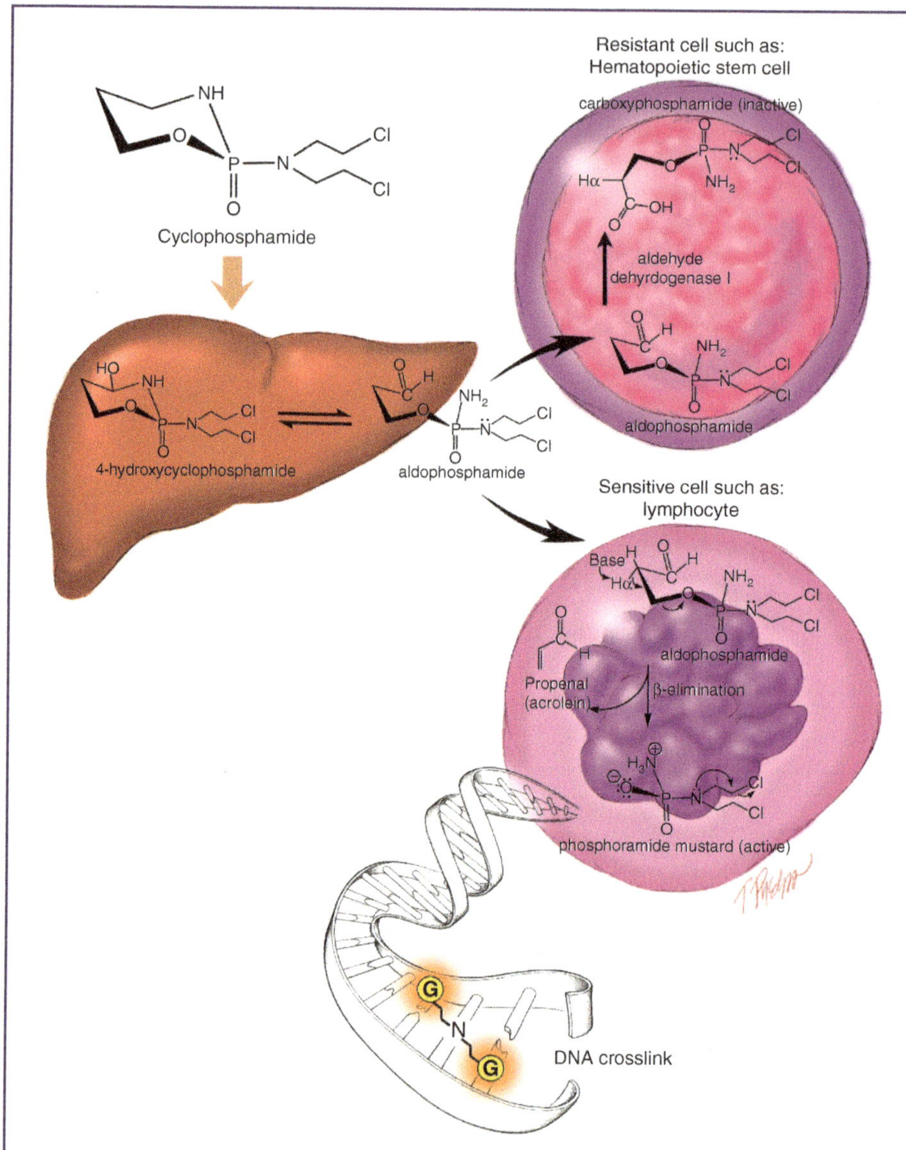

FIGURE 7-5: Cyclophosphamide, the first targeted chemotherapeutic agent. Cyclophosphamide (and ifosfamide) are hydroxylated at C4 in the hepatic microsomal cytochrome P450 system and are converted to 4-hydroxycyclophosphamide and 4-hydroxyifosfamide, respectively. Both of these molecules are in equilibrium with their aldehyde tautomers, aldophosphamide. The protons on Cα of aldo tautomers of cyclophosphamide and ifosfamide are *acidic enough* to promote a base-catalyzed β-elimination reaction to form active metabolites, phosphoramide mustards, and the leaving group acrolein. Acrolein, or propenal, is a very reactive α-β unsaturated aldehyde responsible for hemorrhagic cystitis after administration of cyclophosphamide or ifosfamide. The phosphoramide mustard forms an unstable reactive aziridinium ring, which readily reacts with different nucleophiles (eg, N7 of a guanine base in DNA) forming interstrand and intrastrand crosslinks leading to DNA alkylation and apoptosis of the cells. The role of the β-elimination reaction is critical in the activation of cyclophosphamide and ifosfamide. The inability to undergo β-elimination results in the lack of cytotoxic activity of these agents. Aldophosphamides can be oxidized to carboxyphosphamides by aldehyde dehydrogenases, which are found in high levels within hematopoietic and other stem cells, but not in mature lymphocytes. The protons on Cα attached to carboxyl group are *not acidic enough* that they can be removed under physiologic conditions via initiation of the critical β-elimination reaction necessary for activation of these compounds. The conversion of aldehyde group to carboxyl group by aldehyde dehydrogenase of stem cells culminates in the selective cytotoxic effect of cyclophosphamide against lymphocytes but not stem cells. In recent years, administration of high-dose cyclophosphamide after allogeneic blood or bone marrow transplantation has resulted in reducing the rates of graft-versus-host disease (GVHD) by selective removal of allo-reactive T-cells, but not donor stem cells, which in turn has expanded the donor pool for many patients by allowing successful use of human leukocyte antigen (HLA)-haploidentical grafts.

Source: From Emadi A, Jones RJ, Brodsky RA. Cyclophosphamide and cancer: golden anniversary. *Nat Rev Clin Oncol.* 2009;6(11):638–647.

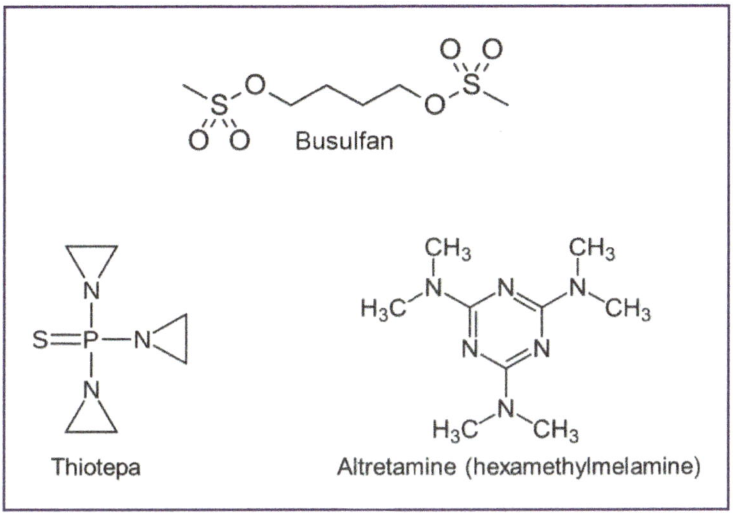

FIGURE 7-6: Alkyl sulfonates and ethylenimines.

ANTIMETABOLITES

- Antimetabolites are a class of drugs that interfere with DNA and RNA growth by substituting for the normal building blocks of RNA and DNA.
- They are classified as *purine analogues, pyrimidine analogues*, and *folic acid analogues.*
- These agents damage cells **during the S phase**.
- They are commonly used to treat leukemias.

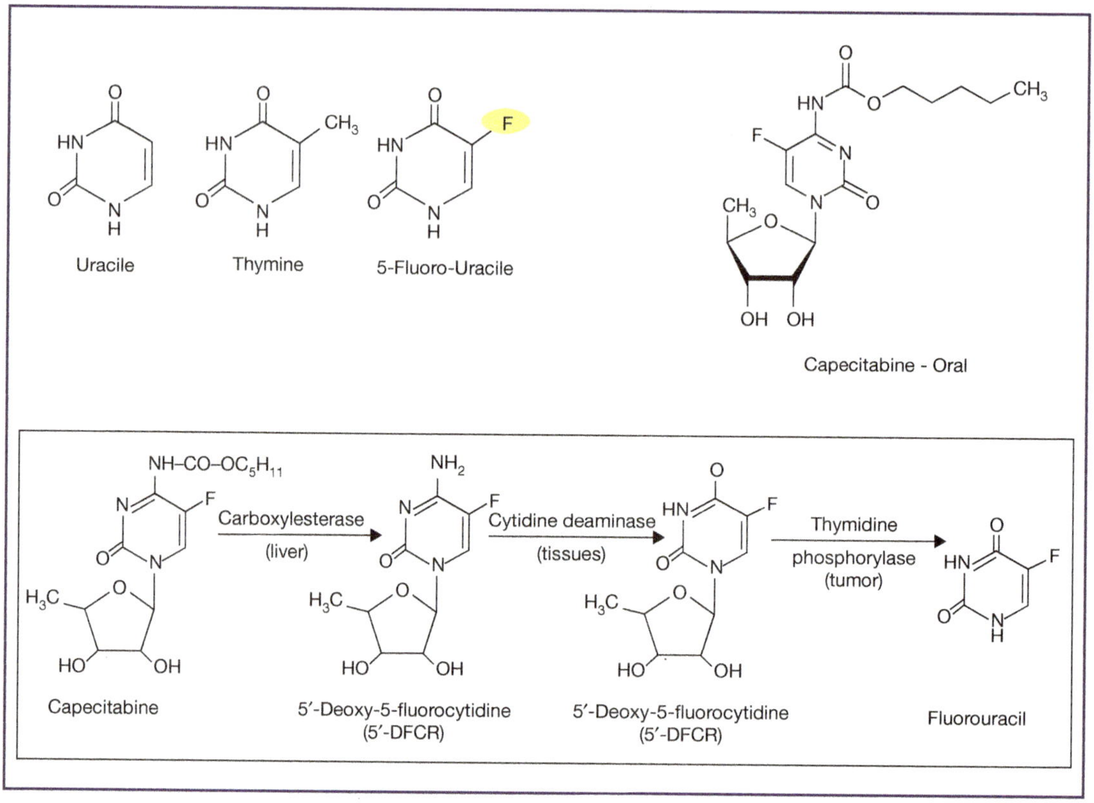

FIGURE 7-7: **The chemical structure of fluoropyrimidines. 5-fluorouracil (5-FU) and capecitabine decrease the biosynthesis of pyrimidine nucleotides by inhibiting thymidylate synthase, the enzyme that catalyzes the rate-limiting step in DNA synthesis. This results in the "thymineless death" of rapidly growing cells. 5-FU cannot be methylated by thymidylate synthase, causing sustained inhibition of the enzyme and decreased production of dTMP. 5-FU also can be incorporated into DNA (via dUMP [deoxyuridine monophosphate] or dTMP [deoxythymidine monophosphate]) or RNA (via UTP), leading to DNA strand breakage and a decrease in protein synthesis. Leucovorin increases binding of 5-FU to thymidylate synthase, thereby increasing 5-FU half life ($t_{1/2}$).**

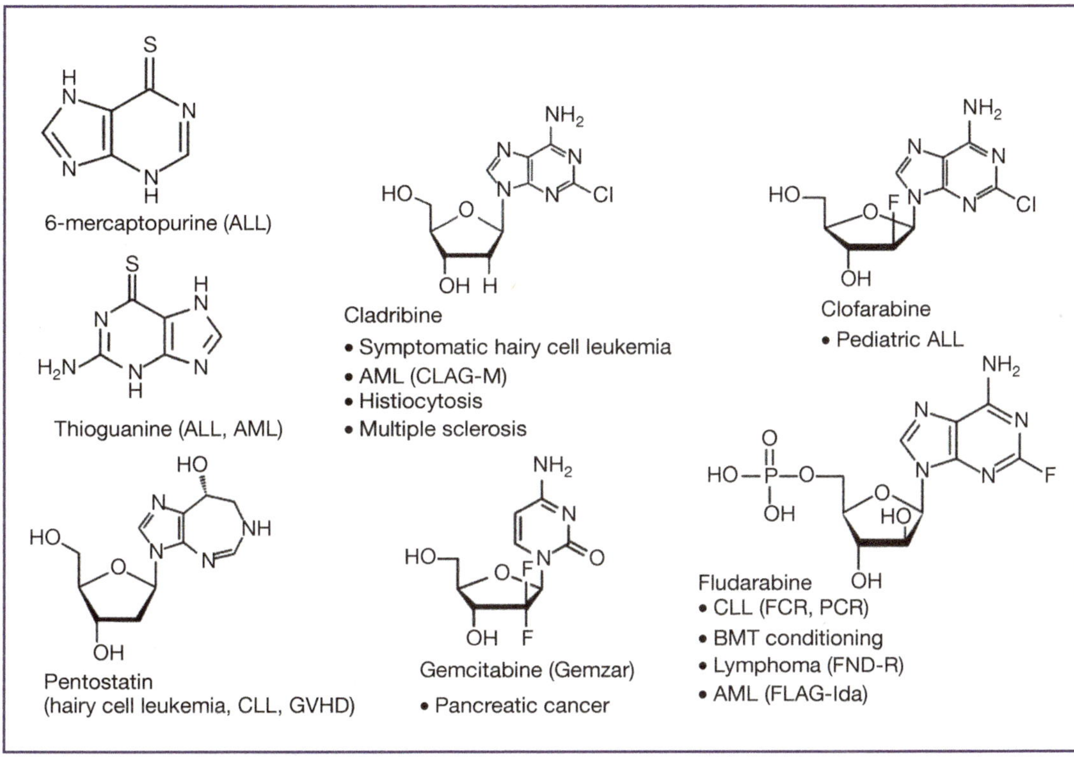

FIGURE 7-8: **Examples of other antimetabolites. 6-Mercaptopurine (6-MP) is an orally available thiopurine analog used in postremission and maintenance therapy in treatment of ALL. 6-MP inhibits the first step in de novo purine synthesis, and when converted to its triphosphate form inhibits DNA and RNA synthesis when incorporated into DNA and RNA. 6-MP is metabolized by the liver. Major side effects include myelosuppression, immunosuppression, gastrointestinal irritation, biliary stasis (hyperbilirubinemia), and transaminitis.**

ALL, acute lymphoblastic leukemia; AML, acute myeloid leukemia; BMT, bone marrow transplantation; CLAG-M, cladribine, ara-C, G-CSF, mitoxantrone; CLL, chronic lymphocytic leukemia; FCR, fludarabine, cyclophosphamide, rituximab; FLAG-Ida, fludarabine, ara-C, G-CSF, idarubicine; FND-R, fludarabine, mitoxantrone, dexamethasone, rituximab; GVHD, graft-versus-host disease; PCR, pentostatin, cyclophosphamide, rituximab.

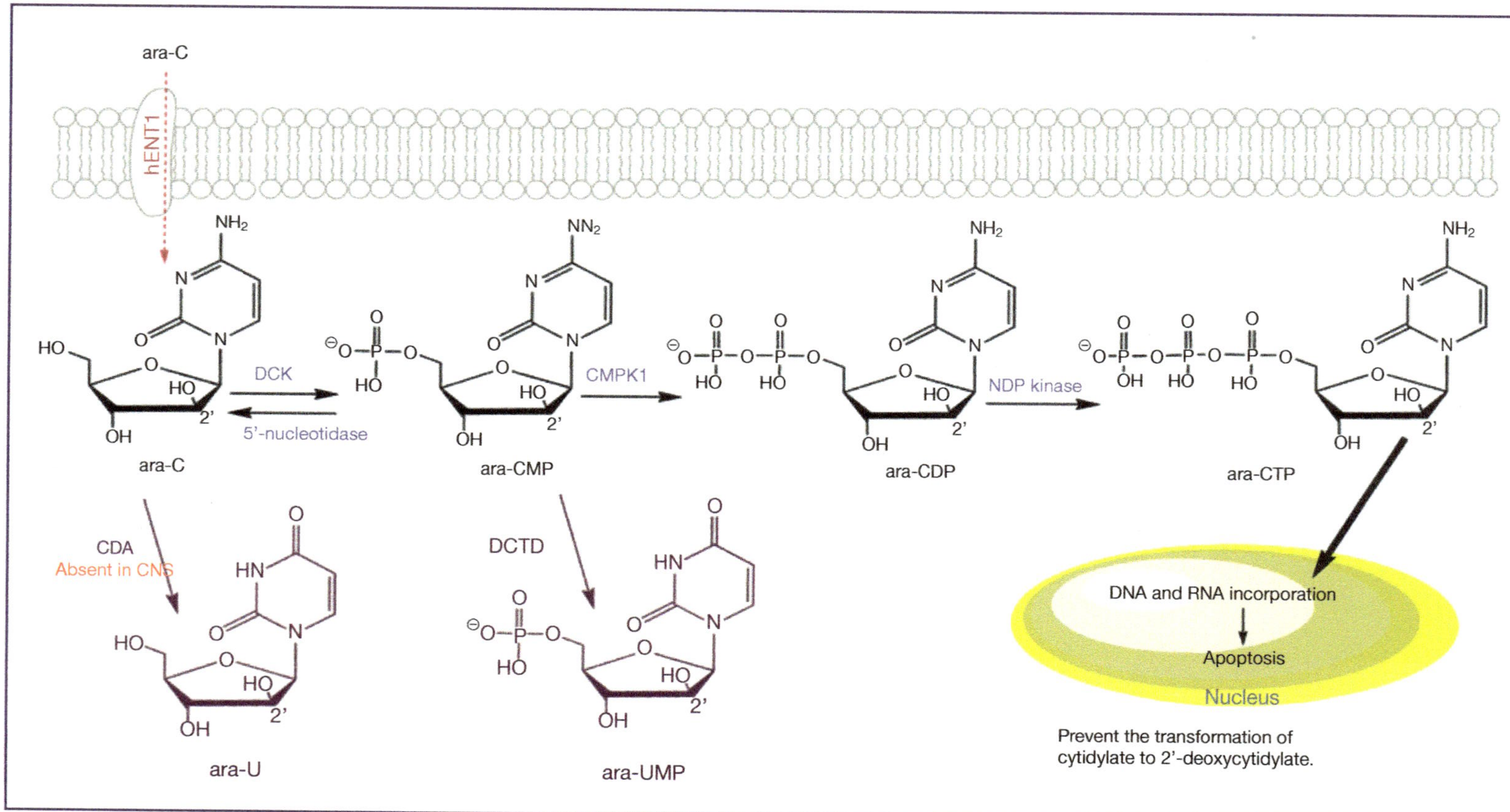

FIGURE 7-9: Cytarabine. Clinical efficacy of cytarabine heavily depends on dose and schedule because of its short biologic half-life. At concentrations less that 1 microM, which is achieved with 100 to 200 mg/m^2 daily, ara-C influx into the cells is strongly correlated with the number of nucleoside transporters (eg, hENT1) per leukemic blast, but at plasma concentrations of more than 10 to 15 microM, which is achieved with high-dose ara-C (2–3 g/m^2 over 2–3 h repeated q12 h for as many as 12 doses), the drug diffuses freely into the cell, and cellular accumulation and retention of ara-CTP are adequate.

Source: From Emadi A, Karp JE. The clinically relevant pharmacogenomic changes in acute myelogenous leukemia. *Pharmacogenomics.* 2012;13(11):1257–1269.

ara-C, cytosine arabinoside or cytarabine; ara-CDP, ara-cytidine-5'-diphosphate; ara-CMP, ara-cytidine-5'-monophosphate; ara-CTP, ara-cytidine-5'-triphosphate; ara-U, uracil arabinoside; ara-UMP, ara-uridine-5'-monophosphate; CDA, cytidine deaminase; CNS, central nervous system; DCK, deoxycytidine kinase; DCTD, deoxycytidylate deaminase; NDP, nucleoside-diphosphate.

Cytarabine has biphasic plasma clearance: a rapid initial phase with a t½ of 10 to 15 min and a second, slower phase with a t½ of 2 to 3 h. By 24 h, nearly 80% of the administered dose is excreted in the urine, almost entirely as ara-U.

Cerebellar dysfunction including dysarthria, dysdiadochokinesia, dysmetria, ataxia, and nystagmus with concomitant cerebral dysfunction after administration of high-dose cytarabine (HiDAC) is the most prominent and most common of all neurologic toxicities associated with cytarabine. Its incidence is approximately 10% to 11% of patients receiving HiDAC, and usually occurs between 3 and 8 days after initiation of HiDAC. CT, MRI, and lumbar puncture (LP) are nearly always normal. Electroencephalogram (EEG) shows slow wave activity.

Renal insufficiency (creatinine clearance <60 mL/min) and age older than 50 years are the two main risk factors of cerebellar toxicity after HiDAC administration.

Based on limited data, it is recommended that cytarabine should be discontinued and never used again after even the first signs of neurologic toxicity. There is no effective therapy for the cerebellar toxicity of cytarabine other than discontinuation of the drug and supportive measures.

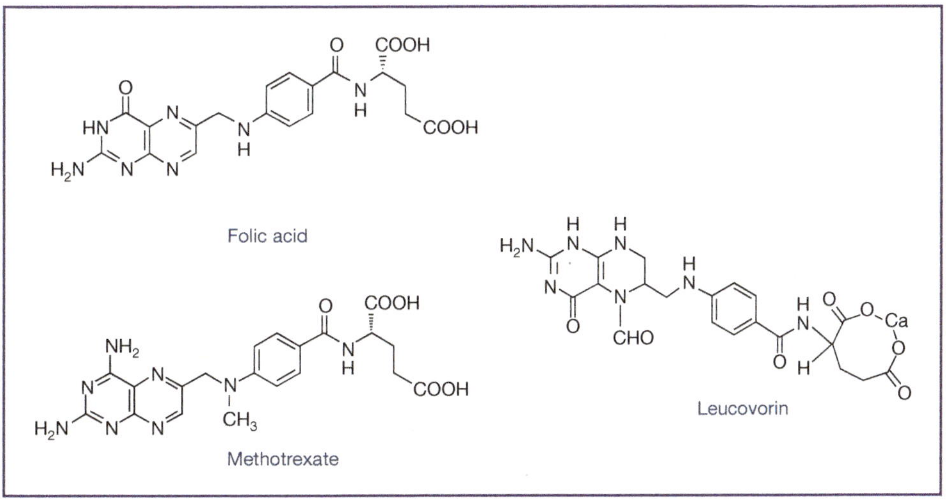

FIGURE 7-10: Antimetabolite folic acid analogues. Methotrexate is an antifolate agent that inhibits dihydrofolate reductase, thereby blocking folate synthesis. Folate depletion by methotrexate prevents the synthesis of purines and thymidine, thus inhibiting DNA and RNA synthesis in tumor cells. Methotrexate is cleared by renal excretion. With high-dose methotrexate, alkalinization of the urine with maintenance of a high urine output is important to prevent methotrexate precipitation in the renal tubules and renal failure. Major toxicities, especially with high-dose methotrexate, include myelosuppression, mucositis, hepatitis, acute renal failure, and rarely seizures. Decreased methotrexate clearance with increased toxicity can result in patients with renal insufficiency, pleural effusions, and ascites as well as those taking medications that decrease renal clearance of methotrexate, including NSAIDs, aspirin, and penicillins. Folinic acid (leucovorin) is given after methotrexate to prevent systemic toxicity from folate depletion. For patients with poor methotrexate clearance despite urine alkalinization, hydration, and diuresis, the dose and frequency of leucovorin can be increased. In refractory cases, carboxypeptidase, a folate-cleaving enzyme, can rapidly lower serum methotrexate concentrations.

NSAIDs, nonsteroidal antiinflammatory drugs.

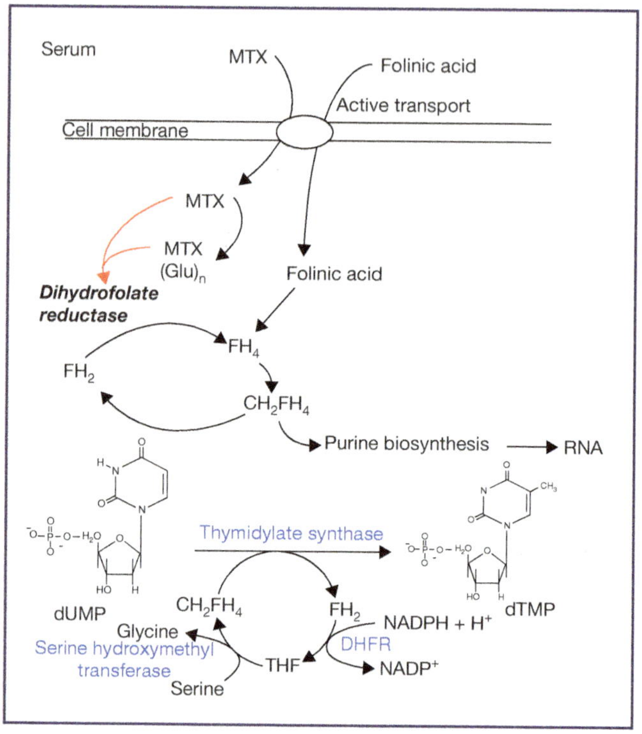

FIGURE 7-11: Folic acid pathway.

CH_2FH_4, methylene etrahydrofolate; DHFR, dihydrofolate reductase; FH_2, dihydrofolate; FH_4, tetrahydrofolate; $(Glu)_n$, poly-glutamate; MTX, methotrexate.

ASPARAGINASE

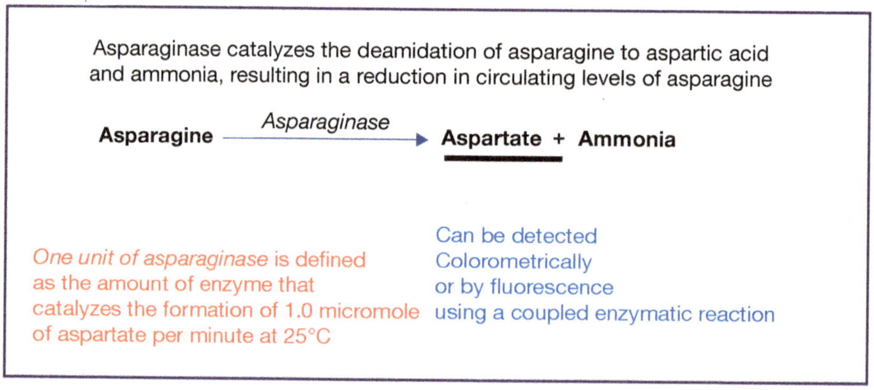

FIGURE 7-12: Asparaginase. Lymphoblasts are unable to synthesize adequate asparagine and are dependent on asparagine from their environment for survival. Normal tissues are able to synthesize asparagine to various degrees. Asparaginases convert asparagine to aspartic acid and ammonia, and to variable degrees, glutamine to glutamic acid and ammonia, depriving lymphoblasts of asparagine. Asparaginases have become an essential part of most ALL treatment regimens.

ALL, acute lymphoblastic leukemia.

Three forms of asparaginase are available for the treatment of ALL: the short-acting native *E. coli* aspararaginase, the short-acting *Erwinia chrysanthemi* asparaginase, and the long-acting pegylated *E. coli* asparaginase.

Major unique toxicities of asparaginase include hypersensitivity, hepatotoxicity, thromboembolism, pancreatitis, hypertriglyceridemia, and hyperglycemia.

Hypersensitivity may occur after sensitization with the first dose of asparaginase. The rates of hypersensitivity are reduced with the use of pegylated asparaginase and may be reduced with the integration of hydrocortisone premedication, high-dose methotrexate, and/or rituximab into regimens. For patients developing hypersensitivity to *E. coli* asparaginase, *Erwinia chrysanthemi* asparaginase is typically substituted to allow continued asparagine depletion.

Hepatotoxicity is common in adult ALL patients treated with asparaginase with rates of Grade 3 to 4 AST, ALT, and bilirubin elevation of about 20% to 50%. Hepatotoxicity is generally self-limited, only rarely leading to fulminant liver failure and death. For life-threatening hepatotoxicity, asparaginase is generally discontinued.

Asparagine depletion can precipitate thromboembolism in about 3% to 16% of patients, including unusual thrombosis such as cerebral venous thrombosis and hepatic vein thrombosis, due to depletion of anticoagulant factors including antithrombin, increased thrombin generation, and increased platelet activation. Strategies to replace antithrombin with recombinant antithrombin have proven feasible and it is generally recommended to avoid replacing fibrinogen unless less than 50 mg/dL given the relatively low risk of bleeding. Some practitioners also use prophylactic-dose anticoagulation although little data exist regarding the risk–benefit of this approach. For CNS thrombosis or hepatic vein thrombosis, asparaginase is generally discontinued although it may be continued safely after institution of therapeutic anticoagulation for other forms of thromboembolism such as central venous catheter-associated thrombosis, deep vein thrombosis, and pulmonary embolism.

Clinically significant pancreatitis occurs in about 3% to 5% of adult ALL patients treated with asparaginase and can be fatal. Asparaginase is generally discontinued permanently in adult patients with symptomatic pancreatitis.

Hypertriglyceridemia is fairly common as well and can generally be managed with fibrates. Hyperglycemia is common with asparaginase exposure and is generally manageable with oral hypoglycemic agents or insulin.

Native *E. coli* asparaginase is now no longer available in the United States and the current NCCN guidelines suggest substituting pegylated asparaginase for native asparaginase despite lack of data supporting the safety and efficacy of pegylated asparaginase in many of these regimens.

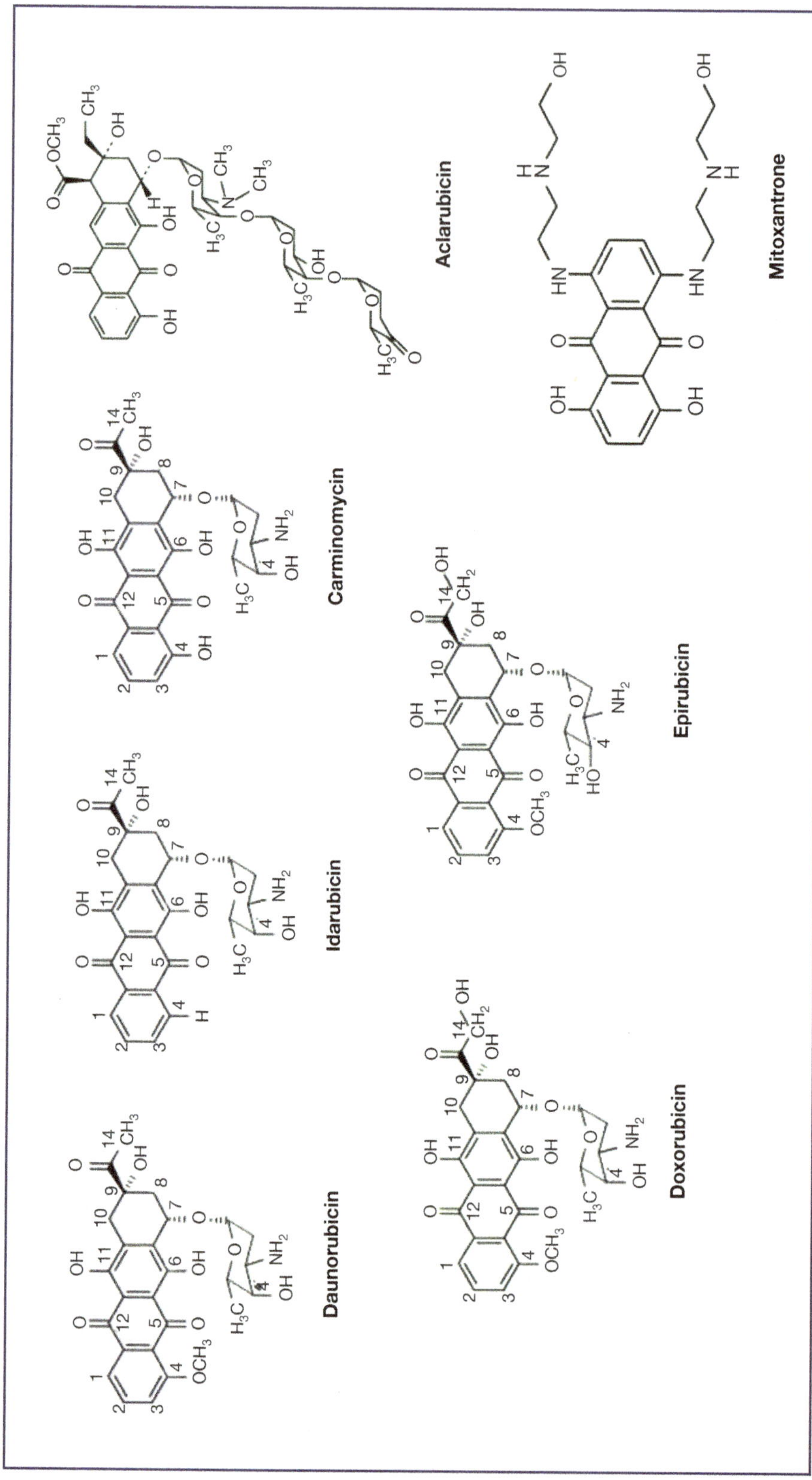

FIGURE 7-13: Anthracyclines are essential components of many therapeutic regimens for treatment of newly diagnosed as well as relapsed or refractory AML and ALL. Anthracyclines and anthracenediones (mitoxantrone) intercalate DNA, inhibit topoisomerase II, and generate reactive oxygen species, causing DNA strand breaks, inhibition of DNA replication, and free radical damage to cell membranes and nucleic acids.

ALL, acute lymphoblastic leukemia; AML, acute myeloid leukemia.

ANTITUMOR ANTIBIOTICS

Anthracyclines

Intravenous administration requires a central venous catheter or a closely monitored peripheral IV catheter as tissue infiltration can cause extensive skin necrosis.

Therapy-related myeloid neoplasms (AML and less commonly MDS) can occur, commonly 1 to 5 years after anthracycline- or anthracenedione-containing therapy.

Myelosuppression is the major expected side effect of these agents.

Anthracyclines and anthracenediones can also cause both acute and chronic cardiac toxicity. Rare reversible acute cardiac toxicities with myopericarditis, QT prolongation, and arrhythmias occurring during or shortly after anthracycline infusion can lead to rapid heart failure and possibly death. Chronic anthracycline cardiac toxicity is irreversible and dependent on a cumulative lifetime dose with rates of congestive heart failure with doxorubicin 3% to 5% at 400 mg/m^2 lifetime dose, increasing to 7% to 26% at 550 mg/m^2. Risk factors for the development of anthracycline-induced cardiomyopathy include cumulative anthracycline dose, advanced age, preexisting cardiovascular disease, and mediastinal radiation. Given the risk of cardiomyopathy with anthracyclines, many practitioners perform screening tests for cardiac function such as an echocardiogram or multigated acquisition (MUGA) scan, especially in older patients and patients with a cardiac disease history or symptoms of underlying cardiac disease.

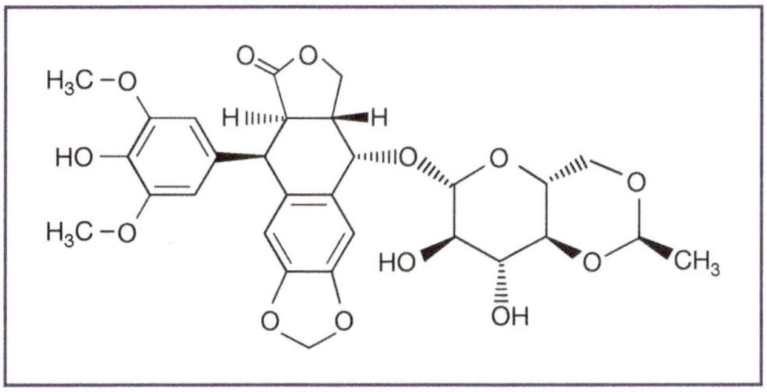

FIGURE 7-14: Etoposide (VP-16). Etoposide is a derivative of podophyllotoxin that has potent antileukemia activity by inhibiting DNA synthesis by forming a complex with topoisomerase II and DNA. Etoposide acts primarily in the G2 and S phases of the cell cycle. Etoposide is used in the MEC (mitomycin, etoposide, cytarabine) regimen for treatment of relapsed AML as well as in induction timed sequential chemotherapy with cytarabine and daunorubicin/idarubicin (AcDVP16) in patients with newly diagnosed AML. It is also used for treatment of refractory testicular cancer as well as small cell and non-small-cell lung cancer.

AML, acute myeloid leukemia.

MITOTIC INHIBITORS

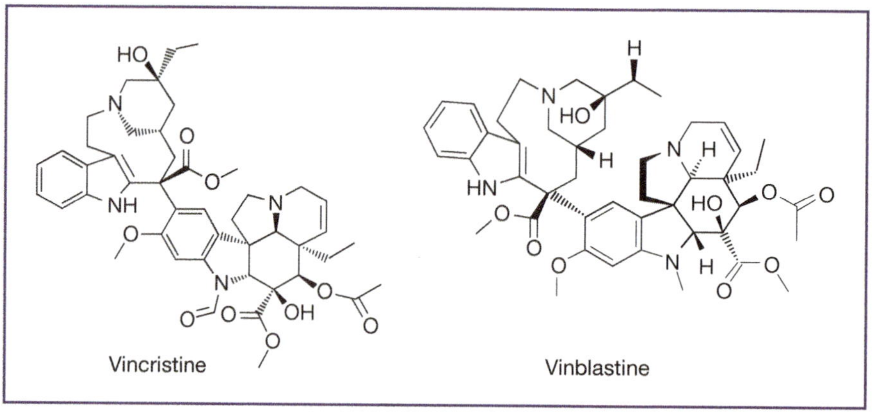

FIGURE 7-15: **Vinca alkaloids. Vincristine is a plant alkaloid that binds beta-tubulin inhibiting microtubule polymerization, leading to arrest of cell division in metaphase, culminating in cell death. Vincristine is metabolized by the liver. The drug can cause dose-dependent sensory-motor and autonomic polyneuropathy, severe constipation, ileus, and hyponatremia. Extravasation of vincristine can cause extensive local tissue necrosis and the drug should be given through a central venous line or a well-monitored peripheral IV catheter.**

CORTICOSTEROIDS

- Corticosteroids have long been a cornerstone of therapy for ALL. The commonly used corticosteroids in ALL therapy are prednisone and dexamethasone.
- Major short-term side effects of corticosteroids include hyperglycemia, hypertension, fluid retention, neuropsychological effects, and immunosuppression. Given the already high risk of infection with ALL therapy, tight glucose control with the use of oral hypoglycemic agents or insulin is recommended to reduce the risk of infection and other complications of hyperglycemia.
- Hypertension is generally manageable with oral antihypertensive medications.
- For patients with significant psychologic side effects compromising patient safety and receipt of therapy, corticosteroids may rarely need to be stopped.
- Avascular necrosis and osteonecrosis can occur as a late complication of corticosteroid exposure. These complications appear more common with dexamethasone rather than with prednisone in the pediatric population although an alternate week dosing schedule appeared to reduce the risk. Avascular necrosis can lead to chronic pain and debility, often requiring joint replacement years after initial treatment. Avascular necrosis incidence increases into late adolescence and young adulthood with rates as high as 20% of young adult patients, then it decreases. Extended corticosteroid administration can also lead to osteopenia and osteoporosis, predisposing patients to fractures with advancing age.

ARSENIC TRIOXIDE

$$\mathrm{R{-}As{=}O} + \left.\begin{matrix}\mathrm{HS{-}CH_2{-}R'_1}\\ \mathrm{HS{-}CH_2{-}R'_2}\end{matrix}\right) \rightleftharpoons \mathrm{R{-}As}\left\langle\begin{matrix}\mathrm{S{-}CH_2{-}R'_1}\\ \mathrm{S{-}CH_2{-}R'_2}\end{matrix}\right) + \mathrm{H_2O}$$

Trivalent arsenic (As^{III}) in As_2O_3 or arsenite ($As[OH]_3$) and pentavalent arsenic (As^{V}) in arsenate ($HAsO_4^{2-}$) are the two biologically significant forms of arsenic. Although As^{V} disrupts cellular processes as a phosphate (HPO_4^{2-}) mimic, the interaction of As^{III} with the thiol (or sulfhydryl) groups (-SH) of

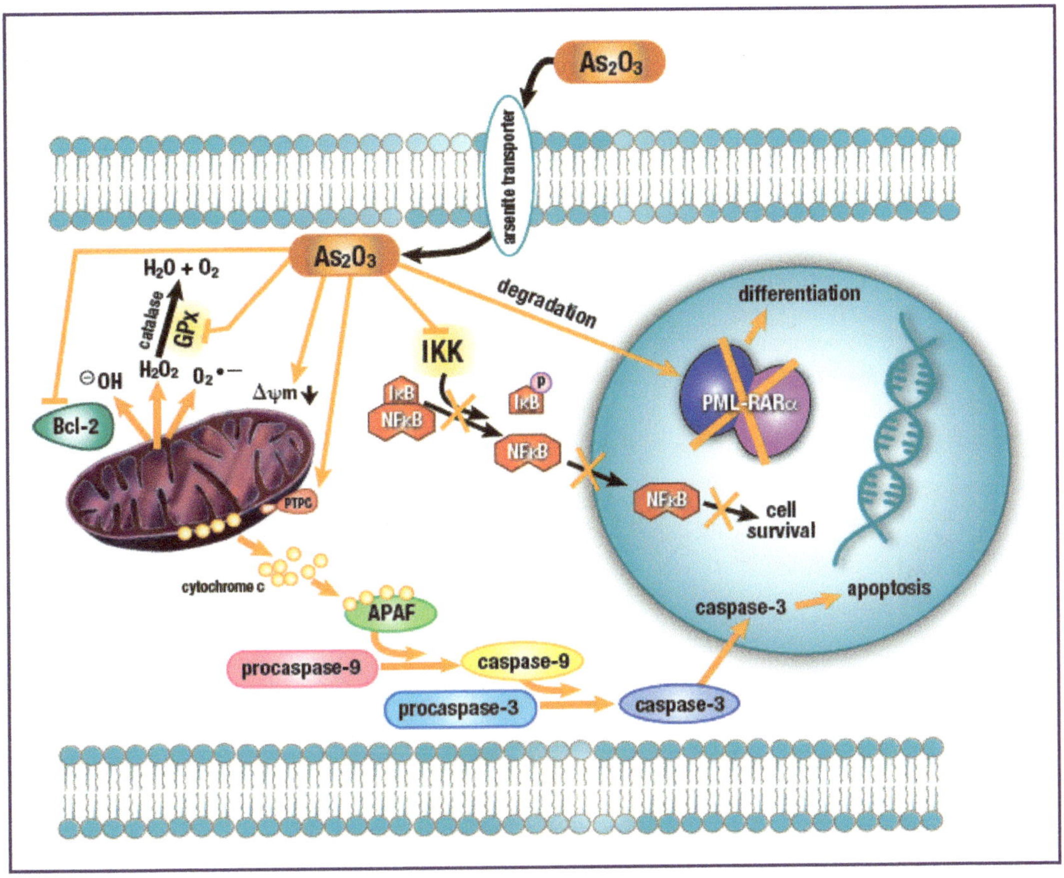

FIGURE 7-16: **Arsenic trioxide (As_2O_3) affects multiple cellular functions via different molecular targets. Although the fundamental mechanism is the favorable chemical reaction between arsenic and thiol groups within a protein, the final outcome depends on the cell type as well as the dose and duration of arsenite exposure. For example, in APL cells, As_2O_3 at low concentrations (<0.5 microM) induces differentiation; at higher concentrations (0.5–2.0 microM) it causes apoptosis.**

Source: From Emadi A, Gore SD. Arsenic trioxide–an old drug rediscovered. *Blood Rev.* 2010;24(4–5):191–199.

APL, acute promyelocytic leukemia.

proteins with a high cysteine content is the basic reaction that underlies the multiple mechanisms of action of this chemotherapeutic agent.

In APL cells, the PML-RARα fusion protein blocks the expression of genes required for normal differentiation. PML contains a cysteine-rich region that is hypothesized to interact with As^{III}, resulting in the degradation of PML-RARα fusion protein. Furthermore, As_2O_3-induced histone acetylation has been reported to promote differentiation via alteration in gene transcription. See also Acute Promyelocytic Leukemia (APL) in Chapter 3.

As_2O_3 induces dose-dependent apoptosis in APL and hematopoietic non-APL as well as tumor and nonmalignant cell lines. The activation of the caspase cascade, the decrease of the mitochondrial membrane potential $\Delta\Psi_m$, and the production of reactive oxygen species (ROS) all play roles in induction of As_2O_3-induced apoptosis. As_2O_3 also promotes apoptosis via down-regulation of Bcl-2 expression by prolongation of the cell cycle and cell cycle arrest of malignant cells and by opening the permeability transition pore complex (PTPC) in mitochondrial membranes by directly binding to thiol groups in the PTPC.

DNA METHYLTRANSFERASE INHIBITORS (A.K.A. HYPOMETHYLATING AGENTS)

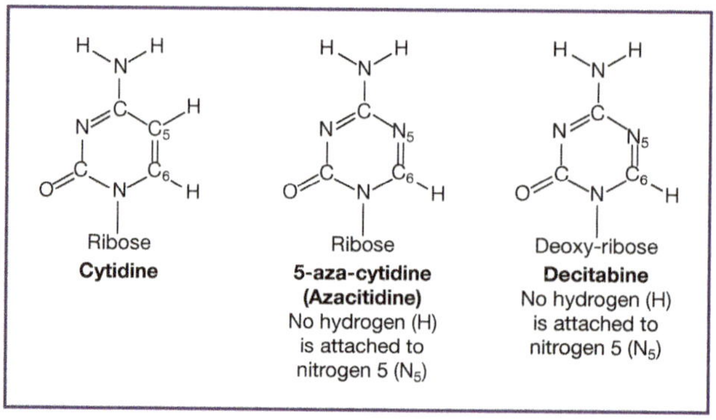

FIGURE 7-17: The chemical structures of cytidine, azacitidine, and decitabine showing their similarities and differences. See also Fundamentals of Epigenetics and Clonal Evolution and Treatment of Secondary AML and MDS/AML in Chapter 3.

AML, acute myeloid leukemia; MDS, myelodysplastic syndrome.

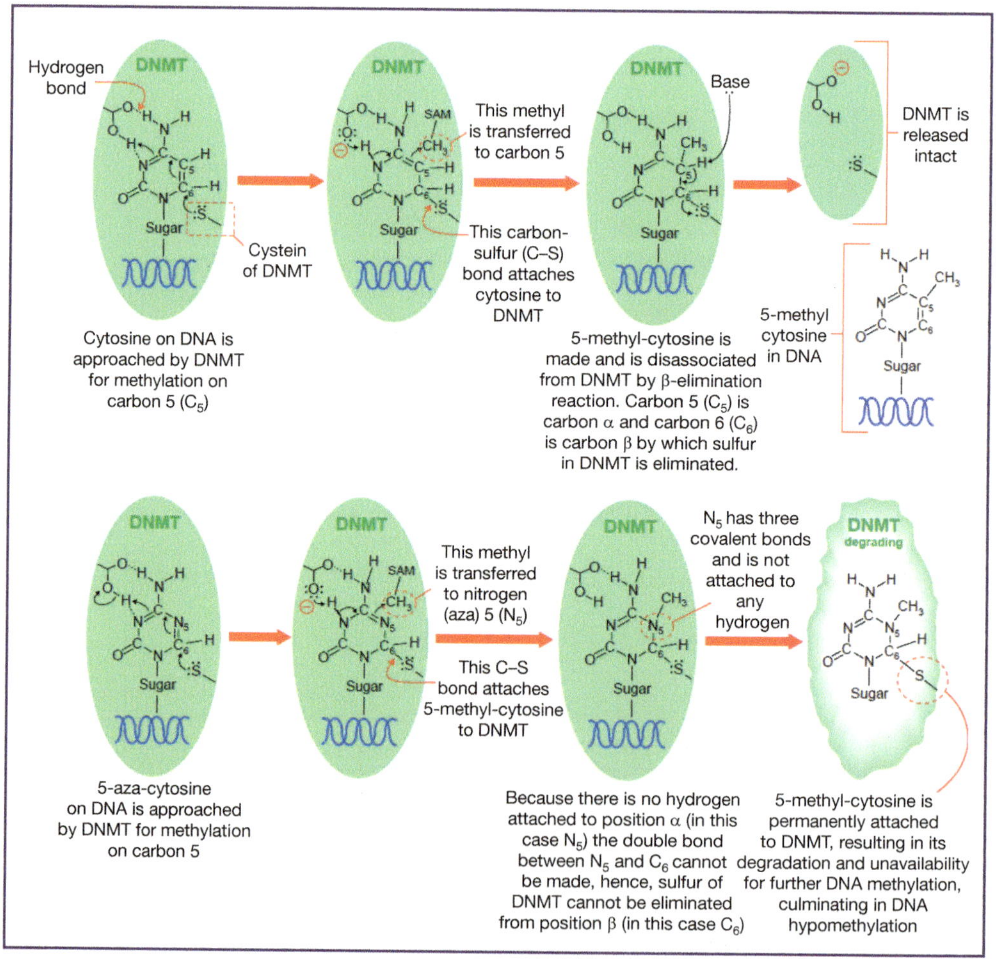

FIGURE 7-18: Top: The chemical reactions result in the formation of 5-methylcytosine and its release from DNA methyltransferase mediated by a β-elimination reaction. Bottom: The mechanism by which 5-aza-cytosine analogues are methylated. Due to the absence of the β-elimination reaction they are not released from DNA methyltransferase, resulting in its degradation and unavailability for future methylation reactions, which culminates in therapeutic hypomethylation of DNA.

DNMT, DNA methyltransferase.

FLT3 INHIBITOR

- On April 28, 2017, FDA approved midostaurin (50 mg orally twice daily with food) for treatment of patients with newly diagnosed AML that is FLT3 mutation-positive as detected by an FDA-approved test, in combination with standard cytarabine and daunorubicin induction and cytarabine consolidation. Midostaurin is not indicated as a single-agent induction therapy for the treatment of patients with AML.
- Midostaurin (100 mg orally twice daily with food) is also approved for treatment of patients with aggressive systemic mastocytosis (ASM), systemic mastocytosis with associated hematological neoplasm (SM-AHN), or mast cell leukemia.
- Patients receiving midostaurin should be monitored for symptoms of interstitial lung disease or pneumonitis. Midostaurin should be discontinued in patients with signs or symptoms of pulmonary toxicity.
- *Mechanism of action:* Midostaurin is a small molecule that inhibits multiple receptor tyrosine kinases including wild-type FLT3, FLT3 mutant kinases (ITD and TKD), KIT (wild-type and D816V mutant), PDGFRα/β, VEGFR2, as well as members of the serine/threonine kinase PKC (protein kinase C) family. Midostaurin inhibits FLT3 receptor signaling and cell proliferation, and induces apoptosis in leukemic cells expressing ITD and TKD mutant FLT3 receptors or overexpressing wild-type FLT3 and PDGF receptors. Midostaurin also inhibits KIT signaling, cell proliferation and histamine release and induces apoptosis in mast cells.
- *Evidence of clinical outcome improvement:*
    - Midostaurin in combination with chemotherapy was investigated in a randomized, double-blind placebo-controlled trial of 717 patients with newly-diagnosed FLT3-mutated AML.
    - Patients were stratified by FLT3 mutation status: TKD, ITD with allelic ratio <70%, and ITD with allelic ratio ≥70%.
    - Patients were randomized (1:1) to receive midostaurin (n = 360) or placebo (n = 357) with food on days 8–21 in combination with daunorubicin (60 mg/m^2 daily on days 1–3)/cytarabine (200 mg/m^2 daily on days 1–7) for up to two cycles of induction and high dose cytarabine (3 g/m^2 every 12 hours on days 1, 3 and 5) for up to four cycles of consolidation, followed by continuous midostaurin or placebo treatment according to initial assignment for up to 12 additional 28-day cycles. Patients who proceeded to hematopoietic stem cell transplantation (SCT) stopped receiving study treatment.
    - The randomized patients had a median age of 47 years (range, 18–60 years), and 88% had a performance status of 0–1. AML was de novo onset in 95%.
    - The percentage of patients with FLT3-ITD allelic ratio <70%, FLT3-ITD allelic ratio ≥70%, and FLT3-TKD mutations were identical (per randomized FLT3 stratum) on both arms (48%, 30%, and 23%, respectively). NPM1 mutations were identified in 55% of patients tested on the midostaurin arm and 60% of patients tested on the placebo arm.
    - A second course of induction was administered to 25% of the patients, 62% initiated at least one cycle of consolidation, 29% initiated maintenance, and 17% completed all 12 planned cycles of maintenance; 21% of the patients underwent SCT in first CR.
    - The overall rate of hematopoietic stem cell transplantation (induction failure, first CR or salvage after relapse) was 59% of patients in the midostaurin plus standard chemotherapy arm compared with 55% in the placebo plus standard chemotherapy arm.
    - Efficacy was established on the basis of overall survival (OS), measured from the date of randomization until death by any cause. The primary analysis was conducted after a minimum follow-up of approximately 3.5 years after the randomization of the last patient.
    - **Midostaurin plus cytarabine and daunorubicin was superior to placebo plus cytarabine and daunorubicin in OS (hazard ratio [HR] 0.77; 95% CI 0.63, 0.95; 2 sided *P* = 0.016).**

Because survival curves plateaued before reaching the median, median survival could not be reliably estimated.

- The analysis of event-free survival (EFS), defined as a failure to obtain a complete remission (CR) within 60 days of initiation of protocol therapy, or relapse, or death from any cause, showed a statistically significant improvement with a median of 8.2 months for midostaurin plus cytarabine and daunorubicin versus 3 months for placebo plus cytarabine and daunorubicin with HR 0.78 (95% CI 0.66, 0.93) and 2 sided $p = 0.005$.
- In an exploratory analysis of EFS defined as a failure to obtain a CR any time during induction, or relapse, or death from any cause with failures assigned as an event on study day 1, the median EFS was 10.6 months for midostaurin plus cytarabine and daunorubicin versus 5.6 months for placebo plus cytarabine and daunorubicin with HR 0.72 (95% CI 0.61, 0.86).

Selected References

Emadi A, Gore SD. Arsenic trioxide–an old drug rediscovered. *Blood Rev.* 2010;24(4–5):191–199.

Emadi A, Jones RJ, Brodsky RA. Cyclophosphamide and cancer: golden anniversary. *Nat Rev Clin Oncol.* 2009;6(11):638–647.

Emadi A, Karp JE. The clinically relevant pharmacogenomic changes in acute myelogenous leukemia. *Pharmacogenomics.* 2012;13(11):1257–1269.

FDA Label for RYDAPT® (midostaurin): https://www.accessdata.fda.gov/drugsatfda_docs/label/2017/207997s000lbl.pdf

8

New Therapeutic Targets for Acute Leukemia

Stem Cells

Craig T. Jordan and Daniel A. Pollyea

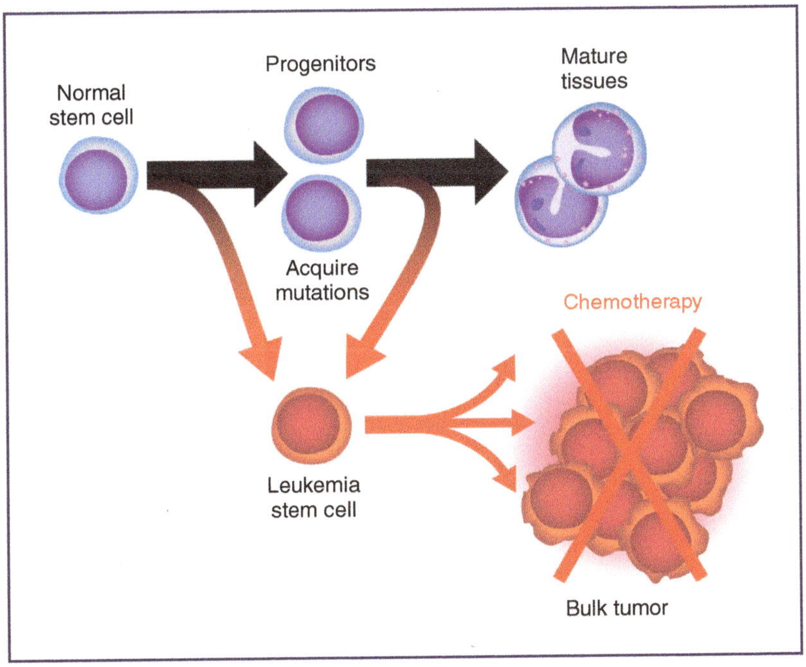

FIGURE 8-1: Genesis of leukemia stem cells (LSCs). LSCs are derived from normal hematopoietic stem cells or early progenitors as a result of the acquisition of leukemogenic mutations. Like their normal hematopoietic stem cell (HSC) brethren, LSCs have the capacity to self-renew and differentiate, producing the bulk disease population that ultimately leads to the deadly complications of AML. The bulk disease population, however, is sufficiently different from the LSCs such that standard chemotherapy approaches, which are typically most effective against rapidly dividing cells, do not have an appreciable impact on the LSC population.

AML, acute myeloid leukemia.

Several cell surface molecules have been described as selectively up-regulated in LSCs in comparison to HSCs. Examples include CD123 (IL3 receptor alpha), IL1 receptor accessory protein (IL1RAP), and TIM3; therapies directed specifically to these molecules are potential ways to eradicate LSCs. In addition, intracellular properties related to metabolism and oxidative stress are also preferentially activated/altered in LSCs, including up-regulation of Bcl-2, NF-kB, and beta-catenin signaling, as are the metabolic enzymes/epigenetic regulators IDH1 and IDH2. Small molecule-based therapies directed toward these targets also have the potential to more effectively eradicate LSCs.

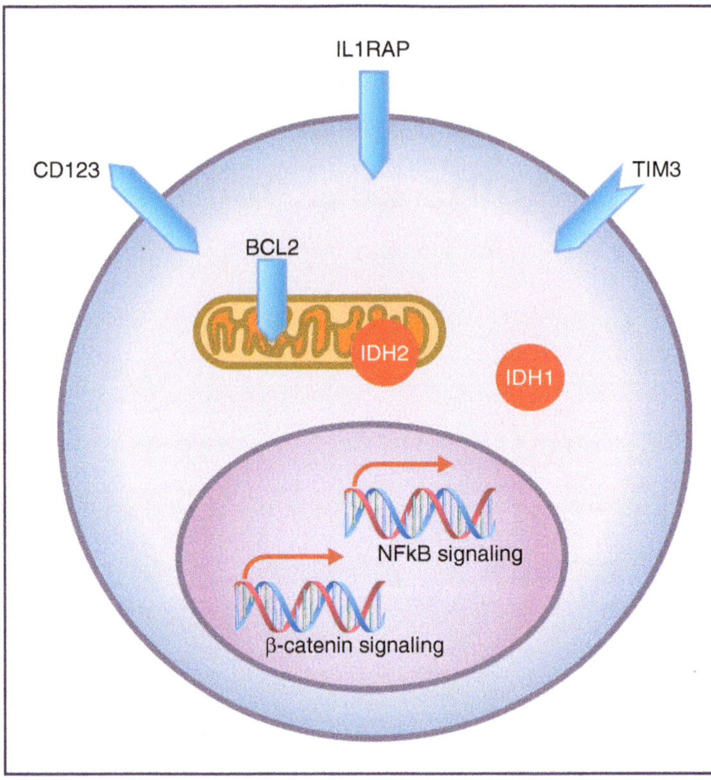

FIGURE 8-2: Therapeutic targeting of LSCs. The therapeutic index to target LSCs but spare the closely related hematopoietic stem cell (HSC) populations is narrow. Great care must be taken to understand the unique features of LSCs so that LSC-directed therapies are not excessively toxic to the hematopoietic system. Because LSCs are derived from HSCs and differentiate to produce the bulk disease, distinctive LSC targets are not necessarily shared by the bulk disease, necessitating that LSC-directed therapies be given with debulking treatments.
LSCs, leukemia stem cells.

Option 1: Before the administration of chemotherapy, the LSC population is likely as homogeneous as it will ever be. Once chemotherapy initiates, iatrogenic splintering of LSCs may occur, making it less likely that an LSC-directed therapy will be effective. Therefore, a rationale to deliver the LSC-directed therapy as the primary treatment, preceding the debulking chemotherapy, may act to maximize the impact of subsequent chemotherapy. The added benefit of this strategy is that it allows for an evaluation of the toxicity of the LSC-directed therapy independent of other therapies, which is of particular interest in the setting of phase 1 studies.

Option 2: Co-administration of the LSC-directed therapy with intensive chemotherapy has the advantage of exploiting any synergy that may exist between the purported LSC targeting therapy and the debulking chemotherapy. Like option 1, this approach also likely targets the LSC population at a relative early stage, before subsequent pathogenesis may make LSCs more difficult to treat. This strategy is not appropriate for instances in which the LSC-targeted therapy may antagonize the debulking therapy.

Option 3: Posttreatment maintenance therapy is an important role to consider for LSC-directed therapies that are well tolerated and ideally orally bioavailable. At this point, the overall disease burden is low, potentially allowing for the impact of a relatively low-intensity therapy to be maximized. The disadvantage of this strategy would be from the increased heterogeneity of the LSC population that occurs after exposure to indiscriminate intensive chemotherapy, potentially muting the impact of a posttreatment maintenance strategy. A further challenge is that well-validated methods to evaluate disease response for patients in remission are not yet readily available.

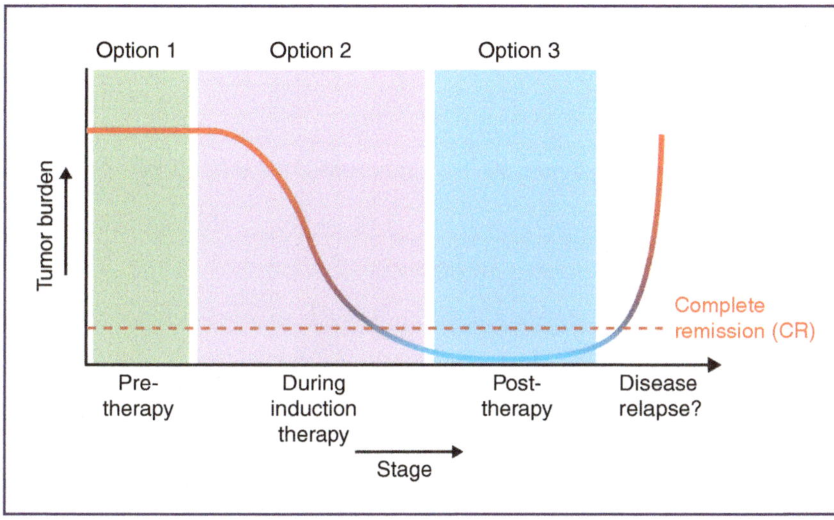

FIGURE 8-3: Clinical strategies for timing of treatment to eradicate leukemia stem cells. Therapies that target leukemia stem cells could conceivably be administered at multiple different time points in the course of a patient's disease. The major examples of these specific windows are listed here as options 1 to 3. The displayed curve is representative of the tumor burden as a function of time. Prior to treatment, the disease is at its apex; with effective treatment, usually intensive chemotherapy, a debulking of the disease, ideally to the level of complete remission, is possible. Patients in the posttreatment setting can remain in a complete remission or have relapsed disease.

Selected References

Askmyr M, Agerstam H, Hansen N, et al. Selective killing of candidate AML stem cells by antibody targeting of IL1RAP. *Blood*. 2013;121(18):3709–3713.

Chan SM, Thomas D, Corces-Zimmerman MR, et al. Isocitrate dehydrogenase 1 and 2 mutations induce BCL-2 dependence in acute myeloid leukemia. *Nat Med*. 2015;21(2):178–184.

Figueroa ME, Abdel-Wahab O, Lu C, et al. Leukemic IDH1 and IDH2 mutations result in a hypermethylation phenotype, disrupt TET2 function, and impair hematopoietic differentiation. *Cancer Cell*. 2010;18(6):553–567.

Guzman ML, Neering SJ, Upchurch D, et al. Nuclear factor-kappaB is constitutively activated in primitive human acute myelogenous leukemia cells. *Blood*. 2001;98(8):2301–2307.

Hamburger AW, Salmon SE. Primary bioassay of human tumor stem cells. *Science*. 1977;197(4302):461–463.

Hope KJ, Jin L, Dick JE. Acute myeloid leukemia originates from a hierarchy of leukemic stem cell classes that differ in self-renewal capacity. *Nat Immunol*. 2004;5(7):738–743.

Ishikawa F, Yoshida S, Saito Y, et al. Chemotherapy-resistant human AML stem cells home to and engraft within the bone-marrow endosteal region. *Nat Biotechnol*. 2007;25(11):1315–1321.

Jan M, Chao MP, Cha AC, et al. Prospective separation of normal and leukemic stem cells based on differential expression of TIM3, a human acute myeloid leukemia stem cell marker. *Proc Natl Acad Sci USA*. 2011;108(12):5009–5014.

Jordan CT, Upchurch D, Szilvassy SJ, et al. The interleukin-3 receptor alpha chain is a unique marker for human acute myelogenous leukemia stem cells. *Leukemia*. 2000;14(10):1777–1784.

Lagadinou ED, Sach A, Callahan K, et al. BCL-2 inhibition targets oxidative phosphorylation and selectively eradicates quiescent human leukemia stem cells. *Cell Stem Cell*. 2013;12:329–341.

Pollyea DA, Gutman JA, Gore L, et al. Targeting acute myeloid leukemia stem cells: a review and principles for the development of clinical trials. *Haematologica*. 2014;99(8):1277–1284.

Reya T, Morrison SJ, Clarke MF, Weissman IL. Stem cells, cancer, and cancer stem cells. *Nature*. 2001;414(6859):105–111.

Salmon SE, Hamburger AW, Soehnlen B, et al. Quantitation of differential sensitivity of human-tumor stem cells to anticancer drugs. *N Engl J Med*. 1978;298(24):1321–1327.

Zhao C, Blum J, Chen A, et al. Loss of beta-catenin impairs the renewal of normal and CML stem cells in vivo. *Cancer Cell*. 2007;12(6):528–541.

Exploiting the DNA Damage Response and Repair Pathways

Ivana Gojo, Keith W. Pratz, and Judith E. Karp

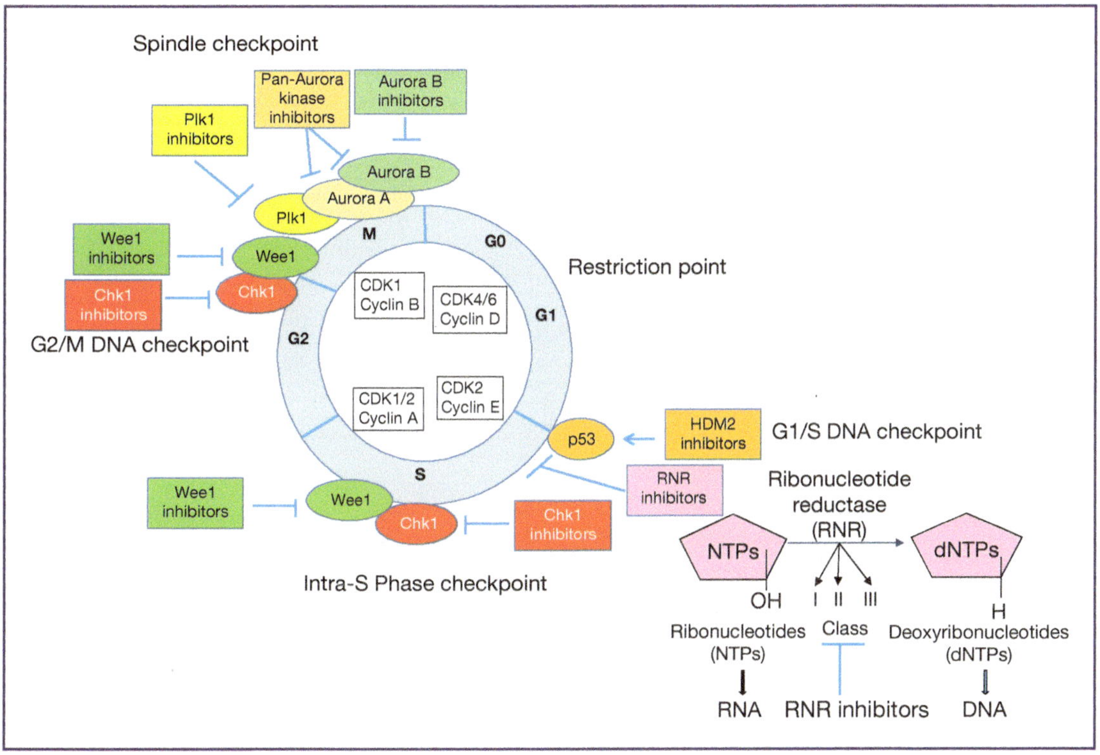

FIGURE 8-4: **Cell cycle checkpoint inhibitors in AML. Cell cycle is controlled by successive activation of cyclin-cyclin dependent kinases (CDKs). Cell cycle checkpoints serve to stop progression of the cell cycle in response to DNA damage, to allow time for DNA repair, and to preserve genomic integrity. The P53-dependent G1/S checkpoint blocks initiation of DNA replication. P53 is frequently altered (mutations or losses) in patients with complex karyotype AML. Inhibitors of HDM2 (RG7112, RO5503781, and MK-8242) are in clinical studies in AML alone or in combination with cytarabine and have a potential to be effective in leukemia cells that retain wild-type p53. Tumors that are defective in p53 function are often defective in arresting cells in G1 in response to DNA damage and rely on an intact S phase and G2 checkpoint. Depending on the type of genotoxic stress, either ataxia-telangectasia mutated (ATM) protein kinase or ataxia-telangiectasia-related (ATR) protein kinase are activated, leading to activation of Chk1 and Wee1 kinases that inactivate Cdk1, resulting in intra S phase and G2/M arrest, allowing time for DNA repair. Inhibition of Chk1 (MK8776) and Wee1 (MK1775) sensitizes leukemia cells to cytarabine cytotoxicity in preclinical studies, and the combination of Chk1 inhibitor and cytarabine is in a phase II testing in AML. Synergistic activity has been described for Chk1 and Wee1 inhibition in leukemia cells. PLK1 and Aurora kinases are critical for centrosome maturation and proper formation of the mitotic spindle, and also play a role in chromosome segregation and cytokinesis. Plk1 inhibitor (Volasertib) and Aurora B kinase inhibitor (AZD1152) have shown promising clinical activity in AML patients when given with low dose cytarabine. In addition, several pan CDK inhibitors (flavopiridol, dinaciclib) have been explored as a therapeutic strategy in AML. Ribonucleotide reductase (RNR) is the enzyme responsible for the conversion of ribonucleotides to 2′-deoxyribonucleotides and thereby provides the precursors needed for both synthesis and repair of DNA. RNR inhibitors target the specific M1 subunit (clofarabine, fludarabine, gemcitabine) and M2 subunit (hydroxyurea, triapine) and have been explored in combination with other cytotoxic agents.**

AML, acute myeloid leukemia.

POLY(ADP-RIBOSE) POLYMERASE (PARP): AN INTRIGUING MOLECULAR TARGET FOR LEUKEMIA

- Family of 19 DNA repair enzymes with pivotal roles in replication, transcription, and preservation of genomic integrity
- Activated in response to DNA single-strand (SS) breaks
- Cells with intact mechanisms to repair DNA double-strand (DS) breaks (eg, Fanconi anemia pathway, BRCA1/2, ATM, Bloom pathways) can circumvent SS breaks
- However, cells with impaired DS repair cannot survive with PARP inhibition

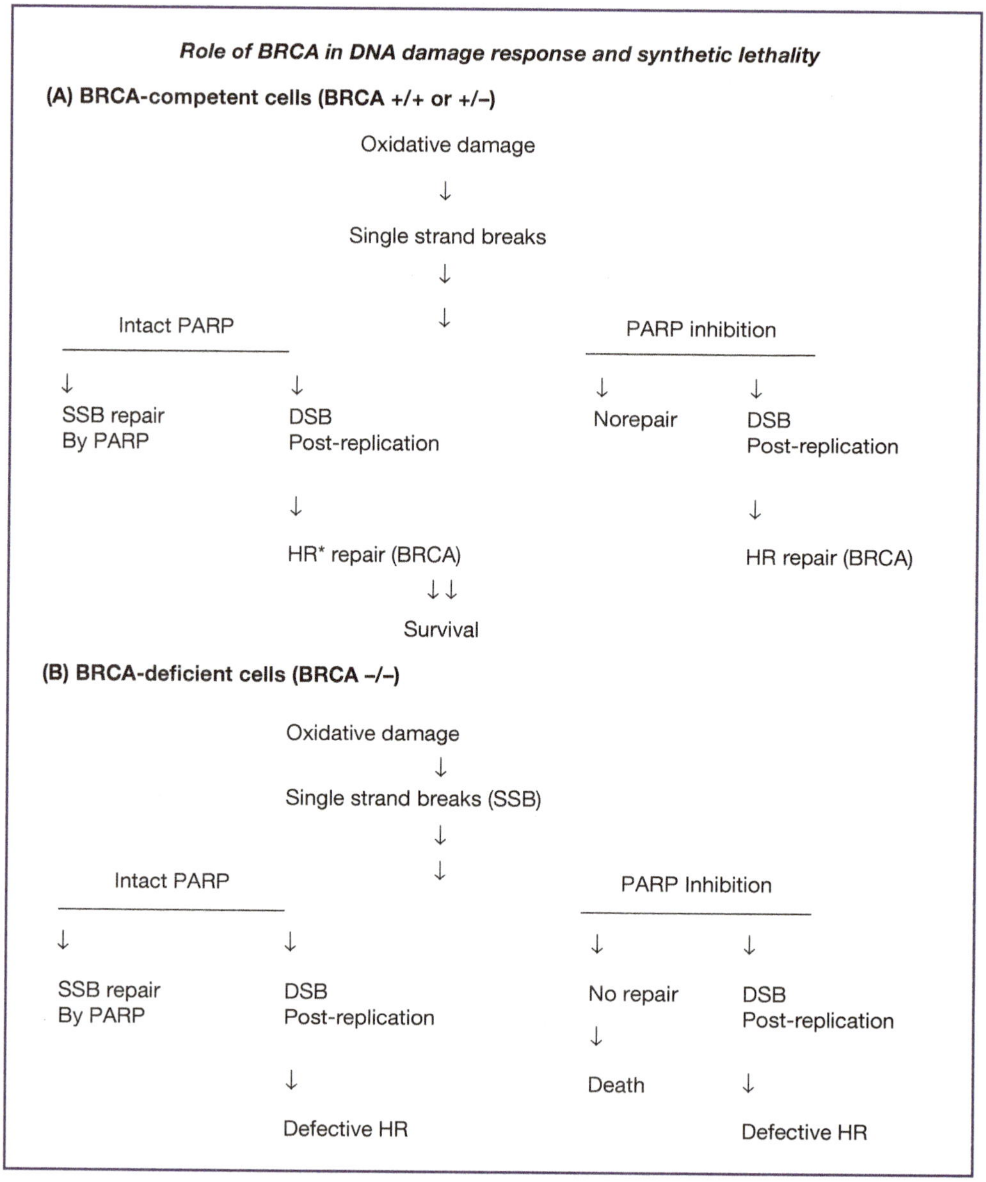

FIGURE 8-5: Synthetic lethality and BRCA pathways.

Source: Adapted from Hoeijmakers JH. DNA damage, aging and cancer. *New Engl J Med.* 2009;361:1475–1485.

DSB, double-strand breaks; HR, homologous recombination.

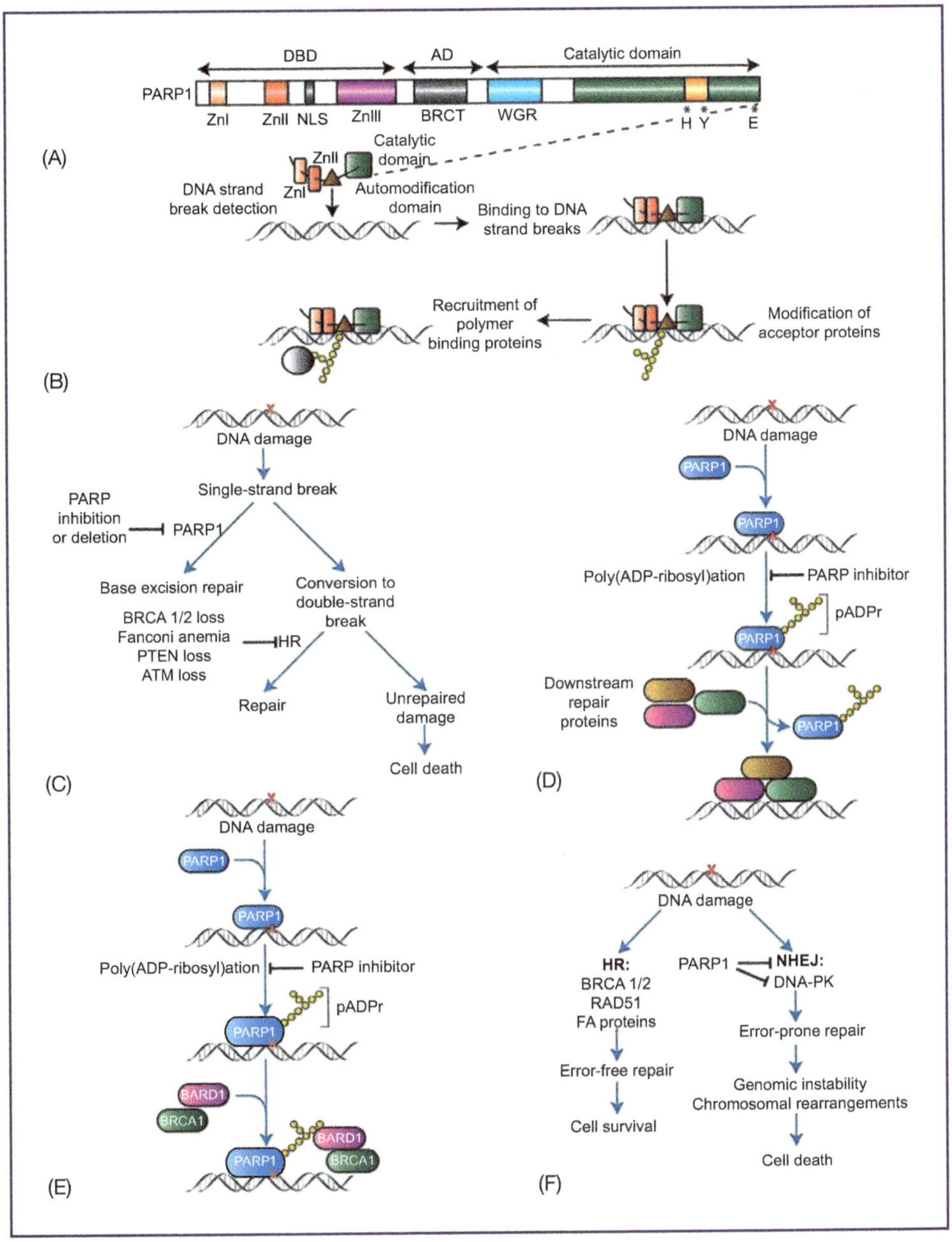

FIGURE 8-6: Summary of poly (ADP-ribose) [pADPr] polymerase 1 (PARP1) structure, function, and proposed contribution to synthetic lethality. (A) Schematic of PARP1 structure. (B) On binding to damaged DNA, PARP1 undergoes conformation change that increases its catalytic activity, leading to cleavage of NAD^+ and addition of ADP-ribose units to various proteins, including its own automodification domain. Resulting pADPr polymers (depicted as chains of yellow circles) alter function of proteins that are modified (eg, by decreasing affinity of PARP1 for damaged DNA) and also recruit additional proteins that bind to polymer noncovalently. (C–F) Models proposed to explain observed synthetic lethality between homologous recombination (HR) deficiency and PARP inhibition. These models emphasize (C) role of PARP1 in base excision repair, (D) recruitment of DNA repair proteins, (E) recruitment of BARD1-BRCA1 complex, and (F) suppression of nonhomologous end joining (NHEJ).

Source: From Scott CL, Swisher EM, Kaufmann SH. Poly(ADP-ribose) polymerase inhibitors: recent advances and future development. *J Clin Oncol*. 2015;33:1397–1406.

AD, automodification domain; BRCT, *BRCA1* C-terminal domain; DBD, DNA binding domain; FA, Fanconi anemia; NLS, nuclear localization signal; PK, protein kinase; WGR, tyrptophan-glycine-arginine-rich domain; Zn, zinc finger.

Table 8-1 Selected therapeutic targets in DNA damage response pathways

TARGET	PHASE OF CELL CYCLE ACTIVITY	SELECTED AGENTS
Cyclin-dependent kinases	all	Flavopiridol, dinaciclib (pan CDK)
	G1	*Palbociclib (CDK4/6)
Ribonucleotide reductase	G1	RR antisense
M1 subunit:		*Clofarabine,*Fludarabine,*Gemcitabine
M2 subunit:		*Hydroxyurea, Triapine
p53	G1	
HDM2**		RG7112, RO5503781, MK8242
Checkpoint kinases (CHK)	S/G2	MK8776
Wee kinase	S/G2	MK1775
PARP	S/G2	*Olaparib, Veliparib, BMN 673, Niraparib, Rucaparib
PARP trapping***		*Temozolomide, *Topotecan
Polo-like kinase (PLK)	M	*Volasertib
Aurora kinases	M	AZD1152

*Approved drug.
**HDM2, human analog of mouse double minute (MDM)2.
***Temozolomide (alkylating agent) and topotecan (topoisomerase I inhibitor) have the capacity to trap PARP at sites of damaged DNA and prevent the activity of downstream intermediaries in the overall PARP-triggered DNA damage response/repair pathway.
CDK, cyclin-dependent kinase

Selected References

Esposito MT, Zhao L, Fung TK, et al. Synthetic lethal targeting of oncogenic transcription factors in acute leukemia by PARP inhibitors. *Nat Med*. 2015;21(12):1481–1490.

Friedenson B. The BRCA1/2 pathway prevents hematologic cancers in addition to breast and ovarian cancers. *BMC Cancer*. 2007;7:152.

Gojo I, Karp JE. New strategies in acute myelogenous leukemia: leukemogenesis and personalized medicine. *Clin Cancer Res*. 2014;20(24):6233–6241.

Hoeijmakers JH. DNA damage, aging and cancer. *New Engl J Med*. 2009;361:1475–1485.

Karp JE, Thomas BM, Greer JM, et al. Phase I pharmacological trial of cytosine arabinoside with the selective checkpoint 1 inhibitor SCH900776 in refractory acute leukemias. *Clin Cancer Res*. 2012;18(24):6723–6731.

Pratz KW, Koh B, Patel AG, et al. Poly(ADP-ribose) polymerase inhibitor hypersensitivity in aggressive myeloproliferative neoplasms. *Clin Cancer Res*. 2016;22(15):3894–3902.

Schenk EL, Koh BD, Flatten K, et al. Effects of selective checkpoint kinase 1 inhibition on cytarabine cytotoxicity in acute myelogenous leukemia. *Clin Cancer Res*. 2012;18(19):5364–5673.

Scott CL, Swisher EM, Kaufmann SH. Poly(ADP-ribose) polymerase inhibitors: recent advances and future development. *J Clin Oncol*. 2015;33:1397–1406.

Targeting Tumor Metabolism for Treatment of Acute Leukemia

Firas El Chaer and Ashkan Emadi

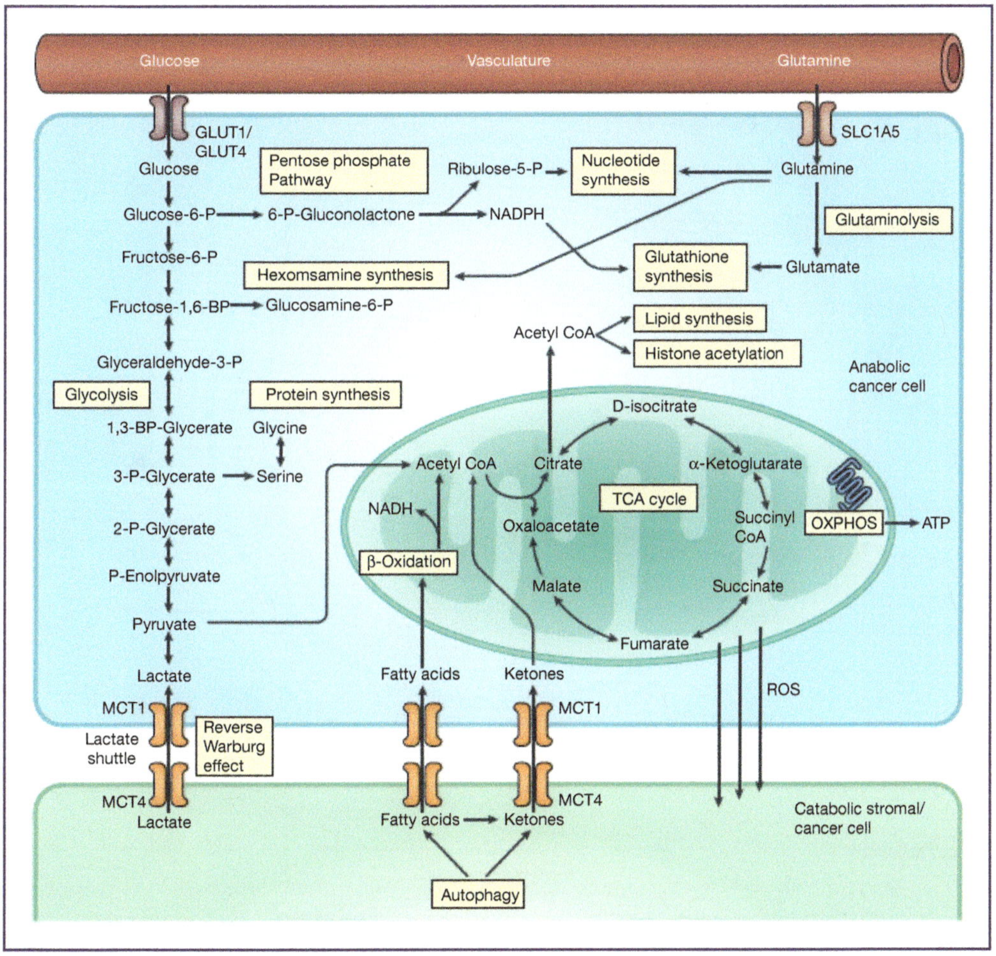

FIGURE 8-7: Metabolic adaptations of cancer/leukemia cells. In contrast to normal cells, rapidly dividing leukemia cells reprogram their nutritional requirements to match an increased metabolic demand. The two main nutrient sources for growth and survival of cancer cells are glucose, a sugar, and glutamine, an amino acid. Glucose and glutamine are used to feed the tricarboxylic acid (TCA) cycle and oxidative phosphorylation (OXPHOS), the pentose phosphate pathway (nucleotide synthesis), the synthesis of hexosamine (involved in the synthesis of glycosylated molecules), amino acids (proteins), and lipids. In addition to glucose and glutamine, neoplastic cells are able to use lactate, free fatty acids, and ketones released by surrounding catabolic cells. These small molecules are utilized to replenish TCA-cycle intermediates. On an important note, increased production of reactive oxygen species (ROS) in metabolically active cells demands the generation of appropriate levels of antioxidants, such as the reduced form of glutathione, which is generated by glutathione reductase using the coenzyme NADPH derived from the pentose phosphate pathway.

Source: **Reprinted by permission from Macmillan Publishers Ltd: Martinez-Outschoorn UE, Peiris-Pagés M, Pestell RG, et al. Cancer metabolism: a therapeutic perspective. *Nat Rev Clin Oncol.* 2017;14(2):113.**

ATP, adenosine triphosphate; BP, bisphosphate; CoA, coenzyme A; GLUT1/GLUT4, glucose transporter 1/4; MCT1, monocarboxylate transporter 1; MCT4, monocarboxylate transporter 4; NADH, nicotinamide adenine dinucleotide (reduced); NADPH, nicotinamide adenine dinucleotide phosphate (reduced); P, phosphate (or phospho); SLC1A5, solute carrier family 1 member 5 (also neutral amino acid transporter B[0]).

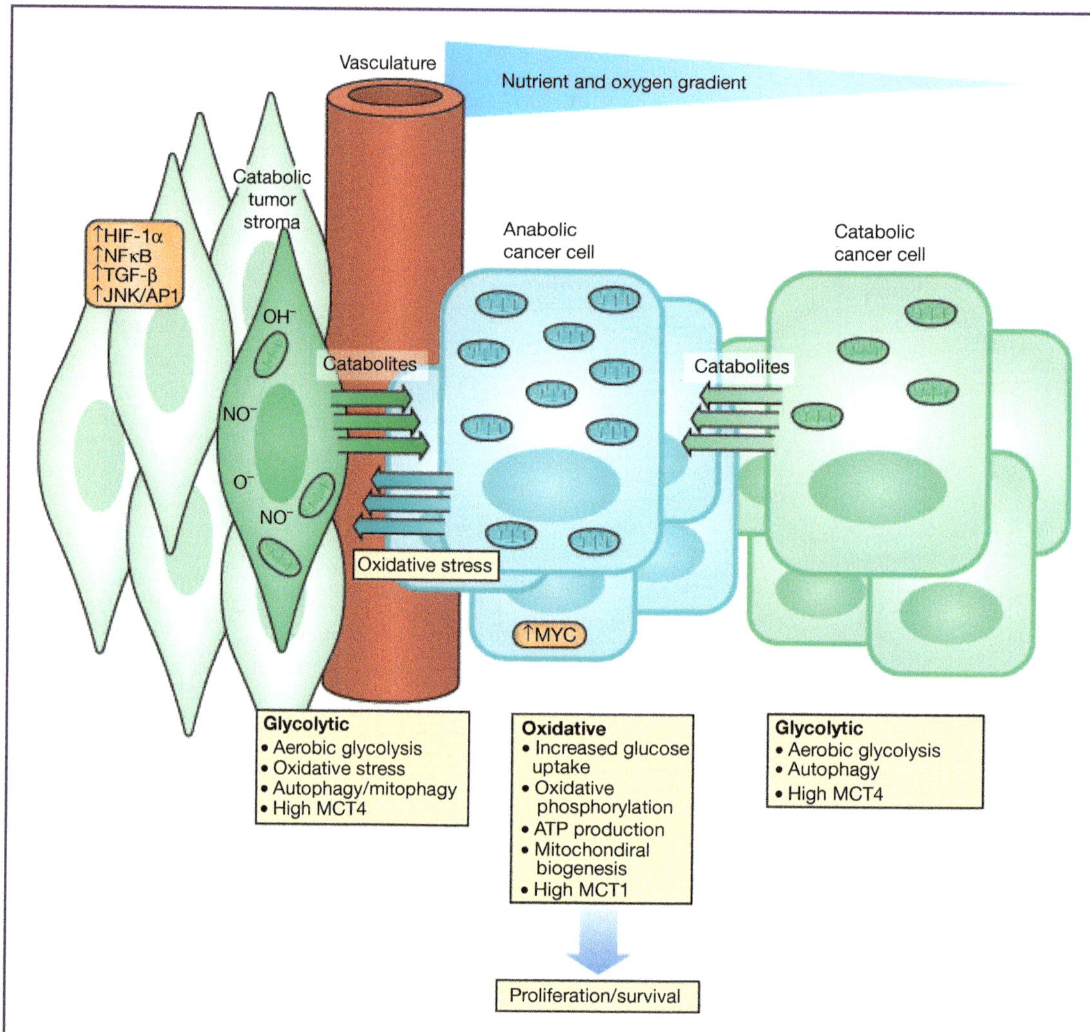

FIGURE 8-8: Metabolic diversity in cancer/leukemia cells. Tumor cells require high catabolite supply to grow and proliferate. In comparison to host cells, through alteration of oncogenes and tumor suppressor genes, cancer cells exhibit distorted metabolism, cell death resistance, and metabolic heterogeneity. Within and among tumors, the cancer cell metabolism depends on the microenvironment and proximity to vasculature. On the one hand, profiting from their easier access to nutrients and oxygen, blood-neighboring cancer cells aerobically generate ATP and up-regulate anabolism. Upon generating this oxidative stress, the surrounding host cells activate glycolysis and autophagy, providing further anabolic material to the tumor. On the other hand, cancer cells located away from the vasculature rely on the anabolic tumor cell population by adopting different metabolic pathways, independent of blood-supplied catabolites. Further examination of this metabolic heterogeneity and study of metabolic target therapies can improve cancer-treatment outcomes.

Source: Reprinted by permission from Macmillan Publishers Ltd: Martinez-Outschoorn UE, Peiris-Pagés M, Pestell RG, et al. Cancer metabolism: a therapeutic perspective. *Nat Rev Clin Oncol.* 2017;14(2):113.

HIF-1α, hypoxia-inducible factor 1α; JNK/AP1, c Jun N terminal kinases/activator protein 1; MCT1, monocarboxylate transporter 1; MCT4, monocarboxylate transporter 4; NFκB, nuclear factor κB; TGF-β, transforming growth factor β.

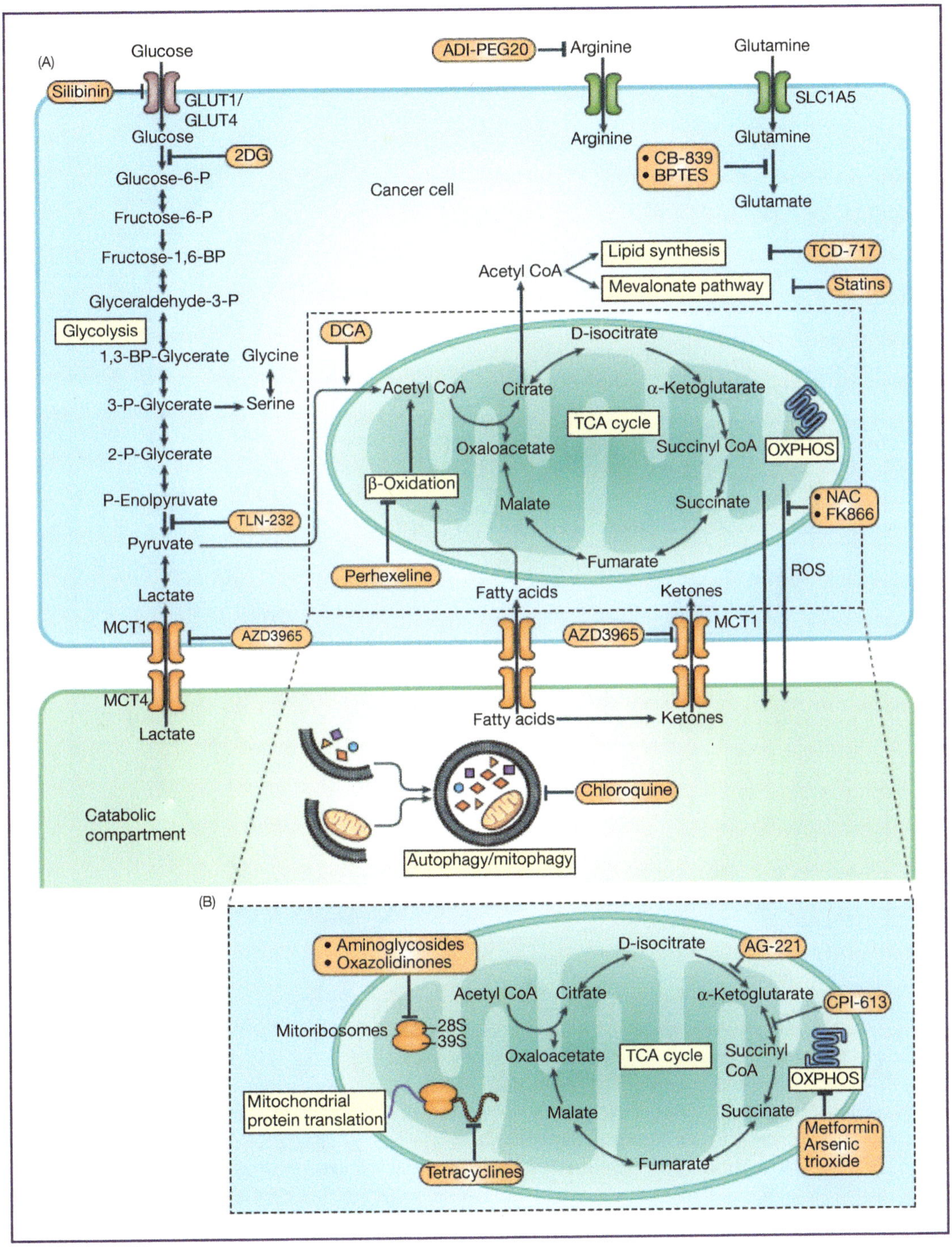

FIGURE 8-9: Examples of agents that target metabolic targets/pathways in cancer/leukemia.

Source: Reprinted by permission from Macmillan Publishers Ltd: Martinez-Outschoorn UE, Peiris-Pagés M, Pestell RG, et al. Cancer metabolism: a therapeutic perspective. *Nat Rev Clin Oncol.* 2017;14(2):113.

BP, bisphosphate; CoA, coenzyme A; GLUT1/GLUT4, glucose transporter 1/4; MCT1, monocarboxylate transporter 1; MCT4, monocarboxylate transporter 4; P, phosphate (or phospho); SLC1A5, solute carrier family 1 member 5 (also neutral amino acid transporter B[0]).

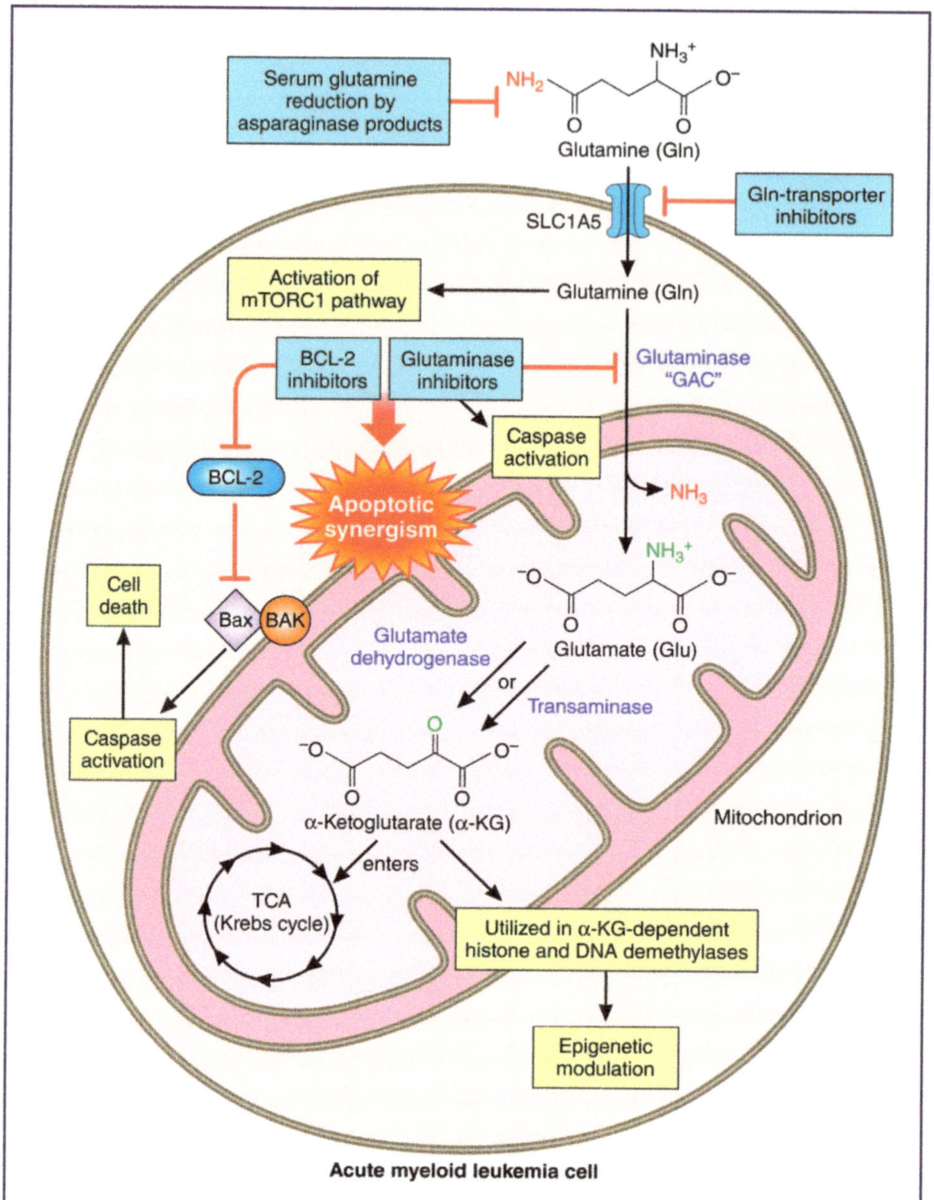

FIGURE 8-10: Glutamine metabolism inhibition for/interference in the treatment of AML. Glutamine, the most abundant amino acid in human cells, constitutes one of the main mitochondrial nutritional sources for cancer cell growth and survival. After entering the cell through SLC1A5, glutaminase C (GAC) removes an amide group from glutamine and converts it to glutamic acid. Then, transaminases or glutamate dehydrogenases transform glutamic acid into α-ketoglutarate (α-KG), a substrate of the Krebs cycle. Purine and pyrimidine synthesis relies on the nitrogen group supplied by this glutaminolysis enzymatic reaction. Moreover, glutamine activates the mammalian target of rapamycin target 1 (mTOR1) pathway, a central regulator of cellular metabolism, utilized in α-KG-dependent histone and DNA demethylases for epigenetic modulation. Glutamine depletion, through asparaginase products or glutamine-transporter inhibitors or glutaminase inhibitors, can result in the apoptosis of AML cells. Interference with glutamine metabolism, pharmacologically or genetically, leads to AML cell death. Glutaminase inhibitors lead to caspase activation and exhibit apoptotic synergism with B-cell lymphoma 2 (BCL-2) inhibitors demonstrating selective antileukemic activity. Targeting glutamine addiction of AML cells, along with other approved and investigational AML treatment strategies, would efficaciously kill AML cells.

Source: From Emadi A. Exploiting AML vulnerability: glutamine dependency. *Blood.* 2015;126(11):1269–1270. Used with permission.

AML, acute myeloid leukemia; SLC1A5, solute carrier family 1 member 5.

Selected References

Emadi A. Exploiting AML vulnerability: glutamine dependency. *Blood*. 2015;126(11):1269–1270.

Martinez-Outschoorn UE, Peiris-Pagés M, Pestell RG, et al. Cancer metabolism: a therapeutic perspective. *Nat Rev Clin Oncol*. 2017;14(2):113.

Mechanisms of Drug Resistance in Acute Leukemia

Maria R. Baer

Acute leukemias are treatable and curable. Treatment may consist of cytotoxic chemotherapy regimens, targeted therapies including kinase inhibitors or immunotherapies, or epigenetic therapies. Unfortunately, acute leukemia response rates and cure rates remain suboptimal, due to resistance of leukemia cells to available therapies. Leukemia cells exhibit multiple mechanisms of drug resistance. Some are drug- or drug class-specific, while others affect response to all drugs. Drug- or drug class-specific mechanisms include impaired drug entry into, or drug retention in, leukemia cells, as well as altered drug metabolism and altered expression or structure of the drug target, while pleiotropic drug resistance mechanisms reflect impaired triggering of cell death response. Acute leukemia recurrence following initial treatment response may be attributable to persistence of drug-resistant leukemia stem cells, with subsequent regrowth of leukemia and drug resistance of leukemia cells at relapse.

Drug uptake

hENT1
Cytarabine
Decitabine
Azacitidine
Cladribine
Clofarabine
Fludarabine
Mercaptopurine

OATP1B1, OATP1B3
Sorafenib
Sunitinib
Imatinib mesylate
Dasatinib
Nilotinib

OCT1
Imatinib mesylate

Drug efflux

ABCB1
Daunorubicin
Etoposide
Vincristine
Dexamethasone
Sorafenib
Creolanib

ABCC4
Cytarabine

ABCC11
Cytarabine

ABCG2
Mitoxantrone
Methotrexate
Mercaptopurine
Fludarabine
Cladribine
Clofarabine
Dasatinib
Sorafenib

FIGURE 8-11: Altered drug transport. Entry of nucleoside analogs into cells is regulated by human equilibrative nucleoside transporters (hENTs), including hENT1, and reduced expression or mutation may confer resistance to substrate drugs. Similarly, the organic anion-transporting polypeptides (OATs) or solute-linked carriers (SLCs) OATP1B1 and OATP1B3 transport fms-like tyrosine 3 (FLT3) inhibitors and BCR-ABL inhibitors. The human organic cation transporter 1 (OCT1; SLC22A1) transports the BCR-ABL inhibitor imatinib into cells. Much work has focused on expression of ATP-binding cassette (ABC) drug efflux proteins on acute leukemia cells, their efflux of chemotherapy drugs and BCR-ABL and FLT3 inhibitors and their role in treatment response. Unfortunately, despite the association of expression and function of resistance-associated ABC proteins on AML cells with adverse treatment response, incorporation of inhibitors of ABC protein-mediated drug transport into treatment regimens did not improve treatment outcomes, nor did substitution of a non-ABC protein substrate chemotherapy drug. Lack of positive impact on outcomes was likely due to the coexistence of additional mechanisms of resistance, so that overcoming drug efflux was not sufficient for overcoming drug resistance.

AML, acute myeloid leukemia; ATP, adenosine triphosphate.

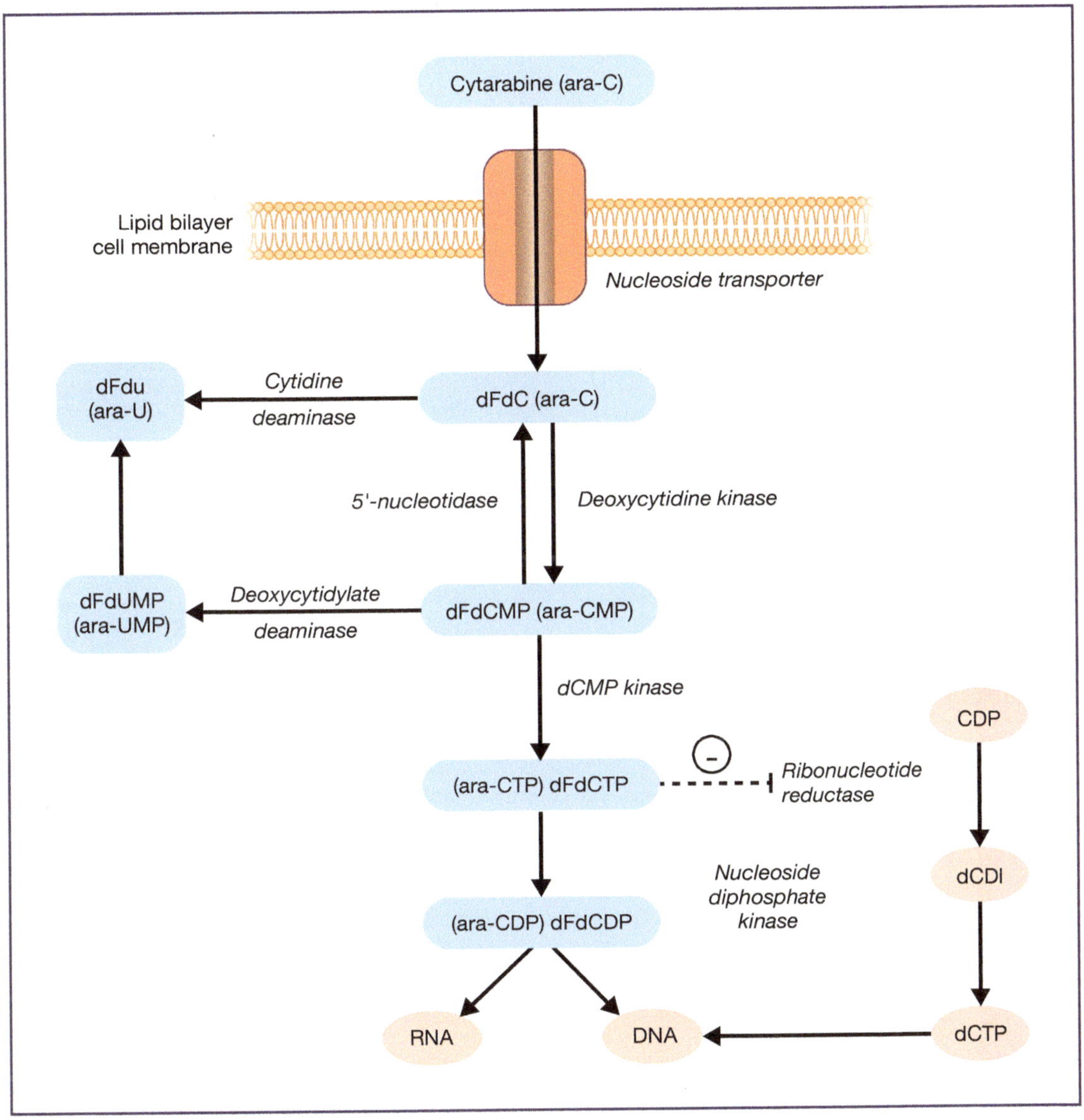

FIGURE 8-12: **Altered drug metabolism. Altered metabolism of several drugs used to treat leukemias is a potential cause of resistance to these drugs. Cytarabine (ara-C) is activated to Ara-CTP by kinases, including deoxycytidine kinase, and deactivated by deaminases, including cytidine deaminase, and ara-C efficacy correlates with ara-CTP levels and with expression of genes involved in cytarabine transport and metabolism. Deoxycytidine kinase also activates the DNA methyltransferase inhibitor decitabine and the antimetabolites cladribine and fludarabine. Efficacy of these drugs is therefore regulated by deoxycytidine kinase expression and activity.**

ara-CDP, ara-cytidine-5′-diphosphate; ara-CMP, ara-cytidine-5′-monophosphate; ara-CTP, ara-cytidine-5′-triphosphate; ara-U, uracil arabinoside; ara-UMP, ara-uridine-5′-monophosphate; CDP, cytidine diphosphate; CMP, common myeloid progenitor; dCTP, deoxycytidine triphosphate.

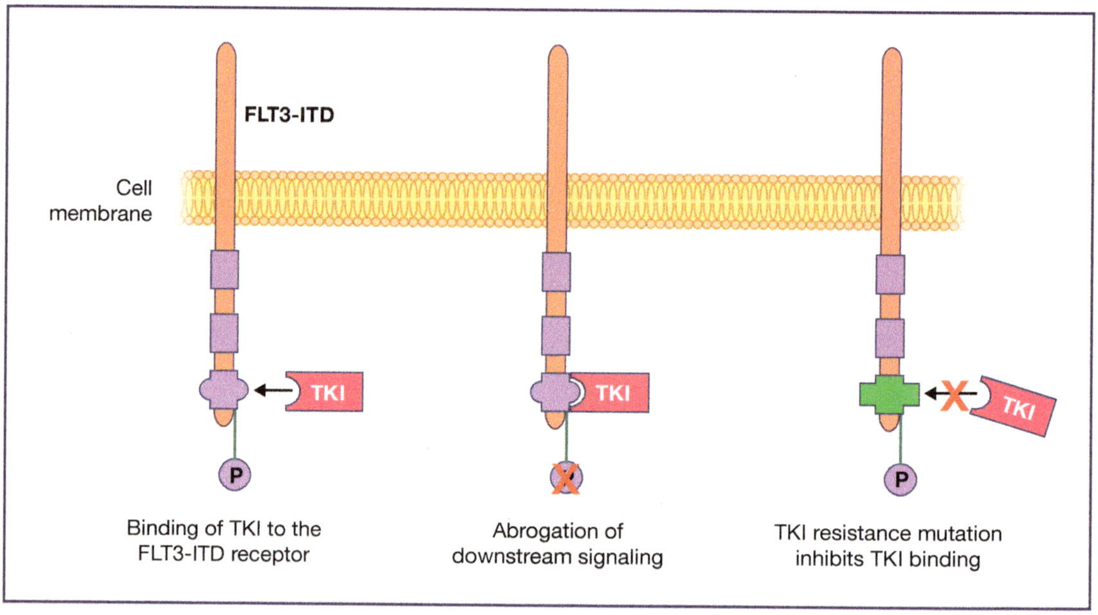

FIGURE 8-13: Altered drug target. Drug resistance may be caused by quantitative or structural changes in the drug target. An example of quantitative change in a drug target is asparaginase resistance in acute lymphoblastic leukemia (ALL) cells caused by increased asparagine synthetase activity. Another example is down-regulation of the microRNA miR29b as a mechanism of resistance to the DNA methyltransferase inhibitor (DNMTi) decitabine. miR29b suppresses the expression of the three DNMT isoforms, DNMT1, DNMT3A, and DNMT3B, explaining the association between high pretreatment miR29b expression and decitabine response. The best-described structural alterations of drug target in leukemia cells are acquired point mutations in BCR-ABL in BCR-ABL-expressing chronic myelogenous leukemia (CML) and ALL cells, resulting in the loss of BCR-ABL inhibitor binding as a mechanism of acquired resistance. Similarly, acquired activating point mutations at D835 in the FLT3 tyrosine kinase domain (TKD) cause resistance to type II FLT3 inhibitors, including quizartinib and sorafenib, which bind to the inactive form of FLT3, but not to type I inhibitors, including midostaurin, crenolanib, and gilteritinib, which bind to FLT3 in active conformation.

FLT3-ITD, FMS-like tyrosine kinase 3 internal tandem duplication; TKI, tyrosine kinase inhibitor.

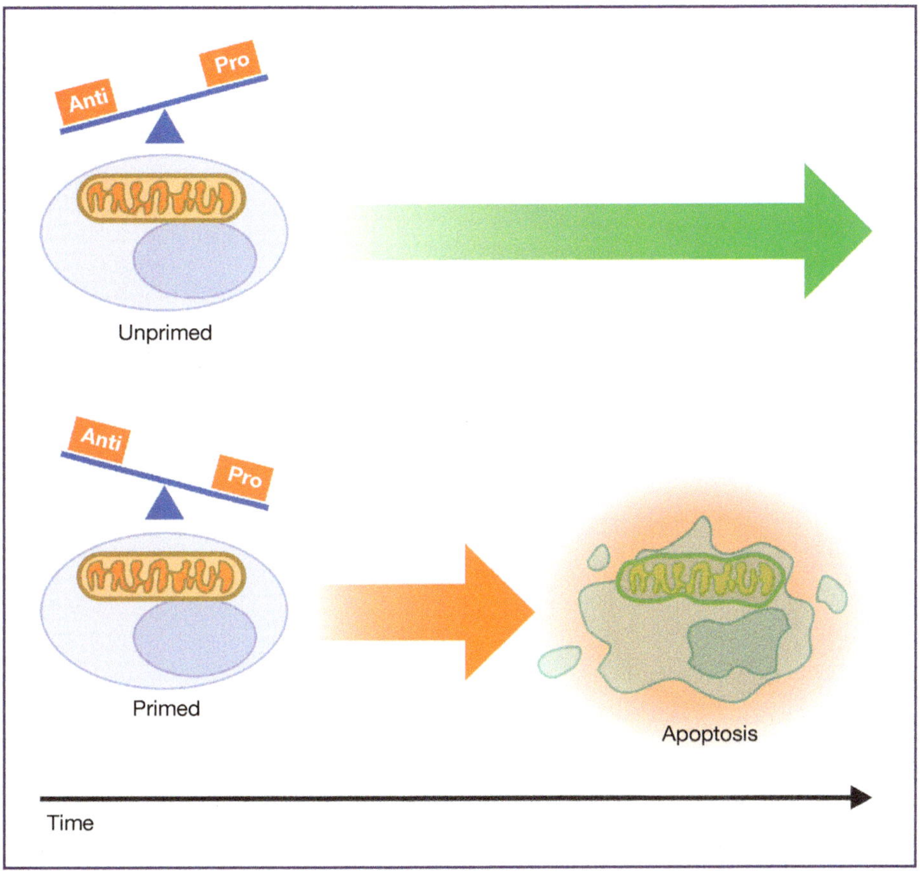

FIGURE 8-14: Impaired triggering of cell death mechanisms. A focus of recent work on drug resistance involves the role of intrinsic priming of leukemia cells to undergo apoptosis in response to drug treatment, reflecting the relative dominance of pro-apoptotic versus anti-apoptotic signals, and the role priming of leukemia cells in relation to normal hematopoietic stem cells has in determination of the therapeutic index. Novel therapeutics are targeting apoptosis and apoptotic priming.

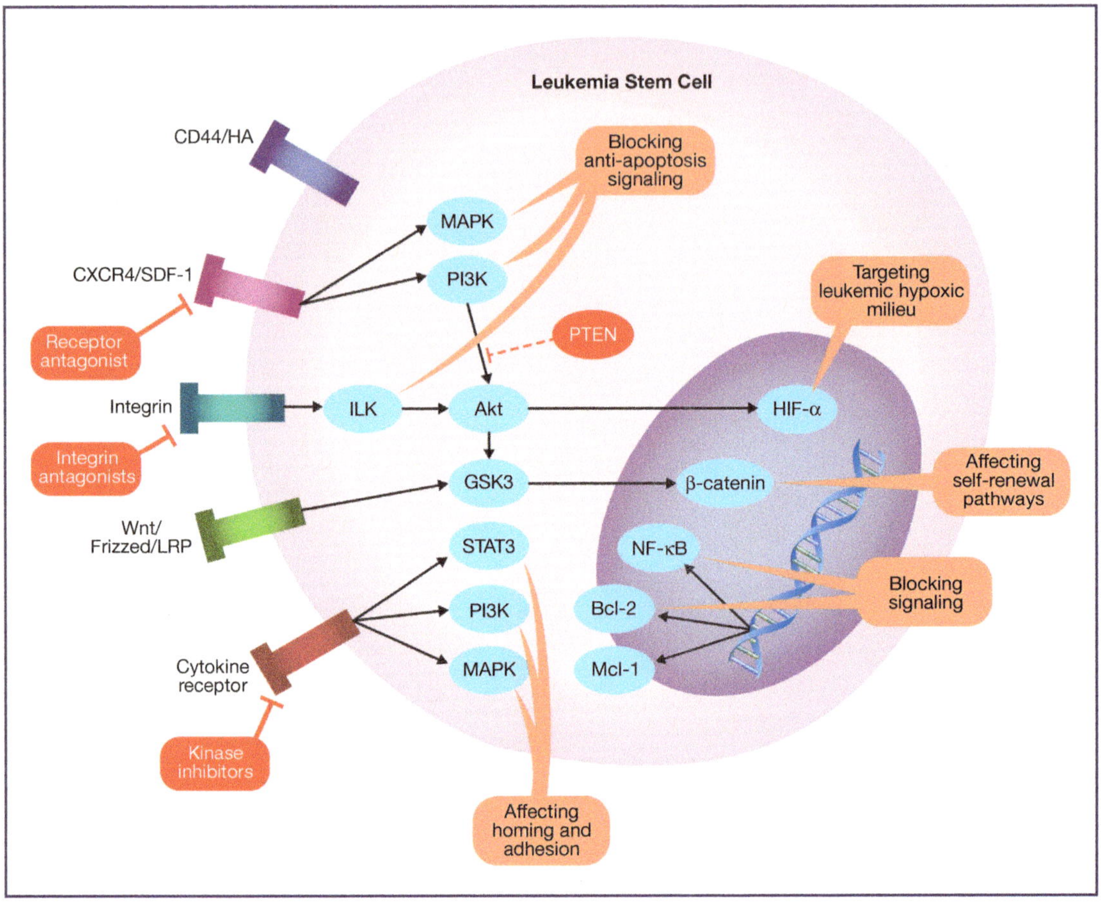

FIGURE 8-15: **Leukemia stem cell drug resistance. Leukemia relapse may be attributable to drug resistance of leukemia stem cells, with subsequent regeneration of leukemia. Properties of leukemia stem cells that are associated with drug resistance include cell cycle quiescence, metabolic quiescence, low cellular oxidative status, homing to the bone marrow microenvironment mediated by expression of the chemokine receptor CXCR4 and of adhesion molecules, and expression of ABC drug efflux proteins. Novel therapeutics are targeting leukemia stem cells.**
MAPK, mitogen-activated protein kinase; Wnt, wingless-type MMTV (mouse mammary tumor virus) integration site.

Selected References

Abraham A, Varatharajan S, Karathedath S, et al. RNA expression of genes involved in cytarabine metabolism and transport predicts cytarabine response in acute myeloid leukemia. *Pharmacogenomics*. 2015;16(8):877–890.

Balasubramanian MN, Butterworth EA, Kilberg MS. Asparagine synthetase: regulation by cell stress and involvement in tumor biology. *Am J Physiol Endocrinol Metab*. 2013;304(8):E789–E799.

Blum W, Garzon R, Klisovic RB, et al. Clinical response and miR-29b predictive significance in older AML patients treated with a 10-day schedule of decitabine. *Proc Natl Acad Sci USA*. 2010;107(16):7473–7478.

Brózik A, Hegedüs C, Erdei Z, et al. Tyrosine kinase inhibitors as modulators of ATP binding cassette multidrug transporters: substrates, chemosensitizers or inducers of acquired multidrug resistance? *Expert Opin Drug Metab Toxicol*. 2011;7(5):623–642.

Cripe LD, Uno H, Paietta EM, et al. Zosuquidar, a novel modulator of P-glycoprotein, does not improve the outcome of older patients with newly diagnosed acute myeloid leukemia: a randomized, placebo-controlled trial of the Eastern Cooperative Oncology Group 3999. *Blood*. 2010;116(20):4077–4085.

Chonghaile TN, Roderick JE, Glenfield C, et al. Maturation stage of T-cell acute lymphoblastic leukemia determines BCL-2 versus BCL-XL dependence and sensitivity to ABT-199. *Cancer Discov*. 2014;4(9):1074–1087.

Etchin J, Montero J, Berezovskaya A, et al. Activity of a selective inhibitor of nuclear export, selinexor (KPT-330), against AML-initiating cells engrafted into immunosuppressed NSG mice. *Leukemia*. 2016;30(1):190–199.

Fukuda Y, Lian S, Schuetz JD. Leukemia and ABC transporters. *Adv Cancer Res*. 2015;125:171–196.

Garzon R, Liu S, Fabbri M, et al. MicroRNA-29b induces global DNA hypomethylation and tumor suppressor gene reexpression in acute myeloid leukemia by targeting directly DNMT3A and 3B and indirectly DNMT1. *Blood*. 2009;113(25):6411–6418.

Gottesman MM, Fojo T, Bates SE. Multidrug resistance in cancer: role of ATP-dependent transporters. *Nat Rev Cancer*. 2002;2(1):48–58.

Herrmann H, Blatt K, Shi J, et al. Small-molecule inhibition of BRD4 as a new potent approach to eliminate leukemic stem–and progenitor cells in acute myeloid leukemia AML. *Oncotarget*. 2012;3(12):1588–1599.

Konopleva MY, Jordan CT. Leukemia stem cells and microenvironment: biology and therapeutic targeting. *J Clin Oncol*. 2011;29(5):591–599.

Lagadinou ED, Sach A, Callahan K, et al. BCL-2 inhibition targets oxidative phosphorylation and selectively eradicates quiescent human leukemia stem cells. *Cell Stem Cell*. 2013;12:329–341.

O'Hare T, Eide CA, Deininger MW. BCR-ABL kinase domain mutations, drug resistance, and the road to a cure for chronic myeloid leukemia. *Blood*. 2007;110(7):2242–2249.

Pan R, Hogdal LJ, Benito JM, et al. Selective BCL-2 inhibition by ABT-199 causes on-target cell death in acute myeloid leukemia. *Cancer Discov*. 2014;4(3):362–375.

Pastor-Anglada M, Pérez-Torras S. Nucleoside transporter proteins as biomarkers of drug responsiveness and drug targets. *Front Pharmacol*. 2015;6:13.

Polillo M, Galimberti S, Baratè C, et al. Pharmacogenetics of BCR/ABL inhibitors in chronic myeloid leukemia. *Int J Mol Sci*. 2015;16(9):22811–22829.

Qin T, Castoro R, El Ahdab S, et al. Mechanisms of resistance to decitabine in the myelodysplastic syndrome. *PLoS One*. 2011;6(8):e23372.

Shaffer BC, Gillet JP, Patel C, et al. Drug resistance: still a daunting challenge to the successful treatment of AML. *Drug Resist Updat*. 2012;15(1–2):62–69.

Smith CC, Wang Q, Chin CS, et al. Validation of ITD mutations in FLT3 as a therapeutic target in human acute myeloid leukaemia. *Nature*. 2012;485(7397):260–263.

Stone RM, Mazzola E, Neuberg D, et al. Phase III open-label randomized study of cytarabine in combination with amonafide L-malate or daunorubicin as induction therapy for patients with secondary acute myeloid leukemia. *J Clin Oncol*. 2015;33(11):1252–1257.

Vo TT, Ryan J, Carrasco R, et al. Relative mitochondrial priming of myeloblasts and normal HSCs determines chemotherapeutic success in AML. *Cell*. 2012;151(2):344–355.

Yamauchi T, Negoro E, Kishi S, et al. Intracellular cytarabine triphosphate production correlates to deoxycytidine kinase/cytosolic 5′-nucleotidase II expression ratio in primary acute myeloid leukemia cells. *Biochem Pharmacol*. 2009;77(12):1780–1786.

Zimmerman EI, Hu S, Roberts JL, et al. Contribution of OATP1B1 and OATP1B3 to the disposition of sorafenib and sorafenib-glucuronide. *Clin Cancer Res*. 2013;19(6):1458–1466.

Microenvironment

Gabriel Ghiaur and Pamela S. Becker

The bone marrow microenvironment is a highly organized structure wherein multiple cellular elements form unique niches with distinct functions and contribution to hematopoiesis. This concept is in stark contrast with the amorphous/liquid samples we obtain from bone marrow aspirates. Malignant cells such as acute leukemia as well as micrometastatic solid tumors take full advantage of protective microenvironments within the bone marrow to evade not only chemotherapy but also radiation and immune attack. In some cases, a deranged microenvironment is believed to be responsible for development of the malignancy. Understanding the complex cross talk between cancer and the bone marrow microenvironment has been recently recognized to offer new therapeutic tools to eliminate minimal residual disease and improve cancer treatment outcomes, particularly in hematologic malignancies.

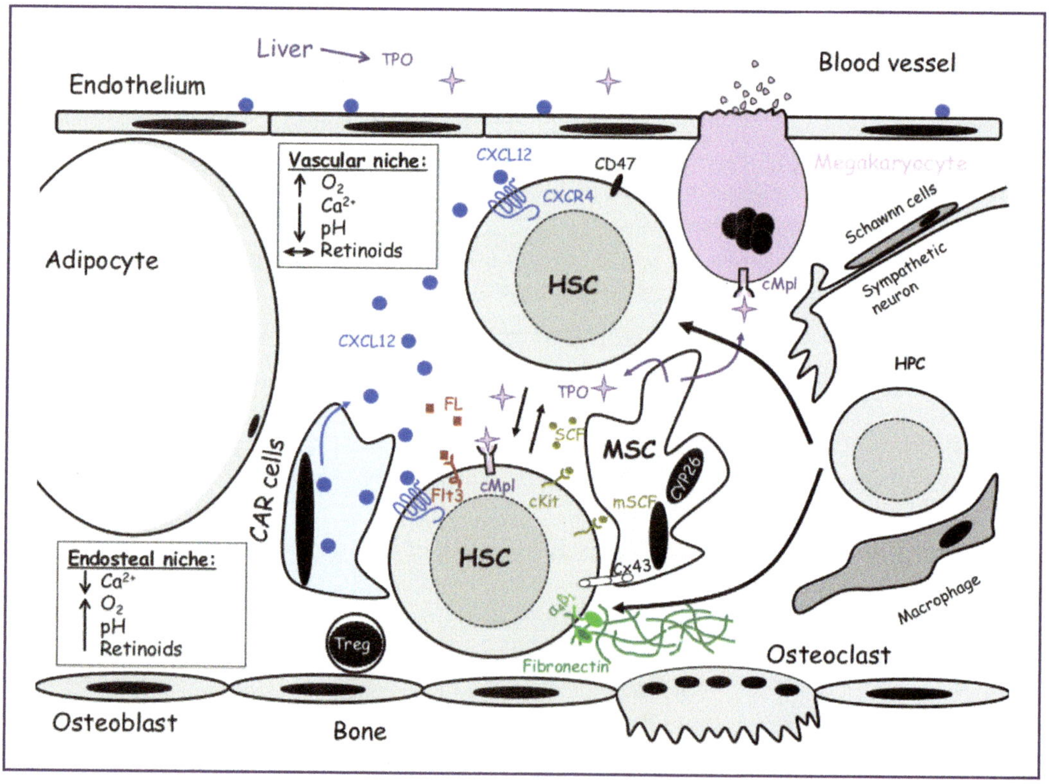

FIGURE 8-16: Hematopoietic stem cell niche in normal bone marrow. The bone marrow microenvironment is a highly organized structure where multiple cellular elements [some hematopoietic: HSC/HPC, macrophages, lymphocytes, megakaryocytes, osteoclasts, and some not: mesenchymal stem cells (MSC), CXCL12 abundant reticular (CAR) cells, nestin positive cells, osteoblasts, adipocytes, endothelial cells, neurons] come together to form unique niches with distinct functions and contributions to hematopoiesis. This is of course in stark contrast with the amorphous/liquid samples we get from bone marrow aspirates. In addition to these cellular elements, special biochemical properties of parts of the bone marrow (ie, relative lower oxygen tension, lower pH, and high concentrations of calcium–closer to the osteoblasts) as well as a repertoire of cytokines/chemokines (SCF, TPO, FLT3 ligand) and extracellular matrix proteins (ie, fibronectin) interact to control HSC behavior in the bone marrow and to match their biological activity to physiological needs.

FLT3, FMS-like tyrosine kinase 3; HPC, hematopoietic progenitor cell; HSC, hematopoietic stem cell; SCF, stem cell factor; TPO, thrombopoietin.

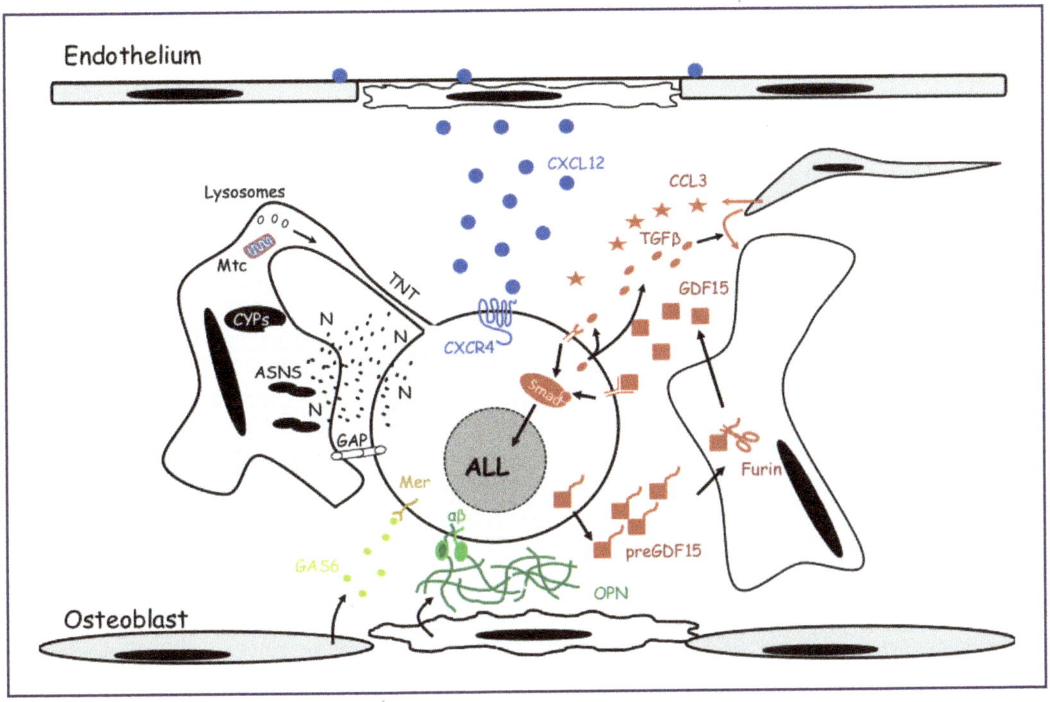

FIGURE 8-17: ALL in the bone marrow niche. In acute lymphoblastic leukemia, the bone marrow microenvironment is initially remodeled to accommodate massive numbers of malignant cells, and subsequently adapts to protect minimal residual disease (MRD). At presentation, patients with ALL have disrupted osteoblast and vascular niches (center osteoblast or endothelial cell with wiggly cell membrane in figure) with relatively low levels of CXCL12, IL7, and osteocalcin. Engagement, likely via integrins ($\alpha_4\beta_1$, $\alpha_5\beta_1$, $\alpha_9\beta_1$) of some leukemia cells by osteopontin (OPN) secreted from osteoblasts, induces dormancy resistance to chemotherapy. Some malignant lymphoblasts activate signaling pathways in the adjacent osteoblasts, resulting in secretion of GAS6, which in turn will ensure survival and resistance from chemotherapy-induced apoptosis of ALL cells downstream of Axl/Mer/Sky receptors. The mesenchymal elements present in the bone marrow niche form tight interactions with ALL cells, including cytoplasm-to-cytoplasm channels via GAP junctions and even larger channels via tunneling nanotubes. The transport of mitochondria, lysosome, reactive oxygen species, and even energy creates true syncytia where lymphoblasts are shielded from biochemical stress. Thus, on the one hand, bone marrow stroma expresses high levels of asparagine synthetase (ASNS) producing asparagine (N)-rich niches; on the other hand, it expresses high levels of drug metabolizing enzymes (CYPs) creating potential drug-free sanctuaries. While most ALL cells are killed with initial therapy, mechanisms mentioned before allow for persistence of MRD. Surviving ALL cells remodel the bone marrow niche to their advantage. By producing CCL3, they attract high numbers of mesenchymal cells, which under the influence of ALL-produced TGFβ will transform so that it can process pre-GDF15 produced by the malignant cells. Mature forms of GDF15 together with TGFβ will converge back on the ALL cells to activate Smad3 and reinforce their resistance to further chemotherapy. Leukemia cells rely on the CXCR4-CXCL12 axis to remain anchored in their niche during various stages of their development. Nevertheless, levels of CXCL12 rise during remission and high levels at diagnosis predict for poor outcome in ALL, making inhibitions of this axis a potential therapeutic target in these situations.

ALL, acute lymphoblastic leukemia; TGFβ, transforming growth factor beta.

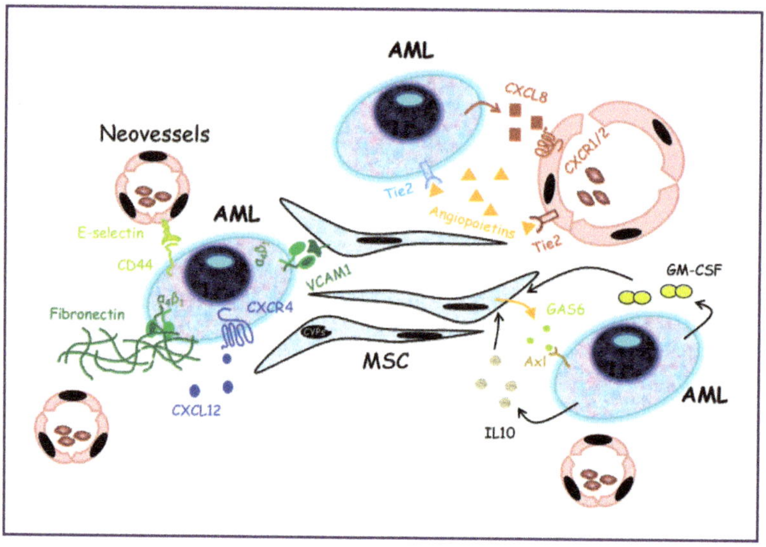

FIGURE 8-18: AML in the bone marrow niche. AML remains protected from chemotherapy in the marrow microenvironment retained via interaction with several receptors, including CXCR4, VLA4, and CD44. Bone marrow homing of both normal HSCs and AML is dependent on CXCR4, a chemokine receptor for CXCL12. Higher CXCR4 expression correlates with poor prognosis in AML. CXCR4 inhibitors can enhance efficacy of chemotherapy in AML. VLA-4 is integrin $\alpha_4\beta_1$, which binds to VCAM-1 on mesenchymal stromal cells (MSCs) or alternatively spliced fibronectin. Adhesion to VLA4 confers chemotherapy resistance. An antibody to CD44 can dislodge and eradicate AML in xenografts. Glycosylated CD44 can serve as an E-selectin ligand. AML blasts express E-selectin ligands and adhesion to E-selectin activates the Wnt survival pathway. In addition, some patients with AML show increased "marrow vascular density" predicting for poor outcome. The mechanism of increased angiogenesis may be secondary to secretion of proangiogenic factors such as CXCL8 from the malignant cells that induce proliferation of endothelial cells. In addition, high levels of angiopoietin 1 or 2 activate endothelial cells and induce proliferation of leukemia blasts via Tie2 receptors. Similar cross talk has been described between AML blasts and mesenchymal elements from the bone marrow microenvironment. In this case, malignant cells secrete IL10 and GM-CSF to induce secretion of Gas6 from stroma, which in turn would induce quiescence and drug resistance via signaling downstream of Axl. Most recently, bone marrow stromal elements have been shown to express drug metabolizing enzymes (CYPs) that can inactivate endogenous as well as pharmacological levels of retinoids and chemotherapy, calling into question whether effective drug levels are routinely achieved in the bone marrow niche.

AML, acute myeloid leukemia; CYP, cytochrome P450; GM-CSF, granulocyte macrophage colony stimulating factor; MSC, mesenchymal stromal cell; VCAM, vascular cell adhesion molecule.

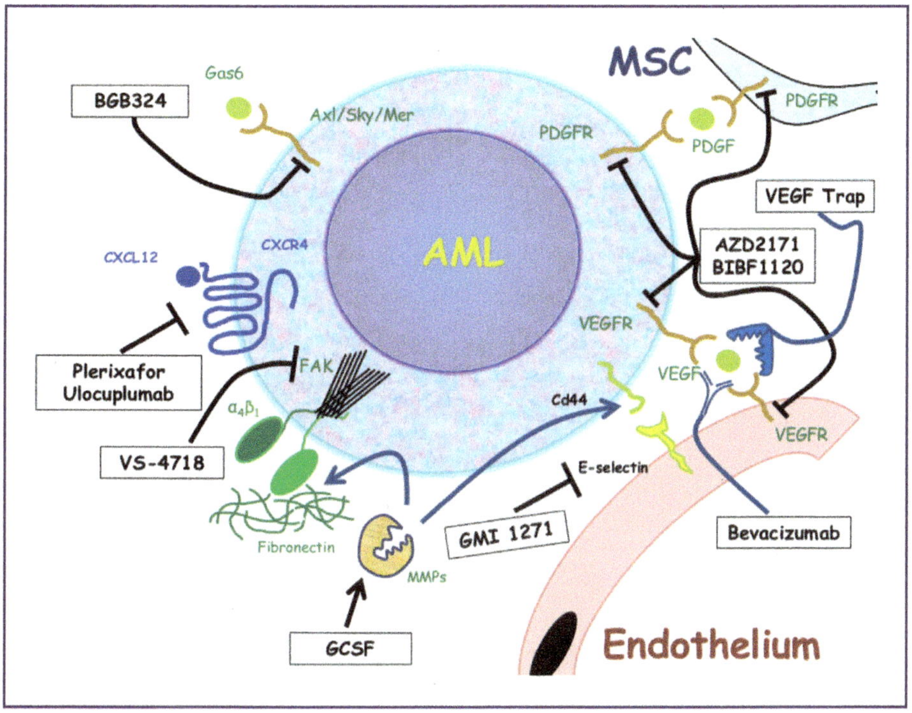

FIGURE 8-19: Strategies to target the bone marrow microenvironment. Several pathways are being targeted to overcome the ability of the microenvironment to promote survival of AML/ALL and cause resistance to chemotherapy. The first drug used to interfere with the CXCR4 pathway was plerixafor, the same drug that is FDA approved for autologous mobilization of peripheral blood stem cells for non-Hodgkin's lymphoma or multiple myeloma. Plerixafor was used in patients with relapsed/refractory AML in combination with MEC chemotherapy and in patients with newly diagnosed AML in combination with 7 + 3 (with high-dose daunorubicin). The novel agent MDX-1338, now known as ulocuplomab, is a humanized monoclonal antibody to CXCR4 that has a longer half-life than plerixafor (days rather than a few hours). Ulocuplomab has been used in combination with MEC for relapsed/refractory patients with AML. Regarding interference with the vascular niche, it has been recognized that AML blasts express VEGF receptors and that AML marrows are highly vascular. The VEGF–VEGFR interaction has been targeted by bevacizumab, an angiogenesis inhibitor that is FDA approved for six solid tumors, and cediranib (AZD2171) that inhibits the VEGFR tyrosine kinases. One signaling axis that is emerging as playing a critical role in quiescence and chemoresistance in both AML and ALL is GAS6-Axl/Sky/Mer. Efforts to target this mechanism are currently in phase 1 clinical trials. Another component of the vascular niche is E-selectin expressed by endothelial cells. AML cells express E-selectin ligands, and an E-selectin inhibitor GMI-1271 is being combined with MEC in a clinical trial for patients with relapsed/refractory AML. Engagement of integrins after adhesion leads to activation of focal adhesion kinase (FAK), the major signal transduction pathway. VS-4718 (aka PND-1186) is a reversible and selective FAK inhibitor that has been shown to disrupt tumors in their three-dimensional environments. Pharmacological levels of G-CSF not only act in combination with chemotherapy to sensitize AML cells but also change the bone marrow microenvironment, resulting in activation of metalloproteases (MMPs) and decreased levels of CXCL12, IL7, and osteocalcin. As a result, leukemic blasts are mobilized out from the bone marrow microenvironment and thus from their protective niche.

ALL, acute lymphoblastic leukemia; AML, acute myeloid leukemia; G-CSF, granulocyte colony stimulating factor; MEC, mitomycin, etoposide, cytarabine; MSC, mesenchymal stromal cell; VEGF, vascular endothelial growth factor.

Table 8-2 Clinical trials targeting the bone marrow microenvironment

TARGETED MECHANISM	TOOL	DISEASE	TYPE OF STUDY	RESULTS	CLINICALTRIALS.GOV
CXCR4-CXCL12	Plerixafor +/– chemo +/– alloBMT	AML/ALL	Phase 1 and 2	NO	NCT02605460
	Plerixafor + MEC	AML (R or R)	Phase 1 and 2	46% response, 39% CR	NCT00512252 NCT00906945 NCT01027923
	Plerixafor + daunorubcin/Ara-C	AML (upfront)	Phase 1	67% CR	
	MDX-1338 (BMS 936564) anti-CXCR4 Ab	AML (R or R)	Phase 1	CR/CRi 51%	NCT01120457
	ALX-0651	Healthy	Phase 1	Safe	NCT01374503
Adhesion	VS-4718 (FAK inhibitor)	AML/ALL	Phase 1	NO	NCT02215629
Angiogenesis					
IMiDs (see immune modulators)					
VEGF	Bevacizumab + mitoxandrone/Ara-C	AML (R or R)	Phase 2	48% response, 33% CR	NCT00015951
	Bevacizumab + Ida/Ara-C	AML (R or R)	Phase 2	NO	NCT00096148
	VEGF trap	AML (R or R)	Phase 2	NO	NCT00601991
TKI that target VEGFR	AZD 2171, BIBF1120, pozapanib (block VEGFR1,2,3; c-Kit, PDGFRα/β)	AML	Phase 1 and 2	NO	NCT00321581 NCT01361334 NCT01555268 NCT01488344
TKI that target Ang1, 2	Trebananib	AML	Phase 1	NO	NCT01555268
Hypoxia	TH-302 & PR104 (prodrugs activated by low O_2)	AML/ALL	Phase 1 and 2	NO	NCT01149915 NCT01037556
Mesenchymal Stroma (See also TKI that target PDGFRα and β)					
Axl-Gas6	BGB324 + Ara-C	AML	Phase 1	NO	NCT02488408
Hedgehog inhibitors	PF04449913	AML/ALL	Phase 1	NO	NCT00953758
	PF04449913 +/– low dose Ara-C, (7 + 3) or decitabine	AML/MDS	Phase 2	NO	NCT01841333 NCT02038777 NCT01546038

(*continued*)

Table 8-2 Clinical trials targeting the bone marrow microenvironment (*continued*)

TARGETED MECHANISM	TOOL	DISEASE	TYPE OF STUDY	RESULTS	CLINICALTRIALS.GOV
	Vismodegib + ribavirin/decitabine	AML	Phase 2	NO	NCT02073838
	Erismodegib + aza	AML	Phase 1b	NO	NCT02129101
Immunomodulators	AS101 (tellurium compound) + induction	AML/MDS	Phase 2	NO	NCT01010373
IMiDs	Lenalidomide, thalidomide, pomalidomide	AML/MDS/ALL	Phase 1 and 2	NO	Over 20 studies
	+/– chemotherapy, allo-BMT, DLI Lenalidomide	Elderly AML	Phase 2	16%–100% response	
	Lenalidomide + Aza	AML (R/R/old)	Phase 1 and 2	22%–28% CR, 41% ORR	
Immune checkpoint inhibitors	PD1 inhibitors (CT-011, Nivolumab)	AML	Phase 2	NO	NCT02532231
	Nivolumab +/– dentritic cell vaccines				NCT01096602
Cytokines	IL12 + IFNα	AML/MDS	Phase 1	NO	NCT00003451
G-CSF (selected recent)	+ Ifosfamide + mitoxantrone + etoposide	R/R ALL	Phase 2	23% CR	
	+ cytarabine + aclarubicin vs. FLAG	Ph neg ALL	Phase 2	50.7% CR	
	+ cytarabine + aclarubicin	AML R/R	Phase 2	60.7% CR	
	In Mito-FLAG	AML R/R	Phase 2	54% CR	
	In FLAG-GO	Upfront CBF AML	Phase 2	95% CR	
	In GCLAC	Upfront AML	Phase 2	76% CR	
	+ idarubicin + cytarabine	Upfront AML	Phase 3	77% vs 81% CR standard vs escalated dose	
GM-CSF	+ daunorubicin + cytarabine timed sequential	Upfront AML	Phase 2	83% CR	
Cytokine receptor	Anti-CD123 (IL-3 receptor)	R/R AML	Phase 1	5% ORR	

ALL, acute lymphoblastic leukemia; AML, acute myeloid leukemia; BMT, bone marrow transplantation; CBF, core binding factor; CR, complete remission; DLI, donor lymphocyte infusion; MDS, myelodysplastic syndrome; ORR, overall response rate; R/R, relapsed/refractory.

Selected References

Alonso S, Su M, Jones JW, et al. Human bone marrow niche chemoprotection mediated by cytochrome P450 enzymes. *Oncotarget*. 2015;6(17):14905–14912.

Ben-Batalla I, Schultze A, Wroblewski M, et al. Axl, a prognostic and therapeutic target in acute myeloid leukemia mediates paracrine crosstalk of leukemia cells with bone marrow stroma. *Blood*. 2013;122(14):2443–2452. doi:10.1182/blood-2013-03-491431

Duan CW, Shi J, Chen J, et al. Leukemia propagating cells rebuild an evolving niche in response to therapy. *Cancer cell*. 2014;25(6):778–793. doi:10.1016/j.ccr.2014.04.015

Ghiaur G, Yegnasubramanian S, Perkins B, et al. Regulation of human hematopoietic stem cell self-renewal by the microenvironment's control of retinoic acid signaling. *Proc Natl Acad Sci USA*. 2013; 110(40):16121–16126. doi:10.1073/pnas.1305937110

Jin L, Hope KJ, Zhai Q, et al. Targeting of CD44 eradicates human acute myeloid leukemic stem cells. *Nat Med*. 2006;12(10):1167–1174. doi:10.1038/nm1483

Matsunaga T, Takemoto N, Sato T, et al. Interaction between leukemic-cell VLA-4 and stromal fibronectin is a decisive factor for minimal residual disease of acute myelogenous leukemia. *Nat Med*. 2003;9(9):1158–1165. doi:10.1038/nm909

Mendez-Ferrer S, Scadden DT, Sanchez-Aguilera A. Bone marrow stem cells: current and emerging concepts. *Ann N Y Acad Sci*. 2015;1335:32–44. doi:10.1111/nyas.12641

Pabst T, Vellenga E, van Putten W, et al. Favorable effect of priming with granulocyte colony-stimulating factor in remission induction of acute myeloid leukemia restricted to dose escalation of cytarabine. *Blood*. 2012;119(23):5367–5373. doi:10.1182/blood-2011-11-389841

Uy GL, Rettig MP, Motabi IH, et al. A phase 1/2 study of chemosensitization with the CXCR4 antagonist plerixafor in relapsed or refractory acute myeloid leukemia. *Blood*. 2012;119(17):3917–3924. doi:10.1182/blood-2011-10-383406

Zeng Z, Shi YX, Samudio IJ, et al. Targeting the leukemia microenvironment by CXCR4 inhibition overcomes resistance to kinase inhibitors and chemotherapy in AML. *Blood*. 2009;113(24):6215–6224. doi:10.1182/blood-2008-05-158311

Immunology

Hanna A. Knaus, Raúl Montiel Esparza, and Ivana Gojo

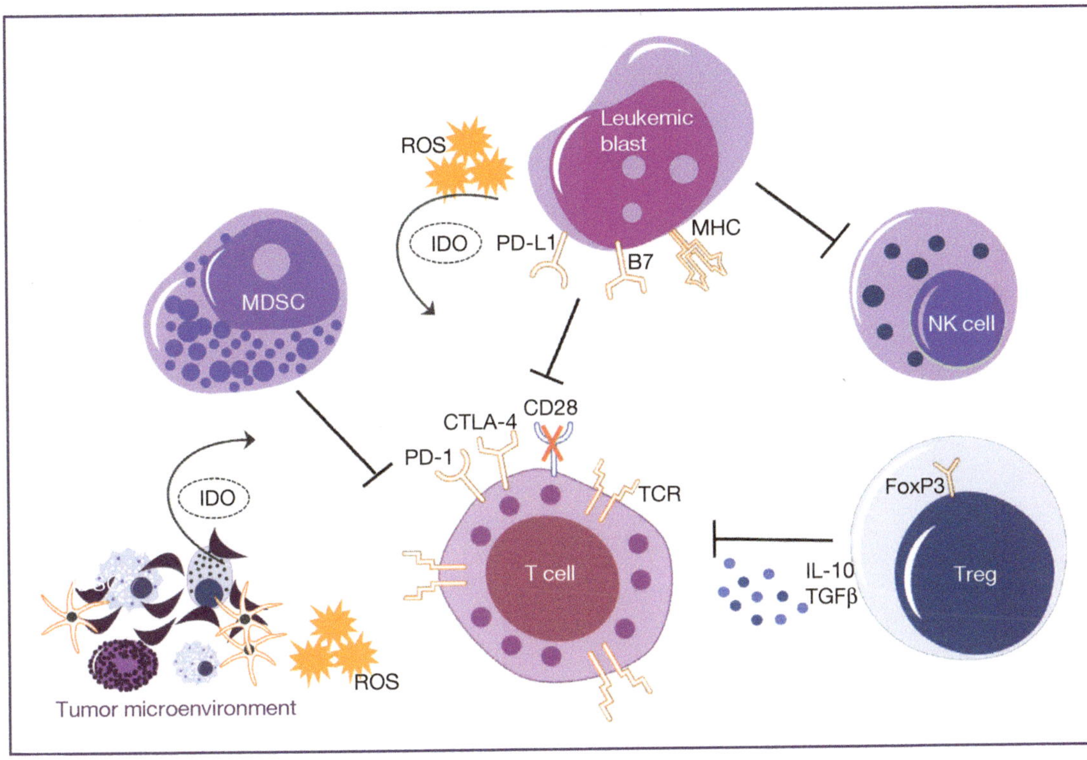

FIGURE 8-20: Dysregulation of the immune system in acute myeloid leukemia.

IDO, indoleamine 2,3 dioxygenase; MDSC, myeloid-derived suppressor cell; MHC, major histocompatibility complex; NK, natural killer; ROS, reactive oxygen species; TCR, T-cell receptor; TGFβ, transforming growth factor beta; Treg, regulatory T cell.

Accumulating evidence suggests that leukemia cells exploit a variety of mechanisms to evade T-cell-mediated immunity, leading to disease progression or relapse. However, multiple mechanisms likely cooperate to create an environment that supports the immune escape of leukemia cells (Figure 8-20).

Although a number of genetic and epigenetic changes within leukemia cells provide antigens that should easily be recognized by T-cells, leukemic blasts have been reported to down-regulate human leukocyte antigen (HLA) molecules and to have altered antigen presentation properties that prevent T-cell activation. Besides antigen presentation, other mechanisms contributing to the dysfunctional T-cell responses in AML include expansion of suppressive immune cell populations, such as regulatory T-cells (Tregs), as well as down-regulation of co-stimulatory receptors on the leukemia cells. Other mechanisms of immune escape include production of immunosuppressive cytokines or reactive oxygen species (ROS) by leukemia cells themselves or within their microenvironment and impaired NK cell function.

Furthermore, enzymes that degrade metabolically important amino acids (eg, tryptophan and arginine) may contribute to altered T-cell immunity. In particular, expression of indoleamine 2,3 dioxygenase (IDO), an enzyme that catalyzes the rate-limiting step of tryptophan degradation along the kynurenine pathway, has been reported in AML blasts and is associated with shortened relapse-free and overall survival (OS). Lastly, up-regulation of inhibitory ligands and their receptors (immune checkpoints) has been described on leukemia cells, serving as critical mechanisms of immune evasion as well as potential therapeutic targets (Figure 8-20).

Table 8-3 Selected immunotherapeutic strategies for treating acute myeloid leukemia

STRATEGY	TARGET	AGENT	STUDIES IN AML
Blocking T-cell inhibitory pathways/immune checkpoints	**CTLA-4** (cytotoxic T-lymphocyte antigen-4)	Ipilimumab	**NCT01757639** • Ipilimumab in relapsed MDS/AML **NCT00060372** • Ipilimumab after allo-HSCT
	PD-1 (programmed death-1)	Nivolumab, MK-3475, CT-011, MEDI0680, BMS-936559, MEDI4736, MPDL3280A	**Berger et al (2008)** • Phase I clinical study of anti-PD1 mAb (CT-011) in patients with advanced hematologic malignancies **NCT01096602** • Anti-PD-1 (CT-011) together with DC/AML vaccine for patients in CR postchemotherapy **NCT01953692** • A Phase Ib multi-cohort trial of MK-3475 in subjects with hematologic malignancies **NCT02397720** • Anti-PD-1 (Nivolumab, BMS-936558) plus 5-azacytidine (Vidaza) for refractory/relapsed AML **NCT02845297** • Phase 2 study of azacitidine plus anti-PD-1 (Pembrolizumab) in relapsed/refractory AML
	LAG-3 (lymphocyte activation gene-3)	BMS-986016, IMP321	No studies in AML.
	TIM-3 (T-cell immunoglobulin domain and mucin domain 3)	mAb, TIM-3 fusion protein	Murine studies showing an additive effect of combined blockade of TIM-3/PD-L1 in improving survival of AML-bearing mice. No clinical studies in AML.
	CD200R–CD200	mAb (anti-CD200)	Human in vitro studies, showing that CD200 is overexpressed in AML cells, increases bone marrow Tregs, and directly inhibits the cytotoxic activity of NK cells. No clinical studies in AML.
Targeting inhibitory enzymes	**IDO** (indoleamine 2,3-dioxygenase)	INCB024360, indoximod, NLG919	IDO overexpressed in AML cells. No clinical studies in AML. Clinical study in MDS (NCT01822691).
Targeting regulatory T-cells (Tregs)	**CD25**	CD25 (basiliximab, daclizumab, denileukin diftitox immunotoxin)	Several clinical studies of anti-CD25 plus vaccine and chemotherapy plus immunomodulatory drugs ongoing in AML: **NCT00975975, NCT01842139, NCT00594308**
Enhancing T-cell proliferation and cytokine secretion	**IMiDs**	immunomodulatory drugs (pomalidomide, lenalidomide, thalidomide)	**NCT02029950** A Phase I study of pomalidomide in AML and high-risk MDS.
Targeting NK cells	**KIR** (killer cell immunoglobulin-like receptors)	Anti-KIR mAb (IPH2101, lirilumab)	Phase I clinical study of anti-KIR mAb as maintenance therapy in older AML patients.

(continued)

Table 8-3 Selected immunotherapeutic strategies for treating acute myeloid leukemia (*continued*)

STRATEGY	TARGET	AGENT	STUDIES IN AML
Enhancing the cytotoxic capacity of T-cells or NK cells against AML blasts	**CD3 x CD123**	CD3 x CD123 DART (dual affinity retargeting)	Preclinical study showing that DART induces a dose-dependent killing of AML cell lines and primary AML blasts in vitro and in vivo.
	CD3 x CD33	CD3 x CD33 BiTe (bispecific T-cell engager), AMG330	Targeting CD33 ex vivo using AMG 330 in primary AML samples led to T-cell recruitment and expansion and antibody-mediated cytotoxicity.
	CD16 x CD33	CD16 x CD33 BiKE (bispecific killer cell engager)	Reversed MDSC immunosuppression of NK cells and induced $CD33^{+}$ MDS and MDSC target cell lysis ex vivo.
	CD123/CD33/CD16	Triplebody (SPM2)	Increased patient's NK cell cytolytic activity against AML cells ex vivo.

allo-HSCT, allogeneic hematopoietic stem cell transplant; AML, acute myeloid leukemia; CR, complete remission; MDS, myelodysplastic syndrome; MDSC, myeloid-derived suppressor cell; NK, natural killer.

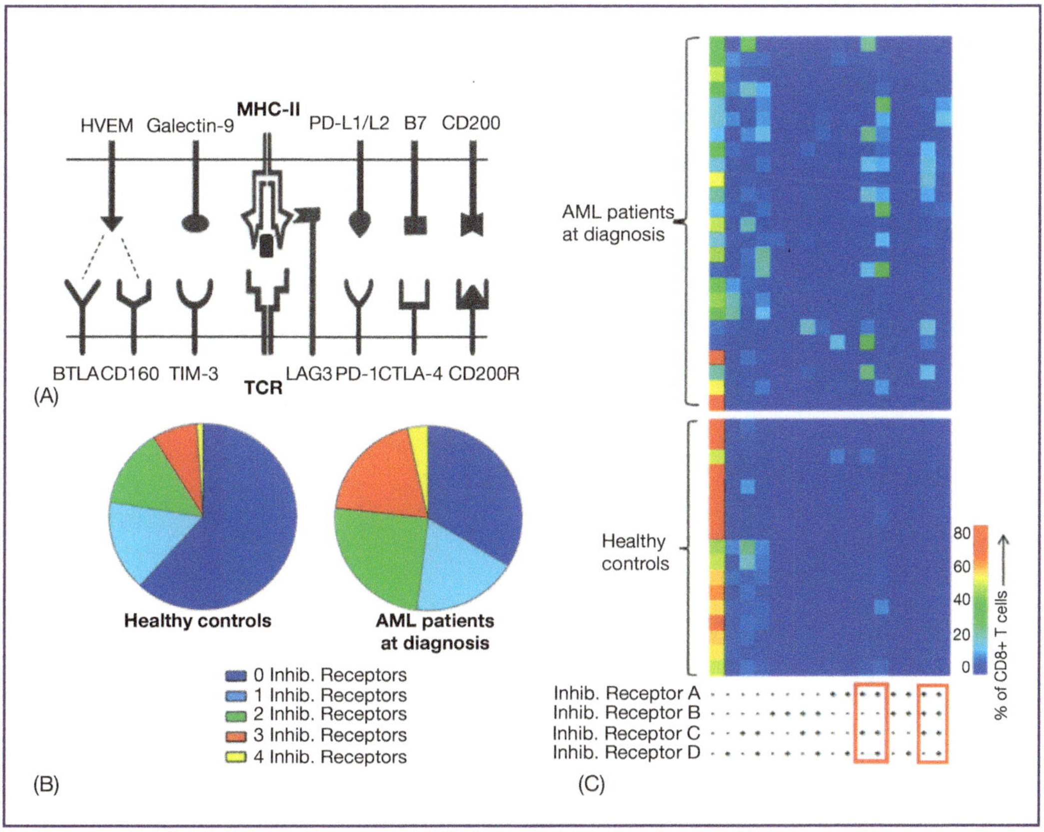

FIGURE 8-21: **$CD8^{+}$ T-cells of AML patients coexpress multiple inhibitory receptors.**
AML, acute myeloid leukemia; HVEM, herpes virus entry mediator; TCR, T-cell receptor.

While engagement of a co-stimulatory receptor such as CD28 strongly amplifies antigen-specific TCR signaling with a resultant increase in lymphocyte proliferation and activation, co-inhibitory receptors serve as immune checkpoints to prevent and limit uncontrolled T-cell responses. In healthy individuals, immune checkpoints are crucial for maintaining self-tolerance, and thus preventing autoimmunity, and for limiting tissue damage when the immune system responds to infection. Tumor cells, however, can hijack these inhibitory pathways as a critical mechanism of immune evasion. Immune checkpoints are initiated by ligand–receptor interactions and inhibit T-cell activation and proliferation. Figure 8-21A shows selected immune checkpoint receptors, including BTLA (B- and T-lymphocyte attenuator) and CD160, that bind to their ligand HVEM (herpes virus entry mediator), CD200R that engages with CD200, CTLA-4 (cytotoxic T-lymphocyte associated antigen 4) that binds the B7 molecules (CD80 and CD86), LAG-3 (lymphocyte activation gene 3) that binds to the MHC complex, PD-1 (programmed cell death-1) that engages with PD-L1 or PD-L2, and TIM-3 (T-cell immunoglobulin and mucin domain-containing protein 3) that binds to galectin 9 on the antigen presenting cell or tumor cell.

Preliminary data from a Johns Hopkins research study, evaluating checkpoint receptor expression in AML, suggests that patients at AML diagnosis co-express significantly higher percentages of multiple inhibitory receptors on CD8$^+$ T-cells than healthy controls (65% vs. 38% for coexpression of four receptors, respectively [Figure 8-21B]). To identify the dominant patterns of checkpoint receptor coexpression in AML patients, a heat-map of immune subsets at play at initial AML diagnosis was generated (Figure 8-21C). Percentage expression of inhibitory molecules on CD8$^+$ T-cells before induction

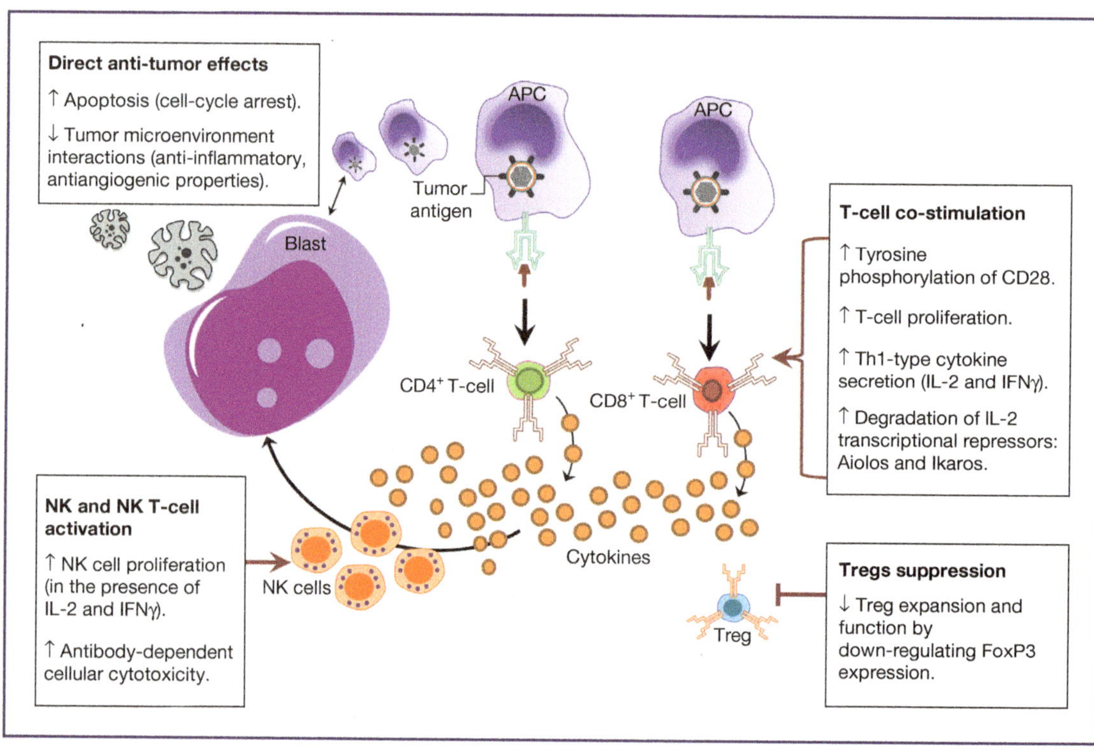

FIGURE 8-22: **Immunomodulatory drugs (IMiDs) as novel therapeutic strategies in acute myeloid leukemia. Lenalidomide and pomalidomide are synthetic compounds derived by modifying the chemical structure of thalidomide. IMiDs' action alone or in combination has shown substantial clinical activities in patients with myeloma, lymphomas, and MDS. Growing evidence suggests IMiDs' ability to enhance immunological activity through the induction of co-stimulatory molecules, activation of T and NK cells, stimulation of antibody-dependent cell-mediated cytotoxicity, inhibition of Tregs, and modulation of co-inhibitory receptors. Their efficacy and potential synergism with other agents still needs to be fully capitalized in other hematological malignancies like AML. Early lymphocyte recovery following induction chemotherapy in AML patients is characterized by complex immune system aberrations and may represent an ideal timing for integration of IMiDs with a goal to unleash their immunomodulatory effects and augment antileukemia immunity.**

APC, antigen-presenting cell; IL-2, interleukin 2; IFNγ, interferon gamma; NK, natural killer; Treg, regulatory T-cell.

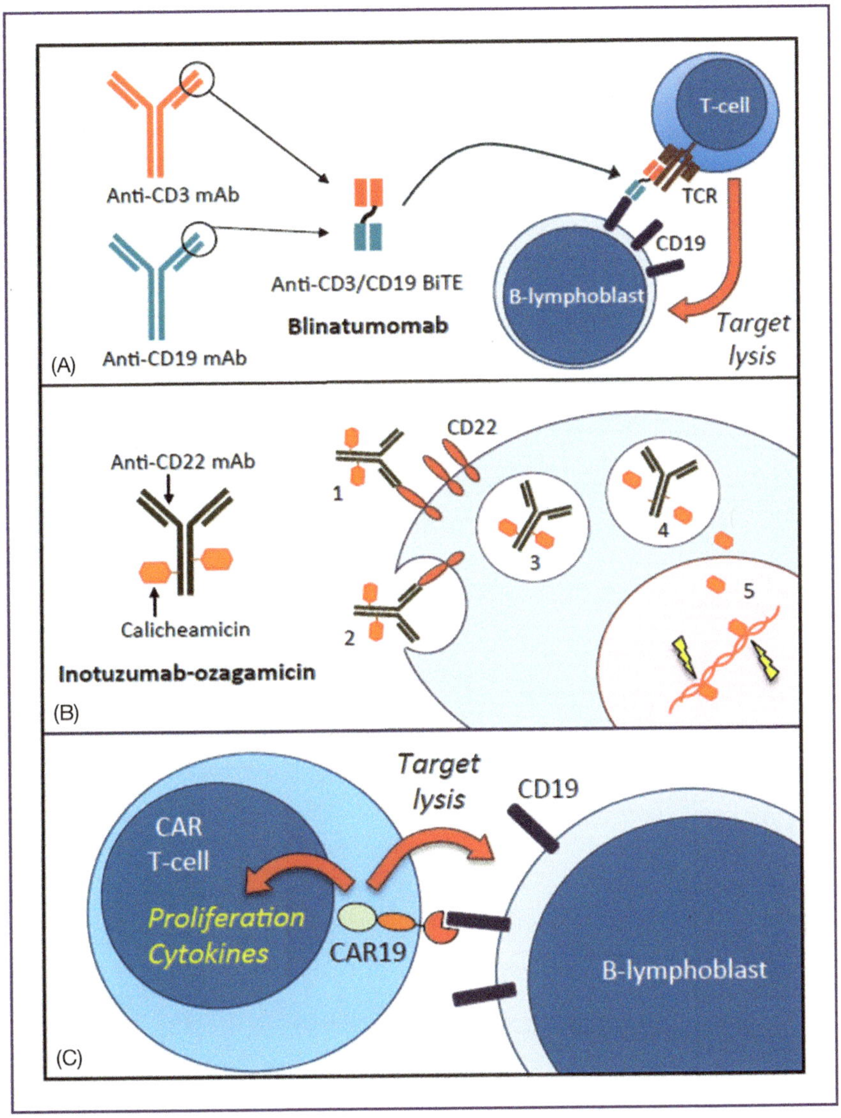

FIGURE 8-23: Targeted treatments for relapsed or refractory adult acute lymphoblastic leukemia. (A) Blinatumomab is a bifunctional T-cell-engaging antibody (BiTE) that joins variable domains from an anti-CD3 monoclonal antibody (red) and anti-CD19 monoclonal antibody (blue) with a peptide linker (black). Blinatumomab engages the CD3 portion of the T-cell receptor (TCR) and CD19 on the surface of lymphoblasts inducing target cell lysis and T-cell proliferation. (B) Inotuzumab-ozagamicin is an antibody–drug conjugate that links the antitumor antibiotic calicheamicin (orange hexagons) to an anti-CD22 monoclonal antibody. Inotuzumab-ozagamicin binds CD22 on the surface of B-lymphoblasts and is internalized into lysosomes where the calicheamicin linker is cleaved releasing free calicheamicin, which binds the minor groove of DNA and causes DNA damage leading to cell death. (C) Chimeric antigen receptor (CAR) T-cells targeting CD19 are created via lentiviral or retroviral introduction of a CAR against CD19 (CAR19) that contains an extracellular single-chain variable fragment (scFv) targeting CD19 (red), a transmembrane domain (black), an intracellular co-stimulatory domain (orange), and a signaling domain (light green) into autologous T-lymphocytes. Interaction of CAR19 T-cells with CD19-expressing B-lymphoblasts leads to CAR T-cell activation with target cell lysis, CAR T-cell proliferation, and cytokine generation.

chemotherapy are shown for each of the 16 phenotypic subsets based on the expression profiles of four different immune checkpoints. Each row represents one person that is grouped into patients (top) and healthy controls (bottom). Importantly, subsets of T-cells coexpressing 2, 3, or 4 inhibitory receptors were highly expressed in leukemic patients but absent in all of the healthy controls.

Selected References

Al-Hussaini M, Rettig MP, Ritchey JK, et al. Targeting CD123 in acute myeloid leukemia using a T-cell-directed dual-affinity retargeting platform. *Blood*. 2016;127(1):122–131.

Aurelius J, Thoren FB, Akhiani AA, et al. Monocytic AML cells inactivate antileukemic lymphocytes: role of NADPH oxidase/gp91(phox) expression and the PARP-1/PAR pathway of apoptosis. *Blood*. 2012;119(24):5832–5837.

Berger R, Rotem-Yehudar R, Slama G, et al. Phase I safety and pharmacokinetic study of CT-011, a humanized antibody interacting with PD-1, in patients with advanced hematologic malignancies. *Clin Cancer Res*. 2008;14(10):3044–3051.

Braciak TA, Wildenhain S, Roskopf CC, et al. NK cells from an AML patient have recovered in remission and reached comparable cytolytic activity to that of a healthy monozygotic twin mediated by the single-chain triplebody SPM-2. *J Trans Med*. 2013;11:289.

Coles SJ, Wang EC, Man S, et al. CD200 expression suppresses natural killer cell function and directly inhibits patient anti-tumor response in acute myeloid leukemia. *Leukemia*. 2011;25(5):792–799.

Costello RT, Sivori S, Marcenaro E, et al. Defective expression and function of natural killer cell-triggering receptors in patients with acute myeloid leukemia. *Blood*. 2002;99(10):3661–3667.

Curti A, Aluigi M, Pandolfi S, et al. Acute myeloid leukemia cells constitutively express the immunoregulatory enzyme indoleamine 2,3-dioxygenase. *Leukemia*. 2007;21(2):353–355.

Galustian C, Meyer B, Labarthe MC, et al. The anti-cancer agents lenalidomide and pomalidomide inhibit the proliferation and function of T regulatory cells. *Cancer Immunol Immunother*. 2009;58(7):1033–1045.

Gandhi AK, Kang J, Havens CG, et al. Immunomodulatory agents lenalidomide and pomalidomide co-stimulate T cells by inducing degradation of T-cell repressors Ikaros and Aiolos via modulation of the E3 ubiquitin ligase complex CRL4(CRBN). *Br J Haematol*. 2014;164(6):811–821.

Gleason MK, Ross JA, Warlick ED, et al. CD16xCD33 bispecific killer cell engager (BiKE) activates NK cells against primary MDS and MDSC CD33+ targets. *Blood*. 2014;123(19):3016–3026.

Gojo I, Karp JE. New strategies in acute myelogenous leukemia: leukemogenesis and personalized medicine. *Clin Cancer Res*. 2014;20(24):6233–6241.

Graf M, Reif S, Hecht K, et al. High expression of costimulatory molecules correlates with low relapse-free survival probability in acute myeloid leukemia (AML). *Ann Hematol*. 2005;84(5):287–297.

Kanakry CG, Hess AD, Gocke CD, et al. Early lymphocyte recovery after intensive timed sequential chemotherapy for acute myelogenous leukemia: peripheral oligoclonal expansion of regulatory T-cells. *Blood*. 2011;117(2):608–617.

Kantarjian H, Thomas D, Jorgensen J, et al. Results of inotuzumab ozogamicin, a CD22 monoclonal antibody, in refractory and relapsed acute lymphocytic leukemia. *Cancer*. 2013;119, 2728–2736.

Knaus HA, Kanakry CG, Luznik L, Gojo I. Immunomodulatory drugs II: immune checkpoint agents in acute leukemia. *Curr Drug Targets*. May 17, 2015 [Epub ahead of print].

Knaus HA, Montiel-Esparza R, Zeidner JF, et al, eds. Tracking effector T-cell dynamics and immune inhibitory receptors in patients with acute myeloid leukemia (AML). *ASH*; Orlando, FL; 2015.

Krupka C, Kufer P, Kischel R, et al. CD33 target validation and sustained depletion of AML blasts in long-term cultures by the bispecific T-cell-engaging antibody AMG 330. *Blood*. 2014;123(3):356–365.

Maude SL, Frey N, Shaw PA, et al. Chimeric antigen receptor T-cells for sustained remissions in leukemia. *N Engl J Med*. 2014;371:1507–1517.

Topp MS, Gökbuget N, Stein AS, et al. Safety and activity of blinatumomab for adult patients with relapsed or refractory B-precursor acute lymphoblastic leukaemia: a multicentre, single-arm, phase 2 study. *Lancet Oncol*. 2015;16(1):57–66.

van Luijn MM, Chamuleau ME, Ossenkoppele GJ, et al. Tumor immune escape in acute myeloid leukemia: class II-associated invariant chain peptide expression as result of deficient antigen presentation. *Oncoimmunology*. 2012;1(2):211–213.

Vey N, Bourhis JH, Boissel N, et al. A phase 1 trial of the anti-inhibitory KIR mAb IPH2101 for AML in complete remission. *Blood*. 2012;120(22):4317–4323.

9

Regulatory Considerations for the Practitioner

Donna Przepiorka and Ann T. Farrell

The rapidly emerging information about the biology of the acute leukemias has led to the discovery of many potential new therapeutic agents. Until such drugs or biologics are approved by the FDA, their use in a clinical investigation requires an Investigational New Drug (IND) application, even for the treatment of only a single patient. Figure 9-1 shows an overview of the types of INDs for use of investigational drugs or investigational biologics in the United States. Most INDs are used for a clinical trial to study the safety and/or effectiveness of a new drug or biologic. Figure 9-2 shows key design elements for each phase of study and lists some points to consider, specifically for clinical trials of new agents for treatment of acute leukemia.

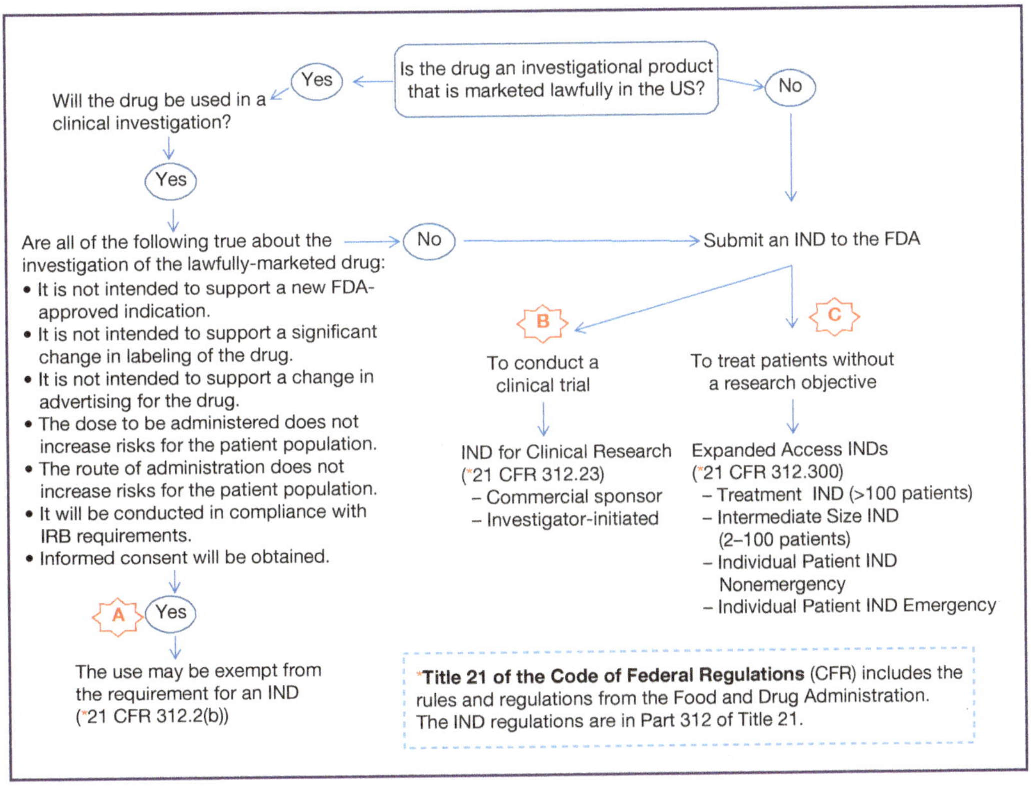

FIGURE 9-1: When is an Investigational New Drug application (IND) needed for treatment of patients with acute leukemia? The blue outlined box identifies the main applicable federal regulations.

FDA, Food and Drug Administration.

Disclaimer: The opinions expressed here are those of the authors and do not represent the official position of the FDA or the United States Government.

Treatment of a patient with acute leukemia using a drug approved for that indication according to the prescribing information does not require an IND. If the planned use of a lawfully marketed drug or biologic is not consistent with that found to be safe and effective as described in the prescribing information, the treatment may still be exempt from the requirement for an IND (Figure 9-1 Point A) if the results will not be used to support a change in labeling or advertising for the agent; the route of administration or dosage level does not pose a significantly increased risk to the patients, given their disease status and the expected risks or benefits of current therapy; and conduct of the plan is in compliance with institutional review board requirements, including informed consent.

Examples of potentially exempt activities include off-label use of an approved drug for treatment of an individual patient with relapsed or refractory acute leukemia and no established therapeutic options, or a clinical trial of a novel combination of approved drugs for the treatment of such patients. There are no submissions to FDA required for exempt activities, but if a practitioner or investigator does submit an IND for an activity that FDA determines is exempt, FDA will notify the individual who submitted the IND but take no further action on the submission thereafter.

If the treatment uses an investigational product or is otherwise not exempt, an IND must be submitted to and approved by FDA prior to initiating any clinical trial to assess its safety and/or effectiveness (Figure 9-1 Point B). The person or entity submitting the IND, also known as the sponsor, is responsible for ensuring that all activities performed under the IND comply with federal regulations. The sponsor may be a commercial organization developing the drug for marketing (commercial IND) (see Figure 9-3), or the individual who will be the investigator conducting the trial (investigator-initiated or research IND).

If there is compelling evidence that an investigational agent is an active treatment, a practitioner might propose to use that agent for treatment of a patient outside of a clinical trial under an Expanded Access IND (Figure 9-1 Point C). Expanded access to investigational products is allowed by regulation when the potential benefit of treatment outweighs the risks for a patient with a serious or immediately life-threatening illness who has no satisfactory alternative treatments, and there is no clinical trial available in which the patient is eligible to participate. Pharmaceutical companies at or near completion of development of an investigational drug or biologic may have an Expanded Access Treatment IND to accommodate therapy of large numbers of patients while pursuing marketing approval.

Commercial organizations or practitioners may also submit an Expanded Access IND for treatment of an individual patient or a small cohort of patients. In addition, when the patient's condition warrants treatment emergently before an IND can be submitted and reviewed, such as may occur with patients who have acute leukemia that has relapsed or is refractory to therapy, FDA may authorize emergency expanded access use based on limited information submitted by telephone or other electronic communications if the sponsor agrees to submit the complete Expanded Access IND within 15 days of authorization.

In order for FDA to determine that the patients who participate in the investigation will not be exposed to unnecessary risks, an IND application must contain sufficient information about manufacturing controls and consistency of the investigational product produced, preclinical studies of the pharmacology and toxicology of the product, a protocol detailing the clinical activities, the qualifications of the investigators, assurance of protection of human subjects, and commitment to comply with the investigational drug regulations. Such information is needed for all types of INDs, although for investigator-initiated INDs and single-patient Expanded Access INDs, the manufacturing and preclinical information is commonly provided by cross-reference to a commercial IND when allowed by the commercial sponsor.

In The Blue Box–Title 21 of the Code of Federal Regulations (CFR) comprises the rules and regulations from the Food and Drug Administration as published in the Federal Register, including the regulations that must be followed by individuals involved in the treatment of patients with acute leukemia using an investigational product. These include regulations on protection of human subjects (Part 50), drugs for human use (Parts 300–369), biologics (Parts 600–680), diagnostic and therapeutic devices (Parts 800–898), and cell therapies (Part 1271). The CFR and additional guidance on FDA regulations and policies are available electronically.

Clinical trials for new drugs for treatment of acute leukemia include three broad designs as outlined in Figure 9-2. The current approach to these studies was based on the experience with cyclic administration of cytotoxic agents for treatment of patients with solid tumors in the outpatient setting. Given the

Usual Design	Considerations for Acute Leukemia
A **Phase 1** **Establish a safe dose and schedule** • Patients: Disease refractory to all therapies • Objective: Determine the maximal tolerated dose (MTD) of the drug • Goal: Dose that causes grade 3–5 toxicities in ≤17% of patients	• Include untreated patients with leukemia having poor-risk genetic markers • Seek the lowest biologically effective dose • Define the acceptable degree of toxicity by the treatment setting (induction vs. maintenance)
B **Phase 2** **Estimate the treatment effect** • Patients: Intended population largely • Objective: Obtain a measure of activity with some degree of certainty • Goal: Quantitative data to support design and conduct of the Phase 3 clinical trial	• When to include target-negative patients • Is drug activity reflected by MRD negativity or by remission without full hematologic recovery • What rate and duration of remission are sufficient to warrant further development
C **Phase 3** **Confirm benefit vs. a comparator** • Patients: Intended population • Objective: Demonstrate clinical benefit • Goal: Show that the drug improves a clinical benefit endpoint in comparison to an acceptable alternative treatment	• Minimize exclusion criteria so that the study patients reflect the breadth of the intended population • If changing populations, ensure that the drug dose and schedule are still applicable • Choose a primary endpoint that reflects the purpose of treatment (cure vs. palliation)

FIGURE 9-2: Design considerations for clinical trials of drugs for acute leukemia.
MRD, minimal residual disease.

observation of a steep dose–response relationship in preclinical studies, cytotoxic cancer drugs were developed to provide the highest dose tolerated by the patient, even if for only a brief period of time.

Many of the new drugs emerging currently, however, inhibit specific molecular targets as described in Chapter 2 rather than being broadly cytotoxic, so there is less basis for using the highest tolerated dose (although safety considerations may still limit dosing). The initial dose-escalation trial (Figure 9-2 Point A) might therefore be guided by objective measurement of a biomarker to identify the lowest dose maximally inhibiting the molecular target in order to avoid potentially toxic doses higher than needed for efficacy. This is especially important for use of drugs in the maintenance setting, since limited long-term tolerability would likely lead to noncompliance and loss of efficacy.

For clinical trials used to obtain an estimate of the treatment effect (Figure 9-2 Point B), an important consideration is the actual measure of clinical activity. Complete remission with hematological recovery is an established measure of drug activity for studies in patients with acute leukemia. As reviewed in Chapter 5, a deeper response, such as complete remission with no evidence of minimal residual disease by highly sensitive assays, may provide a better measure of lasting activity of the treatment. A lesser degree of response, such as complete remission with partial hematologic recovery and transfusion independence, may be of value in the palliative setting, but whether that is a sufficient response for a population traditionally treated for cure or extended long-term survival has not been determined.

Randomized trials comparing the effect of the new drug or biologic to a control (Figure 9-2 Point C) are used to demonstrate clinical benefit. These studies may change the standard of care in clinical practice or be used to support a marketing application for a new treatment. In order for the results of such a study to be generalizable to the broad population of patients with active leukemia and concurrent comorbidities, minimizing exclusions to only those for whom it is clear that use of the drug would not be safe should be considered. If the drug was originally developed for patients with relapsed or refractory leukemia and is now proposed for study of treatment of minimal residual disease, one might also need to reevaluate whether the established regimen is appropriate for the new population with regard to safety and dose-schedule. Additionally, although survival is the critical outcome when the goal of treatment is cure, alternative endpoints might be considered for more advanced disease where patients may seek only a palliative option.

Commercial development of a new drug or biologic for marketing usually follows a sequence of steps, each building on the knowledge learned in the previous steps. Figure 9-3 shows an overview of the drug development pathway. A major goal of drug development is to obtain the data used to establish the instructions for safe use of the new drug or biologic as displayed in the prescribing information. Figure 9-4 shows the breadth of information about a drug that can be found in the prescribing information and how it is organized to allow rapid review by practitioners.

There are four broad steps in the commercial development of drugs for acute leukemia—preclinical testing, clinical testing, application for approval, and postmarketing surveillance. The first step, preclinical testing (Figure 9-3 Point A), includes in vitro testing to determine the actions of the drug as well as animal studies to establish potential toxic effects induced by the drug in vivo. The latter is especially important in estimating a safe starting dose for studies in humans and in determining what special monitoring might be needed to ensure safe use in clinical trials. Proof-of-concept testing per se (ie, is the drug cytotoxic to leukemia cells in vitro?) is not required prior to initiation of a clinical trial, but if a new drug is expected to have toxicity and there is no basis for an expectation that patients with leukemia will derive any benefit, a clinical trial for treatment of leukemia might not be considered acceptable.

The second broad step in development includes clinical testing (Figure 9-3 Point B). The early phase clinical trials establish a safe dose with sufficient activity to warrant further development (Phase 1) and to refine an estimate of the degree of activity (Phase 2), while the later phase trials establish whether the treatment as described in the protocol is safe and effective in the intended population (Phase 3). Design

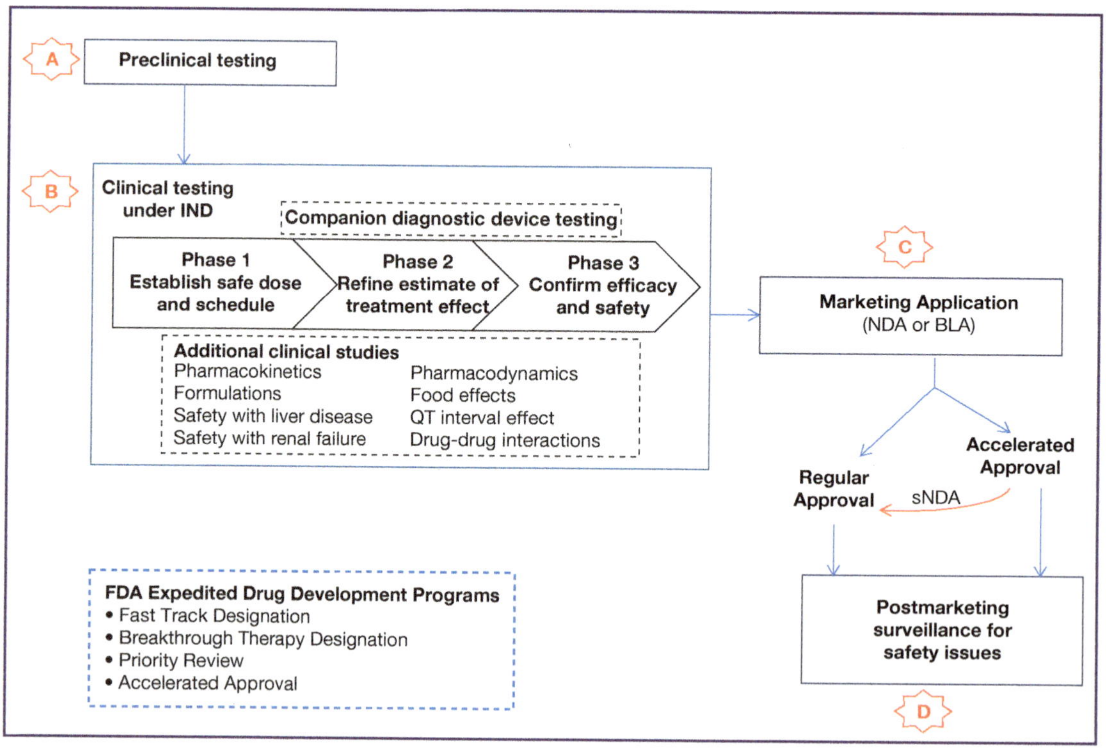

FIGURE 9-3: Overview of commercial development of drugs for treatment of acute leukemia. The blue outline box identifies pathways for expedited development programs.

BLA, biologics license application; NDA, new drug application.

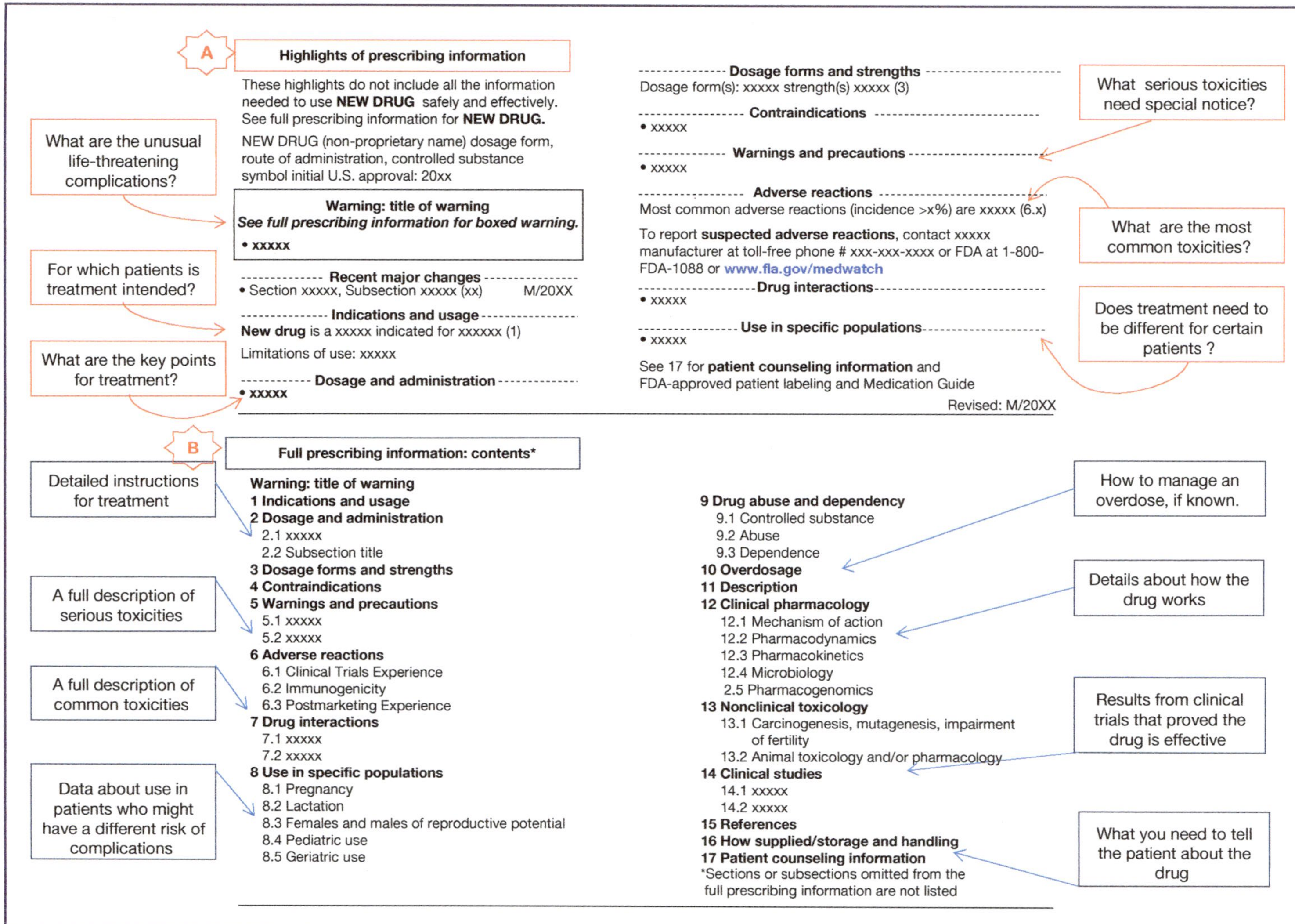

FIGURE 9-4: What information is in the prescribing information?

issues specific to acute leukemia are highlighted in Figure 9-2. The second broad step also includes clinical studies to ensure that information is available to support the instructions for safe use in the prescribing information (Figure 9-4). These additional clinical studies may look at the effects of the drug on the heart, pharmacokinetic or metabolic interactions with other drugs, effects of taking the medicine with food, and whether the dose needs to be modified in patients with liver or kidney disease.

Since many of the new drugs target specific mutations in acute leukemia cells that may be present in only a subpopulation of the patients as described in Chapter 2, a diagnostic test may be needed in order to identify which patients have the mutation that make the leukemia susceptible to the drug. Such diagnostic tests may be considered devices that must also be approved by FDA. Testing of the device to support its approval may occur concurrently with development of the drug.

The third step involves submission of the marketing application, a New Drug Application (NDA) for drugs or a Biologics License Application (BLA) for biologics, to the FDA for review (Figure 9-3 Point C). Approval is based on an assessment of the balance of risks from using the new drug versus the benefit derived from treatment as demonstrated in the clinical studies. Regular approval generally requires a demonstration of a direct clinical benefit, such as improvement in the quantity or quality of life. For acute leukemia, the accepted efficacy endpoint for regular approval is survival when the goal of treatment is cure or extension of long-term survival. There are no drugs approved in the modern era for palliative treatment of acute leukemia, so the accepted measure of clinical benefit in this setting is not yet established.

Accelerated approval is a mechanism by which FDA can grant marketing approval on the basis of a surrogate clinical endpoint for which there is evidence that the surrogate is reasonably likely to predict that patients would derive a direct clinical benefit from the treatment. This mechanism allows for approval decisions to be made much sooner in the development of a drug, expediting the time to marketing and availability to the public. Since there is still some uncertainty about clinical benefit with approval based on a surrogate, use of accelerated approval is limited to drugs for serious or life-threatening diseases and when the drug appears to provide benefit over available therapies, such as treatments for poor-prognosis acute leukemia or relapsed acute leukemia. Durable complete remission with hematological recovery is an accepted surrogate endpoint that has been used for accelerated approvals of new drugs for acute leukemia. If a marketing application is granted accelerated approval, additional clinical trials to confirm the predicted benefit still need to be conducted in order to gain regular approval at a later time.

At the time of approval of a new drug, the extent of the data about safety is limited by the relatively small number of patients and the relatively short duration of treatment as experienced in the clinical studies under IND. Consequently, once a new drug is approved for use by practitioners, new safety issues may emerge in the postmarketing period (Figure 9-3 Point D). Commercial sponsors are required to report to the FDA any new information about the safety of their drugs on a regular basis during the entire life of the drug. In addition, FDA maintains a web-based reporting system, MedWatch, through which practitioners or patients may voluntarily report new serious safety issues that they observe.

In The Blue Box–In addition to accelerated approval, the FDA has other programs designed to expedite drug development for conditions that are serious like acute leukemia, so that much needed effective drugs can be available for public use as quickly as possible. Fast Track Designation indicates that there are nonclinical or clinical data demonstrating the potential to address an unmet medical need. Breakthrough Designation indicates that there is preliminary clinical evidence that the drug may demonstrate a substantial improvement in a clinically significant endpoint over available therapies. Neither the Fast Track Designation nor the Breakthrough Therapy Designation is an indication that the drug is effective. Rather, the designations indicate that the FDA is committed to advising and working with the sponsor to ensure the most efficient pathway for successful development of the product. Lastly, for drugs that do show a significant improvement in safety or effectiveness in clinical trials, the marketing applications may receive Priority Review, which shortens the time between submission and approval by 4 months.

The prescribing information, also known as the package insert, is designed to include the information needed by a practitioner for safe use of the drug for treatment of patients in the intended population.

The content of the prescribing information is based on the results of the clinical trials and ancillary studies as described in the drug development scheme in Figure 9-3. The first page of the prescribing information has two parts–the highlights on the top half and the table of contents on the bottom.

The highlights of the prescribing information (Figure 9-4 Point A) display key information about the identity, safety, and intended use of the drug. The indication statement describes what the drug is used for and in what specific population it has been shown to be safe and effective for that use. For drugs granted accelerated approval, the indication statement will state so and describe the basis for the approval. The key elements of dosage and administration are displayed in the highlights, but the detailed instructions for use are provided within the full contents.

A boxed warning is displayed prominently in the highlights when serious complications of the treatment need to be considered in patient selection or when special monitoring or other actions are required to mitigate a serious or life-threatening risk. Additional safety information in the highlights includes a bulleted listing of warnings with concise instructions to prevent the hazard or manage the complication, and a list of the most common adverse reactions.

The table of contents (Figure 9-4 Point B) outlines the detailed information contained within the full prescribing information. The contents include detailed instructions for treatment including when dose modifications are needed (Sections 2 and 5), what is known about safe use of the drug in special populations such as children or the elderly (Section 8), and how to treat an overdose if that is known (Section 10).

Section 14 summarizes the results of the clinical trials used to demonstrate the efficacy of the drug, including the endpoints used as the basis for the approval. Relevant safety data (Section 6) from clinical trials are tabulated in the section on adverse reactions, and the safety information that emerged from postmarket surveillance is also provided. The most important points about the drug that the practitioner should discuss with the patient are outlined in the Patient Counseling Information (Section 17).

The National Library of Medicine maintains DailyMed, an online public database of prescribing information and Medication Guides for drugs and biologics marketed in the United States. The FDA-approved version of the prescribing information for most drugs can also be found in PDF format at Drugs@FDA.

Selected References

Appelbaum FR, Rosenblum D, Arceci RJ, et al. End points to establish the efficacy of new agents in the treatment of acute leukemia. *Blood*. 2007;109(5):1810–1816.

DailyMed. http://dailymed.nlm.nih.gov/dailymed/index.cfm

Drugs@FDA. http://www.accessdata.fda.gov/scripts/cder/drugsatfda

Electronic Code of Federal Regulations. Title 21. www.ecfr.gov/cgi-bin/text-idx?SID=db5b7c2022447b69f2d5471396e58ac6&mc=true&tpl=/ecfrbrowse/Title21/21tab_02.tpl

Expanded Access: Information for physicians. http://www.fda.gov/NewsEvents/PublicHealthFocus/ExpandedAccessCompassionateUse/ucm429624.htm

Guidance for Industry. Expanded access to investigational drugs for treatment use—Qs & As. http://www.fda.gov/downloads/drugs/guidancecomplianceregulatoryinformation/guidances/ucm351261.pdf

Guidance for Industry. Expedited programs for serious conditions–drugs and biologics. http://www.fda.gov/downloads/drugs/guidancecomplianceregulatoryinformation/guidances/ucm358301.pdf

Guidance for Industry. IND Exemptions for studies of lawfully marketed drug or biological products for the treatment of cancer. http://www.fda.gov/downloads/drugs/guidancecomplianceregulatoryinformation/guidances/ucm071717.pdf

Guidances (Drugs). http://www.fda.gov/Drugs/GuidanceComplianceRegulatoryInformation/Guidances/default.htm

Investigational New Drug (IND) Application. http://www.fda.gov/Drugs/DevelopmentApprovalProcess/HowDrugsareDevelopedandApproved/ApprovalApplications/InvestigationalNewDrugINDApplication/default.htm

MedWatch. https://www.accessdata.fda.gov/scripts/medwatch/index.cfm?action=reporting.home

Index